CLINICAL PRACTICE PROTOCOLS IN
ONCOLOGY NURSING

DEBRA S. PRESCHER-HUGHES, RN, BSN, OCN

Private Practice
Denver, Colorado

CYNTHIA J. ALKHOUDAIRY, RN, BSN, OCN

Private Practice
Denver, Colorado

JONES AND BARTLETT PUBLISHERS

Sudbury, Massachusetts

BOSTON   TORONTO   LONDON   SINGAPORE

OLSON LIBRARY
NORTHERN MICHIGAN UNIVERSITY
MARQUETTE, MI 49855

World Headquarters
Jones and Bartlett Publishers
40 Tall Pine Drive
Sudbury, MA 01776
978-443-5000
info@jbpub.com
www.jbpub.com

Jones and Bartlett Publishers Canada
6339 Ormindale Way
Mississauga, Ontario L5V 1J2
CANADA

Jones and Bartlett Publishers International
Barb House, Barb Mews
London W6 7PA
UK

Jones and Bartlett's books and products are available through most bookstores and online booksellers. To contact Jones and Bartlett Publishers directly, call 800-832-0034, fax 978-443-8000, or visit our website, www.jbpub.com.

Substantial discounts on bulk quantities of Jones and Bartlett's publications are available to corporations, professional associations, and other qualified organizations. For details and specific discount information, contact the special sales department at Jones and Bartlett via the above contact information or send an email to specialsales@jbpub.com.

Library of Congress Cataloging-in-Publication Data
Not available at time of printing.

6048

Production Credits
Executive Publisher: Christopher Davis
Production Director: Amy Rose
Associate Editor: Kathy Richardson
Production Editor: Renée Sekerak
Associate Marketing Manager: Laura Kavigian
Manufacturing Buyer: Therese Connell
Cover Design: Kristin E. Ohlin
Text Design and Composition: Auburn Associates, Inc.
Printing and Binding: Courier Companies–Stoughton
Cover Printing: Courier Companies–Stoughton

The authors, editor, and publisher have made every effort to provide accurate information. However, they are not responsible for errors, omissions, or for any outcomes related to the use of the contents of this book and take no responsibility for the use of the products described. Treatments and side effects described in this book may not be applicable to all patients; likewise, some patients may require a dose or experience a side effect that is not described herein. The reader should confer with his or her own physician regarding specific treatments and side effects. Drugs and medical devices are discussed that may have limited availability controlled by the Food and Drug Administration (FDA) for use only in a research study or clinical trial. The drug information presented has been derived from reference sources, recently published data, and pharmaceutical research data. Research, clinical practice, and government regulations often change the accepted standard in this field. When consideration is being given to use of any drug in the clinical setting, the healthcare provider or reader is responsible for determining FDA status of the drug, reading the package insert, reviewing prescribing information for the most up-to-date recommendations on dose, precautions, and contraindications, and determining the appropriate usage for the product. This is especially important in the case of drugs that are new or seldom used.

Printed in the United States of America
10 09 08 07 06   10 9 8 7 6 5 4 3 2 1

Dedication

We as oncology nurses care for people who face the reality of life and death on a daily basis. Early in my career as an oncology nurse I asked Dr. Richard Hesky, a well respected oncologist in our community with whom I have worked for the last 23 years, how he dealt with the loss of his patients. His answer was one I will never forget. "Deb, you have to remember that we did not cause the cancer. We may not be able to cure it, but we can make the time that they have left the best they can possibly have."

Through our knowledge, skills, love, and support we are somehow able to give patients the care and encouragement that make it possible to get through another day. The death of a patient, family member, or close friend can shake us to our very core; but the inevitable growth from the loss enables us to be stronger, more caring, and even better oncology nurses.

To my good friend Linda Vandendriessche-Johnson, who lost her loving husband Allan to gastric cancer and three years later her 21-year-old son Michael to Ewing's sarcoma, my sincere sympathy, always. Her ability to continue living life to its fullest with her children Gina, Mark, and David has been an inspiration to many. I can't thank her enough for renewing my desire to make the time our patients have living with their cancer the best it can possibly be.

Debra S. Prescher-Hughes

Disclaimer

The authors have attempted to ensure that the information is current and accurate. Due to the vast amount of information regarding each chemotherapy agent, we have included only the major side effects of these agents. We do not proclaim to have included every reaction to these agents and referencing to the package insert, other references, the manufacturer or a pharmacist, for more comprehensive information may not be included in this text.

Under no circumstances can the authors be held liable for the use and application of the information of any of the contents of this book. The ultimate responsibility in administering chemotherapy is in the hands of the physicians and nurses on the basis of their professional licenses, their level of expertise, and experience.

About the Authors

Debra S. Prescher-Hughes obtained her Associates Degree in Nursing at Rochester Community College, Rochester Minnesota in 1975. She worked as a staff nurse at St. Mary's Hospital, Rochester Minnesota, a Mayo Clinic Affiliate from 1975 through 1977. She worked as a PRN nurse while obtaining her Bachelor of Science in Nursing at Metropolitan State College in Denver, Colorado. After graduation she worked at St. Joseph Hospital, Denver, Colorado, on the oncology unit, and was charge nurse for one year and worked for Kaiser Permanente for two years. In 1986, she opened an oncology practice with Dr. Richard Hesky in Denver. Over the years that practice has grown into a three doctor practice, Hesky-Fisher-Luknic, MDs, with a staff of 15 employees.

In addition to her responsibilities with the practice, Ms. Prescher-Hughes is a nationally recognized speaker providing education programs for oncology nurses, administrative staff, and patients. She is on multiple speaker's bureaus including, Genentech, Novartis, Solvay, AstraZeneca, Roche, Wyeth, Abraxis Oncology, and Pfizer.

She is a member of the Oncology Nursing Society and her local chapter is the Metro Denver ONS. She is Oncology Certified through the ONS.

Cynthia J. Shryock (Alkhoudairy) earned a Bachelor's Degree in Business Administration in 1983 from the University of Colorado in Boulder, Colorado, an Associates Degree in Nursing in 1985 from Arapahoe Community College in Littleton, Colorado, and a Bachelor of Science in Nursing in 1987 from the University of Colorado Health Sciences Center in Denver, Colorado. She has been an Oncology Certified Nurse since 1999 and is a member of the Oncology Nursing Society. Her local chapter is the Metro Denver ONS.

Cynthia worked as a Graduate Nurse at the Hospice of St. John during her nurse's training and as a staff nurse and later, Charge Nurse of Oncology at St. Joseph Hospital in Denver, Colorado from 1985–1997. She moved to the private practice with Drs Hesky, Fisher, and Luknic in 1997, and continues to work in the growing practice that just added its fourth doctor, Deborah Cook.

Preface

Developing Practice Protocols

Protocols are the recipes for an efficient and well run oncology practice, (the term protocol used in this article does not mean research protocols but is the term used for the guidelines for administering commonly used chemotherapy regimens). Without practice protocols you may be spending precious time hunting for articles, calling the pharmaceutical representative or the manufacturer, looking for protocol on the internet and/or checking the compendia in order to obtain the appropriate information for the treatment that has been ordered for your patients. In addition, your nurses will be hastily looking up the drugs and their side effects. They need to know how to mix them, how to dilute the drugs, how to administer the drug and the amount time that it will take to administer those drugs. They also need to know if the drugs need to be administered via a pump or with special tubing and if anti-emetics or other supportive drugs are required. They need to know if there is a specific order in which the drugs should be administered. Is there adequate patient education material available and are the nurses familiar with that information? These are the obstacles your practice may face if you do not have evidence based practice protocols in place. Additionally there is strong evidence that reducing variability improves patient safety.

Clinical Practice Protocols in Oncology Nursing has been a work in progress for over 20 years. There were no "Cliff Notes" for Chemotherapy Administration. I kept thinking that there must be something out there, perhaps a cheat sheet that would make my job easier. I discussed the idea with our doctors, pharmaceutical representatives and anyone who would listen. I thought, "Someone should put this information together." But no one had. Finally, I realized that I could be that someone. I convinced one of my nurses, Cindy Shryock (Alkhoudairy) to write the book with me and she has been a tremendous asset to this project. Developing practice protocols has been a time consuming task, but they have made our practice more efficient and eliminated the hassle of looking for a protocol at the last minute. I feel that these protocols have improved our patient safety and saved our practice money by improving our efficiencies. Today when reimbursement is diminishing, experienced nurses are in short supply, and nursing salaries are increasing, practice protocols are a must. We need an avenue to obtain accurate information quickly.

In our practice, as the nurse manager, I was assigned the task of developing our practice protocols, our own "chemotherapy recipe book" so to speak. Most books that have been published give us the "ingredients" of the protocol but not the "how to" of mixing, stability, or how long to administer the drugs. We started with a list of the most commonly used protocols and then gathered the necessary information to mix and administer the chemotherapy agents. Over time we have expanded the practice protocols to include the major side effects of the chemotherapy agents and any supportive drugs that may be necessary to support the patient through their treatments. These protocols not only include the administration piece, but they also serve as the physician orders for a particular patient. Additionally, we included the frequency of the visits and the number of visits that will be required to complete the chemotherapy course. This information adds another dimension to the protocol as it will give the necessary information for scheduling patients' appointments, this frees nurses who, in many practices have had that responsibility, from the administrative tasks. By including all of this information, we have provided a one page summary for the entire practice.

In the evolution of *Clinical Practice Protocols in Oncology Nursing*, I realized that reimbursement is an issue that everyone in the practice needs to be conscious. Therefore, we added a chapter on billing and reimbursement. Risë Cleland, a good friend and colleague of mine volunteered to write this chapter providing information regarding "Reimbursement, What Nurses Need to Know." As you can see by her biography, she has an incredible amount of experience and is very knowledgeable in this area of oncology.

These protocols have evolved to make our practice protocols comprehensive tools for efficient and safe chemotherapy administration. Not only have we included the *how to's* for nurses, but we have also included a tool for the support staff to determine the length of time for the patient's appointment and to obtain the appropriate number of referrals and authorization from the insurance companies. *Clinical Practice Protocols in Oncology Nursing* was written with nurses in mind, but they may also be an easy tool for your physicians and/or residents for writing chemotherapy orders that could become a part of the patient's permanent record. A CD-ROM is included to allow you to customize the protocols to your particular preferences in fluids, fluid volume, antiemetics, antidiarrheal medications, and other supportive drugs so that the protocol you print out on your letterhead is truly the protocol for your practice.

We hope that these protocols will be as valuable to your practice as they have been to ours and that perhaps the efficiencies of having the necessary information so readily available will improve your patient care and allow you to spend more quality time with your patients.

Debra S. Prescher-Hughes, RN, BSN, OCN

Acknowledgments

The writing of this book began with the idea of providing nurses with a resource that would allow them to have the necessary information to not only administer chemotherapy accurately and safely, but to also have enough information at their finger tips to help educate their patients as to the side effects of those treatments. All of the information in this book was obtained from common chemotherapy treatments with the appropriate references in medical and nursing literature. Providing a resource that contains all of that information in one location makes the protocols a very valuable resource. By adding the infusion time, chair time, and treatment schedules in addition to the insurance piece and making the entire form a part of the permanent record, I feel we have created a tool that is useful to the entire office.

This book would not have been possible without the help of many wonderful friends and colleagues. First of all, we would like to thank Dr. Richard Hesky, Dr. Kerry Fisher, and Dr. Alice Luknic for allowing us to publish these protocols that originated, in a less elaborate form, as the practice protocols used in our office. Over the past 20 years while working with these doctors, we have developed a very collaborative practice with quality patient care as our focus and I thank them for the opportunity they have provided.

I would also like to acknowledge our oncology nurses, Jennifer Anthony, Becky Brown, Cleo Morgan, and Janelle Wagner for taking on more work when Cindy and I were collecting information we needed for the book. They are an awesome group of nurses and make working fun. I want to thank our entire staff, Jean Stahlecker, Renea Lockwood, Vanessa Mitchell, Sara Collins, Aimee Allen, Laura Hund, Jane Sellers, Darrin Garcia, and Michelle Lewis for their support, understanding, and the prompt delivery of phone calls and messages that were so important especially during our deadlines. Our entire office staff was extremely tolerant with us when we had worked into the late evening hours and came back to work the next day a little overtired and sometimes a little grumpy. You are the best!

A special thank you to Cindy Shryock (Alkhoudairy), my co-author, for buying into my idea and working so hard to make this a book a reality. This would not have happened without you. Risë Cleland, a good friend and colleague, was very generous in providing us with information on reimbursement that will be invaluable to so many practices caring for cancer patients.

I also need to express our appreciation to our pharmaceutical representatives who were so diligent in helping us obtain the references for our protocols. Their efforts lightened our load tremendously. We have so many representatives that it would be impossible to name them all, but you know who you are. Thanks to all of you.

A thank you to Connie Yarbro who introduced me to our editors at Jones and Bartlett. I don't think Chris Davis really understood the depth of information we were attempting to put together, but he stuck with us. Renée Sekerak, our production editor is destined to sainthood after working with us over the past two years. She has been incredibly tolerant of two rookie authors and we couldn't have accomplished this without her.

Last but not least I want to thank my husband Patrick, my children Andrew, Katie, her husband Rob, and our youngest son Tim for allowing me to spend so much of my time behind a computer and on the Internet, writing and editing this book. After 20 years of thinking about the book I finally put the wheel in motion in 2005, the year Tim graduated from high school and my daughter Katie married Rob. What was I thinking? They were all so very supportive and I thank them for encouraging me to undertake this important project. I love you guys!

Contents

ANAL CANCER

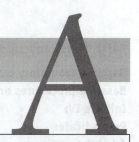

5-Fluorouracil: 1000 mg/m^2/day IV continuous infusion on days 1–4 and 29–32

Mitomycin: 15 mg/m^2 IV on day 1

Radiation therapy: 200 cGy/day on days 1–5, 8–12, and 5–19 (total dose, 3000 cGy)

Chemotherapy is given concurrently with radiation therapy[1,2]

5-Fluorouracil: 750 mg/m^2/day IV continuous infusion on days 1–5 and 29–33

Mitomycin: 15 mg/m^2 IV on day 1

Radiation therapy: 180 cGy/day over 5-week period (total dose, 4500 cGy)

Chemotherapy is given concurrently with radiation therapy. If partial or complete response occurs, a boost of 1500–2000 cGy is given[1,3]

5-Fluorouracil: 250 mg/m^2/day IV continuous infusion on days 1–5 of each week of radiation therapy

Cisplatin: 4 mg/m^2/day IV continuous infusion on days 1–5 of each week of radiation therapy

Radiation therapy: Total dose, 5500 cGy over 6 weeks

Chemotherapy is given concurrently with radiation therapy[1,4]

Metastatic Disease and/or Salvage Chemotherapy

5-Fluorouracil: 1000 mg/m^2/day IV continuous infusion on days 1–5

Cisplatin: 100 mg/m^2 IV on day 2

Repeat cycle every 21–28 days.[1,5]

5-FU + Mitomycin + Radiation Therapy (Wayne State Regimen)

Baseline laboratory tests:	CBC: Chemistry and carcinoembryonic antigen (CEA)
Baseline procedures or tests:	Central line placement
Initiate IV:	0.9% sodium chloride
Premedicate:	5-HT$_3$ and dexamethasone 10 in 100 cc of normal saline (NS)
Administer:	**Fluorouracil** _____ mg (1000 mg/m^2/day) IV continuous infusion days 1–4 and 29–32

- Available in solution as 50 mg/mL.
- No dilution required. Can be further diluted with 0.9% sodium chloride or 5% dextrose and water (D5W).

AND

Mitomycin _____ mg (15 mg/m^2) IV on day 1

- Potent vesicant
- Available in 5-, 20-, and 40-mg vials for IV use.
- Dilute with sterile water to give a final concentration of 0.5 mg/mL.
- Reconstituted solution is stable for 14 days if refrigerated or 7 days at room temperature.

Radiation therapy:	200 cGy/day on days 1–5, 8–12, and 15–19 (total dose, 3000 cGy)

- Chemotherapy is given concurrently with radiation therapy.

Major Side Effects

- Bone Marrow Depression: Dose limiting and cumulative toxicity, with leukopenia being more common than thrombocytopenia. Nadir counts are delayed at 4–6 weeks.
- Gastrointestinal Toxicities: Nausea and vomiting usually mild to moderate. Mucositis and diarrhea can be severe and dose limiting.
- Skin: Mitomycin causes tissue necrosis and chemical thrombophlebitos if extravasated. Local tissue irritation progressing to desquamation can occur in radiation (XRT) fields. Do not use oil-based lotions or creams in radiation field. Hyperpigmentation, photosensitivity, and nail changes may occur. Hand-foot syndrome can be dose limiting.
- Ocular: Photophobia, increased lacrimation, acute and chronic conjunctivitis, blepharitis, and blurred vision.
- Pulmonary: Interstitial pneumonitis. Presents with dyspnea, non-productive cough, and interstitial infiltiates on CXR.
- Hemolytic-uremic Syndrome: Hematocrit < 25%, platelets < 100 × 10^3/mm^3, and renal failure (serum creatinine > 1.6 mg/dL). Rare event (< 2%).
- Reproductive: Pregnancy category D. Breast feeding should be avoided.

Initiate antiemetic protocol:	Mild to moderately emetogenic protocol.
Supportive drugs:	☐ pegfilgrastim (Neulasta) ☐ filgrastim (Neupogen)
	☐ epoetin alfa (Procrit) ☐ darbepoetin alfa (Aranesp)
Treatment schedule:	Chair time 1 hour on days 1 and 29. Total cycle 32 days.
Estimated number of visits:	Five visits per treatment course.

Dose Calculation by: 1. _____ 2. _____

_____
Physician

_____
Date

_____
Patient Name

_____
ID Number

_____
Diagnosis

_____ / _____ / _____
Ht   Wt   M^2

5-FU + Mitomycin + Radiation Therapy (EORTC Regimen)

Baseline laboratory tests:	CBC: Chemistry and CEA
Baseline procedures or tests:	Central line placement
Initiate IV:	0.9% sodium chloride
Premedicate:	5-HT$_3$ and dexamethasone 10 in 100 cc of NS
Administer:	**Fluorouracil** _____ mg (750 mg/m^2/day) IV continuous infusion days 1–5 and 29–33

- Available in solution as 50 mg/mL.
- No dilution required. Can be further diluted with 0.9% sodium chloride or D5W.

AND

Mitomycin _____ mg (15 mg/m^2) IV bolus on day 1

- Available in 5-, 20-, and 40-mg vials for IV use.
- Potent vesicant
- Dilute with sterile water to give a final concentration of 0.5 mg/mL. Reconstituted solution stable for 14 days refrigerated or 7 days at room temperature.

Radiation therapy:	180 cGy/day over 5 week period. Total dose, 4500 cGy over 5 weeks

- Chemotherapy is given concurrently with radiation therapy.
- If partial or complete response seen, a boost of 1500–2000 cGy is given.

Major Side Effects

- Bone Marrow Depression: Dose limiting, and cumulative toxicity with leukopenia more common than thrombocytopenia. Nadir counts are delayed at 4–6 weeks.
- Gastrointestinal (GI) Toxicities: Nausea and vomiting usually mild to moderate. Mucositis and diarrhea can be severe and dose limiting.
- Skin: Mitomycin causes tissue necrosis if extravasated. Local tissue irritation progressing to desquamation can occur in XRT fields. Do not use oil-based lotions or creams in radiation field. Hyperpigmentation, photosensitivity, and nail changes may occur. Hand-foot syndrome can be dose limiting.
- Ocular: Photophobia, increased lacrimation, acute and chronic conjunctivitis, blepharitis, and blurred vision.
- Pulmonary: Interstitial pneumonitis. Presents with dyspnea, non-productive cough, and interstitial infiltiates on CXR.
- Hemolytic-uremic syndrome: Hematocrit < 25%, platelets < 100 × 10^3/mm^3, and renal failure (serum creatinine > 1.6 mg/dL). Rare event (< 2%).
- Reproductive: Pregnancy category D. Breast feeding should be avoided.

Initiate antiemetic protocol:	Mild to moderately emetogenic protocol.
Supportive drugs:	☐ pegfilgrastim (Neulasta) ☐ filgrastim (Neupogen)
	☐ epoetin alfa (Procrit) ☐ darbepoetin alfa (Aranesp)
Treatment schedule:	Chair time 1 hour on days 1 and 29. Total cycle 33 days.
Estimated number of visits:	Four visits per treatment course.

Dose Calculation by: 1. _____   2. _____

Physician _____   Date _____

Patient Name _____   ID Number _____

Diagnosis _____   Ht _____ / Wt _____ / M^2 _____

5-FU + Cisplatin + Radiation Therapy (MD Anderson Regimen)

Baseline laboratory tests:	CBC: Chemistry (including Mg^{2+}) and CEA
Baseline procedures or tests:	Central line placement
Initiate IV:	0.9% sodium chloride
Premedicate:	5-HT$_3$ and dexamethasone 10–20 mg in 100 cc of NS
Administer:	**Fluorouracil** _____mg (250 mg/m²/day) IV continuous infusion days 1–5 of each week of radiation therapy

- Available in solution as 50 mg/mL.
- No dilution required. Can be further diluted with 0.9% sodium chloride or D5W.

AND

Cisplatin _____mg (4 mg/m²/day) IV continuous infusion days 1–5 of each week of radiation therapy

- Available in solution as 1 mg/mL.
- Do not use aluminum needles because precipitate will form.
- Further dilute solution with 250 cc or more NS.
- Stable for 96 hours when protected from light and only 6 hours if not protected from light.

Radiation therapy:	Total dose 5500 cGy over 6 weeks

- Chemotherapy is given concurrently with radiation therapy.

Major Side Effects

- Hypersensitivity Reactions: Facial edema, wheezing, bronchospasm, and hypotension possible with cisplatin.
- Bone Marrow Depression: Neutropenia, thrombocytopenia, and anemia are dose related. Can be dose limiting for daily × 5 or weekly regimens.
- GI Toxicities: Moderate to severe nausea and vomiting may be acute or delayed. Mucositis and diarrhea can be severe and dose limiting. Metallic taste to food.
- Renal: Nephrotoxicity is dose related and dose limiting with cisplatin and presents at 10–20 days. Usually reversible.
- Electrolyte Imbalance: Decreases Mg^{2+}, K^+, Ca^{2+}, Na^+, and P levels. Inappropriate secretion of antidiuretic hormone (SIADH).
- Skin: Alopecia. Local tissue irritation progressing to desquamation can occur in radiation field. Do not use oil-based lotions or creams in radiation field. Hyperpigmentation, photosensitivity, and nail changes may occur. Hand-foot syndrome can be dose limiting.
- Ototoxicity: High frequency hearing loss and tinnitus.
- Ocular: Photophobia, increased lacrimation, acute and chronic conjunctivitis, blepharitis, and blurred vision.
- Reproductive: Pregnancy category D. Breast feeding should be avoided. Azoospermia, impotence, and sterility.

Initiate antiemetic protocol:	Moderately to highly emetogenic protocol.
Supportive drugs:	☐ pegfilgrastim (Neulasta) ☐ filgrastim (Neupogen)
	☐ epoetin alfa (Procrit) ☐ darbepoetin alfa (Aranesp)
Treatment schedule:	Chair time 2 hours on day 1 of each week of radiation therapy.
Estimated number of visits:	Twelve visits per treatment course.

Dose Calculation by: 1. _____   2. _____

_____   _____
Physician   Date

_____   _____
Patient Name   ID Number

_____   _____ / _____ / _____
Diagnosis   Ht   Wt   M²

Metastatic Disease and/or Salvage Chemotherapy

5-FU and Cisplatin

Baseline laboratory tests:	CBC: Chemistry (including Mg^{2+}) and CEA
Baseline procedures or tests:	Central line placement
Initiate IV:	0.9% sodium chloride
Premedicate:	5-HT_3 and dexamethasone 10–20 mg in 100 cc of NS
Administer:	**Fluorouracil** _____ mg (1000 mg/m²/day) IV continuous infusion on days 1–5

- Available in solution as 50 mg/mL.
- No dilution required. Can be further diluted with 0.9% sodium chloride or D5W.

AND

Cisplatin _____ mg (100 mg/m²) IV on day 2

- Available in solution 1 mg/mL.
- Do not use aluminum needles because precipitate will form.
- Further dilute solution with 250 cc or more of NS.
- Stable for 96 hours when protected from light and only 6 hours when not protected from light.

Major Side Effects

- Bone Marrow Depression: Neutropenia, thrombocytopenia, and anemia are dose related. Can be dose limiting for daily × 5 or weekly regimens.
- GI Toxicities: Moderate to severe nausea and vomiting, may be acute or delayed. Mucositis and diarrhea can be severe and dose limiting.
- Renal: Nephrotoxicity is dose related and dose limiting with cisplatin and presents at 10–20 days. Usually reversible.
- Electrolyte Imbalance: Decreases Mg^{2+}, K^+, Ca^{2+}, Na^+, and P levels. Inappropriate secretion of antidiuretic hormone (SIADH).
- Skin: Hyperpigmentation, photosensitivity, and nail changes may occur. Hand-foot syndrome can be dose limiting.
- Ototoxicity: High frequency hearing loss and tinnitus.
- Ocular: Photophobia, increased lacrimation, acute and chronic conjunctivitis, blepharitis, and blurred vision.
- Reproductive: Pregnancy category D. Breast feeding should be avoided. Azoospermia, impotence, and sterility.

Initiate antiemetic protocol:	Moderately to highly emetogenic protocol.
Supportive drugs:	☐ pegfilgrastim (Neulasta) ☐ filgrastim (Neupogen)
	☐ epoetin alfa (Procrit) ☐ darbepoetin alfa (Aranesp)
Treatment schedule:	Chair time 1 hour on day 1 and 3 hours on day 2. Repeat every 21–28 days as tolerated or until disease progression.
Estimated number of visits:	Two visits per cycle. Ask for three cycles worth of visits.

Dose Calculation by: 1. _____   2. _____

_____
Physician

_____
Date

_____
Patient Name

_____
ID Number

_____
Diagnosis

_____ / _____ / _____
Ht   Wt   M²

BILIARY TRACT CANCER

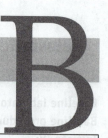

Gemcitabine: 1250 mg/m^2 IV on days 1 and 8
Cisplatin: 75 mg/m^2 IV on day 1
Repeat cycle every 21 days.[1,2]

Gemcitabine: 1000 mg/m^2 IV on days 1 and 8
Capecitabine: 650 mg/m^2 PO bid on days 1–14
Repeat cycle every 21 days.[1,7]

Gemcitabine + Cisplatin

Baseline laboratory tests:	CBC: Chemistry panel, LFTs, creatinine clearance, and CA 19-9
Baseline procedures or tests:	N/A
Initiate IV:	0.9% sodium chloride
Premedicate:	5-HT$_3$ and dexamethasone 10–20 mg in 100 cc of NS
Administer:	**Gemcitabine** _____ mg (1250 mg/m^2) IV on days 1 and 8

- Available in 1-g or 200-mg vials; reconstitute with 0.9% sodium chloride USP (5 cc for 200 mg, 25 cc for 1 g). Further dilute in 0.9% sodium chloride.
- Reconstituted solution is stable for 24 hours at room temperature. DO NOT refrigerate, because precipitate will form.

Cisplatin _____ mg (75 mg/m^2) IV on days 1 and 15

- Available in solution 1 mg/mL.
- Do not use aluminum needles, because precipitate will form.
- Further dilute solution with 250 cc or more 0.9% sodium chloride.
- Stable for 96 hours when protected from light and only 6 hours when not protected from light.

Major Side Effects

- Hypersensitivity Reaction: Facial edema, wheezing, bronchospasm, and hypotension possible with cisplatin.
- Hematologic: Leukopenia, thrombocytopenia, and anemia, with grade 3 and 4 thrombocytopenia more common in elderly patients. Myelosuppression is dose limiting. Nadir occurs in 10–14 days, with recovery at 21 days. Prolonged infusion time (> 60 minutes) of gemcitabine is associated with higher toxicities.
- GI Symptoms: Moderate to severe nausea and vomiting; may be acute or delayed. Diarrhea and/or mucositis. Metallic taste to food.
- Flulike Syndrome: Fever in absence of infection 6–12 hours after treatment common. Fever, malaise, chills, headache, and myalgias.
- Renal: Nephrotoxicity is dose related and dose limiting with cisplatin and occurs at 10–20 days. Usually reversible.
- Neurotoxicity: Sensory neuropathy; dose related.
- Electrolyte imbalance: Decreased Mg^{2+}, K, Ca^{2+}, Na$^+$, and P. Inappropriate secretion of antidiuretic hormone (SIADH).
- Hepatic: Elevation of serum transaminase and bilirubin levels.
- Skin: Pruritic, maculopapular skin rash, usually involving trunk and extremities. Edema occurs in 30% of patients. Alopecia.
- Ototoxicity: High frequency hearing loss and tinnitus.
- Use in Pregnancy: Embryotoxic; women of childbearing potential should avoid becoming pregnant during treatment.

Initiate antiemetic protocol:	Moderately to highly emetogenic protocol.
Supportive drugs:	☐ pegfilgrastim (Neulasta) ☐ filgrastim (Neupogen)
	☐ epoetin alfa (Procrit) ☐ darbepoetin alfa (Aranesp)
Treatment schedule:	Chair time 3 hours on days 1 and 15, and 1 hour on day 8. Repeat cycle every 21 days.
Estimated number of visits:	Three visits per cycle. Request three cycles worth of visits.

Dose Calculation by: 1. _____ 2. _____

_____
Physician

_____
Date

_____
Patient Name

_____
ID Number

_____
Diagnosis

_____ / _____ / _____
Ht   Wt   M^2

Gemcitabine + Capecitabine

Baseline laboratory tests:	CBC: Chemistry panel, LFTs, creatinine clearance, and CA 19-9
Baseline procedures or tests:	N/A
Initiate IV:	0.9% sodium chloride
Premedicate:	Oral phenothiazine
	OR
	5-HT$_3$ and dexamethasone 10 mg in 100 cc of NS
Administer:	**Gemcitabine** _____ mg (1000 mg/m^2) IV days 1 and 8

- Available in 1-g or 200-mg vials, reconstitute with 0.9% sodium chloride USP (5 cc for 200 mg, 25 cc for 1 g). Further dilute in 0.9% sodium chloride.
- Reconstituted solution is stable for 24 hours at room temperature. DO NOT refrigerate, because precipitate will form.

Capecitabine _____ mg (650 mg/m^2) PO bid on days 1–14

- Available in 150 mg and 500 mg tablets.
- Administer within 30 minutes of a meal with plenty of water.
- Monitor international normalized ratios (INRs) closely in patients taking warfarin; may increase INR

Major Side Effects

- Hematologic: Leukopenia, thrombocytopenia, and anemia, with grades 3 and 4 thrombocytopenia more common in elderly patients. Myelosuppression is dose limiting. Nadir occurs in 10–14 days with recovery at 21 days. Prolonged infusion time (> 60 minutes) of gemcitabine is associated with higher toxicities.
- GI Symptoms: Mild-to-moderate nausea and vomiting (70%), diarrhea and/or mucositis (15%–20%). Diarrhea occurs in up to 40%, with 12% being grade 3–4. Stomatitis is common, 3% of which is severe.
- Flulike Syndrome: Fever in absence of infection 6–12 hours after treatment common. Fever, malaise, chills, headache, and myalgias.
- Hepatic: Elevation of serum transaminase and bilirubin levels. Dose modifications may be required if hyperbilirubinemia occurs.
- Renal Insufficiency: Capecitabine contraindicated in patients with creatinine clearance < 30 mL/min. Dose reduction to 75% should be made with baseline creatinine clearance of 30–50 mL/min.
- Skin: Hand-foot syndrome (15%–20%). Pruritic, maculopapular skin rash, usually involving trunk and extremities. Edema occurs in 30% of patients. Alopecia is rare.
- Use in Pregnancy: Embryotoxic; women of childbearing potential should avoid becoming pregnant during treatment.

Initiate antiemetic protocol:	Mildly to moderately emetogenic protocol.
Supportive drugs:	☐ pegfilgrastim (Neulasta) ☐ filgrastim (Neupogen)
	☐ epoetin alfa (Procrit) ☐ darbepoetin alfa (Aranesp)
Treatment schedule:	Chair time 1 hour days 1 and 8. Repeat cycle every 3 weeks on, 1 week off until disease progression.
Estimated number of visits:	Three visits per cycle. Request 4 cycles worth of visits.

Dose Calculation by: 1. _____ 2. _____

_____
Physician

_____
Date

_____
Patient Name

_____
ID Number

_____
Diagnosis

_____ / _____ / _____
Ht   Wt   M^2

BLADDER CANCER

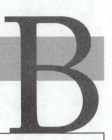

Combination Regimens

Ifosfamide: 1500 mg/m^2 IV on days 1, 2, and 3
Paclitaxel: 200 mg/m^2 IV over 3 hours on day 1
Cisplatin: 70 mg/m^2 IV on day 1
Repeat cycle every 21 days.[1,8] Granulocyte colony stimulating factor
(G-CSF) support is recommended. Regimen can also be administered
every 28 days.

Gemcitabine: 1000 mg/m^2 IV on days 1, 8, and 15
Cisplatin: 75 mg/m^2 IV on day 1
Repeat cycle every 28 days.[1,9]

Methotrexate: 30 mg/m^2 IV on days 1, 15, and 22
Vinblastine: 3 mg/m^2 IV on days 2, 15, and 22
Doxorubicin: 30 mg/m^2 IV on day 2
Cisplatin: 70 mg/m^2 IV on day 2
Repeat cycle every 28 days.[1,10]

Cisplatin: 100 mg/m^2 IV on day 2 (give 12 hours after methotrexate)
Methotrexate: 30 mg/m^2 IV on days 1 and 8
Vinblastine: 4 mg/m^2 IV on days 1 and 8
Repeat cycle every 21 days.[1,11]

Cyclophosphamide: 650 mg/m^2 IV on day 1
Doxorubicin: 50 mg/m^2 IV on day 1
Cisplatin: 100 mg/m^2 IV on day 2
Repeat cycle every 21–28 days.[1,12]

Paclitaxel: 225 mg/m^2 IV over 3 hours on day 1

Carboplatin: Area under the curve (AUC) of 6, IV on day 1, given 15 minutes after paclitaxel

Repeat cycle every 21 days.[1,13]

Cyclophosphamide: 400 mg/m^2 IV on day 1

Doxorubicin: 40 mg/m^2 IV on day 1

Cisplatin: 75 mg/m^2 IV on day 1

Repeat cycle every 21 days.[1,14]

Cisplatin: 70 mg/m^2 IV on day 2

Methotrexate: 30 mg/m^2 IV on days 1, 15, and 22

Vinblastine: 3 mg/m^2 IV on days 2, 15, and 22

Repeat cycle every 28 days for two cycles.[1,15] Radiation therapy to be given after two cycles of induction chemotherapy at a total dose of 45 cGy in 180cGy fractions combined with cisplatin 70 mg/m^2 IV on days 1 and 2 of radiation therapy.

Single-Agent Regimens

Gemcitabine: 1200 mg/m^2 IV on days 1, 8, and 15

Repeat cycle every 28 days.[1,16]

Paclitaxel: 250 mg/m^2 IV over 24 hours on day 1

Repeat cycle every 21 days.[1,17]

OR

Paclitaxel: 80 mg/m^2 IV weekly for 3 weeks

Repeat cycle every 4 weeks.[1,18]

Combination Regimens

Ifosfamide + Paclitaxel + Cisplatin (ITP)

Baseline laboratory tests:	CBC: Chemistry (including Mg^{2+})
Baseline procedures or tests:	N/A
Initiate IV:	0.9% sodium chloride
Premedicate:	5-HT_3 and dexamethasone 10–20 mg in 100 cc of NS (days 1–3)
	Diphenhydramine 25–50 mg and cimetidine 300 mg in 100 cc of NS (day 1 only)

Administer:

Ifosfamide _____ mg (1500 mg/m²) IV on days 1, 2, and 3

- Available as powder in 1- and 3-mg single dose vials.
- Reconstitute powder with sterile water for injection. Discard unused portion after 8 hours.
- May further dilute in D5W or 0.9% sodium chloride.

Paclitaxel _____ mg (200 mg/m²) IV over 3 hours on day 1

- Available in solution 6 mg/mL.
- Final concentration is $\leq$ 1.2 mg/mL
- **Use non-PVC tubing and containers and 0.22-micron inline filter to administer.**

Cisplatin _____ mg (70 mg/m²) IV on day 1

- Available in solution 1 mg/mL.
- Do not use aluminum needles because precipitate will form.
- Further dilute solution with 250 cc or more of NS.
- Stable for up to 27 hours at room temperature in 0.3–1.2 mg/mL solutions.

Major Side Effects

- Hypersensitivity Reaction: Paclitaxel: Usually seen in the first 2–3 minutes of infusion. Characterized by generalized skin rash, flushing, erythema, hypotension, dyspnea and/or bronchospasm. Premedicate as described. Cisplatin: Facial edema, wheezing, bronchospasm, and hypotension is possible.
- Bone Marrow Depression: Neutropenia, thrombocytopenia, and anemia are cumulative and dose related. Can be dose limiting. G-CSF support recommended. Give paclitaxel before cisplatin to decrease severity of myelosuppression.
- GI Toxicities: Moderate to severe nausea and vomiting may be acute or delayed. Mucositis and/or diarrhea common.
- Renal: Nephrotoxicity is dose related and dose limiting with cisplatin and presents at 10–20 days. Hemorrhagic cystitis dysuria and increased urinary frequency occurs with ifosfamide. Uroprotection with mesna and hydration mandatory.
- Electrolyte Imbalance: Decreases Mg^{2+}, K^+, Ca^{2+}, Na^+, and P. Inappropriate secretion of antidiuretic hormone (SIADH).
- Neurotoxicity: Sensory neuropathy with numbness and paresthesias. Is dose-related and dose limiting.
- Central Nervous System (CNS): Somnolence, confusion, depressive psychosis, or hallucinations.
- Alopecia: Total loss of body hair occurs in nearly all patients.
- Ototoxicity: High frequency hearing loss and tinnitus.
- Reproduction: Ifosfamide is mutagenic, teratogenic, carcinogenic, and excreted in breast milk. Also causes amenorrhea, oligospermia, and infertility. Paclitaxel is embryotoxic.

Initiate antiemetic protocol:	Moderately to highly emetogenic protocol.

Supportive drugs:

☐ pegfilgrastim (Neulasta) ☐ filgrastim (Neupogen)
☐ epoetin alfa (Procrit) ☐ darbepoetin alfa (Aranesp)

Treatment schedule:	Chair time 7 hours on day 1, and 3 hours on days 2 and 3. Repeat cycle every 28 days.
Estimated number of visits:	Four visits per cycle. Request three cycles worth of visits.

Dose Calculation by: 1. _____   2. _____

_____   _____
Physician   Date

_____   _____
Patient Name   ID Number

_____   _____/_____/_____
Diagnosis   Ht   Wt   M²

Gemcitabine + Cisplatin

Baseline laboratory tests:	CBC: Chemistry panel (including Mg^{2+}) and liver function tests (LFTs)
Baseline procedures or tests:	N/A
Initiate IV:	0.9% sodium chloride
Premedicate:	5-HT$_3$ and dexamethasone 10–20 mg in 100 cc of NS
Administer:	**Gemcitabine** _____ mg (1000 mg/m²) IV on days 1, 8, and 15

- Available in 1-g or 200-mg vials; reconstitute with 0.9% sodium chloride USP (5 cc for 200 mg, 25 cc for 1 g). Further dilute in 0.9% sodium chloride.
- Reconstituted solution is stable 24 hours at room temperature. Do not refrigerate, because precipitate will form.

Cisplatin _____ mg (75 mg/m²) IV on day 1. Do not use aluminum needles, because precipitate will form.

- Available in solution 1 mg/mL.
- Further dilute solution with 250 cc or more of 0.9% sodium chloride.
- Stable for 96 hours when protected from light and only 6 hours when not protected from light.

Major Side Effects

- Hypersensitivity Reaction: Facial edema, wheezing, bronchospasm, and hypotension is possible with cisplatin.
- Hematologic: Leukopenia, thrombocytopenia and anemia, with grade 3 and 4 thrombocytopenia being more common in elderly patients. Myelosuppression is dose limiting. Nadir occurs in 10–14 days, with recovery at 21 days. Prolonged infusion time (> 60 minutes) is associated with higher toxicities from Gemcitabine.
- GI Symptoms: Moderate-to-severe nausea and vomiting, may be acute or delayed. Diarrhea and/or mucositis. Metallic taste.
- Flulike Syndrome: Fever in absence of infection 6–12 hours after treatment common. Fever, malaise, chills, headache, and myalgias.
- Renal: Nephrotoxicity is dose related and dose limiting with cisplatin and occurs at 10–20 days.
- Neurotoxicity: Sensory neuropathy, dose related. Usually reversible.
- Electrolyte Imbalance: Decreases serum values of magnesium, potassium, calcium, sodium, and phosphorus. Inappropriate secretion of antidiuretic hormone (SIADH).
- Hepatic: Elevation levels of serum transaminases and bilirubin.
- Skin: Pruritic, maculopapular skin rash, usually involving trunk and extremities. Edema is seen in 30% of patients. Alopecia.
- Ototoxicity: High frequency hearing loss and tinnitus.
- Use in Pregnancy: Embryotoxic, women of child-bearing potential should avoid becoming pregnant during treatment.

Initiate antiemetic protocol:	Moderately to highly emetogenic protocol.
Supportive drugs:	☐ pegfilgrastim (Neulasta) ☐ filgrastim (Neupogen)
	☐ epoetin alfa (Procrit) ☐ darbepoetin alfa (Aranesp)
Treatment schedule:	Chair time 3 hours on day 1, and 1 hour on days 8 and 15. Repeat cycle every 28 days.
Estimated number of visits:	Four visits per cycle. Request three cycles worth of visits.
Dose Calculation by:	1. _____ 2. _____

_____

Physician

_____

Patient Name

_____

Diagnosis

_____

Date

_____

ID Number

_____ / _____ / _____

Ht   Wt   M²

Methotrexate + Vinblastine + Doxorubicin + Cisplatin (MVAC)

Baseline laboratory tests:	CBC: Chemistry (including Mg^{2+})
Baseline procedures or tests:	Multigated angiogram (MUGA) scan
Initiate IV:	0.9% sodium chloride
Premedicate:	5-HT_3 and dexamethasone 20 mg in 100 cc of NS.
Administer:	**Methotrexate** _____mg (30 mg/m²) IV on days 1, 15, and 22

- Available as solution in 5-, 50-, 100-, and 200-mg vials.
- May further dilute in 0.9% sodium chloride.
- Reconstituted solution stable 24 hours at room temperature.
- Use with caution in patients on warfarin due to increased anticoagulation effects.
- Have patients discontinue folic acid supplements while taking drug.

Vinblastine _____mg (3 mg/m²) IV on days 2, 15, and 22

- Potent vesicant
- Available in 10-mg, 1-mg/mL vials. Store in refrigerator until use.

Doxorubicin _____mg (30 mg/m²) IV on day 2

- Potent vesicant
- Available as a 2-mg/mL solution.
- Doxorubicin will form a precipitate if it is mixed with heparin or 5-FU.

Cisplatin _____mg (70 mg/m²) IV on day 2

- Available in solution as 1 mg/mL
- Do not use aluminum needles, because precipitate will form.
- Further dilute solution with 250–1000 cc of NS.
- Stable for 24 hours at room temperature.

Major Side Effects

- Hypersensitivity Reaction: Facial edema, wheezing, bronchospasm, and hypotension is possible with cisplatin.
- Bone Marrow Toxicity: Myelosuppression can be severe.
- GI Toxicities: Nausea and vomiting are moderate to severe and can be acute or delayed. Mucositis can be severe. Constipation, abdominal pain, or paralytic ileus. Metallic taste.
- Cardiovascular: Cardiomyopathy can occur with cumulative doses of doxorubicin. Hypertension, stroke, myocardial infarction, and Raynaud's syndrome seen with vinblastine.
- Renal: Acute renal failure, azotemia, urinary retention, and uric acid nephropathy. Red-orange colored urine for 24–48 hours after doxorubicin.
- Electrolyte Imbalance: Decreased Mg^{2+}, K^+, Ca^{2+}, Na^+, and P. Inappropriate secretion of antidiuretic hormone (SIADH).
- Pulmonary: Pneumonitis.
- Hepatic: Dose reduction of doxorubicin necessary in presence of liver dysfunction.
- Skin: Extravasation of vesicants causes severe tissue destruction. Rash, hyperpigmentation, photosensitivity, and radiation recall occur. Alopecia.
- Neurotoxicity: Peripheral sensory neuropathy, paresthesias.
- Ototoxicity: High-frequency hearing loss and tinnitus with cisplatin.
- Reproduction: Pregnancy category D. Breast feeding should be avoided.

Initiate antiemetic protocol:	Moderately to highly emetogenic protocol.
Supportive drugs:	☐ pegfilgrastim (Neulasta)　　　☐ filgrastim (Neupogen)
	☐ epoetin alfa (Procrit)　　　　☐ darbepoetin alfa (Aranesp)
Treatment schedule:	Chair time 1 hour on days 1, 15, and 22, and 3 hours on day 2. Repeat cycle every 28 days.
Estimated number of visits:	Four visits per cycle. Request four cycles worth of visits.[19–20]

Dose Calculation by: 1. _____   2. _____

_____   _____
Physician   Date

_____   _____
Patient Name   ID Number

_____   _____/_____   /   _____
Diagnosis   Ht   Wt M^2

Cisplatin + Methotrexate + Vinblastine (CMV)

Baseline laboratory tests:	CBC: Chemistry (including Mg^{2+})
Baseline procedures or tests:	None
Initiate IV:	0.9% sodium chloride
Premedicate:	5-HT_3 and dexamethasone 20 mg in 100 cc of NS.
Administer:	**Cisplatin** _____mg (100 mg/m^2) IV on day 2 (give 12 hours after methotrexate)

- Available in solution 1 mg/mL.
- Do not use aluminum needles, because precipitate will form.
- Available in solution as 1 mg/mL.
- Further dilute solution in 250 cc or more of NS.
- Stable for 96 hours when protected from light and only 6 hours when not protected from light.

Methotrexate _____mg (30 mg/m^2) IV on days 1 and 8

- Available as solution in 5-, 50-, 100-, and 200-mg vials.
- May further dilute in 0.9% sodium chloride.
- Use with caution in patients taking warfarin due to increased anticoagulation effects.
- Have patients discontinue folic acid supplements while taking drug.

Vinblastine _____mg (4 mg/m^2) IV on days 1 and 8

- Potent vesicant
- Available in 10-mg vials; store in refrigerator until use.

Major Side Effects

- Hypersensitivity Reaction: Facial edema, wheezing, bronchospasm, and hypotension is possible with cisplatin.
- Bone Marrow Depression: Myelosuppression can be severe.
- GI Toxicities: Nausea and vomiting are moderate to severe and can be acute or delayed. Mucositis can be severe. Constipation, abdominal pain, or paralytic ileus. Metallic taste.
- Renal: Acute renal failure, azotemia, urinary retention, and uric acid nephropathy.
- Electrolyte Imbalance: Decreased Mg^{2+}, K^+, Ca^{2+}, Na^+, and P. Inappropriate secretion of antidiuretic hormone (SIADH).
- Pulmonary: Pneumonitis.
- Skin: Extravasation of vesicants causes severe tissue destruction. Rash, hyperpigmentation, photosensitivity, and radiation recall occur. Alopecia.
- Neurotoxicity: Peripheral sensory neuropathy, paresthesias.
- Ototoxicity: High-frequency hearing loss and tinnitus with cisplatin.
- Reproduction: Pregnancy category D. Breast feeding should be avoided.

Initiate antiemetic protocol:	Moderately to highly emetogenic protocol.
Supportive drugs:	☐ pegfilgrastim (Neulasta) ☐ filgrastim (Neupogen)
	☐ epoetin alfa (Procrit) ☐ darbepoetin alfa (Aranesp)
Treatment schedule:	Chair time 1 hour on days 1 and 8, and 3 hours on day 2. Repeat cycle every 21 days.
Estimated number of visits:	Three visits per cycle. Request four cycles worth of visits.

Dose Calculation by: 1. _____   2. _____

_____
Physician

_____
Date

_____
Patient Name

_____
ID Number

_____
Diagnosis

_____ / _____ / _____
Ht   Wt   M^2

Cyclophosphamide + Doxorubicin + Cisplatin (CISCA)

Baseline laboratory tests:	CBC, Chemistry (including Mg^{2+})
Baseline procedures or tests:	MUGA scan
Initiate IV:	0.9% sodium chloride
Premedicate:	5-HT$_3$ and dexamethasone 20 mg in 100 cc of NS.
Administer:	**Cyclophosphamide** _____ mg (650 mg/m^2) IV on day 1

- Available in 100-, 200-, 500-, 1000-, and 2000-mg vials.
- Dilute with sterile water and shake well to ensure that solution is completely dissolved.
- Reconstituted solution stable for 24 hours at room temperature, 6 days refrigerated.

Doxorubicin _____ mg (50 mg/m^2) IV on day 1

- Potent vesicant
- Available as a 2 mg/mL solution.
- Doxorubicin will form a precipitate if it is mixed with heparin or 5-FU.

Cisplatin _____ mg (100 mg/m^2) IV on day 2

- Do not use aluminum needles, because precipitate will form.
- Available in solution as 1 mg/mL.
- Further dilute solution with 250 cc or more of NS.
- Stable for 96 hours when protected from light and only 6 hours when not protected from light.

Major Side Effects

- Hypersensitivity Reaction: Facial edema, wheezing, bronchospasm, and hypotension is possible with cisplatin. Cyclophosphamide can cause rhinitis and irritation of nose and throat.
- Bone Marrow Depression: Leukopenia, thrombocytopenia, and anemia all seen; may be severe.
- GI Toxicities: Nausea and vomiting are moderate to severe and can be acute or delayed. Stomatitis occurs in some patients but is not dose limiting. Metallic taste.
- Cardiac: Acutely, pericarditis-myocarditis syndrome may occur. With high cumulative doses of doxorubicin (> 550 mg/m^2), cardiomyopathy may occur.
- Renal/bladder toxicities: Nephrotoxicity is dose related with cisplatin and presents at 10–20 days. Hemorrhagic cystitis, dysuria, and urinary frequency.
- Hepatic: With cyclophosphamide, dose reduction of doxorubicin necessary in presence of liver dysfunction.
- Electrolyte Imbalance: Decreased Mg^{2+}, K^+, Ca^{2+}, Na^+, and P. Inappropriate secretion of antidiuretic hormone (SIADH).
- Skin: Extravasation of doxorubicin causes severe tissue destruction. Hyperpigmentation, photosensitivity and radiation recall occur. Complete alopecia.
- Neurotoxicity: Dose-limiting toxicity, usually in the form of peripheral sensory neuropathy. Paresthesias and numbness in a classic "stocking-glove" pattern.
- Ototoxicity: High-frequency hearing loss and tinnitus with cisplatin.
- Secondary Malignancies: Increased risk with cyclophosphamide.
- Reproduction: Pregnancy category D. Breast feeding should be avoided.

Initiate antiemetic protocol:	Moderately to severely emetogenic protocol.
Supportive drugs:	☐ pegfilgrastim (Neulasta) ☐ filgrastim (Neupogen) ☐ epoetin alfa (Procrit) ☐ darbepoetin alfa (Aranesp)
Treatment schedule:	Chair time 2 hours on day 1 and 3 hours on day 2. Repeat cycle every 21–28 days.
Estimated number of visits:	Three visits per cycle. Request four cycles worth of visits.

Dose Calculation by: 1. _____   2. _____

_____
Physician   Date

_____
Patient Name   ID Number

_____ / _____ / _____
Diagnosis   Ht   Wt   M²

Paclitaxel and Carboplatin

Baseline laboratory tests:	CBC: Chemistry (including Mg^{2+})
Baseline procedures or tests:	N/A
Initiate IV:	0.9% sodium chloride
Premedicate:	5-HT$_3$ and dexamethasone 10–20 mg in 100 cc of NS
	Diphenhydramine 25–50 mg and cimetidine 300 mg in 100 cc of NS

Administer: **Paclitaxel** _____ mg (225 mg/m^2) IV over 3 hours on day 1

- Available in solution as 6 mg/mL.
- Final concentration is $\leq$ 1.2 mg/mL.
- Stable for up to 27 hours at room temperature in 0.3–1.2 mg/mL solutions.
- **Use non-PVC containers and tubing with 0.22-micron inline filter to administer.**

Carboplatin _____ mg (AUC of 6) IV on day 1 (give 15 minutes after paclitaxel)

- Available in solution as 10 mg/mL or as lyopholized powder.
- Reconstitute sterile water for injection, 5% dextrose of 0.99 sodium chloride solution.
- Do not use aluminum needles, because precipitate will form.
- Reconstituted solution stable for 8 hours at room temperature.
- Give carboplatin **after** paclitaxel to decrease toxicities.

Major Side Effects

- Hypersensitivity Reaction: Paclitaxel, usually seen in the first 2–3 minutes of infusion. Characterized by generalized skin rash, flushing, erythema, hypotension, dyspnea, and/or bronchospasm. Premedicate as described. Increased risk of hypersensitivity reactions in patients receiving more than seven courses of carboplatin therapy.
- Bone Marrow Depression: Neutropenia, thrombocytopenia, and anemia are cumulative and dose related. Can be dose limiting. G-CSF support recommended.
- GI Toxicities: Nausea and vomiting are moderate to severe and may be acute or delayed. Mucositis and/or diarrhea common.
- Renal: Nephrotoxicity less common than with cisplatin and rarely symptomatic. Dose reduction required in presence of renal dysfunction.
- Electrolyte Imbalance: Decreases Mg^{2+}, K^+, Ca^{2+}, and Na^+.
- Neurotoxicity: Sensory neuropathy with numbness and paresthesias; dose related. Can be dose limiting.
- Alopecia: Total loss of body hair occurs in nearly all patients.
- Reproduction: Pregnancy category D. Breast feeding should be avoided. Amenorrhea, azoospermia, impotence, and sterility.

Initiate antiemetic protocol:	Moderately to highly emetogenic protocol.
Supportive drugs:	☐ pegfilgrastim (Neulasta) ☐ filgrastim (Neupogen)
	☐ epoetin alfa (Procrit) ☐ darbepoetin alfa (Aranesp)
Treatment schedule:	Chair time 5 hours on day 1. Repeat cycle every 21 days until progression.
Estimated number of visits:	Two visits per cycle. Request six cycles worth of visits.

Dose Calculation by: 1. _____ 2. _____

_____
Physician

_____
Patient Name

_____
Diagnosis

_____
Date

_____
ID Number

_____ / _____ / _____
Ht   Wt   M^2

Cyclophosphamide + Doxorubicin + Cisplatin (CAP)

Baseline laboratory tests:	CBC: Chemistry (including Mg^{2+})
Baseline procedures or tests:	MUGA scan
Initiate IV:	0.9% sodium chloride
Premedicate:	$5\text{-}HT_3$ and dexamethasone 10–20 mg in 100 cc of NS
Administer:	**Cyclophosphamide** _____mg (400 mg/m^2) IV on day 1

- Available in 100-, 200-, 500-, 1000-, and 2000-mg vials.
- Dilute with sterile water. Shake well to ensure that all particles completely dissolve.
- Reconstituted solution is stable for 24 hours at room temperature and for 6 days refrigerated.

Doxorubicin _____mg (40 mg/m^2) IV on day 1

- **Potent vesicant**
- Available as a 2 mg/mL solution.
- Doxorubicin will form a precipitate if it is mixed with heparin or 5-FU.

Cisplatin _____mg (75/m^2) IV over 1–3 hours on day 1

- Available in solution as 1 mg/mL.
- Do not use aluminum needles, because precipitate will form.
- Further dilute solution with 250 cc or more of NS.
- Stable for 96 hours when protected from light and only 6 hours when not protected from light.

Major Side Effects

- Hypersensitivity Reaction: Facial edema, wheezing, bronchospasm, and hypotension possible with cisplatin. Cyclophosphamide can cause rhinitis and irritation of nose and throat.
- Bone Marrow Depression: Neutropenia, thrombocytopenia, and anemia occur equally in many patients. Leukopenia and thrombocytopenia are dose related.
- GI Toxicities: Nausea and vomiting are moderate to severe. May be acute (first 24 hours) or delayed (> 24 hours). Mucositis. Metallic taste.
- GU: Nephrotoxicity is dose related with cisplatin and presents at 10–20 days. Bladder toxicity in the form of hemorrhagic cystitis, dysuria, and increased urinary frequency.
- Electrolyte Imbalance: Decreases Mg^{2+}, K^+, Ca^{2+}, Na^+, and P.
- Cardiotoxicity: Acutely, pericarditis or myocarditis can occur. Later, cardiomyopathy in the form of congestive heart failure may occur.
- Neurotoxicity: Dose-limiting toxicity, usually in the form of peripheral sensory neuropathy. Paresthesias and numbness in a classic "stocking-glove" pattern.
- Ototoxicity: High-frequency hearing loss and tinnitus.
- Skin: Extravasation of doxorubicin causes severe tissue damage. Hyperpigmentation, photosensitivity, and radiation recall occur. Alopecia.
- Reproduction: Pregnancy category D. Breast feeding should be avoided. Azoospermia, impotence, and sterility.

Initiate antiemetic protocol:	Moderately to highly emetogenic protocol.
Supportive drugs:	☐ pegfilgrastim (Neulasta) ☐ filgrastim (Neupogen)
	☐ epoetin alfa (Procrit) ☐ darbepoetin alfa (Aranesp)
Treatment schedule:	Chair time 4 hours on day 1. Repeat cycle every 21 days.
Estimated number of visits:	Two visits per cycle. Request six cycles worth of visits.

Dose Calculation by: 1. _____   2. _____

_____

Physician   Date

_____

Patient Name   ID Number

_____   _____/_____ /_____

Diagnosis   Ht   Wt M^2

Cisplatin + Methotrexate + Vinblastine + XRT (CMV + Radiation Therapy)

Baseline laboratory tests:	CBC: Chemistry (including Mg^{2+})
Baseline procedures or tests:	N/A
Initiate IV:	0.9% sodium chloride
Premedicate:	5-HT_3, and dexamethasone 20 mg in 100 cc of NS
Administer:	**Cisplatin** _____mg (70 mg/m²) IV on day 2

- Available in solution as 1 mg/mL
- Do not use aluminum needles, because precipitate will form.
- Further dilute solution in 250 cc or more of NS.
- Stable for 96 hours when protected from light and only 6 hours when not protected from light.

Methotrexate _____mg (30 mg/m²) IV on days 1, 15, and 22

- Available as solution in 5-, 50-, 100- and 200-mg vials.
- May further dilute in 0.9% sodium chloride.
- Use with caution in patients taking warfarin due to increased anticoagulation effects.
- Have patients discontinue taking folic acid supplements while taking drug.

Vinblastine _____mg (3 mg/m²) IV on days 2, 15, and 22

- **Potent vesicant**
- Available in 10-mg vials; store in refrigerator until use.

Repeat cycle every 28 days for two cycles. Radiation therapy to be given after two cycles of induction chemotherapy at a dose of 45 cGy in 180 cGy fractions combined with cisplatin 70 mg/m² on days 1 and 2 of radiation therapy.

Major Side Effects	- Hypersensitivity Reaction: Facial edema, wheezing, bronchospasm, and hypotension possible with cisplatin.

- Bone Marrow Depression: Myelosuppression can be severe.
- GI Toxicities: Nausea and vomiting are moderate to severe and can be acute or delayed. Mucositis can be severe. Constipation, abdominal pain, or paralytic ileus. Metallic taste.
- Renal: Acute renal failure, azotemia, urinary retention, and uric acid nephropathy.
- Fluid/electrolyte Imbalance: Decreased Mg^{2+}, K^+, Ca^{2+}, Na^+, and P. Inappropriate secretion of antidiuretic hormone (SIADH).
- Pulmonary: Pneumonitis.
- Skin: Extravasation of vesicants causes severe tissue destruction. Rash, hyperpigmentation, photosensitivity, and radiation recall occur. Alopecia. Local tissue irritation to desquamation can occur in radiation trials. Do not use oil-based lotions or creams in radiation field.
- Neurotoxicity: Peripheral sensory neuropathy, paresthesia.
- Reproduction: Pregnancy category D. Breast feeding should be avoided. Azoospermia, impotence, and sterility.

Initiate antiemetic protocol:	Moderately to highly emetogenic protocol.
Supportive drugs:	☐ pegfilgrastim (Neulasta) ☐ filgrastim (Neupogen)
	☐ epoetin alfa (Procrit) ☐ darbepoetin alfa (Aranesp)
Treatment schedule:	Chair time 1 hour on days 1, 15, and 22, and 3 hours on day 2. Repeat cycle every 28 days for 2 cycles, then begin radiation therapy as dsecribed above.
Estimated number of visits:	Five visits per cycle. Request four cycles worth of visits.

Dose Calculation by: 1. _____   2. _____

_____

Physician

_____

Patient Name

_____

Diagnosis

_____

Date

_____

ID Number

_____/_____/_____

Ht   Wt   M^2

Single-Agent Regimens

Gemcitabine

Baseline laboratory tests:	CBC: Chemistry panel, and LFTs
Baseline procedures or tests:	N/A
Initiate IV:	0.9% sodium chloride
Premedicate:	Oral phenothiazine
	OR
	5-HT$_3$ and dexamethasone 10 mg in 100 cc of NS

Administer: **Gemcitabine** _____mg (1200 mg/m^2) IV on days 1, 8, and 15

- Available in 1-g or 200-mg vials, reconstitute with 0.9% sodium chloride USP (5 cc for 200 mg, 25 cc for 1 g). Further dilute in 0.9% sodium chloride.
- Reconstituted solution is stable 24 hours at room temperature. Do not refrigerate, because precipitate will form.

Major Side Effects

- Hematologic: Leukopenia (63%), thrombocytopenia (36%), and anemia (73%), with grades 3 and 4 thrombocytopenia being more common in elderly patients. Myelosuppression is dose limiting. Nadir occurs in 10–14 days, with recovery at 21 days. Prolonged infusion time (> 60 minutes) is associated with higher toxicities.
- GI Symptoms: Mild-to-moderate nausea and vomiting (70%), diarrhea, and/or mucositis (15%–20%).
- Flulike Syndrome (20%): Fever in absence of infection 6–12 hours after treatment (40%). Fever, malaise, chills, headache, and myalgias.
- Pulmonary: Mild dyspnea and drug induced pneumonitis.
- Hepatic: Transient elevation of serum transaminases and bilirubin.
- Skin: Pruritic, maculopapular skin rash, usually involving trunk and extremities. Edema occurs in 30% of patients. Alopecia is rare.
- Reproduction: Pregnancy category D. Breast feeding should be avoided..

Initiate antiemetic protocol:	Mildly to moderately emetogenic protocol.
Supportive drugs:	☐ pegfilgrastim (Neulasta) ☐ filgrastim (Neupogen)
	☐ epoetin alfa (Procrit) ☐ darbepoetin alfa (Aranesp)
Treatment schedule:	Chair time 1 hour on days 1, 8, and 15. Repeat cycle every 28 days.
Estimated number of visits:	Three visits per cycle. Request three cycles worth of visits.

Dose Calculation by: 1. _____   2. _____

_____   _____
Physician   Date

_____   _____
Patient Name   ID Number

_____   _____/_____/_____
Diagnosis   Ht   Wt   M^2

Paclitaxel

Baseline laboratory tests:	CBC: Chemistry
Baseline procedures or tests:	Central line placement
Initiate IV:	0.9% sodium chloride
Premedicate:	5-HT$_3$ and dexamethasone 10–20 mg in 100 cc of NS
	Diphenhydramine 25–50 mg and cimetidine 300 mg in 100 cc of NS

Administer: **Paclitaxel** _____mg (250 mg/m^2) IV over 24 hours on day 1

- Available in solution as 6 mg/mL.
- Final concentration is ≤ 1.2 mg/mL.
- Stable for up to 27 hours at room temperature in 0.3–1.2 mg/mL solutions.
- **Use non-PVC containers and tubing with 0.22-micron inline filter for administration.**

Major Side Effects

- Hypersensitivity reaction: Occurs in 20%–40% of patients. Characterized by generalized skin rash, flushing, erythema, hypotension, dyspnea, and/or bronchospasm. Usually occurs within the first 2–3 minutes of infusion and almost always within the first 10 minutes. Premedicate as described.
- Bone Marrow Depression: Dose-limiting neutropenia with nadir at days 8–10 and recovery by days 15–21. Decreased incidence of neutropenia with 3-hour schedule when compared with 24-hour schedule. G-CSF support recommended.
- GI Toxicity: Mucositis and/or diarrhea seen in 30–40% of patients. Mucositis more common with 24-hour schedule. Mild to moderate nausea and vomiting, usually of brief duration.
- Neurotoxicity: Sensory neuropathy with numbness and paresthesias; dose related and dose limiting. More frequent with longer infusions and at doses > 175 mg/m^2.
- Hepatic: Transient elevations in serum transaminases, bilirubin, and alkaline phosphatase.
- Skin: Onycholysis with weekly dosing. Alopecia, total loss of body hair in nearly all patients.
- Reproductive: Pregnancy category D. Breast feeding should be avoided.

Initiate antiemetic protocol:	Mildly to moderately emetogenic protocol.
Supportive drugs:	☐ pegfilgrastim (Neulasta) ☐ filgrastim (Neupogen)
	☐ epoetin alfa (Procrit) ☐ darbepoetin alfa (Aranesp)
Treatment schedule:	Chair time 1 hour. Repeat every 21 days as tolerated or until disease progression.
Estimated number of visits:	Three visits per cycle. Request four cycles worth of visits.

Dose Calculation by: 1. _____   2. _____

_____   _____
Physician   Date

_____   _____
Patient Name   ID Number

_____   _____/_____/_____
Diagnosis   Ht   Wt   M^2

OR

Paclitaxel

Baseline laboratory tests:	CBC: Chemistry
Baseline procedures or tests:	Central line placement
Initiate IV:	0.9% sodium chloride
Premedicate:	5-HT$_3$ and dexamethasone 10–20 mg in 100 cc of NS
	Diphenhydramine 25–50 mg and cimetidine 300 mg in 100 cc of NS
Administer:	**Paclitaxel** _____ mg (80 mg/m^2) IV over 24 hours on day 1

- Available in solution as 6 mg/mL.
- Final concentration is ≤ 1.2 mg/mL.
- Stable for up to 27 hours at room temperature in 0.3–1.2 mg/mL solutions.
- **Use non-PVC containers and tubing with 0.22-micron inline filter for administration.**

Major Side Effects

- Hypersensitivity Reaction: Occurs in 20%–40% of patients. Characterized by generalized skin rash, flushing, erythema, hypotension, dyspnea, and/or bronchospasm. Usually occurs within the first 2–3 minutes of infusion and almost always within the first 10 minutes. Premedicate as described.
- Bone Marrow Depression: Dose-limiting neutropenia with nadir at days 8–10 and recovery by days 15–21. Decreased incidence of neutropenia with 3-hour schedule when compared with 24-hour schedule. G-CSF support recommended.
- GI Toxicity: Mucositis and/or diarrhea seen in 30–40% of patients. Mucositis more common with 24-hour schedule. Mild to moderate nausea and vomiting, usually of brief duration.
- Neurotoxicity: Sensory neuropathy with numbness and paresthesias; dose related and dose limiting. More frequent with longer infusions and at doses > 175 mg/m^2.
- Hepatic: Transient elevations in serum transaminases, bilirubin, and alkaline phosphatase.
- Skin: Onycholysis with weekly dosing. Alopecia, is complete in nearly all patients.
- Reproductive: Pregnancy category D. Breast feeding should be avoided.

Initiate antiemetic protocol:	Mildly to moderately emetogenic protocol.
Supportive drugs:	☐ pegfilgrastim (Neulasta) ☐ filgrastim (Neupogen)
	☐ epoetin alfa (Procrit) ☐ darbepoetin alfa (Aranesp)
Treatment schedule:	Chair time 1 hour. Repeat every 21 days as tolerated or until disease progression.
Estimated number of visits:	Three visits per cycle. Request four cycles worth of visits.

Dose Calculation by: 1. _____   2. _____

_____

Physician

_____

Patient Name

_____

Diagnosis

_____

Date

_____

ID Number

_____ / _____ / _____

Ht   Wt   M^2

BONE METASTASIS

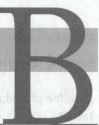

Zometa 4-mg dose adjusted for baseline creatinine clearance on day 1
Repeat cycle every 21–28 days.[1,21-25]

Pamidronate 90 mg IV on day 1
Repeat cycle every 21–28 days.[1,27]

Zometa

Baseline laboratory tests:	CBC: serum creatinine (check before each dose)
	Calculate baseline creatinine clearance.
Baseline procedures or tests:	N/A
Initiate IV:	Normal saline
Premedicate:	Calcium supplement 500 mg and vitamin D 400 IU PO daily
	• **DO NOT** give when treating hypercalcemia
Administer:	**Zometa** _____mg (4 mg adjusted for baseline creatinine clearance)
	In 100 cc of NS over a minimum of 15 minutes day 1

• Available in 4-mg vials (reconstitute with 5 mL of sterile water for injection) or in 5 mL solution.

• Further dilute in 100 cc of D5W or NS.

Patient's baseline creatinine clearance _____. (Cockcroft-Gault formula)

Dosing Adjustments for Creatinine Clearance

Baseline creatinine clearance (mL/min)	Zoledronic acid (Zometa) dose (mg)	Volume of 5-mL zoledronic acid concentrate (mL)
> 60	4.0	5.0
50–60	3.5	4.4
40–49	3.3	4.1
30–39	3.0	3.8

Major Side Effects

• Renal Toxicity: Deterioration of renal function (increase of 0.5 mg/dL for patients with normal baseline creatinine or increase of 1.0 mg/dL for patients with an abnormal baseline creatinine). **Treatment should be held for renal deterioration.** Treatment may be resumed at the same dose when the creatinine returns to within 10% of baseline value.

• Flulike Symptoms: Fever occurs in 44% of patients. Chills, bone pain, and/or arthralgias and myalgias also occur.

• GI Toxicities: Nausea and vomiting are usually mild. Diarrhea, constipation, abdominal pain, and anorexia reported.

• Bone Marrow Toxicity: Anemia can occur but not significant.

• Fluid/electrolyte Balance: Hypocalcemia, hypophosphatemia, hypomagnesemia, or increased blood urea nitrogen (BUN) and serum creatinine.

• Osteonecrosis of the Jaw: Most reported cases are in cancer patients attendant to a dental procedure. It is prudent to avoid dental surgery because recovery may be prolonged. Discontinue therapy if osteonecrosis occurs.

• Reproduction: Do not use in pregnancy.

Initiate antiemetic protocol:	Mildly to moderately emetogenic protocol.
Supportive drugs:	☐ epoetin alfa (Procrit) ☐ darbepoetin alfa (Aranesp)
	☐ oprelvekin (Neumega) ☐ filgrastim (Neupogen)
	☐ pegfilgrastim (Neulasta) ☐ Other _____
Treatment schedule:	Chair time 1 hour. Repeat cycle every 3–4 weeks in patients with multiple myeloma and metastatic bone lesions from solid tumors.
	Hypercalcemia of malignancy may give every 7 days prn.
Estimated number of visits:	One visit per cycle. Request 12 cycles worth of visits.

Dose Calculation by: 1. _____   2. _____

_____

Physician

_____

Patient Name

_____

Diagnosis

_____

Date

_____

ID Number

_____ / _____ / _____

Ht   Wt   M^2

Pamidronate

Baseline laboratory tests:	CBC: Chemistry panel (including Mg^{2+})
Baseline procedures or tests:	N/A
Initiate IV:	Normal saline
Premedicate:	None required
Administer:	Bone metastases

Pamidronate 90 mg in 250 cc of NS or D5W IV over 2 hours

Repeat cycle every 3–4 weeks.

OR

Multiple Myeloma

Pamidronate 90 mg in 500 cc of NS or D5W over 4 hours

Repeat cycle every 4 weeks.

- Available in 90-mg vial (as powder for reconstitution or in 10mL solution).
- Reconstitute powder with 10 mL of sterile water for injection.
- Reconstituted solution stable for 24 hours at room temperature.
- Store reconstituted drug in refrigerator.

Major Side Effects

- Flulike Symptoms: Fever occurs in 44% of patients. Chills, bone pain, and/or arthralgias and myalgias also occur.
- GI Toxicities: Nausea, vomiting, abdominal discomfort, constipation, and anorexia may occur rarely. GI hemorrhage rare.
- Bone Marrow Toxicity: Myelosuppression occurs but not significant.
- Fluid/electrolyte Balance: Hypocalcemia, hypercalcemia, hypokalemia, hypophosphatemia, hypomagnesemia, or increased BUN and serum creatinine levels.
- Renal: Renal dysfunction, renal failure. Use with extreme caution in patients with renal impairment.
- CV Toxicities: Atrial fibrillation, tachycardia, hypertension, fluid overload.
- Skin: Infusion-site reaction, pain at infusion site.
- Reproduction: Do not use in pregnancy.

Initiate antiemetic protocol: Mildly emetogenic protocol.

Supportive drugs:

☐ epoetin alfa (Procrit)   ☐ darbepoetin alfa (Aranesp)

☐ oprelvekin (Neumega)   ☐ filgrastim (Neupogen)

☐ pegfilgrastim (Neulasta)   ☐ Other _____

Treatment schedule: Chair time 2 hours. Repeat cycle every 3–4 weeks.

OR

Chair time 4 hours. Repeat cycle every 4 weeks.

Estimated number of visits: One visit per cycle. Request 12 cycles worth of visits.[19–20]

Dose Calculation by: 1. _____   2. _____

_____   _____
Physician   Date

_____   _____
Patient Name   ID Number

_____   _____/ _____/ _____
Diagnosis   Ht   Wt M^2

BRAIN CANCER

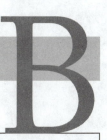

ADJUVANT THERAPY
Combination Regimens

Temozolomide + Radiation Therapy..33

Radiation therapy: 200 cGy/day for 5 days per week for total of 6 weeks

Temozolomide: 75 mg/m² PO for 6 weeks with radiation therapy, followed by 150 mg/m² PO on days 1–5

Repeat cycle every 28 days.[20] If drug is well tolerated, dose can be increased to 200 mg/m.[21,27]

PCV..34

Procarbazine: 60 mg/m² PO on days 8–21
Lomustine: 130 mg/m² PO on day 1
Vincristine: 1.4 mg/m² IV on days 8 and 29
Repeat cycle every 8 weeks for six cycles.[1,28]

Single-Agent Regimens

BCNU..35

BCNU: 220 mg/m² IV on day 1
Repeat cycle every 6–8 weeks for 1 year.[1,29]
OR
BCNU: 75–100 mg/m² IV on days 1 and 2
Repeat cycle every 6–8 weeks.[1,29]

ADVANCED DISEASE
Combination Regimens

PCV..36

Procarbazine: 75 mg/m² PO on days 8–21
Lomustine: 130 mg/m² PO on day 1
Vincristine: 1.4 mg/m² IV on days 8 and 29
Repeat cycle every 8 weeks.[1,30]

31

Single-Agent Regimens

BCNU: 200 mg/m^2 IV on day 1
Repeat cycle every 6–8 weeks.[1,30]

Procarbazine: 150 mg/m^2 PO daily divided into 3 doses
Repeat daily.[1,31]

Temozolomide: 150 mg/m^2 PO on days 1–5
Repeat cycle every 28 days.[20] If drug is well tolerated, dose can be
increased to 200 mg/m.[21,32]

Irinotecan: 350 mg/m^2 IV over 90 minutes on day 1
Repeat cycle every 3 weeks.[1,33]
OR
Irinotecan: 125 mg/m^2 IV weekly for 4 weeks
Repeat cycle every 6 weeks.[1,34]

ADJUVANT THERAPY
Combination Regimens

Temozolomide + Radiation Therapy

Baseline laboratory tests:	CBC: Chemistry and LFTs
Baseline procedures or tests:	N/A
Initiate IV:	N/A
Premedicate:	Oral phenothiazine or 5-HT$_3$
Administer:	**Temozolomide:** 75 mg/m^2 PO for 6 weeks with radiation therapy, followed by 150 mg/m^2 PO on days 1–5. Repeat cycle every 28 days.

* If well tolerated, can increase dose to 200 mg/m^2 on days 1–5 (after radiation therapy).
* Available in 5-, 20-, 100-, and 250-mg capsules for oral use.
* Store at room temperature; protect from light and moisture.
* Take with full glass of water on an empty stomach.

Radiation therapy:	200 cGy/day for 5 days per week for total of 6 weeks.
Major Side Effects	

* Bone Marrow Depression: Myelosuppression is dose-limiting toxicity, with leukopenia more frequent than thrombocytopenia. Elderly patients are at increased risk for myelo-suppression. Nadir day 28–29. Anemia may also occur. Does not usually require G-CSF administration.
* GI Toxicities: Nausea and vomiting occur in 75% of patients, usually mild to moderate and occurring on day 1. Diarrhea, constipation, and/or anorexia may affect up to 40% of patients.
* Skin: Rash, itching, and alopecia may occur and are mild.
* Central Nervous System Effects: Fatigue, headache, ataxia, and dizziness.
* Reproductive: Pregnancy category D. Breast feeding should be avoided.

Initiate antiemetic protocol:	Mildly to moderately emetogenic protocol.
Supportive drugs:	☐ pegfilgrastim (Neulasta) ☐ filgrastim (Neupogen)
	☐ epoetin alfa (Procrit) ☐ darbepoetin alfa (Aranesp)
	☐ loperamide (Imodium) ☐ diphenoxylate/atropine sulfate (Lomotil)
Treatment schedule:	No chair time. Repeat every 28 days as tolerated or until disease progression.
Estimated number of visits:	One to four visits per month.

Dose Calculation by: 1. _____   2. _____

_____
Physician

_____
Date

_____
Patient Name

_____
ID Number

_____
Diagnosis

_____ / _____ / _____
Ht   Wt   M^2

Procarbazine + Lomustine + Vincristine (PCV)

Baseline laboratory tests:	CBC: Chemistry and LFTs
Baseline procedures or tests:	N/A
Initiate IV:	Normal saline prior to vincristine.
Premedicate:	Oral 5-HT$_3$
Administer:	**Procarbazine** _____mg (60 mg/m^2) PO on days 8–21

- Available in 50-mg capsules
- Avoid exposure to moisture.

Lomustine _____mg (130 mg/m^2) PO on day 1

- Available in 10-, 30-, and 100-mg capsules
- Administer on an empty stomach at bedtime.

Vincristine _____mg (1.4 mg/m^2) IV on days 8 and 29

- **Vesicant**
- Available in 1-, 2-, and 5-mg vials; refrigerate until use.

Major Side Effects

- Food and Drug Interactions: **Alcohol.** Antabuse-like reaction may result if alcohol is consumed. **Tyramines:** Foods containing high amounts of tyramine should be avoided (dark beer, wine, cheese, bananas, yogurt, and pickled and smoked foods). **CNS depressants:** Synergistic effect. **Tricyclic antidepressants:** May result in CNS excitation.
- Bone Marrow Suppression with Procarbazine: Myelosuppression is the major dose-limiting toxicity. Nadir is delayed, occurs at 4–6 weeks, and persists for 1–3 weeks.
- GI Toxicities: Nausea and vomiting may be a dose-limiting toxicity. Severe nausea may occur 2–6 hours after lomustine is taken. Constipation, abdominal pain, and paralytic ileus.
- CNS: 10%–30% of patients experience lethargy, depression, frequent nightmares, insomnia, nervousness, or hallucinations. Tremors and convulsions are less common. Crosses blood-brain barrier.
- Neurotoxicities. Peripheral neuropathies occur as a result of toxicity to nerve fibers. Absent deep-tendon reflexes, numbness, weakness, myalgias, cramping, and late, severe motor difficulties.
- Respiratory: Interstitial pneumonitis.
- Flulike Syndrome: Fever chills, sweating, lethargy, myalgias, and arthralgias commonly occur.
- Skin Toxicities: Rarely occurs as alopecia, pruritus, rash, and hyperpigmentation.
- Reproduction: Impotence, amenorrhea, azoospermia. Pregnancy category D.

Initiate antiemetic protocol:	Moderately to highly emetogenic protocol.
Supportive drugs:	☐ pegfilgrastim (Neulasta) ☐ filgrastim (Neupogen)
	☐ epoetin alfa (Procrit) ☐ darbepoetin alfa (Aranesp)
Treatment schedule:	Chair time 1 hour on days 8 and 29. Repeat cycle every 8 weeks for 6 cycles.
Estimated number of visits:	Every 2 weeks for 1 year.

Note: Preauthorize as oral chemotherapy under prescription benefits or as chemotherapy under major medical coverage.

Dose Calculation by: 1. _____   2. _____

_____
Physician

_____
Patient Name

_____
Diagnosis

_____
Date

_____
ID Number

_____/ _____/ _____
Ht   Wt   M^2

Single-Agent Regimens

BCNU (Carmustine)

Baseline laboratory tests:	CBC: Chemistry and LFTs
Baseline procedures or tests:	Pulmonary function tests
Initiate IV:	0.9% sodium chloride
Premedicate:	5-HT$_3$ and dexamethasone 10–20 mg in 100 cc of NS
Administer:	BCNU _____ mg (220 mg/m^2) IV over 1–2 hours on day 1

OR

BCNU _____ mg (75–100 mg/m^2) over 1–2 hours on days 1 and 2

- Each package contains 100 mg of carmustine and a 3-mL vial of sterile diluent.
- Add sterile alcohol (provided with drug) to vial, then sterile water as directed.
- Reconstituted solution stable for 8 hours at room temperature or 24 hours refrigerated.
- Further dilute in 100–250 cc of D5W or NS.

Major Side Effects

- Bone Marrow Depression: Myelosuppression involving all blood elements is delayed and cumulative. Nadir typically occurs at 4–6 weeks and lasts 1–3 weeks. Cimetidine may increase myelosuppression, avoid if possible.
- GI Toxicities: Severe nausea and vomiting may occur 2 hours after administration and last 4–6 hours.
- Pulmonary Toxicities: Uncommon at low doses. Interstitial lung disease and pulmonary fibrosis in the form of an insidious cough, dyspnea, pulmonary infiltrates, and/or respiratory failure may develop in cumulative doses > 1400 mg/m^2 or in patients with a prior history of lung disease.
- Renal Toxicity: Increase in BUN occurs in 10% of patients and is usually reversible. Decreased kidney size, progressive azotemia, and renal failure have occurred in larger cumulative doses over long periods.
- Hepatic Toxicities: Transient elevations in serum transaminase levels in up to 90% of patients within 1 week of therapy.
- Skin: Facial flushing and a burning sensation at the IV injection site. Skin contact with drug may cause brownish discoloration and pain. Drug is an irritant, avoid extravasation.
- Ocular Toxicities: Infarcts of optic nerve fiber, retinal hemorrhage, and neuroretinitis have been associated with high-dose therapy.
- Reproduction: Pregnancy category D. Impotence, sterility, and infertility seen.

Initiate antiemetic protocol:	Mildly emetogenic protocol.
Supportive drugs:	☐ pegfilgrastim (Neulasta) ☐ filgrastim (Neupogen)
	☐ epoetin alfa (Procrit) ☐ darbepoetin alfa (Aranesp)
Treatment schedule:	Chair time 3 hours on day 1 OR 3 hours on days 1 and 2. Repeat cycle every 6–8 weeks for 1 year.
Estimated number of visits:	One visit per cycle. Request 6 months worth of visits.

Dose Calculation by: 1. _____ 2. _____

_____
Physician

_____
Date

_____
Patient Name

_____
ID Number

_____
Diagnosis

_____ / _____ / _____
Ht   Wt   M^2

ADVANCED DISEASE
Combination Regimens

Procarbazine + Lomustine + Vincristine (PCV)

Baseline laboratory tests:	CBC: Chemistry and LFTs
Baseline procedures or tests:	N/A
Initiate IV:	N/A
Premedicate:	Oral 5-HT$_3$
Administer:	**Procarbazine** _____ mg (75 mg/m^2) PO on days 8–21

- Available in 50-mg capsules
- Avoid exposure to moisture.

Lomustine _____ mg (130 mg/m^2) PO on day 1
- Available in 10-, 30-, and 100-mg capsules
- Administer on an empty stomach at bedtime.

Vincristine _____ mg (1.4 mg/m^2) IV on days 8 and 29
- Vesicant
- Available in 1-, 2-, and 5-mg vials; refrigerate until use.

Major Side Effects

- Drug and Food Interactions with Procarbazine: **Alcohol:** Antabuse-like reaction may result if alcohol consumed. **Tyramines:** Foods containing high amounts of tyramine should be avoided (dark beer, wine, cheese, yogurt, and pickled and smoked foods). **CNS depressants:** Synergistic effect. **Tricyclic antidepressants:** May result in CNS excitation.
- Bone Marrow Suppression: Myelosuppression is the major dose-limiting toxicity. Nadir is delayed, occurs at 4–6 weeks, and persists for 1–3 weeks.
- GI Toxicities: Nausea and vomiting may be a dose-limiting toxicity. Severe nausea may occur 2–6 hours after taking lomustine. Constipation, abdominal pain, and paralytic ileus.
- CNS: Some patients experience lethargy, depression, frequent nightmares, insomnia, nervousness, or hallucinations. Tremors and convulsions are less common. Crosses blood-brain barrier.
- Neurotoxicities. Peripheral neuropathies occur as a result of toxicity to nerve fibers. Absent deep tendon reflexes, numbness, weakness, myalgias, cramping, and later, severe motor difficulties.
- Flulike Syndrome: Fever chills, sweating, lethargy, myalgias, and arthralgias commonly occur.
- Skin Toxicities: Rarely occurs as alopecia, pruritus, rash, and hyperpigmentation.
- Reproduction: Impotence, amenorrhea, azoospermia. Pregnancy category D.

Initiate antiemetic protocol:	Moderately to highly emetogenic protocol.
Supportive drugs:	☐ pegfilgrastim (Neulasta) ☐ filgrastim (Neupogen)
	☐ epoetin alfa (Procrit) ☐ darbepoetin alfa (Aranesp)
Treatment schedule:	Chair time 1 hour on days 8 and 29. Repeat cycle every 8 weeks.
Estimated number of visits:	Every 2 weeks for 1 year.

Dose Calculation by: 1. _____ 2. _____

Physician _____

Date _____

Patient Name _____

ID Number _____

Diagnosis _____

Ht _____ / Wt _____ / M^2 _____

Single-Agent Regimens

BCNU (Carmustine)

Baseline laboratory tests:	CBC: Chemistry and LFTs
Baseline procedures or tests:	Pulmonary function tests
Initiate IV:	0.9% sodium chloride
Premedicate:	5-HT$_3$ and dexamethasone 10–20 mg in 100 cc of NS
Administer:	BCNU _____mg (200 mg/m^2) IV over 1–2 hours on day 1

- Each package contains carmustine 100 mg and a 3-mL vial of sterile diluent.
- Add sterile alcohol (provided with drug) to vial, then sterile water as directed.
- Reconstituted solution stable for 8 hours at room temperature or 24 hours refrigerated.
- Further dilute in 100–250 cc of D5W or NS

Major Side Effects

- Bone Marrow Depression: Myelosuppression involving all blood elements is delayed and cumulative. Nadir typically occurs at 4–6 weeks and lasts 1–3 weeks. Cimetidine may increase myelosuppression, avoid if possible.
- GI toxicities: Severe nausea and vomiting may occur 2 hours after administration and last 4–6 hours.
- Pulmonary toxicities: Uncommon at low doses. Interstitial lung disease and pulmonary fibrosis in the form of an insidious cough, dyspnea, pulmonary infiltrates, and/or respiratory failure may develop at cumulative doses > 1400 mg/m^2 or in patients with a prior history of lung disease.
- Renal Toxicity: Increase in BUN occurs in 10% of patients and is usually reversible. Decreased kidney size, progressive azotemia, and renal failure have occurred in larger cumulative doses over long periods.
- Hepatic Toxicities: Transient elevations in serum transaminase levels in up to 90% of patients within 1 week of therapy.
- Skin: Facial flushing and a burning sensation at the IV injection site. Skin contact with drug may cause brownish discoloration and pain. Drug is irritant, avoid extravasation.
- Ocular Toxicities: Infarcts of optic nerve fiber, retinal hemorrhage, and neuroretinitis have been associated with high-dose therapy.
- Reproduction: Impotence, amenorrhea, and azoospermia. Pregnancy category D.

Initiate antiemetic protocol:	Moderately to highly emetogenic protocol.
Supportive drugs:	☐ pegfilgrastim (Neulasta) ☐ filgrastim (Neupogen)
	☐ epoetin alfa (Procrit) ☐ darbepoetin alfa (Aranesp)
Treatment schedule:	Chair time 3 hours on day 1. Repeat cycle every 6–8 weeks.
Estimated number of visits:	Four visits per cycle. Request 6 months worth of visits.

Dose Calculation by: 1. _____   2. _____

_____   _____

Physician   Date

_____   _____

Patient Name   ID Number

_____ / _____ / _____

_____   Ht   Wt   M^2

Diagnosis

Procarbazine

Baseline laboratory tests:	CBC: Chemistry and LFTs
Baseline procedures or tests:	N/A
Initiate IV:	N/A
Premedicate:	Oral 5-HT$_3$
Administer:	**Procarbazine** _____mg (150 mg/m^2) PO daily divided into three doses

- Available in 50-mg capsules.
- Avoid exposure to moisture.

Major Side Effects

- Drug and Food Interactions: **Alcohol**. Antabuse-like reaction may result if alcohol is consumed. **Tyramines**: Foods containing high amounts of tyramine should be avoided (e.g., beer, wine, cheese, brewer's yeast, chicken livers, and bananas). **CNS depressants**: Synergistic effect with barbiturates, antihistamines, narcotics, hypotensive agents, and phenothiazines. **Tricyclic antidepressants**: May result in CNS excitation, hypertension, tremors, palpitations, and, in severe cases, hypertensive crisis and/or angina.

- Bone Marrow Suppression: Myelosuppression is the major dose-limiting toxicity. Thrombocytopenia occurs in 50% of patients, with nadir occurring in 4 weeks and recovery in 4–6 weeks. Leukopenia usually occurs after thrombocytopenia. Anemias may be due to bone marrow depression or hemolysis.

- GI Toxicities: Nausea and vomiting occur in 70% of patients and may be a dose-limiting toxicity. Diarrhea is uncommon but rarely may be protracted and thus would be an indication for dose reduction.

- CNS: 10%–30% of patients experience lethargy, depression, frequent nightmares, insomnia, nervousness, or hallucinations. Tremors and convulsions are less common. Crosses blood-brain barrier.

- Neurotoxicities: 10% of patients exhibit paresthesias, decrease in deep tendon reflexes. Foot drop and ataxia occasionally reported. Reversible when drug is discontinued.

- Flulike Syndrome: Fever, chills, sweating, lethargy, myalgias, and arthralgias commonly occur.

- Skin Toxicities: Rarely occurs as alopecia, pruritus, rash, hyperpigmentation.

- Reproduction: Drug is teratogenic. Causes azoospermia. Causes cessation of menses, although may be reversible. Pregnancy category D.

Initiate antiemetic protocol:	Moderately to highly emetogenic protocol.
Supportive drugs:	☐ pegfilgrastim (Neulasta) ☐ filgrastim (Neupogen)
	☐ darbepoetin alfa (Aranesp) ☐ epoetin alfa (Procrit)
	☐ loperamide (Imodium) ☐ diphenoxylate/atropine sulfate (Lomotil)
Treatment schedule:	No chair time. Repeat daily as tolerated or until disease progression.
Estimated number of visits:	One visit per month.

Dose Calculation by: 1. _____   2. _____

_____   _____
Physician   Date

_____   _____
Patient Name   ID Number

_____   _____ / _____ / _____
Diagnosis   Ht   Wt   M^2

Temozolomide

Baseline laboratory tests:	CBC: Chemistry and LFTs
Baseline procedures or tests:	N/A
Initiate IV:	N/A
Premedicate:	Oral phenothiazine or 5-HT$_3$
Administer:	**Temozolomide** _____ mg (150 mg/m^2) PO on days 1–5

- If well tolerated, can increase dose to 200 mg/m^2 on days 1–5
- Available in 5-, 20-, 100-, and 250-mg capsules for oral use
- Store at room temperature; protect from light and moisture.
- Take with full glass of water on an empty stomach.

Major Side Effects

- Bone Marrow Depression: Myelosuppression is dose-limiting toxicity, with leukopenia more frequent than thrombocytopenia. Elderly patients are at increased risk for myelosuppression. Nadir day 28–29. Anemia may also occur. Does not usually require G-CSF administration.
- GI Toxicities: Nausea and vomiting occur in 75% of patients, usually mild to moderate and occurring on day 1. Diarrhea, constipation, and/or anorexia may affect up to 40% of patients.
- Skin: Rash, itching, and alopecia may occur and are mild.
- Central Nervous System Effects: Fatigue, lethargy, headache, ataxia, and dizziness.
- Reproductive: Pregnancy category D. Breast feeding should be avoided.

Initiate antiemetic protocol:	Mildly to moderately emetogenic protocol.
Supportive drugs:	☐ pegfilgrastim (Neulasta) ☐ filgrastim (Neupogen)
	☐ epoetin alfa (Procrit) ☐ darbepoetin alfa (Aranesp)
	☐ loperamide (Imodium) ☐ diphenoxylate/atropine sulfate (Lomotil)
Treatment schedule:	No chair time. Repeat every 28 days as tolerated or until disease progression.
Estimated number of visits:	One visit per month.

Dose Calculation by: 1. _____   2. _____

_____
Physician

_____
Date

_____
Patient Name

_____
ID Number

_____
Diagnosis

_____ / _____ / _____
Ht   Wt   M^2

Irinotecan

Baseline laboratory tests:	CBC: Chemistry panel
Baseline procedures or tests:	N/A
Initiate IV:	D5W
Premedicate:	5-HT$_3$ and 20 mg of dexamethasone in 100 cc of D5W
	Atropine 0.25–1.0 mg IV unless contraindicated
Administer:	**Irinotecan** _____ mg (125 mg/m^2) IV in 500 cc of D5W weekly for 4 weeks
	OR
	Irinotecan _____ mg (350 mg/m^2) IV in 500 cc of D5W over 90 minutes day 1

- Available in 100-mg/5 mL single-use vials.
- Store unopened vials at room temperature and protect from light.
- Dilute and mix drug in D5W (preferred) or 0.9% sodium chloride to a final concentration of 0.12–1.1 mg/mL.
- The drug is commonly diluted in 500 cc of D5W.
- Reconstituted drug is stable for 24 hours at room temperature. When diluted in D5W, it is stable for 48 hours when refrigerated and protected from light.

Major Side Effects

- Bone Marrow Depression: Dose limiting, grade 3–4 neutropenia in 17%. Nadir in 6–9 days.
- GI Toxicities: Early diarrhea, most likely a cholinergic effect, can be managed with atropine before therapy. Late diarrhea observed in 22% of patients can be severe and should be treated aggressively with loperamide. Nausea and vomiting occurs in 35%–60% of patients, with 17% experiencing grade 3–4 nausea and 13% experiencing grade 3–4 vomiting.
- Pulmonary Toxicities: Range from transient dyspnea to pulmonary infiltrates, fever, increased cough, and decreased DLCO in a small number of patients.
- Hepatic: Transient elevations in serum transaminases, alkaline, phosphatase, and bilirubin.
- Reproductive: Pregnancy category D. Breast feeding should be avoided.
- Alopecia: Mild.

Initiate antiemetic protocol:	Moderately to highly emetogenic protocol.
Supportive drugs:	☐ pegfilgrastim (Neulasta) ☐ filgrastim (Neupogen)
	☐ epoetin alfa (Procrit) ☐ darbepoetin alfa (Aranesp)
	☐ loperamide (Imodium) ☐ diphenoxylate/atropine sulfate (Lomotil)
Treatment schedule:	Chair time 3 hours weekly for 4 weeks. Repeat cycle every 6 weeks. Repeat one cycle every 3 weeks for 350 mg/m^2 OR weekly for 125 mg/m^2 dose.
Estimated number of visits:	Four visits per cycle OR two visits per cycle. Request three cycles worth of visits.

Dose Calculation by: 1. _____   2. _____

_____

Physician

_____

Date

_____

Patient Name

_____

ID Number

_____

Diagnosis

_____ / _____ / _____

Ht   Wt   M^2

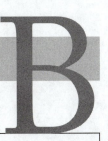

NEOADJUVANT THERAPY
Combination Regimens

Doxorubicin: 60 mg/m^2 IV on day 1

Cyclophosphamide: 600 mg/m^2 IV on day 1

Docetaxel: 100 mg/m^2 IV on day 1

Repeat cycle every 21 days for a total of four cycles, followed by surgery.[1,35]

ADJUVANT THERAPY
Combination Regimens

Doxorubicin: 60 mg/m^2 IV on day 1

Cyclophosphamide: 600 mg/m^2 IV on day 1

Repeat cycle every 21 days for a total of four cycles.[1,36]

Doxorubicin: 60 mg/m^2 IV on day 1

Cyclophosphamide: 600 mg/m^2 IV on day 1

Repeat cycle every 21 days for a total of four cycles, followed by

Paclitaxel: 175 mg/m^2 IV on day 1

Repeat cycle every 21 days for a total of four cycles.[1,37]

Doxorubicin: 60 mg/m^2 IV on day 1

Cyclophosphamide: 600 mg/m^2 IV on day 1

Repeat cycle every 21 days for a total of four cycles, followed by

Paclitaxel: 80 mg/m^2 IV on day 1

Trastuzumab: 4 mg/kg IV loading dose, then 2mg/kg IV weekly

Repeat cycle weekly for a total of 12 weeks, followed by

Trastuzumab: 2m/kg IV weekly

Repeat for 40 weeks.[1,38]

A followed by T followed by C (Dose-Dense Therapy) 51

Doxorubicin: 60 mg/m^2 IV on day 1
Repeat cycle every 2 weeks for four cycles, followed by
Paclitaxel: 175 mg/m^2 IV on day 1
Repeat cycle every 2 weeks for four cycles, followed by
Cyclophosphamide: 600 mg/m^2 IV on day 1
Repeat cycle every 2 weeks for four cycles.
Administer Filgrastim 5 µg/kg SC on days 3–10 of each weekly cycle.[1,39]

CAF 53

Cyclophosphamide: 600 mg/m^2 IV on day 1
Doxorubicin: 60 mg/m^2 IV on day 1
5-Fluorouracil: 600 mg/m^2 IV on day 1
Repeat cycle every 21 days for a total of six cycles.[1,40]
OR
Cyclophosphamide: 100 mg/m^2 PO on days 1–14
Doxorubicin: 30 mg/m^2 IV on days 1 and 8
5-Fluorouracil: 500 mg/m^2 IV on days 1 and 8
Repeat cycle every 28 days for a total of six cycles.[1,41]

CMF (Bonadonna Regimen) 57

Cyclophosphamide: 100 mg/m^2/day PO on days 1–14
Methotrexate: 40 mg/m^2 IV on days 1 and 8
5-Fluorouracil: 600 mg/m^2 IV on days 1 and 8
Repeat cycle every 28 days for a total of six cycles.[1,42]

CMF (IV Regimen) 59

Cyclophosphamide: 600 mg/m^2 IV on day 1
Methotrexate: 40 mg/m^2 IV on day 1
5-Fluorouracil: 600 mg/m^2 IV on day 1
Repeat cycle every 21 days for a total of six cycles.[1,43]

Doxorubicin + CMF 61

Doxorubicin: 75 mg/m^2 IV on day 1
Repeat cycle every 21 days for a total of four cycles.
THEN
Cyclophosphamide: 600 mg/m^2 IV on day 1
Methotrexate: 40 mg/m^2 IV on day 1
5-Fluorouracil: 600 mg/m^2 IV on day 1
Repeat cycle every 21 days for a total of eight cycles.[1,44]

FEC **63**

5-Fluorouracil: 500 mg/m^2 IV on day 1
Epirubicin: 100 mg/m^2 IV on day 1
Cyclophosphamide: 500 mg/m^2 IV on day 1
Repeat cycle every 21 days for a total of six cycles.[1,45]

CMFP **65**

Cyclophosphamide: 100 mg/m^2 PO on days 1–14
Methotrexate: 40 mg/m^2 IV on days 1 and 8
5-Fluorouracil: 600 mg/m^2 IV on days 1 and 8
Prednisone: 20 mg PO qid on days 1–7
Repeat cycle every 28 days.[1,46]

Single-Agent Regimens

Tamoxifen **67**

Tamoxifen: 20 mg PO daily for 5 years in patients with estrogen
receptor positive tumors or estrogen receptor status unknown
Repeat daily for 5 years.[1,47]

Anastrozole (Arimidex) **68**

Anastrozole: 1 mg PO daily. Repeat daily for 5 years in patients with ER+
tumors or ER status unknown.[1,48]

Tamoxifen + Letrozole **69**

Tamoxifen: 20 mg PO daily for 5 years in patients with ER+ tumors,
  followed by
Letrozole: 2.5 mg PO daily for 5 years.[1,49]

Tamoxifen + Exemestane **71**

Tamoxifen: 20 mg PO daily for 2–3 years in patients with ER+ tumors,
  followed by
Exemestane: 25 mg PO daily for the remainder of 5 years.[1,50]

NEOADJUVANT THERAPY
Combination Regimens

Doxorubicin+Cyclophosphamide + Docetaxel (ACT)

Baseline laboratory tests:	CBC: Chemistry, LFTs, and CA 27-29
Baseline procedures or tests:	MUGA scan
Initiate IV:	0.9% sodium chloride
Premedicate:	Dexamethasone 8 mg bid for 3 days, starting the day before treatment
	5-HT$_3$ and dexamethasone 10–20 mg in 100 cc of NS
	Diphenhydramine 25–50 mg and cimetidine 300 mg in 100 cc of NS

Administer:

Doxorubicin _____mg (60 mg/m^2) IV on day 1

- Potent vesicant
- Available as a 2-mg/mL solution.
- Doxorubicin will form a precipitate if it is mixed with heparin or 5-FU.

Cyclophosphamide _____mg (600 mg/m^2) IV on day 1

- Available in 100-, 200-, 500-, 1000-, and 2000-mg vials.
- Dilute with sterile water and shake well to ensure that solution is completely dissolved.
- Reconstituted solution stable for 24 hours at room temperature, and 6 days refrigerated.

Administer:

Docetaxel _____mg (100 mg/m^2) IV on day 1

- Comes in 20- or 80-mg packs with own diluent. Do not shake.
- Reconstituted vials stable at room temperature or for 8 hours refrigerated.
- Further dilute in 250 cc of D5W or NS.
- **Use non-PVC containers and tubing to administer.**

Major Side Effects

- Hypersensitivity Reactions: Severe hypersensitivity reactions with docetaxel in 2%–3% of patients. Premedication with dexamethasone recommended. Cyclophosphamide can cause rhinitis and irritation of nose and throat.
- Bone Marrow Depression: Leukopenia, thrombocytopenia, and anemia all seen; may be severe and dose limiting.
- GI Toxicities: Nausea and vomiting are moderate to severe and can be acute or delayed. Stomatitis and diarrhea occur in some patients but is not dose limiting.
- Cardiac: Acutely, pericarditis-myocarditis syndrome may occur. With high cumulative doses > 550 mg/m^2 of doxorubicin cardiomyopathy may occur. Cyclophosphamide may increase the risk of doxorubicin-induced cardiotoxicity.
- Hepatic: Use doxorubicin and docetaxel with caution in patients with abnormal liver function. Dose reduction is required in the presence of liver dysfunction.
- Neuropathy: Peripheral neuropathy with sensory alterations are paresthesias in a glove and stocking distribution, and numbness.
- Fluid Balance: Fluid retention syndrome: weight gain, peripheral and/or generalized edema, pleural effusion, and ascites. Premedication with dexamethasone effective in preventing or minimizing occurrences.
- Bladder Toxicities: Hemorrhagic cystitis, dysuria, and urinary frequency. Red-orange discoloration of urine; resolves by 24–48 hours.
- Skin: Extravasation of doxorubicin causes severe tissue destruction. Hyperpigmentation, photosensitivity, and radiation recall occur. Maculopapular rash and dry, itchy skin. Complete alopecia.
- Reproduction: Amenorrhea with ovarian failure. Pregnancy category D.

Initiate antiemetic protocol:	Moderately to highly emetogenic protocol.
Supportive drugs:	☐ pegfilgrastim (Neulasta) ☐ filgrastim (Neupogen)
	☐ epoetin alfa (Procrit) ☐ darbepoetin alfa (Aranesp)
Treatment schedule:	Chair time 3–4 hours on day 1. Repeat cycle every 21 days for four cycles followed by surgery.

Estimated number of visits: Two visits per cycle. Request four cycles worth of visits.

Dose Calculation by: 1. _____   2. _____

_____   _____
Physician   Date

_____   _____
Patient Name   ID Number

_____   _____/_____/_____
Diagnosis   Ht   Wt   M^2

ADJUVANT THERAPY
Combination Regimens

Doxorubicin + Cyclophosphamide (AC)

Baseline laboratory tests:	CBC: Chemistry, LFTs, and CA 27-29
Baseline procedures or tests:	MUGA scan
Initiate IV:	0.9% sodium chloride
Premedicate:	5-HT$_3$ and dexamethasone 20 mg in 100 cc of NS.
Administer:	**Doxorubicin** _____ mg (60 mg/m^2) IV on day 1

- **Potent vesicant**
- Available as a 2-mg/mL solution.
- Doxorubicin will form a precipitate if it is mixed with heparin or 5-FU.

Cyclophosphamide _____ mg (600 mg/m^2) IV on day 1

- Available in 100-, 200-, 500-, 1000-, and 2000-mg vials.
- Dilute with sterile water and shake well to ensure that solution is completely dissolved.
- Reconstituted solution stable for 24 hours at room temperature, and 6 days refrigerated.

Major Side Effects

- Hypersensitivity Reaction: Cyclophosphamide can cause rhinitis and irritation of nose and throat.
- Bone Marrow Depression: Leukopenia, thrombocytopenia, and anemia all seen; may be severe.
- GI Toxicities: Nausea and vomiting are moderate to severe and can be acute or delayed. Stomatitis and diarrhea occur in some patients but is not dose limiting.
- Cardiac: Acutely, pericarditis-myocarditis syndrome may occur. With high cumulative doses > 550 mg/m^2 of doxorubicin cardiomyopathy may occur. Cyclophosphamide may increase the risk of doxorubicin-induced cardiotoxicity.
- Hepatic: Use with caution in patients with abnormal liver function. Dose reduction is required in the presence of liver dysfunction.
- Bladder Toxicities: Hemorrhagic cystitis, dysuria, and urinary frequency with cyclophosphamide. Red-orange discoloration of urine; resolves by 24–48 hours.
- Secondary Malignancies: Increased risk with cyclophosphamide.
- Skin: Extravasation of doxorubicin causes severe tissue destruction. Hyperpigmentation, photosensitivity, and radiation recall occur. Complete alopecia. Inappropriate secretion of antidiuretic hormone (SIADH).
- Reproduction: Amenorrhea with ovarian failure. Sterility may be permanent. Pregnancy category D.

Initiate antiemetic protocol:	Moderately to mildly emetogenic protocol.
Supportive drugs:	☐ pegfilgrastim (Neulasta) ☐ filgrastim (Neupogen)
	☐ epoetin alfa (Procrit) ☐ darbepoetin alfa (Aranesp)
Treatment schedule:	Chair time 2 hours on day 1. Repeat cycle every 21 days.
Estimated number of visits:	Two per cycle. Request four cycles worth of visits.

Dose Calculation by: 1. _____   2. _____

_____
Physician

_____
Date

_____
Patient Name

_____
ID Number

_____
Diagnosis

_____ / _____ / _____
Ht   Wt   M^2

Doxorubicin + Cyclophosphamide Followed by Paclitaxel (AC followed by T)

Baseline laboratory tests:	CBC: Chemistry, LFTs, and CA 27-29
Baseline procedures or tests:	MUGA scan
Initiate IV:	0.9% sodium chloride
Premedicate:	5-HT$_3$ and dexamethasone 20 mg in 100 cc of NS.
Administer:	**Doxorubicin** _____mg (60 mg/m^2) IV on day 1

- **Potent vesicant**
- Available as a 2-mg/mL solution.
- Doxorubicin will form a precipitate if it is mixed with heparin or 5-FU.

Cyclophosphamide _____mg (600 mg/m^2) IV on day 1

- Available in 100-, 200-, 500-, 1000-, and 2000-mg vials.
- Dilute with sterile water and shake well to ensure that solution is completely dissolved.
- Reconstituted solution stable for 24 hours at room temperature, and 6 days refrigerated.

Repeat cycle every 21 days for a total of four cycles, followed by four cycles paclitaxel.

Premedicate:	5-HT$_3$ and dexamethasone 10–20 mg in 100 cc of NS.
	Diphenhydramine 25–50 mg and cimetidine 300 mg in 100 cc of NS.
Administer:	**Paclitaxel** _____mg (175 mg/m^2) IV over 3 hours on day 1

- Available in solution as 6 mg/mL.
- Final concentration is $\leq$ 1.2 mg/mL.
- Stable for up to 27 hours at room temperature in 0.3–1.2 mg/mL solutions.
- **Use non-PVC containers and tubing with 0.22-micron inline filter for administration.**

Major Side Effects

- Hypersensitivity Reaction: With paclitaxel occurs in 20%–40% of patients. Characterized by generalized skin rash, flushing, erythema, hypotension, dyspnea, and/or bronchospasm. Usually occurs within the first 2–3 minutes of infusion and almost always within the first 10 minutes. Premedicate as described. Cyclophosphamide can cause rhinitis and irritation of nose and throat.
- Bone Marrow Depression: Dose-limiting neutropenia with nadir at days 8–10 and recovery by days 15–21. Decreased incidence of neutropenia with 3-hour schedule when compared with 24-hour schedule. G-CSF support recommended.
- Neurotoxicity: Dose-related sensory neuropathy with numbness and paresthesias. More frequent with longer infusions and at doses > 175 mg/m^2.
- GI Toxicities: Nausea and vomiting are moderate to severe and can be acute or delayed. Mucositis and diarrhea occur in 10% of patients but is not dose limiting.
- Cardiac: Acutely, pericarditis-myocarditis syndrome may occur. With high cumulative doses > 550 mg/m^2 of doxorubicin cardiomyopathy may occur. Cyclophosphamide may increase the risk of doxorubicin-induced cardiotoxicity.
- Hepatic: Use with caution in patients with abnormal liver function. Dose reduction is required in the presence of liver dysfunction.
- Bladder Toxicities: Hemorrhagic cystitis, dysuria, and urinary frequency with cyclophosphamide. Red-orange discoloration of urine; resolves by 24–48 hours.
- Inappropriate secretion of antidiuretic hormone (SIADH).
- Skin: Extravasation of doxorubicin causes severe tissue destruction. Hyperpigmentation, photosensitivity, and radiation recall occur. Complete alopecia.
- Secondary Malignancies: Increased risk with cyclophosphamide.
- Reproduction: Amenorrhea and ovarian failure. Sterility may be permanent. Pregnancy category D. Breast feeding should be voided.

Initiate antiemetic protocol:	Moderately to highly emetogenic protocol.
Supportive drugs:	☐ pegfilgrastim (Neulasta) ☐ filgrastim (Neupogen)
	☐ epoetin alfa (Procrit) ☐ darbepoetin alfa (Aranesp)
Treatment schedule:	Chair time 2 hours on day 1 for AC. 4–5 hours day 1 for paclitaxel. Repeat AC cycle every 21 days for a total of four cycles, followed by paclitaxel every 21 days for four cycles.

Estimated number of visits: Two visits per cycle. Request eight cycles worth of visits

Dose Calculation by: 1. _____   2. _____

_____   _____
Physician   Date

_____   _____
Patient Name   ID Number

_____   _____ / _____ / _____
Diagnosis   Ht   Wt   M²

Doxorubicin + Cyclophosphamide Followed by Paclitaxel + Trastuzumab (AC followed by T + Trastuzumab)

Baseline laboratory tests:	CBC: Chemistry, LFTs, and CA 27-29
Baseline procedures or tests:	MUGA scan, FISH for HER2
Initiate IV:	0.9% sodium chloride
Premedicate:	5-HT$_3$ and dexamethasone 20 mg in 100 cc of NS
Administer:	**Doxorubicin** _____mg (60 mg/m^2) IV on day 1

- Potent vesicant
- Available as a 2-mg/mL solution.
- Doxorubicin will form a precipitate if it is mixed with heparin or 5-FU.

Cyclophosphamide _____mg (600 mg/m^2) IV on day 1

- Available in 100-, 200-, 500-, 1000-, and 2000-mg vials.
- Dilute with sterile water and shake well to ensure that solution is completely dissolved.
- Reconstituted solution stable for 24 hours at room temperature, and 6 days refrigerated.

Repeat cycle every 21 days for a total of four cycles, followed by four cycles paclitaxel + trastuzumab.

Premedicate:	5-HT$_3$ and dexamethasone 10–20 mg in 100 cc of NS.
	Diphenhydramine 25–50 mg and cimetidine 300 mg in 100 cc of NS.
Administer:	**Paclitaxel** _____mg (80 mg/m^2) IV over 1 hour on day 1

- Final concentration is ± 1.2 mg/mL.
- **Use non-PVC containers and tubing with 0.22-micron inline filter for administration.**

Trastuzumab _____mg (4 m/kg) loading dose IV in 250 cc of NS over 90 minutes day 1 week 1 only. Then,

Trastuzumab _____mg (2 mg/kg) IV in 250 cc of NS over 30 minutes weekly week 2–12 followed by:

Trastuzumab _____mg (2 m/kg) IV in 250 cc of NS over 30 minutes weekly × 40 weeks

- Available as a lyophilized, sterile powder in 440-mg multiuse vials for IV use.
- Requires refrigeration. DO NOT FREEZE.
- Reconstitute with 20 mL of bacteriostatic water for injection, USP, containing 1.1% benzyl alcohol, which is supplied with each vial. DO NOT SHAKE.
- Reconstituted solution contains 21 mg/mL. Stable 28 days refrigerated.
- Further dilute desired dose in 250 cc of NS.

Major Side Effects

- Hypersensitivity Reaction: With paclitaxel occurs in 20%–40% of patients. Characterized by generalized skin rash, flushing, erythema, hypotension, dyspnea, and/or bronchospasm. Usually occurs within the first 2–3 minutes of infusion and almost always within the first 10 minutes. Premedicate as described. Trastuzumab: Fever, chills, viricaria, flushing, fatigue, headache, bronchospasm, dyspnea, angioendema, and hypotension seen in 40–50% of patients. Usually mild to moderate and most often in first dose only.
- Bone Marrow Depression: Dose-limiting neutropenia with nadir at days 8–10 and recovery by days 15–21. Decreased incidence of neutropenia with 3-hour schedule when compared with 24-hour schedule. G-CSF support recommended.
- Neurotoxicity: Dose-related sensory neuropathy with numbness and paresthesias. More frequent with longer infusions and at doses > 175 mg/m^2.
- GI Toxicities: Nausea and vomiting are moderate to severe and can be acute or delayed. Mucositis and diarrhea occur in 10% of patients but is not dose limiting.
- Cardiac: Acutely, pericarditis-myocarditis syndrome may occur. With high cumulative doses > 550 mg/m^{2}of doxorubicin cardiomyopathy may occur. Cyclophosphamide may increase the risk of doxorubicin-induced cardiotoxicity. Risk to cardiotoxicity with trastuzumab significantly increased when used in combination with anthracycline/cyclophosphamide regimen.

- Hepatic: Use with caution in patients with abnormal liver function. Dose reduction is required in the presence of liver dysfunction.
- Bladder Toxicities: Hemorrhagic cystitis, dysuria, and urinary frequency with cyclophosphamide. Red-orange discoloration of urine; resolves by 24–48 hours.
- Inappropriate secretion of antidiuretic hormone (SIADH).
- Skin: Extravasation of doxorubicin causes severe tissue destruction. Hyperpigmentation, photosensitivity, and radiation recall occur. Complete alopecia, loss of total body hair, occurs in nearly all patients. Hair may return when on trastuzumab alone.
- Secondary Malignancies: Increased risk with cyclophosphamide.
- Reproduction: Amenorrhea and ovarian failure. Sterility may be permanent. Pregnancy category D. Breast feeding should be avoided.

Initiate antiemetic protocol:	Moderately to highly emetogenic protocol.
Supportive drugs:	☐ pegfilgrastim (Neulasta) ☐ filgrastim (Neupogen)
	☐ epoetin alfa (Procrit) ☐ darbepoetin alfa (Aranesp)
Treatment schedule:	Chair time 2 hours on day 1 for AC. 3 hours day 1 for paclitaxel and trastuzumab, 1 hour for trastuzumab alone. Repeat AC cycle every 21 days for a total of four cycles, followed by paclitaxel and trastuzumab weekly for 12 weeks; followed by trastuzumab weekly × 40 weeks.
Estimated number of visits:	Two visits per cycle. Request eight cycles worth of visits.

Dose Calculation by: 1. _____ 2. _____

_____

Physician _____ Date _____

Patient Name _____ ID Number _____

Diagnosis _____ Ht _____ / Wt _____ / M^2 _____

Doxorubicin → Paclitaxel → Cyclophosphamide A → T → C (Dose-Dense Therapy)

Baseline laboratory tests:	CBC: Chemistry and CA 27-29
Baseline procedures or tests:	MUGA scan
Initiate IV:	0.9% sodium chloride
Premedicate:	5-HT$_3$ and dexamethasone 10–20 mg in 100 cc of NS.
Administer:	**Doxorubicin** _____ mg (60 mg/m^2) IV on day 1

- **Potent vesicant**

- Available as a 2-mg/mL solution.

- Doxorubicin will form a precipitate if it is mixed with heparin or 5-FU.

Repeat cycle every 2 weeks for four cycles, followed by

Premedicate:	5-HT$_3$ and dexamethasone 10–20 mg in 100 cc of NS.
	Diphenhydramine 25–50 mg and cimetidine 300 mg in 100 cc of NS.
Administer:	**Paclitaxel** _____ mg (175 mg/m^2) IV over 3 hours on day 1

- Available in solution as 6 mg/mL.

- Final concentration is ≤ 1.2 mg/mL.

- Stable for up to 27 hours at room temperature in 0.3–1.2 mg/mL solutions.

- **Use non-PVC containers and tubing with 0.22-micron inline filter for administration.**

Repeat cycle every 2 weeks for four cycles. Followed by:

Premedicate:	5-HT$_3$ and dexamethasone 10–20 mg in 100 cc of NS.
Administer:	**Cyclophosphamide** _____ 600 mg/m^2 IV day 1. Repeat cycle every 2 weeks for four cycles

- Available in 100-, 200-, 500-, 1000-, and 2000-mg vials.

- Dilute with sterile water and shake well to ensure that solution is completely dissolved.

- Reconstituted solution stable for 24 hours at room temperature, and 6 days refrigerated.

Administer:	**Filgastrim** _____ 5 µg/kg SC on days 3–10 of each 2-week cycle

Major Side Effects

- Hypersensitivity Reaction: Occurs in 20%–40% of patients. Characterized by generalized skin rash, flushing, erythema, hypotension, dyspnea, and/or bronchospasm. Usually occurs within the first 2–3 minutes of infusion and almost always within the first 10 minutes. Premedicate as described. Cyclophosphamide can cause rhinitis and irritation of nose and throat.

- Bone Marrow Depression: Dose-limiting neutropenia with nadir at days 8–10 and recovery by days 15–21. Decreased incidence of neutropenia with 3-hour schedule when compared with 24-hour schedule. G-CSF support recommended.

- GI Toxicities: Nausea and vomiting are moderate to severe with doxorubicin and cyclophosphamide. May be acute or delayed with cyclophosphamide. Usually mild to moderate with paclitaxel. Mucositis and diarrhea seen.

- Cardiac: Acutely, pericarditis-myocarditis syndrome may occur. With high cumulative doses > 550 mg/m^2 of doxorubicin cardiomyopathy may occur. Cyclophosphamide may increase risk of doxorubicin-induced cardiotoxicity.

- Hepatic: Use with caution in patients with abnormal liver function. Dose reduction required in the presence of liver dysfunction.

- Skin: Extravasation of doxorubicin causes severe tissue destruction. Hyperpigmentation, photosensitvity, and radiation recall occur. Complete alopecia.

- Neurotoxicity: Dose-related sensory neuropathy with numbness and paresthesias. More frequent with longer infusions and at doses > 175 mg/m^2.

- Bladder Toxicities: Hemorrhagic cystitis, dysuria, and urinary frequency with cyclophosphamide. Can be prevented with adequate hydration. Red-orange discoloration of urine; resolves by 24–48 hours.

- Secondary Malignancies: Increased risk with cyclophosphamide.

- Reproductive: Amenorrhea and ovarian failure. Sterility may be permanent. Pregnancy category D. Breast feeding should be avoided.

Initiate antiemetic protocol:	Moderately to highly emetogenic protocol.

Supportive drugs: ☐ pegfilgrastim (Neulasta)   ☐ filgrastim (Neupogen)

                                   ☐ epoetin alfa (Procrit)   ☐ darbepoetin alfa (Aranesp)

Treatment schedule: Chair time for AC 1 hour every 2 weeks. Repeat cycle every 2 weeks for four cycles. **Follow with:** Paclitaxel 3–4 hours day 1 every 2 weeks for 4 weeks; followed by cyclophosphamide 2 hours every 2 weeks for 4 weeks.

Estimated number of visits: One visit per cycle. Request 12 cycles worth of visits.

Dose Calculation by: 1. _____   2. _____

_____ _____

Physician   Date

_____ _____

Patient Name   ID Number

_____ _____ / _____ / _____

Diagnosis   Ht   Wt   M^2

Cyclophosphamide + Doxorubicin + 5-Flourouracil (CAF)

Baseline laboratory tests:	CBC: Chemistry, LFTs, and CA 27-29
Baseline procedures or tests:	MUGA scan
Initiate IV:	0.9% sodium chloride
Premedicate:	5-HT$_3$ and dexamethasone 20 mg in 100 cc of NS.
Administer:	**Cyclophosphamide** _____mg (600 mg/m^2) IV on day 1

- Available in 100-, 200-, 500-, 1000-, and 2000-mg vials.
- Dilute with sterile water and shake well to ensure that solution is completely dissolved.
- Reconstituted solution stable for 24 hours at room temperature, and 6 days refrigerated.

Doxorubicin _____mg (60 mg/m^2) IV on day 1

- Potent vesicant
- Available as a 2-mg/mL solution.
- Doxorubicin will form a precipitate if it is mixed with heparin or 5-FU.

5-Flourouracil _____mg (600 mg/m^2) IV on day 1

- Available in solution as 50 mg/mL.
- No dilution required.
- May further dilute with NS or D5W.

Major Side Effects

- Hypersensitivity Reaction: Cyclophosphamide can cause rhinitis and irritation of nose and throat.
- Bone Marrow Depression: Leukopenia, thrombocytopenia, and anemia all seen; may be severe.
- GI Toxicities: Nausea and vomiting are moderate to severe and can be acute or delayed. Stomatitis and diarrhea can be severe and dose limiting.
- Cardiac: Acutely, pericarditis-myocarditis syndrome may occur. With high cumulative doses > 550 mg/m^2, cardiomyopathy may occur. Cyclophosphamide may increase the risk of doxorubicin-induced cardiotoxicity.
- Hepatic: Use with caution in patients with abnormal liver function. Dose reduction is required in the presence of liver dysfunction.
- Bladder Toxicities: Hemorrhagic cystitis, dysuria, and urinary frequency with cyclophosphamide. Red-orange discoloration of urine; resolves by 24–48 hours.
- Inappropriate secretion of antidiuretic hormone (SIADH).
- Skin: Extravasation of doxorubicin causes severe tissue destruction. Hyperpigmentation, photosensitivity, nail changes, and radiation recall occur. Complete alopecia. Hand-foot syndrome can be dose limiting.
- Ocular: Photophobia, increased lacrimation, acute and chronic conjunctivitis, blepharitis, and blurred vision.
- Secondary Malignancies: Increased risk with cyclophosphamide.
- Reproduction: Amenorrhea with ovarian failure. Sterility may be permanent. Pregnancy category D. Breast feeding should be avoided.

Initiate antiemetic protocol:	Moderately to highly emetogenic protocol.
Supportive drugs:	☐ pegfilgrastim (Neulasta) ☐ filgrastim (Neupogen) ☐ epoetin alfa (Procrit) ☐ darbepoetin alfa (Aranesp)
Treatment schedule:	Chair time 2 hours on day 1. Repeat cycle every 21 days for a total of six cycles.
Estimated number of visits:	Two visits per cycle. Request six cycles worth of visits.

Dose Calculation by: 1. _____   2. _____

_____

Physician   Date

_____   / _____ / _____

Patient Name   ID Number

_____   / _____ / _____

Diagnosis   Ht   Wt   M^2

Cyclophosphamide + Doxorubicin + 5-Flourouracil (CAF–Oral)

Baseline laboratory tests:	CBC: Chemistry, LFTs, and CA 27-29
Baseline procedures or tests:	MUGA scan
Initiate IV:	0.9% sodium chloride
Premedicate:	5-HT$_3$ and dexamethasone 20 mg in 100 cc of NS.
Administer:	

Cyclophosphamide _____ mg (100 mg/m^2/day) PO on days 1–14

- Available in 25- and 50-mg tablets
- Administer in morning or early afternoon to allow adequate excretion time.
- Take with meals.

Doxorubicin _____ mg (30 mg/m^2) IV on days 1 and 8

- **Potent vesicant**
- Available as a 2-mg/mL solution.
- Doxorubicin will form a precipitate if it is mixed with heparin or 5-FU.

5-Flourouracil _____ mg (500 mg/m^2) IV on days 1 and 8

- Available in solution as 50 mg/mL.
- No dilution required.
- May further dilute with NS or D5W.

Major Side Effects

- Hypersensitivity Reaction: Cyclophosphamide can cause rhinitis and irritation of nose and throat.
- Bone Marrow Depression: Leukopenia, thrombocytopenia, and anemia; may be severe.
- GI Toxicities: Nausea and vomiting are moderate to severe and can be acute or delayed. Stomatitis and diarrhea can be severe and dose limiting.
- Cardiac: Acutely, pericarditis-myocarditis syndrome may occur. With high cumulative doses > 550 mg/m^2, cardiomyopathy may occur. Cyclophosphamide may increase the risk of doxorubicin-induced cardiotoxicity.
- Hepatic: Use with caution in patients with abnormal liver function. Dose reduction is required in the presence of liver dysfunction.
- Bladder Toxicities: Hemorrhagic cystitis, dysuria, and urinary frequency with cyclophosphamide. Red-orange discoloration of urine; resolves by 24–48 hours.
- Inappropriate secretion of antidiuretic hormone (SIADH).
- Skin: Extravasation of doxorubicin causes severe tissue destruction. Hyperpigmentation, photosensitivity, nail changes, and radiation recall occur. Complete alopecia. Hand-foot syndrome can be dose limiting.
- Ocular: Photophobia, increased lacrimation, acute and chronic conjunctivitis, blepharitis, and blurred vision.
- Secondary Malignancies: Increased risk with cyclophosphamide.
- Reproduction: Amenorrhea with ovarian failure. Sterility may be permanent. Pregnancy category D. Breast feeding should be avoided.

Initiate antiemetic protocol:	Moderately to highly emetogenic protocol.
Supportive drugs:	☐ pegfilgrastim (Neulasta) ☐ filgrastim (Neupogen)
	☐ epoetin alfa (Procrit) ☐ darbepoetin alfa (Aranesp)
Treatment schedule:	Chair time 1 hour on days 1 and 8. Repeat cycle every 28 days for a total of six cycles.
Estimated number of visits:	Three visits per cycle. Request six cycles worth of visits.

Dose Calculation by: 1. _____   2. _____

_____

Physician   Date

_____

Patient Name   ID Number

_____/_____/_____/_____

Diagnosis   Ht   Wt   M²

Cyclophosphamide + Methotrexate + 5-Flourouracil (CMF-Bonadonna Regimen)

Baseline laboratory tests:	CBC: Chemistry, LFTs, and CA 27-29
Baseline procedures or tests:	None
Initiate IV:	0.9% sodium chloride
Premedicate:	5-HT$_3$ and dexamethasone 20 mg in 100 cc of NS on days 1 and 8
	Oral 5-HT$_3$ or phenothiazine days 2–7 and 9–14

Administer:

Cyclophosphamide _____mg (100 mg/m^2/day) PO on days 1–14

- Available in 25- and 50-mg tablets.
- Administer in morning or early afternoon to allow adequate excretion time.
- Administer with meals.

Methotrexate _____mg (40 mg/m^2) IV on days 1 and 8

- Available in 50-, 100-, 200-, and 1000-mg single-use reconstituted vials.
- May dilute further in NS.
- Reconstituted solution is stable for 24 hours at room temperature.

5-Flourouracil _____mg (600 mg/m^2) IV on days 1 and 8

- Available in solution as 50 mg/mL.
- No dilution required.
- Can be further diluted with NS or D5W

Major Side Effects

- Hypersensitivity Reaction: Cyclophosphamide can cause rhinitis and irritation of nose and throat.
- Bone Marrow Depression: Leukopenia can be severe, thrombocytopenia is less frequent, and anemia is mild.
- GI Toxicities: Nausea and vomiting are moderate to severe and occur within 24 hours of administration. Mucositis and diarrhea can be severe; dose dependent.
- Renal: Acute renal failure, azotemia, urinary retention, and uric acid nephropathy have been observed with methotrexate.
- Hepatic: Hepatotoxicity is rare.
- Pulmonary Toxicity: Rare; onset is insidious (fever, cough) and appears as interstitial pneumonitis, which may progress to fibrosis. May respond to steroids.
- Bladder Toxicities: Hemorrhagic cystitis, dysuria, and urinary frequency with cyclophosphamide.
- Hormonal: SIADH
- Ocular: Photophobia, increased lacrimation, acute and chronic conjunctivitis, blepharitis, and blurred vision.
- Skin: Complete alopecia in 50% of patients, diffuse thinning in others. Hyperpigmentation of nails and skin, banding of nails, and radiation recall may occur. Photosensitivity, sunburn-like rash. Hand-foot syndrome can be dose limiting.
- Secondary Malignancies: Increased risk with cyclophosphamide.
- Reproductive: Amenorrhea with ovarian failure. Sterility may be permanent. Pregnancy category D. Breast feeding should be avoided.

Initiate antiemetic protocol:	Moderately to highly emetogenic protocol.	
Supportive drugs:	☐ pegfilgrastim (Neulasta)	☐ filgrastim (Neupogen)
	☐ epoetin alfa (Procrit)	☐ darbepoetin alfa (Aranesp)
Treatment schedule:	Chair time 1 hour on days 1 and 8. Repeat cycle every 28 days for six cycles.	
Estimated number of visits:	Three visits per cycle. Request six cycles worth of visits.	

Dose Calculation by: 1. _____ 2. _____

_____
Physician

Date

_____
Patient Name

ID Number

_____   /   /
Diagnosis   Ht   Wt   M²

Cyclophosphamide + Methotrexate + 5-Flourouracil (CMF-IV Regimen)

Baseline laboratory tests:	CBC: Chemistry, LFTs, and CA 27-29
Baseline procedures or tests:	None
Initiate IV:	0.9% sodium chloride
Premedicate:	5-HT$_3$ and dexamethasone 20 mg in 100 cc of NS.
Administer:	**Cyclophosphamide** _____mg (600 mg/m^2) IV on day 1

* Available in 100-, 200-, 500-, 1000-, and 2000-mg vials.
* Dilute with sterile water and shake well to ensure that solution is completely dissolved.
* Reconstituted solution stable for 24 hours at room temperature, and 6 days refrigerated.

Methotrexate _____mg (40 mg/m^2) IV on day 1

* Available in 50-, 100-, 200-, and 1000-mg single-use reconstituted vials.
* May dilute further in NS.
* Reconstituted solution is stable for 24 hours at room temperature.

5-Flourouracil _____mg (600 mg/m^2) IV on day 1

* Available in solution as 50 mg/mL.
* No dilution required.
* Can be further diluted with NS or D5W

Major Side Effects

* Hypersensitivity Reaction: Cyclophosphamide can cause rhinitis and irritation of nose and throat.
* Bone Marrow Depression: Leukopenia can be severe, thrombocytopenia is less frequent, and anemia is mild.
* GI Toxicities: Nausea and vomiting are moderate to severe and occur within 24 hours of administration. Mucositis and diarrhea can be severe; dose dependent.
* Renal: Acute renal failure, azotemia, urinary retention, and uric acid nephropathy have been observed with methotrexate.
* Hepatic: Hepatotoxicity is rare.
* Pulmonary Toxicity: Rare; onset is insidious (fever, cough) and appears as interstitial pneumonitis, which may progress to fibrosis. May respond to steroids.
* Bladder Toxicities: Hemorrhagic cystitis, dysuria, and urinary frequency with cyclophosphamide.
* Hormonal: SIADH
* Ocular: Photophobia, increased lacrimation, acute and chronic conjunctivitis, blepharitis, and blurred vision.
* Skin: Complete alopecia in 50% of patients, diffuse thinning in others. Hyperpigmentation of nails and skin, banding of nails, and radiation recall may occur. Photosensitivity, sunburn-like rash. Hand-foot syndrome can be dose limiting.
* Secondary Malignancies: Increased risk with cyclophosphamide.
* Reproductive: Amenorrhea with ovarian failure. Sterility may be permanent. Pregnancy category D. Breast feeding should be avoided.

Initiate antiemetic protocol:	Moderately to highly emetogenic protocol.
Supportive drugs:	☐ pegfilgrastim (Neulasta) ☐ filgrastim (Neupogen)
	☐ epoetin alfa (Procrit) ☐ darbepoetin alfa (Aranesp)
Treatment schedule:	Chair time 2 hours on day 1. Repeat cycle every 21 days for six cycles.
Estimated number of visits:	Two visits per cycle. Request six cycles worth of visits.

Dose Calculation by: 1. _____   2. _____

_____

Physician _____   Date _____

Patient Name _____   ID Number _____

Diagnosis _____   Ht _____ / _____ Wt _____ / _____ M² _____

Doxorubicin + CMF

Baseline laboratory tests:	CBC: Chemistry and CA 27-29
Baseline procedures or tests:	MUGA scan
Initiate IV:	0.9% sodium chloride
Premedicate:	5-HT$_3$ and dexamethasone 10–20 mg in 100 cc of NS.
Administer:	**Doxorubicin** _____ mg (75 mg/m^2) IV on day 1

- **Potent vesicant**
- Available as a 2-mg/mL solution.
- Doxorubicin will form a precipitate if it is mixed with heparin or 5-FU.

Repeat cycle every 21 days for four cycles; follow by:

Premedicate:	5-HT$_3$ and dexamethasone 20 mg in 100 cc of NS.
Administer:	**Cyclophosphamide** _____ mg (600 mg/m^2) IV on day 1

- Available in 100-, 200-, 500-, 1000-, and 2000-mg vials.
- Dilute with sterile water and shake well to ensure that solution is completely dissolved.
- Reconstituted solution stable for 24 hours at room temperature, and 6 days refrigerated.

Methotrexate _____ mg (40 mg/m^2) IV on day 1

- Available in 50-, 100-, 200-, and 1000-mg single-use reconstituted vials.
- May dilute further in NS.
- Reconstituted solution is stable for 24 hours at room temperature.

5-Flourouracil _____ mg (600 mg/m^2) IV on day 1

- Available in solution as 50 mg/mL.
- No dilution required.
- Can be further diluted with NS or D5W.

Major Side Effects

- Hypersensitivity Reaction: Cyclophosphamide can cause rhinitis and irritation of nose and throat.
- Bone Marrow Depression: WBC and platelet nadir 10–14 days after drug dose, with recovery from days 15–21. Myelosuppression may be severe but is less severe with weekly dosing.
- GI Toxicities: Nausea and vomiting are moderate to severe and can occur within 24 hours of administration. Mucositis and diarrhea can be severe; dose dependent.
- Cardiac: Acutely, pericarditis-myocarditis syndrome may occur. With high cumulative doses > 550 mg/m^2, cardiomyopathy may occur. Increased risk of cardiotoxicity when doxorubicin is given with trastuzumab (Herceptin) or mitomycin.
- Renal: Acute renal failure, azotemia, urinary retention, and uric acid nephropathy have been observed with methotrexate.
- Hepatic: Hepatotoxicity is rare.
- Pulmonary Toxicity: Rare; onset is insidious (fever, cough) and appears as interstitial pneumonitis, which may progress to fibrosis. May respond to steroids.
- Bladder Toxicities: Hemorrhagic cystitis, dysuria, and urinary frequency with cyclophosphamide.
- Hormonal: SIADH.
- Ocular: Photophobia, increased lacrimation, acute and chronic conjunctivitis, blepharitis, and blurred vision.
- Skin: Extravasation of doxorubicin causes severe tissue destruction. Hyperpigmentation, photosensitivity, and radiation recall occur with doxorubicin. Complete alopecia occurs with doses > 50 mg/m^2. Hyperpigmentation of nails and skin, banding of nails, and radiation recall may occur with 5-Fluorouracil. Photosensitivity with a sunburn-like rash. Hand-foot syndrome can be dose limiting.
- Secondary Malignancies: Increased risk with cyclophosphamide.
- Reproductive: Amenorrhea with ovarian failure. Sterility may be permanent. Pregnancy category D. Breast feeding should be avoided.

Initiate antiemetic protocol: Moderately to highly emetogenic protocol.

Supportive drugs: ☐ pegfilgrastim (Neulasta)   ☐ filgrastim (Neupogen)
☐ epoetin alfa (Procrit)   ☐ darbepoetin alfa (Aranesp)

Treatment schedule: Chair time 1 hour on day 1 for doxorubicin. Repeat cycle every 21 days for four cycles; followed by chair time 2 hours for CMF every 21 days for a total of eight cycles.

Estimated number of visits: Two visits per cycle. Request twelve cycles worth of visits.

Dose Calculation by: 1. _____   2. _____

_____

Physician   Date

_____

Patient Name   ID Number

_____

Diagnosis   Ht _____ / Wt _____ / M^2 _____

5-Fluorouracil + Epirubicin + Cyclophosphamide (FEC)

Baseline laboratory tests:	CBC: Chemistry, LFTs, and CA 27-29
Baseline procedures or tests:	MUGA scan
Initiate IV:	0.9% sodium chloride
Premedicate:	5-HT$_3$ and dexamethasone 20 mg in 100 cc of NS.
Administer:	**5-Flourouracil** _____mg (500 mg/m^2) IV on day 1

- Available in solution as 50 mg/mL.
- No dilution required.
- May further dilute with NS or D5W

Epirubicin _____mg (100 mg/m^2) IV on day 1

- **Vesicant**
- Drug is provided as a preservative-free, ready-to-use solution (2 mg/mL).
- Use within 24 hours of penetration of rubber stopper; discard unused portion.
- Store unopened vials in refrigerator.

Cyclophosphamide _____mg (500 mg/m^2) IV on day 1

- Available in 100-, 200-, 500-, 1000-, and 2000-mg vials.
- Dilute with sterile water and shake well to ensure that solution is completely dissolved.
- Reconstituted solution stable for 24 hours at room temperature, and 6 days refrigerated.

Major Side Effects

- Hypersensitivity Reaction: Cyclophosphamide can cause rhinitis and irritation of nose and throat.
- Bone Marrow Depression: Leukopenia, thrombocytopenia, and anemia all seen; may be severe.
- GI Toxicities: Nausea and vomiting are moderate to severe. Mucositis and diarrhea can be severe and dose limiting.
- Cardiac: Cardiotoxicity is dose related, is cumulative, and may occur during or months to years after cessation of therapy. Cyclophosphamide may increase the risk of cardiotoxicity.
- Hepatic: Use with caution in patients with abnormal liver function. Dose reduction is required in the presence of liver dysfunction.
- Bladder Toxicities: Hemorrhagic cystitis, dysuria, and urinary frequency, preventable with adequate hydration. Red-orange discoloration of urine; resolves by 24–48 hours.
- Skin: Extravasation of epirubicin causes severe tissue destruction. Epirubicin may cause "flare" reaction or streaking along vein during peripheral administration. If this occurs, slow drug administration time and flush more. Hyperpigmentation, photosensitivity, nail changes, and radiation recall occur. Complete alopecia. Hand-foot syndrome can be dose limiting.
- Inappropriate secretion of antidiuretic hormone (SIADH).
- Ocular: Photophobia, increased lacrimation, acute and chronic conjunctivitis, blepharitis, and blurred vision.
- Secondary Malignancies: Increased risk with cyclophosphamide.
- Reproductive: Amenorrhea with ovarian failure. Sterility may be permanent. Pregnancy category D. Breast feeding should be avoided.

Initiate antiemetic protocol:	Moderately to highly emetogenic protocol.
Supportive drugs:	☐ pegfilgrastim (Neulasta) ☐ filgrastim (Neupogen)
	☐ epoetin alfa (Procrit) ☐ darbepoetin alfa (Aranesp)
Treatment schedule:	Chair time 2 hours on day 1. Repeat cycle every 21 days for a total of six cycles.
Estimated number of visits:	Two visits per cycle. Request six cycles worth of visits.

Dose Calculation by: 1. _____   2. _____

_____

Physician   Date

_____

Patient Name   ID Number

_____   /   /

Diagnosis   Ht   Wt M^2

CMFP

Baseline laboratory tests:	CBC: Chemistry, LFTs, and CA 27-29
Baseline procedures or tests:	None
Initiate IV:	0.9% sodium chloride
Premedicate:	5-HT$_3$ and dexamethasone 20 mg in 100 cc of NS on days 1 and 8
	Oral 5-HT$_3$ or phenothiazine days 2–7 and 9–14
Administer:	**Cyclophosphamide** _____mg (100 mg/m^2/day) PO on days 1–14

- Available in 25- and 50-mg tablets
- Administer in morning or early afternoon to allow adequate excretion time.
- Administer with meals.

Methotrexate _____mg (40 mg/m^2) IV on days 1 and 8

- Available in 50-, 100-, 200-, and 1000-mg single-use reconstituted vials.
- May dilute further in NS.
- Reconstituted solution is stable for 24 hours at room temperature.

5-Flourouracil _____mg (600 mg/m^2) IV on days 1 and 8

- Available in solution as 50 mg/mL.
- No dilution required.
- Can be further diluted with NS or D5W.

Prednisone: 20 mg PO qid on days 1–7

Major Side Effects	

- Hypersensitivity Reaction: Cyclophosphamide can cause rhinitis and irritation of nose and throat.
- Bone Marrow Depression: Leukopenia can be severe, thrombocytopenia is less frequent, and anemia is mild.
- GI Toxicities: Nausea and vomiting are moderate to severe and occur within 24 hours of administration. Mucositis and diarrhea can be severe; dose dependent.
- Renal: Acute renal failure, azotemia, urinary retention, and uric acid nephropathy have been observed with methotrexate.
- Hepatic: Hepatotoxicity is rare.
- Pulmonary Toxicity: Rare; onset is insidious (fever, cough) and appears as interstitial pneumonitis, which may progress to fibrosis. May respond to steroids.
- Bladder Toxicities: Hemorrhagic cystitis, dysuria, and urinary frequency. Preventable with adequate hydration with cyclophosphamide.
- Hormonal: SIADH.
- Ocular: Photophobia, increased lacrimation, acute and chronic conjunctivitis, blepharitis, and blurred vision
- Skin: Complete alopecia in 50% of patients, diffuse thinning in others. Hyperpigmentation of nails and skin, banding of nails, and radiation recall may occur. Photosensitivity, sunburn-like rash. Hand-foot syndrome can be dose limiting.
- Steroid Effects: Hyperglycemia, insomnia, emotional lability, agitation, fluid retention, and perceptual alterations related to cataracts or glaucoma with long-term use.
- Secondary Malignancies: Increased risk with cyclophosphamide.
- Reproductive: Amenorrhea with ovarian failure. Sterility may be permanent. Pregnancy category D. Breast feeding should be avoided.

Initiate antiemetic protocol:	Moderately to highly emetogenic protocol.	
Supportive drugs:	☐ pegfilgrastim (Neulasta)	☐ filgrastim (Neupogen)
	☐ epoetin alfa (Procrit)	☐ darbepoetin alfa (Aranesp)
Treatment schedule:	Chair time 1 hour on days 1 and 8. Repeat cycle every 28 days for six cycles.	
Estimated number of visits:	Three visits per cycle. Request six cycles worth of visits.	

Dose Calculation by: 1. _____ 2. _____

_____   _____

Physician   Date

_____   _____

Patient Name   ID Number

_____   _____/_____/_____

Diagnosis   Ht   Wt M^2

Single-Agent Regimens

Tamoxifen (Nolvadex)

Baseline laboratory tests:	CBC: Chemistry, LFTs, and CA 27-29
Baseline procedures or tests:	ER/PR testing
Initiate IV:	N/A
Premedicate:	Oral phenothiazine or 5-HT$_3$ if nausea occurs
Administer:	**Tamoxifen** 20 mg PO daily

- Available in 10- and 20-mg tablets
- Monitor (prothrombin time) PT/INR closely in patients taking warfarin; increases PT/INR

Major Side Effects

- GI Toxicities: Nausea and vomiting rarely observed.
- Tumor Flare: Usually occurs within the first 2 weeks of beginning of therapy. May observe increased bone pain, urinary retention, back pain with spinal cord compression and/or hypercalcemia.
- CV Toxicities: Deep vein thrombosis, pulmonary embolism, and superficial phlebitis are rare cardiovascular complications of tamoxifen therapy. Incidence of thromboembolic events may be increased when tamoxifen is given concomitantly with chemotherapy.
- Fluid/electrolyte Imbalance: Fluid retention and peripheral edema observed in about 30% of patients.
- Hormonal Effects: Menstrual irregularity, hot flashes, milk production in breasts, vaginal discharge, and bleeding. Usually not severe enough to discontinue therapy.
- Gynecological: Increased incidence of endometrial hyperplasia, polyps, and endometrial cancer.
- Sensory/perception Alteration: Headache, lethargy, and dizziness occur rarely. Visual disturbances, including cataract, retinopathy, and decreased visual acuity, have been described.
- Myelosuppression: Mild, transient leukopenia and thrombocytopenia occur rarely.
- Laboratory Values: Elevations in serum triglyceride levels.
- Reproductive: Pregnancy category D. Breast feeding should be avoided.

Initiate antiemetic protocol:	Mildly emetogenic protocol.
Treatment schedule:	No chair time. Daily dosing for 5 years.
Estimated number of visits:	One visit every 2–3 months first year, then every 6–12 months for remaining 4 years. Request 12 months worth of visits at a time.

Dose Calculation by: 1. _____   2. _____

_____
Physician

_____
Date

_____
Patient Name

_____
ID Number

_____
Diagnosis

_____/_____/_____
Ht   Wt   M^2

Anastrozole (Arimidex)

Baseline laboratory tests:	CBC: Chemistry panel, LFTs, and CA 27-29
Baseline procedures or tests:	ER/PR testing
Initiate IV:	N/A
Premedicate:	Oral phenothiazine or 5-HT$_3$ if nausea occurs
Administer:	**Anastrozole** 1 mg PO daily

- Available as a 1-mg, white, film-coated tablet for oral use.
- Take orally with or without food, at approximately the same time daily.

Major Side Effects

- Hormonal: Hot flashes, and vaginal dryness may occur.
- CV Toxicities: Thrombophlebitis may occur but is uncommon. Mild swelling of arms or legs may occur.
- GI Toxicities: Mild nausea and vomiting. Mild constipation or diarrhea can also occur.
- Skin: Dry, scaling skin rash.
- Flulike Syndrome: Presents in the form of fever, malaise, and myalgias.
- Musculoskeletal: Arthralgias occur in 10%–15% of patients and involve hands, knees, hips, lower back, and shoulders. Early morning stiffness is usual presentation.
- CNS Toxicity: Headaches are mild and occur in about 13% of patients. Decreased energy and weakness are common.
- Reproductive: Pregnancy category D. Breast feeding should be avoided.

Initiate antiemetic protocol:	Mildly emetogenic protocol.
Treatment schedule:	No chair time. Daily dosing for 5 years with ER+ tumors or with ER status unknown.
Estimated number of visits:	One visit every 2–3 months first year, then every 6–12 months for remaining 4 years. Request 12 months worth of visits at a time.

Dose Calculation by: 1. _____   2. _____

_____

Physician   Date

_____

Patient Name   ID Number

_____

Diagnosis   Ht _____/_____ Wt _____/_____ M^2

Tamoxifen + Letrozole

Tamoxifen (First Five Years)

Baseline laboratory tests:	CBC: Chemistry, LFTs, and CA 27-29
Baseline procedures or tests:	ER/PR testing
Initiate IV:	N/A
Premedicate:	Oral phenothiazine or $5\text{-}HT_3$ if nausea occurs
Administer:	**Tamoxifen** 20 mg PO daily for 5 years.

- Available in 10- and 20-mg tablets
- Monitor PT/INR closely in patients taking warfarin; increases PT/INR

Followed by letrozole 2.5 mg PO daily for 5 years

Major Side Effects

- GI Toxicities: Nausea and vomiting rarely observed.
- Tumor Flare: Usually occurs within the first 2 weeks of beginning of therapy. May observe increased bone pain, urinary retention, back pain with spinal cord compression and/or hypercalcemia.
- CV Toxicities: Deep vein thrombosis, pulmonary embolism, and superficial phlebitis are rare cardiovascular complications of tamoxifen therapy. Incidence of thromboembolic events may be increased when tamoxifen is given concomitantly with chemotherapy.
- Fluid/electrolyte Imbalance: Fluid retention and peripheral edema observed in about 30% of patients.
- Hormonal Effects: Menstrual irregularity, hot flashes, milk production in breasts, vaginal discharge, and bleeding. Usually not severe enough to discontinue therapy.
- Gynecological: Increased incidence of endometrial hyperplasia, polyps, and endometrial cancer.
- Sensory/perception Alteration: Headache, lethargy, and dizziness occur rarely. Visual disturbances, including cataract, retinopathy, and decreased visual acuity, have been described.
- Myelosuppression: Mild, transient leukopenia and thrombocytopenia occur rarely.
- Laboratory Values: Elevations in serum triglyceride levels.
- Reproductive: Pregnancy category D. Breast feeding should be avoided.

Initiate antiemetic protocol:	Mildly emetogenic protocol.
Treatment schedule:	No chair time. Daily dosing for 5 years followed by letrozole 2.5 mg PO daily for 5 years.
Estimated number of visits:	One visit every 2–3 months first year, then every 6–12 months remaining 4 years. Request 12 months worth of visits at a time.

Dose Calculation by: 1. _____ 2. _____

_____

Physician

_____

Date

_____

Patient Name

_____

ID Number

_____

Diagnosis

_____ / _____ / _____

Ht   Wt M^2

Letrozole (Second Five Years) (Femara)

Baseline laboratory tests:	CBC: Chemistry panel, LFTs, and CA 27-29
Baseline procedures or tests:	ER/PR testing (already done prior to starting tamoxifen)
Initiate IV:	N/A
Premedicate:	Oral phenothiazine or 5-HT$_3$ if nausea occurs
Administer:	**Letrozole** 2.5 mg PO daily

- Available as a 2.5-mg tablet for oral use.
- Food does not interfere with oral absorption.

Major Side Effects

- Musculoskeletal: Most common side effects. Musculoskeletal pain (back, arms, legs) and arthralgias.
- Hormonal: Hot flashes occur in approximately 6% of patients.
- CV Toxicities: Thromboembolic events are rare and less common than with megestrol acetate. Chest pain reported in some patients.
- GI Toxicities: Mild nausea with vomiting and anorexia occurring less frequently. Mild constipation or diarrhea can also occur.
- Hepatic: Mild elevation in serum transaminase and serum bilirubin levels. Most often seen in patients with known metastatic disease in the liver.
- CNS Toxicity: Headaches and fatigue are mild.
- Reproductive: Pregnancy category D. Breast feeding should be avoided.

Initiate antiemetic protocol:	Mildly emetogenic protocol.
Treatment schedule:	No chair time. Daily dosing for 5 years.
Estimated number of visits:	One visit every 6–12 months during treatment. Request 12 months worth of visits at a time.

Dose Calculation by: 1. _____   2. _____

_____   _____

Physician   Date

_____   _____

Patient Name   ID Number

_____   _____ / _____ / _____

Diagnosis   Ht   Wt   M^2

Tamoxifen + Exemestane

Tamoxifen (First 2–3 Years)

Baseline laboratory tests:	CBC: Chemistry, LFTs, and CA 27-29
Baseline procedures or tests:	ER/PR testing
Initiate IV:	N/A
Premedicate:	Oral phenothiazine or 5-HT$_3$ if nausea occurs
Administer:	**Tamoxifen** 20 mg PO daily

- Available in 10- and 20-mg tablets
- Monitor PT/INR closely in patients taking warfarin; increases PT/INR

Followed by exemestane 25 mg PO daily for remainder of 5 years.

Major Side Effects	• GI Toxicities: Nausea and vomiting rarely observed.

- Tumor Flare: Usually occurs within the first 2 weeks of beginning of therapy. May observe increased bone pain, urinary retention, back pain with spinal cord compression and/or hypercalcemia.
- CV Toxicities: Deep vein thrombosis, pulmonary embolism, and superficial phlebitis are rare cardiovascular complications of tamoxifen therapy. Incidence of thromboembolic events may be increased when tamoxifen is given concomitantly with chemotherapy.
- Fluid/electrolyte Imbalance: Fluid retention and peripheral edema observed in about 30% of patients.
- Hormonal Effects: Menstrual irregularity, hot flashes, milk production in breasts, vaginal discharge, and bleeding. Usually not severe enough to discontinue therapy.
- Gynecological: Increased incidence of endometrial hyperplasia, polyps, and endometrial cancer.
- Sensory/perception Alteration: Headache, lethargy, and dizziness occur rarely. Visual disturbances, including cataract, retinopathy, and decreased visual acuity, have been described.
- Myelosuppression: Mild, transient leukopenia and thrombocytopenia occur rarely.
- Laboratory Values: Elevations in serum triglyceride levels.
- Reproductive: Pregnancy category D. Breast feeding should be avoided.

Initiate antiemetic protocol:	Mildly emetogenic protocol.
Treatment schedule:	No chair time. Daily dosing for 2–3 years in ER + tumors, followed by exemestane 25 mg PO daily for remainder of 5 years.
Estimated number of visits:	One visit every 2–3 months first year, every 6–12 months thereafter. Request 12 months worth of visits at a time.

Dose Calculation by: 1. _____ 2. _____

Physician _____   Date _____

Patient Name _____   ID Number _____

Diagnosis _____   Ht _____ / Wt _____ / M^2 _____

Exemestane (Remainder of 5 years) (Aromasin)

Baseline laboratory tests:	CBC: Chemistry panel, LFTs, and CA 27-29
Baseline procedures or tests:	ER/PR testing (already done prior to tamoxifen)
Initiate IV:	N/A
Premedicate:	Oral phenothiazine or 5-HT$_3$ if nausea occurs
Administer:	**Exemestane** 25 mg PO daily

- Available as a 25-mg tablet for oral use.
- Take once daily after a meal.

Major Side Effects

- Hot Flashes: Hot flashes, increased sweating, and pain reported.
- GI Toxicities: Mild-to-moderate nausea, increased appetite, and weight gain reported.
- CNS Toxicity: Depression and insomnia occurred in 13% and 11%, respectively. Headache and fatigue also seen.
- Reproductive: Pregnancy category D. Breast feeding should be avoided.

Initiate antiemetic protocol:	Mildly emetogenic protocol.
Treatment schedule:	No chair time. Daily dosing for remainder of 5 years.
Estimated number of visits:	One visit every 6–12 months during treatment.

Dose Calculation by: 1. _____   2. _____

_____   _____
Physician   Date

_____   _____
Patient Name   ID Number

_____   _____/_____/_____
Diagnosis   Ht   Wt   M^2

METASTATIC BREAST CANCER

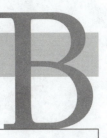

Combination Regimens

AC 79

Doxorubicin: 60 mg/m^2 IV on day 1
Cyclophosphamide: 600 mg/m^2 IV on day 1
Repeat cycle every 21 days.[36]

AT...80

Doxorubicin: 50 mg/m^2 IV on day 1
Paclitaxel: 150 mg/m^2 IV over 24 hours on day 1
Repeat cycle every 21 days.[51]
OR
Doxorubicin: 60 mg/m^2 IV on day 1
Repeat cycle every 21 days up to a maximum of eight cycles, followed by
Paclitaxel: 175 mg/m^2 IV on day 1
Repeat cycle every 21 days until disease progression.[51]
OR
Paclitaxel: 175 mg/m^2 IV on day 1
Repeat cycle every 21 days until disease progression, followed by
Doxorubicin: 60 mg/m^2 IV on day 1
Repeat cycle every 21 days up to a maximum of eight cycles.[51]

CAF...82

Cyclophosphamide: 600 mg/m^2 IV on day 1
Doxorubicin: 60 mg/m^2 IV on day 1
5-Fluorouracil: 600 mg/m^2 IV on day 1
Repeat cycle every 21 days.[40]

CEF 84

Cyclophosphamide: 75 mg/m^2/day PO on days 1–14
Epirubicin: 60 mg/m^2 IV on days 1 and 8
5-Fluorouracil: 500 mg/m^2 IV on days 1 and 8
Repeat cycle every 28 days.[52]

CMF (Bonadonna Regimen) 86

Cyclophosphamide: 100 mg/m^2/day PO on days 1–14
Methotrexate: 40 mg/m^2 IV on days 1 and 8
5-Fluorouracil: 500 mg/m^2 IV on days 1 and 8
Repeat cycle every 28 days.[42]

CMF (IV Bolus) 88

Cyclophosphamide: 600 mg/m^2 IV on day 1
Methotrexate: 40 mg/m^2 IV on day 1
5-Fluorouracil: 600 mg/m^2 IV on day 1
Repeat cycle every 21 days.[43]

Capecitabine + Docetaxel (XT) 90

Capecitabine: 1250 mg/m^2 PO bid on days 1–14
Docetaxel: 75 mg/m^2 IV on day 1
Repeat cycle every 21 days.[53]
May decrease dose of capecitabine to 850–1000 mg/m^2 PO bid on days 1–14 to reduce the risk of toxicity without compromising clinical efficacy.

Capecitabine + Paclitaxel (XP) 92

Capecitabine: 825 mg/m^2 PO bid on days 1–14
Paclitaxel: 175 mg/m^2 IV on day 1
Repeat cycle every 21 days.[54]

Capecitabine + Navelbine (XN) 93

Capecitabine: 1000 mg/m^2 PO bid on days 1–14
Navelbine: 25 mg/m^2 IV on days 1 and 8
Repeat cycle every 21 days.[54]

Docetaxel + Doxorubicin 94

Docetaxel: 75 mg/m^2 IV on day 1
Doxorubicin: 50 mg/m^2 IV on day 1
Repeat cycle every 21 days.[55]

FEC-100 95

5-Fluorouracil: 500 mg/m^2 IV on day 1
Epirubicin: 100 mg/m^2 IV on day 1
Cyclophosphamide: 500 mg/m^2 IV on day 1
Repeat cycle every 21 days.[56]

Paclitaxel + Vinorelbine 97

Paclitaxel: 135 mg/m^2 IV over 3 hours on day 1, starting 1 hour after vinorelbine

Vinorelbine: 30 mg/m^2 IV over 20 minutes on days 1 and 8

Repeat cycle every 28 days.[57]

Vinorelbine + Doxorubicin 98

Vinorelbine: 25 mg/m^2 IV on days 1 and 8

Doxorubicin: 50 mg/m^2 IV on day 1

Repeat cycle every 21 days.[58]

Trastuzumab + Paclitaxel 99

Trastuzumab: 4 mg/kg IV loading dose, then 2 mg/kg weekly

Paclitaxel: 175 mg/m^2 IV over 3 hours on day 1

Repeat cycle every 21 days.[59]

OR

Trastuzumab: 4 mg/kg IV loading dose, then 2 mg/kg weekly

Paclitaxel: 80 mg/m^2 IV weekly

Repeat cycle every 4 weeks.[60]

Trastuzumab + Docetaxel 101

Trastuzumab: 4 mg/kg IV loading dose, then 2 mg/kg IV on days 8 and 15

Docetaxel: 35 mg/m^2 IV on days 1, 8, and 15

The first cycle is administered weekly for 3 weeks, with 1 week rest. For subsequent cycles,

Trastuzumab: 2 mg/kg IV weekly

Docetaxel: 35 mg/m^2 IV weekly

Repeat cycle every 4 weeks.[61]

Gemcitabine + Paclitaxel 103

Gemcitabine: 1250 mg/m^2 IV on days 1 and 8

Paclitaxel: 175 mg/m^2 IV on day 1

Repeat cycle every 21 days.[62]

Carboplatin + Paclitaxel 104

Carboplatin: AUC of 6, IV on day 1

Paclitaxel: 200 mg/m^2 over 3 hours IV on day 1

Repeat cycle every 21 days.[63]

Carboplatin + Docetaxel..**105**

Carboplatin: AUC of 6, IV on day 1
Docetaxel: 75 mg/m^2 IV on day 1
Repeat cycle every 21 days.[64]

Mitomycin + Vinblastine **106**

Mitomycin: 20 mg/m^2 IV on day 1
Vinblastine: 1.4–2 mg/m^2 IV continuous infusion on days 1–5
Repeat cycle every 6–8 weeks.[65]

Single-Agent Regimens

Tamoxifen (Nolvadex) **107**

Tamoxifen: 20 mg PO daily[66]

Toremifene Citrate (Fareston) **108**

Toremifene: 60 mg PO daily[67]

Exemestane (Aromasin) **109**

Exemestane: 25 mg PO daily[68]

Anastrozole (Arimidex) **110**

Anastrozole: 1 mg PO daily[69]

Letrozole (Femara) **111**

Letrozole: 2.5 mg PO daily[70]

Fulvestrant (Faslodex) **112**

Fulvestrant: 250 mg IM on day 1
Repeat injection every month.[71]

Megestrol (Megace) **113**

Megestrol: 40 mg PO qid[72]

Trastuzumab (Herceptin) **114**

Trastuzumab: 4 mg/kg IV loading dose, then 2 mg/kg IV weekly

Repeat cycle weekly for a total of 10 weeks. In the absence of disease
  progression, continue weekly maintenance dose of 2 mg/kg.[73]

OR

Trastuzumab (Herceptin) **115**

Trastuzumab: 8 mg/kg IV loading dose, then 6 mg/kg IV every 3 weeks
  until disease progression.[73a]

Capecitabine **116**

Capecitabine: 1250 mg/m^2 PO bid for 2 weeks, followed by 1 week rest
  period

Repeat cycle every 21 days.[74] May decrease dose to 850–1000 mg/m^2 PO
  bid on days 1–14 to reduce the risk of toxicity without compromising
  clinical efficacy.

Docetaxel **117**

Docetaxel: 100 mg/m^2 IV on day 1

Repeat cycle every 21 days.[75]

OR

Docetaxel: 35–40 mg/m^2 IV weekly for 6 weeks

Repeat cycle every 8 weeks.[76]

Paclitaxel **118**

Paclitaxel: 175 mg/m^2 IV over 3 hours on day 1

Repeat cycle every 21 days.[77]

OR

Paclitaxel: 80–100 mg/m^2 IV weekly for 3 weeks

Repeat cycle every 4 weeks.[78]

Vinorelbine **119**

Vinorelbine: 30 mg/m^2 IV on day 1

Repeat cycle every 7 days.[79]

Doxorubicin **120**

Doxorubicin: 20 mg/m^2 IV on day 1

Repeat cycle every 7 days.[80]

Gemcitabine **121**

Gemcitabine: 725 mg/m^2 IV weekly for 3 weeks
Repeat cycle every 28 days.[81]

Liposomal Doxorubicin (Doxil) **122**

Liposomal doxorubicin: 45–60 mg/m^2 IV on day 1
Repeat cycle every 21–28 days.[82]

Paclitaxel Protein-bound Particles for Injectable Suspension (Abraxane) **123**

Paclitaxel protein-bound particles for injectable suspension: 260mg/m^2 IV day 1.

Repeat cycle every 3 weeks.[83]

OR

Paclitaxel protein-bound particles for injectable suspension: 100 mg/m^2 IV weekly for 3 weeks or weekly.

Repeat cycle every 4 weeks or weekly.[84]

Combination Regimens

Doxorubicin + Cyclophosphamide (AC)

Baseline laboratory tests:	CBC: Chemistry, LFTs, and CA 27-29
Baseline procedures or tests:	MUGA scan
Initiate IV:	0.9% sodium chloride
Premedicate:	5-HT$_3$ and dexamethasone 20 mg in 100 cc of NS.
Administer:	**Doxorubicin** _____ mg (60 mg/m^2) IV on day 1

- **Potent vesicant**
- Available as a 2-mg/mL solution.
- Doxorubicin will form a precipitate if it is mixed with heparin or 5-FU.

Cyclophosphamide _____ mg (600 mg/m^2) IV on day 1

- Available in 100-, 200-, 500-, 1000-, and 2000-mg vials
- Dilute with sterile water and shake well to ensure that solution is completely dissolved.
- Reconstituted solution stable for 24 hours at room temperature, and 6 days refrigerated.

Major Side Effects

- Hypersensitivity Reaction: Cyclophosphamide can cause rhinitis and irritation of nose and throat.
- Bone Marrow Depression: Leukopenia, thrombocytopenia, and anemia; may be severe.
- GI Toxicities: Nausea and vomiting are moderate to severe and can be acute or delayed. Stomatitis and diarrhea occur in some patients but is not dose limiting.
- Cardiac: Acutely, pericarditis-myocarditis syndrome may occur. With high cumulative doses > 550 mg/m^2 of doxorubicin, cardiomyopathy may occur. Cyclophosphamide may increase the risk of doxorubicin-induced cardiotoxicity.
- Hepatic: Use with caution in patients with abnormal liver function. Dose reduction is required in the presence of liver dysfunction.
- Bladder Toxicities: Hemorrhagic cystitis, dysuria, and urinary frequency with cyclophosphamide. Red-orange discoloration of urine; resolves by 24–48 hours.
- Inappropriate secretion of antidiuretic hormone (SIADH).
- Skin: Extravasation of doxorubicin causes severe tissue destruction. Hyperpigmentation, photosensitivity, and radiation recall occur. Complete alopecia.
- Secondary Malignancies: Increased risk with cyclophosphamide.
- Reproductive: Amenorrhea with ovarian failure. Sterility may be permanent. Pregnancy category D. Breast feeding should be avoided.

Initiate antiemetic protocol:	Moderately to highly emetogenic protocol.
Supportive drugs:	☐ pegfilgrastim (Neulasta) ☐ filgrastim (Neupogen)
	☐ epoetin alfa (Procrit) ☐ darbepoetin alfa (Aranesp)
Treatment schedule:	Chair time 2 hours on day 1. Repeat cycle every 21 days until progression of disease.
Estimated number of visits:	Two visits per cycle. Request four cycles worth of visits.

Dose Calculation by: 1. _____ 2. _____

_____

Physician   Date

_____

Patient Name   ID Number

_____

Diagnosis   Ht _____ / Wt _____ / M^2 _____

Doxorubicin + Paclitaxel (AT)

Baseline laboratory tests:	CBC: Chemistry and CA 27-29
Baseline procedures or tests:	Central line placement for continuous infusion and MUGA scan
Initiate IV:	0.9% sodium chloride
Premedicate:	5-HT$_3$ and dexamethasone 10–20 mg in 100 cc of NS
	Diphenhydramine 25–50 mg and cimetidine 300 mg in 100 cc of NS

Administer:

Doxorubicin _____ mg (50 mg/m^2) IV on day 1

Paclitaxel _____ mg (150 mg/m^2) IV over 24 hours on day 1

Repeat cycle every 21 days.

OR

Doxorubicin _____ mg (60 mg/m^2) IV on day 1

Repeat cycle every 21 days up to a maximum of eight cycles, followed by

Paclitaxel _____ mg (175 mg/m^2) IV on day 1

Repeat cycle every 21 days until disease progression.

OR

Paclitaxel _____ mg (175 mg/m^2) IV on day 1

- Available in solution as 6 mg/mL.
- Final concentration is $\leq$ 1.2 mg/mL
- Stable for up to 27 hours at room temperature in 0.3–1.2 mg/mL solutions.
- **Use non-PVC containers and tubing with 0.22-micron inline filter for administration.**

Repeat cycle every 21 days until disease progression, followed by

Doxorubicin _____ mg (60 mg/m^2) IV on day 1

- **Potent vesicant**
- Available as a 2-mg/mL solution.
- Doxorubicin will form precipitate if it is mixed with heparin or 5-FU.

Repeat cycle every 21 days up to a maximum of eight cycles.

Major Side Effects

- Hypersensitivity Reaction: Occurs in 20%–40% of patients receiving paclitaxel. Characterized by generalized skin rash, flushing, erythema, hypotension, dyspnea, and/or bronchospasm. Usually occurs within the first 2–3 minutes of infusion and almost always within the first 10 minutes. Premedicate as described.
- Bone Marrow Depression: Dose-limiting neutropenia. Use G-CSF support. Thrombocytopenia and anemia also seen.
- GI Toxicities: Nausea and vomiting are mild to moderate. Stomatitis can occur but is not dose limiting.
- Hepatic: Use with caution in patients with impaired liver function, dose reduct.
- Cardiotoxicities: Acutely, pericarditis-myocarditis. Later, cardiomyopathy.
- Neurotoxicity: Sensory neuropathy with numbness/paresthesias; dose related and dose limiting.
- Bladder Toxicities: Red-orange discoloration of urine; resolves by 24–48 hours.
- Skin: Extravasation of doxorubicin causes severe tissue destruction. Hyperpigmentation, photosensitivity, and radiation recall occur. Alopecia.
- Reproductive: Amenorrhea with ovarian failure. Sterility may be permanent. Pregnancy category D. Breast feeding should be avoided.

Initiate antiemetic protocol:	Mildly to moderately emetogenic protocol.
Supportive drugs:	☐ pegfilgrastim (Neulasta) ☐ filgrastim (Neupogen)
	☐ epoetin alfa (Procrit) ☐ darbepoetin alfa (Aranesp)
Treatment schedule:	Chair time: **1.** 1 hour on day 1; repeat every 21 days. **2.** 1 hour on day 1; repeat every 21 days up to maximum of 8. Then 4 hours on day 1; repeat every 21 days until disease progression. **3.** 4 hours on day 1; repeat every 21 days until disease progression, then chair time 1 hour on day 1, repeated every 21 days up to a maximum of eight cycles.

Estimated number of visits: 1. Two visits per cycle. Request four cycles worth of visits. 2. Two visits per cycle. Request eight cycles worth of visits. 3. Two visits per cycle. Request eight cycles worth of visits.

Dose Calculation by: 1. _____   2. _____

_____   _____
Physician   Date

_____   _____
Patient Name   ID Number

_____/_____/_____
Diagnosis   Ht   Wt   M²

Cyclophosphamide + Doxorubicin + 5-Flourouracil (CAF)

Baseline laboratory tests:	CBC: Chemistry, LFTs, and CA 27-29
Baseline procedures or tests:	MUGA scan
Initiate IV:	0.9% sodium chloride
Premedicate:	5-HT$_3$ and dexamethasone 20 mg in 100 cc of NS.
Administer:	**Cyclophosphamide** _____ mg (600 mg/m^2) IV on day 1

- Available in 100-, 200-, 500-, 1000-, and 2000-mg vials
- Dilute with sterile water and shake well to ensure that solution is completely dissolved.
- Reconstituted solution stable for 24 hours at room temperature, and 6 days refrigerated

Doxorubicin _____ mg (60 mg/m^2) IV on day 1

- Potent vesicant
- Available as a 2-mg/mL solution.
- Doxorubicin will form a precipitate if it is mixed with heparin or 5-FU.

5-Flourouracil _____ mg (600 mg/m^2) IV on day 1

- Available in solution as 50 mg/mL.
- No dilution required.
- May further dilute with NS or D5W.

Major Side Effects

- Hypersensitivity Reaction: Cyclophosphamide can cause rhinitis and irritation of nose and throat.
- Bone Marrow Depression: Leukopenia, thrombocytopenia, and anemia; may be severe.
- GI Toxicities: Nausea and vomiting are moderate to severe and can be acute or delayed. Stomatitis and diarrhea can be severe and dose limiting.
- Cardiac: Acutely, pericarditis-myocarditis syndrome may occur. With high cumulative doses > 550 mg/m^2 of doxorubicin, cardiomyopathy may occur. Cyclophosphamide may increase the risk of doxorubicin-induced cardiotoxicity.
- Hepatic: Use with caution in patients with abnormal liver function. Dose reduction of doxorubicin is required in the presence of liver dysfunction.
- Bladder Toxicities: Hemorrhagic cystitis, dysuria, and urinary frequency. Red-orange discoloration of urine; resolves by 24–48 hours.
- Inappropriate secretion of antidiuretic hormone (SIADH).
- Skin: Extravasation of doxorubicin causes severe tissue destruction. Hyperpigmentation, photosensitivity, nail changes, and radiation recall occur. Complete alopecia. Hand-foot syndrome can be dose limiting.
- Ocular: Photophobia, increased lacrimation, acute and chronic conjunctivitis, blepharitis, and blurred vision.
- Secondary Malignancies: Increased risk with cyclophosphamide.
- Reproductive: Amenorrhea with ovarian failure. Sterility may be permanent. Pregnancy category D. Breast feeding should be avoided.

Initiate antiemetic protocol:	Moderately to highly emetogenic protocol.
Supportive drugs:	☐ pegfilgrastim (Neulasta) ☐ filgrastim (Neupogen)
	☐ epoetin alfa (Procrit) ☐ darbepoetin alfa (Aranesp)
Treatment schedule:	Chair time 2 hours on day 1. Repeat cycle every 21 days until disease progression.
Estimated number of visits:	Two visits per cycle. Request six cycles worth of visits.

Dose Calculation by: 1. _____   2. _____

_____
Physician

_____
Date

_____
Patient Name

_____
ID Number

_____
Diagnosis

_____/_____/_____
Ht   Wt   M^2

Cyclophosphamide + Epirubicin + 5-Fluorouracil (CEF)

Baseline laboratory tests:	CBC: Chemistry, LFTs, and CA 27-29
Baseline procedures or tests:	MUGA scan
Initiate IV:	0.9% sodium chloride
Premedicate:	5-HT$_3$ and dexamethasone 20 mg in 100 cc of NS.
	Oral 5-HT$_3$ or phenothiazine before taking cyclophosphamide days 2–7 and 9–14
Administer:	**Cyclophosphamide** _____mg (75 mg/m^2/day) PO days 1–14

- Available in 25- and 50-mg tablets
- Administer in morning or early afternoon to allow adequate excretion time.
- Administer with meals.

Epirubicin _____mg (60 mg/m^2) IV on days 1 and 8

- **Vesicant**
- Drug is provided as a preservative-free solution (2 mg/mL)
- Use within 24 hours of penetration of rubber stopper; discard unused portion.
- Store unopened vials in refrigerator.

5-Flourouracil _____mg (500 mg/m^2) IV on days 1 and 8

- Available in solution as 50 mg/mL.
- No dilution required.
- May further dilute with NS or D5W.

Major Side Effects	

- Hypersensitivity Reaction: Cyclophosphamide can cause rhinitis and irritation of nose and throat.
- Bone Marrow Depression: Leukopenia, thrombocytopenia, and anemia all seen; may be severe.
- GI Toxicities: Nausea and vomiting are moderate to severe. Mucositis and diarrhea can be severe and dose limiting.
- Cardiac: Cardiotoxicity is dose related, is cumulative, and may occur during months to years after cessation of therapy. Cyclophosphamide may increase the risk of cardiotoxicity.
- Hepatic: Use with caution in patients with abnormal liver function. Dose reduction is required in the presence of liver dysfunction.
- Bladder Toxicities: Hemorrhagic cystitis, dysuria, and urinary frequency. Red-orange discoloration of urine; resolves by 24–48 hours.
- Skin: Extravasation of epirubicin causes severe tissue destruction. Epirubicin may cause "flare" reaction or streaking along vein during peripheral administration. If occurs, slow drug administration time and flush more. Hyperpigmentation, photosensitivity, nail changes, and radiation recall occur. Complete alopecia. Hand-foot syndrome can be dose limiting.
- Inappropriate secretion of antidiuretic hormone (SIADH).
- Ocular: Photophobia, increased lacrimation, acute and chronic conjunctivitis, blepharitis, and blurred vision.
- Secondary Malignancies: Increased risk with cyclophosphamide.
- Reproductive: Amenorrhea with ovarian failure. Sterility may be permanent. Pregnancy category D. Breast feeding should be avoided.

Initiate antiemetic protocol:	Moderately to highly emetogenic protocol.
Supportive drugs:	☐ pegfilgrastim (Neulasta) ☐ filgrastim (Neupogen)
	☐ epoetin alfa (Procrit) ☐ darbepoetin alfa (Aranesp)
Treatment schedule:	Chair time 1 hour on days 1 and 8. Repeat cycle every 28 days.
Estimated number of visits:	Three visits per cycle. Request four cycles worth of visits.

Dose Calculation by: 1. _____   2. _____

_____
Physician   Date

_____
Patient Name   ID Number

_____
Diagnosis   Ht   Wt   M²

Cyclophosphamide + Epirubicin + 5-Fluorouracil (CEF)

Baseline laboratory tests:	CBC: Chemistry, LFTs, and CA 27-29
Baseline procedures or tests:	MUGA scan
Initiate IV:	0.9% sodium chloride
Premedicate:	5-HT$_3$ and dexamethasone 20 mg in 100 cc of NS.
	Oral 5-HT$_3$ or phenothiazine before taking cyclophosphamide days 2–7 and 9–14
Administer:	**Cyclophosphamide** _____ mg (75 mg/m^2/day) PO days 1–14

- Available in 25- and 50-mg tablets
- Administer in morning or early afternoon to allow adequate excretion time.
- Administer with meals.

Epirubicin _____ mg (60 mg/m^2) IV on days 1 and 8

- **Vesicant**
- Drug is provided as a preservative-free solution (2 mg/mL)
- Use within 24 hours of penetration of rubber stopper; discard unused portion.
- Store unopened vials in refrigerator.

5-Flourouracil _____ mg (500 mg/m^2) IV on days 1 and 8

- Available in solution as 50 mg/mL.
- No dilution required.
- May further dilute with NS or D5W.

Major Side Effects

- Hypersensitivity Reaction: Cyclophosphamide can cause rhinitis and irritation of nose and throat.
- Bone Marrow Depression: Leukopenia, thrombocytopenia, and anemia all seen; may be severe.
- GI Toxicities: Nausea and vomiting are moderate to severe. Mucositis and diarrhea can be severe and dose limiting.
- Cardiac: Cardiotoxicity is dose related, is cumulative, and may occur during months to years after cessation of therapy. Cyclophosphamide may increase the risk of cardiotoxicity.
- Hepatic: Use with caution in patients with abnormal liver function. Dose reduction is required in the presence of liver dysfunction.
- Bladder Toxicities: Hemorrhagic cystitis, dysuria, and urinary frequency. Red-orange discoloration of urine; resolves by 24–48 hours.
- Skin: Extravasation of epirubicin causes severe tissue destruction. Epirubicin may cause "flare" reaction or streaking along vein during peripheral administration. If occurs, slow drug administration time and flush more. Hyperpigmentation, photosensitivity, nail changes, and radiation recall occur. Complete alopecia. Hand-foot syndrome can be dose limiting.
- Inappropriate secretion of antidiuretic hormone (SIADH).
- Ocular: Photophobia, increased lacrimation, acute and chronic conjunctivitis, blepharitis, and blurred vision.
- Secondary Malignancies: Increased risk with cyclophosphamide.
- Reproductive: Amenorrhea with ovarian failure. Sterility may be permanent. Pregnancy category D. Breast feeding should be avoided.

Initiate antiemetic protocol:	Moderately to highly emetogenic protocol.
Supportive drugs:	☐ pegfilgrastim (Neulasta) ☐ filgrastim (Neupogen)
	☐ epoetin alfa (Procrit) ☐ darbepoetin alfa (Aranesp)
Treatment schedule:	Chair time 1 hour on days 1 and 8. Repeat cycle every 28 days.
Estimated number of visits:	Three visits per cycle. Request four cycles worth of visits.

Dose Calculation by: 1. _____   2. _____

_____

Physician

_____

Patient Name

_____

Diagnosis

_____

Date

_____

ID Number

_____ / _____ / _____

Ht   Wt   M²

Cyclophosphamide + Methotrexate + 5-Flourouracil (CMF-Bonadonna Regimen)

Baseline laboratory tests:	CBC: Chemistry, LFTs, and CA 27-29
Baseline procedures or tests:	None
Initiate IV:	0.9% sodium chloride
Premedicate:	5-HT$_3$ and dexamethasone 20 mg in 100 cc of NS on days 1 and 8
	Oral 5-HT$_3$ or phenothiazine days 2–7 and 9–14

Administer:

Cyclophosphamide _____mg (100 mg/m^2/day) PO on days 1–14

- Available in 25- and 50-mg tablets
- Administer in morning or early afternoon to allow adequate excretion time.
- Administer with meals.

Methotrexate _____mg (40 mg/m^2) IV on days 1 and 8

- Available in 50-, 100-, 200-, and 1000-mg single-use reconstituted vials
- May dilute further in NS
- Reconstituted solution is stable for 24 hours at room temperature.

5-Flourouracil _____mg (500 mg/m^2) IV on days 1 and 8

- Available in solution as 50 mg/mL.
- No dilution required.
- Can be further diluted with NS or D5W.

Major Side Effects

- Hypersensitivity Reaction: Cyclophosphamide can cause rhinitis and irritation of nose and throat.
- Bone Marrow Depression: Leukopenia can be severe, thrombocytopenia is less frequent, and anemia is mild.
- GI Toxicities: Nausea and vomiting are moderate to severe and occur within 24 hours of administration. Mucositis and diarrhea can be severe; dose dependent.
- Renal: Acute renal failure, azotemia, urinary retention, and uric acid nephropathy have been observed with methotrexate.
- Hepatic: Hepatotoxicity is rare.
- Pulmonary Toxicity: Rare; onset is insidious (fever, cough) and appears as interstitial pneumonitis, which may progress to fibrosis. May respond to steroids.
- Bladder Toxicities: Hemorrhagic cystitis, dysuria, and urinary frequency with cyclophosphamide.
- Hormonal: SIADH.
- Ocular: Photophobia, increased lacrimation, acute and chronic conjunctivitis, blepharitis, and blurred vision.
- Skin: Complete alopecia in 50% of patients, diffuse thinning in others. Hyperpigmentation of nails and skin, banding of nails, and radiation recall may occur. Photosensitivity, sunburn-like rash. Hand-foot syndrome can be dose limiting.
- Secondary Malignancies: Increased risk with cyclophosphamide.
- Reproductive: Amenorrhea with ovarian failure. Sterility may be permanent. Pregnancy category D. Breast feeding should be avoided.

Initiate antiemetic protocol:	Moderately to highly emetogenic protocol.
Supportive drugs:	☐ pegfilgrastim (Neulasta) ☐ filgrastim (Neupogen)
	☐ epoetin alfa (Procrit) ☐ darbepoetin alfa (Aranesp)
Treatment schedule:	Chair time 1 hour on days 1 and 8. Repeat cycle every 28 days until disease progression.
Estimated number of visits:	Three visits per cycle. Request six cycles worth of visits.

Dose Calculation by: 1. _____ 2. _____

_____

Physician   Date

_____

Patient Name   ID Number

_____   ____/____ ____/____ _____

Diagnosis   Ht   Wt   M²

Cyclophosphamide + Methotrexate + 5-Flourouracil (IV Bolus)

Baseline laboratory tests:	CBC: Chemistry, LFTs, and CA 27-29
Baseline procedures or tests:	None
Initiate IV:	0.9% sodium chloride
Premedicate:	5-HT$_3$ and dexamethasone 20 mg in 100 cc of NS.
Administer:	**Cyclophosphamide** _____mg (600 mg/m^2) IV on day 1

- Available in 100-, 200-, 500-, 1000-, and 2000-mg vials.
- Dilute with sterile water and shake well to ensure that solution is completely dissolved.
- Reconstituted solution stable for 24 hours at room temperature, and 6 days refrigerated.

Methotrexate _____mg (40 mg/m^2) IV on day 1

- Available in 50-, 100-, 200-, and 1000-mg single-use reconstituted vials.
- May dilute further in NS.
- Reconstituted solution is stable for 24 hours at room temperature.

5-Flourouracil _____mg (600 mg/m^2) IV on day 1

- Available in solution as 50 mg/mL.
- No dilution required.
- Can be further diluted with NS or D5W.

Major Side Effects

- Hypersensitivity Reaction: Cyclophosphamide can cause rhinitis and irritation of nose and throat.
- Bone Marrow Depression: Leukopenia can be severe, thrombocytopenia is less frequent, and anemia is mild.
- GI Toxicities: Nausea and vomiting are moderate to severe and occur within 24 hours of administration. Mucositis and diarrhea can be severe; dose dependent.
- Renal: Acute renal failure, azotemia, urinary retention, and uric acid nephropathy have been observed with methotrexate.
- Hepatic: Hepatotoxicity is rare.
- Pulmonary Toxicity: Rare; onset is insidious (fever, cough) and appears as interstitial pneumonitis, which may progress to fibrosis. May respond to steroids.
- Bladder Toxicities: Hemorrhagic cystitis, dysuria, and urinary frequency with cyclophosphamide.
- Hormonal: SIADH.
- Ocular: Photophobia, increased lacrimation, acute and chronic conjunctivitis, blepharitis, and blurred vision.
- Skin: Complete alopecia in 50% of patients, diffuse thinning in others. Hyperpigmentation of nails and skin, banding of nails, and radiation recall may occur. Photosensitivity, sunburn-like rash. Hand-foot syndrome, can be dose limiting.
- Secondary Malignancies: Increased risk with cyclophosphamide.
- Reproductive: Amenorrhea with ovarian failure. Sterility may be permanent. Pregnancy category D. Breast feeding should be avoided.

Initiate antiemetic protocol:	Moderately to highly emetogenic protocol.
Supportive drugs:	☐ pegfilgrastim (Neulasta) ☐ filgrastim (Neupogen)
	☐ epoetin alfa (Procrit) ☐ darbepoetin alfa (Aranesp)
Treatment schedule:	Chair time 2 hours on day 1. Repeat cycle every 21 days until disease progression.
Estimated number of visits:	Two visits per cycle. Request six cycles worth of visits.

Dose Calculation by: 1. _____ 2. _____

_____

Physician   Date

_____   _____

Patient Name   ID Number

_____   _____/_____/_____

Diagnosis   Ht   Wt   M²

Capecitabine + Docetaxel (XT)

Baseline laboratory tests:	CBC: Chemistry, bilirubin, LFTs, creatinine clearance, and CA 27-29
Baseline procedures or tests:	N/A
Initiate IV:	Normal saline.
Premedicate:	Dexamethasone 8 mg bid for 3 days, starting the day before treatment
	Oral phenothiazine or 5-HT$_3$

Administer:

Capecitabine _____mg (1250 mg/m^2) PO bid on days 1–14

- May decrease dose to 850–1000 mg/m^2 PO bid on days 1–14 to reduce the risk of toxicity without compromising efficacy.
- Available in 150- and 500-mg tablets.
- Administer within 30 minutes of a meal with plenty of water.
- Monitor international normalized ratios (INRs) closely in patients taking warfarin; may increase INR.

Docetaxel _____mg (75 mg/m^2) IV on day 1

- Available in 20- or 80-mg packs with own diluent. Do not shake.
- Reconstituted vials stable at room temperature or refrigerated for 8 hours.
- Further dilute in 250 cc of D5W or NS.
- **Use non-PVC containers and tubing to administer.**

Major Side Effects

- Hypersensitivity Reactions: Severe hypersensitivity reactions with docetaxel in 2%–3% of patients. Premedication with dexamethasone recommended.
- Bone Marrow Depression: Neutropenia is dose limiting. Thrombocytopenia and anemia also occur.
- GI Toxicities: Nausea and vomiting are usually mild to moderate. Diarrhea is common, can be severe. Stomatitis is common, can be severe.
- Neuropathy: Peripheral neuropathy with sensory alterations are paresthesias in a glove and stocking distribution, and numbness.
- Fluid Balance: Fluid retention syndrome: weight gain, peripheral and/or generalized edema, pleural effusion, and ascites. Premedication with dexamethasone effective in preventing or minimizing occurrences.
- Renal Insufficiency: Capecitabine is contraindicated in patients with baseline creatinine clearance < 30 mL/min. A dose reduction to 75% of capecitabine should be made with baseline creatinine clearance of 30–50 mL/min.
- Skin: Hand-foot syndrome (palmar-plantar erythrodysesthesia) characterized by tingling, numbness, pain, erythema, dryness, rash, swelling, increased pigmentation, and/or pruritus of the hands and feet. Less frequent in reduced doses. Nail changes, rash, dry, pruritic skin seen. Alopecia common.
- Ocular: Blepharitis, tear-duct stenosis, acute and chronic conjunctivitis.
- Hepatic: Elevations in serum bilirubin, alkaline phosphatase, and hepatic transaminase (aspartate transaminase, alanine transaminase) levels. Dose modifications may be required if hyperbilirubinemia occurs.
- Reproductive: Pregnancy category D. Breast feeding should be avoided.

Initiate antiemetic protocol:	Mildly to moderately emetogenic protocol.

Supportive drugs:

☐ pegfilgrastim (Neulasta)   ☐ filgrastim (Neupogen)

☐ epoetin alfa (Procrit)   ☐ darbepoetin alfa (Aranesp)

☐ loperamide (Imodium)   ☐ diphenoxylate/atropine sulfate (Lomotil)

Treatment schedule:	Chair time 2 hours on day 1. Repeat cycle every 21 days until disease progression.
Estimated number of visits:	Two visits per cycle. Request four cycles worth of visits.

Dose Calculation by: 1. _____ 2. _____

_____

Physician

_____

Patient Name

_____

Diagnosis

_____

Date

_____

ID Number

_____ / _____ / _____

Ht   Wt   M^2

Capecitabine + Paclitaxel (XP)

Baseline laboratory tests: CBC: Chemistry, bilirubin, LFTs, creatinine clearance, and CA 27-29

Baseline procedures or tests: N/A

Initiate IV: 0.9% sodium chloride

Premedicate: 5-HT$_3$ and dexamethasone 10–20 mg in 100 cc of NS

Diphenhydramine 25–50 mg and cimetidine 300 mg in 100 cc of NS

Oral phenothiazine or 5-HT$_3$ before capecitabine on days 2–14

Administer: **Capecitabine** _____mg (825 mg/m^2) PO bid on days 1–14

- Available in 150- and 500-mg tablets.
- Administer within 30 minutes of a meal with plenty of water.
- Monitor INRs closely in patients taking warfarin; may increase INR.

Paclitaxel _____mg (175 mg/m^2) IV over 3 hours on day 1

- Available in solution as 6 mg/mL.
- Final concentration is $\leq$ 1.2 mg/mL.
- Stable for up to 27 hours at room temperature in 0.3–1.2 solutions.
- **Use non-PVC containers and tubing with 0.22-micron inline filter for administration.**

Major Side Effects

- Hypersensitivity Reaction: Occurs in 20%–40% of patients. Characterized by generalized skin rash, flushing, erythema, hypotension, dyspnea, and/or bronchospasm. Usually occurs within the first 2–3 minutes of paclitaxel infusion and almost always within the first 10 minutes. Premedicate as described.
- GI Toxicities: Nausea and vomiting, usually mild to moderate and of short duration. Diarrhea and stomatitis can be severe.
- Hepatic: Elevations in serum bilirubin, alkaline phosphatase, and hepatic transaminase levels. Dose modifications may be required for hyperbilirubinemia.
- Renal Insufficiency: Capecitabine is contraindicated in patients with baseline creatinine clearance < 30 mL/min. A dose reduction to 75% of capecitabine should be made with baseline creatinine clearance of 30–50 mL/min.
- Skin: Hand-foot syndrome (palmar-plantar erythrodysesthesia) characterized by tingling, numbness, pain, erythema, dryness, rash, swelling, increased pigmentation, and/or pruritus of the hands and feet.
- Bone Marrow Depression: Dose-limiting neutropenia. Use G-CSF support.
- Neurotoxicity: Sensory neuropathy with numbness and paresthesias; dose related. More frequent with longer paclitaxel infusions and at doses > 175 mg/m^2.
- Ocular: Blepharitis, tear-duct stenosis, acute and chronic conjunctivitis.
- Alopecia: Loss of total body hair occurs in nearly all patients.
- Reproductive: Pregnancy category D. Breast feeding should be avoided.

Initiate antiemetic protocol: Mildly emetogenic protocol.

Supportive drugs: ☐ pegfilgrastim (Neulasta)   ☐ filgrastim (Neupogen)

☐ epoetin alfa (Procrit)   ☐ darbepoetin alfa (Aranesp)

Treatment schedule: Chair time 4 hours on day 1. Repeat every 21 days as tolerated or until disease progression.

Estimated number of visits: Two visits per cycle. Request three cycles worth of visits.

Dose Calculation by: 1. _____ 2. _____

_____
Physician

_____
Patient Name

_____
Diagnosis

_____
Date

_____
ID Number

_____/ _____/ _____
Ht   Wt   M^2

Capecitabine + Navelbine (XN)

Baseline laboratory tests:	CBC: Chemistry, bilirubin, LFTs, creatinine clearance, and CA 27-29
Baseline procedures or tests:	N/A
Initiate IV:	0.9% sodium chloride
Premedicate:	Oral phenothiazine or 5-HT$_3$
Administer:	**Capecitabine** _____ mg (1000 mg/m^2) PO bid on days 1–14

- Available in 150- or 500-mg tablets
- Administer within 30 minutes of a meal with plenty of water.
- Monitor INRs closely in patients taking warfarin; may increase INR.

Navelbine _____ mg (25 mg/m^2) IV on days 1 and 8

- Vesicant
- Available in 1- or 5-mL single-use vials at a concentration of 10 mg/mL.
- Further dilute in syringe or IV bag to concentration of 1.5–3.0 mg/mL.
- Reconstituted solution is stable for 24 hours refrigerated.

Major Side Effects

- Hypersensitivity Reaction: Cyclophosphamide can cause rhinitis and irritation of nose and throat.
- Bone Marrow Depression: Leukopenia is dose-limiting toxicity. Nadir at 7–10 days. Severe thrombocytopenia and anemia are uncommon.
- GI Toxicities: Nausea and vomiting are mild to moderate. Stomatitis and diarrhea can be severe.
- Hepatic: Elevations in LFT results. Dose modifications may be required if hyperbilirubinemia occurs.
- Renal Insufficiency: Capecitabine is contraindicated in patients with baseline creatinine clearance < 30 mL/min. A dose reduction to 75% of capecitabine should be made with baseline creatinine clearance of 30–50 mL/min.
- Hormonal: SIADH.
- Skin: Extravasation of vinorelbine may cause local tissue injury and inflammation. Hand-foot syndrome can be dose limiting. Alopecia observed in some patients.
- Neurotoxicity: Usually mild and occurs much less frequently than with other vinca alkaloids.
- Ocular: Blepharitis, tear-duct stenosis, acute and chronic conjunctivitis.
- Reproductive: Pregnancy category D. Breast feeding should be avoided.

Initiate antiemetic protocol:	Mildly to moderately emetogenic protocol.
Supportive drugs:	☐ pegfilgrastim (Neulasta) ☐ filgrastim (Neupogen)
	☐ epoetin alfa (Procrit) ☐ darbepoetin alfa (Aranesp)
Treatment schedule:	Chair time 1 hour on days 1 and 8. Repeat cycle every 21 days until disease progression.
Estimated number of visits:	Three visits per cycle. Request four cycles worth of visits.

Dose Calculation by: 1. _____   2. _____

_____
Physician

_____
Patient Name

_____
Diagnosis

_____
Date

_____
ID Number

_____ / _____ / _____
Ht   Wt   M^2

Docetaxel + Doxorubicin

Baseline laboratory tests: CBC: Chemistry and CA 27-29

Baseline procedures or tests: MUGA scan

Initiate IV: 0.9% sodium chloride

Premedicate: Dexamethasone 8 mg bid for 3 days, starting the day before treatment

HT$_3$ and dexamethasone 10–20 mg in 100 cc of NS

Diphenhydramine 25–50 mg and cimetidine 300 mg in 100 cc of NS

Administer: **Docetaxel** _____mg (75 mg/m^2) IV on day 1

- Comes in 20- or 80-mg packs with own diluent. Do not shake.
- Reconstituted vials stable at room temperature or for 8 hours refrigerated.
- Further dilute in 250 cc of D5W or NS.
- **Use non-PVC containers and tubing to administer.**

Doxorubicin _____mg (50 mg/m^2) IV on day 1

- **Potent vesicant**
- Available as a 2-mg/mL solution.
- Doxorubicin will form a precipitate if it is mixed with heparin or 5-FU.

Major Side Effects
- Hypersensitivity Reaction: Severe hypersensitivity reactions with docetaxel in 2%–3% of patients. Premedication with dexamethasone recommended.
- Bone Marrow Depression: Dose-limiting neutropenia. Use G-CSF support. Thrombocytopenia and anemia also occur.
- GI Toxicities: Nausea and vomiting are moderate to severe. Stomatitis can occur but is not dose limiting.
- Cardiotoxicities: Acutely, pericarditis-myocarditis syndrome may occur; later, with high cumulative doses (> 550 mg/m^2) cardiomyopathy may occur.
- Neurotoxicity: Peripheral neuropathy—sensory alterations are paresthesias in a glove and stocking distribution and numbness.
- Fluid Balance: Fluid retention syndrome: weight gain, edema, pleural effusion, and ascites. Premedication with dexamethasone effective in preventing or minimizing occurrences.
- Hepatic: Use doxorubicin with caution in patients with liver dysfunction. Dose reduction necessary.
- Bladder Toxicities: Red-orange discoloration of urine; resolves by 24–48 hours.
- Skin: Extravasation of doxorubicin causes severe tissue destruction. Hyperpigmentation, nail changes, rash, dry, pruritic skin, photosensitivity, and radiation recall occur. Alopecia.
- Reproductive: Pregnancy category D. Breast feeding should be avoided.

Initiate antiemetic protocol: Mildly emetogenic protocol.

Supportive drugs:
☐ pegfilgrastim (Neulasta) ☐ filgrastim (Neupogen)

☐ epoetin alfa (Procrit) ☐ darbepoetin alfa (Aranesp)

Treatment schedule: Chair time 2 hours. Repeat cycle every 21 days until disease progression.

Estimated number of visits: Two visits per cycle. Request four cycles worth of visits.

Dose Calculation by: 1. _____ 2. _____

_____

Physician

_____

Date

_____

Patient Name

_____

ID Number

_____

Diagnosis

_____/ _____/ _____

Ht   Wt   M^2

5-Fluorouracil + Epirubicin + Cyclophosphamide (FEC-100)

Baseline laboratory tests:	CBC: Chemistry, LFTs, and CA 27-29
Baseline procedures or tests:	MUGA scan
Initiate IV:	0.9% sodium chloride
Premedicate:	5-HT$_3$ and dexamethasone 20 mg in 100 cc of NS.

Administer:

5-Flourouracil _____ mg (500 mg/m^2) IV on day 1

- Available in solution as 50 mg/mL.
- No dilution required.
- May further dilute with NS or D5W

Epirubicin _____ mg (100 mg/m^2) IV on day 1

- **Vesicant**
- Drug is provided as a preservative-free solution (2 mg/mL).
- Use within 24 hours of penetration of rubber stopper; discard unused portion.
- Store unopened vials in refrigerator.

Cyclophosphamide _____ mg (500 mg/m^2) IV on day 1

- Available in 100-, 200-, 500-, 1000-, and 2000-mg vials
- Dilute with sterile water and shake well to ensure that solution is completely dissolved.
- Reconstituted solution stable for 24 hours at room temperature, and 6 days refrigerated.

Major Side Effects

- Hypersensitivity Reaction: Cyclophosphamide can cause rhinitis and irritation of nose and throat.
- Bone Marrow Depression: Leukopenia, thrombocytopenia, and anemia all occur; may be severe.
- GI Toxicities: Nausea and vomiting are moderate to severe. Mucositis and diarrhea can be severe and dose limiting.
- Cardiac: Cardiotoxicity is dose related, is cumulative, and may occur during months to years after cessation of therapy. Cyclophosphamide may increase the risk of cardiotoxicity.
- Hepatic: Use with caution in patients with abnormal liver function. Dose reduction is required in the presence of liver dysfunction.
- Bladder Toxicities: Hemorrhagic cystitis, dysuria, and urinary frequency with cyclophosphamide. Red-orange discoloration of urine; resolves by 24–48 hours.
- Skin: Extravasation of epirubicin causes severe tissue destruction. Epirubicin may cause "flare" reaction or streaking along vein during peripheral administration. If this occurs, slow drug administration time and flush more. Hyperpigmentation, photosensitivity, nail changes, and radiation recall occur. Complete alopecia. Hand-foot syndrome can be dose limiting.
- Inappropriate secretion of antidiuretic hormone (SIADH).
- Ocular: Photophobia, increased lacrimation, conjunctivitis, and blurred vision.
- Secondary Malignancies: Increased risk with cyclophosphamide.
- Reproductive: Amenorrhea with ovarian failure. Sterility may be permanent. Pregnancy category D. Breast feeding should be avoided.

Initiate antiemetic protocol:	Moderately to highly emetogenic protocol.
Supportive drugs:	☐ pegfilgrastim (Neulasta) ☐ filgrastim (Neupogen)
	☐ epoetin alfa (Procrit) ☐ darbepoetin alfa (Aranesp)
Treatment schedule:	Chair time 2 hours on day 1. Repeat cycle every 21 days until disease progression.
Estimated number of visits:	Two visits per cycle. Request six cycles worth of visits.

Dose Calculation by: 1. _____ 2. _____

_____

Physician

_____

Patient Name

_____

Diagnosis

_____

Date

_____

ID Number

_____ / _____ / _____

Ht   Wt   M²

Paclitaxel + Vinorelbine

Baseline laboratory tests:	CBC: Chemistry and CA 27-29
Baseline procedures or tests:	N/A
Initiate IV:	0.9% sodium chloride
Premedicate:	5-HT$_3$ and dexamethasone 10–20 mg in 100 cc of NS
	Diphenhydramine 25–50 mg and cimetidine 300 mg in 100 cc of NS

Administer:

Vinorelbine _____ mg (30 mg/m^2) IV over 20 minutes on days 1 and 8

- **Vesicant**
- Available in 1- or 5-mL single-use vials at a concentration of 10 mg/mL.
- Further dilute in syringe or IV bag to concentration of 1.5–3.0 mg/mL.
- Reconstituted solution is stable for 24 hours refrigerated.

Paclitaxel _____ mg (135 mg/m^2) IV over 3 hours on day 1; start 1 hour after vinorelbine

- Available in solution as 6 mg/mL.
- Final concentration is $\leq$ 1.2 mg/mL.
- Stable for up to 27 hours at room temperature in 0.3–1.2 mg/mL solutions.
- **Use non-PVC containers and tubing with 0.22-micron inline filter for administration.**

Major Side Effects

- Hypersensitivity Reaction: Occurs in 20%–40% of patients. Characterized by generalized skin rash, flushing, erythema, hypotension, dyspnea, and/or bronchospasm. Usually occurs within the first 2–3 minutes of paclitaxel infusion and almost always within the first 10 minutes. Premedicate as described. Hypersensitivity reaction to vinorelbine presents as dyspnea and bronchospasm.
- Bone Marrow Depression: Dose-limiting neutropenia. G-CSF support recommended. Thrombocytopenia and anemia also occur.
- GI Toxicities: Nausea and vomiting are mild. Stomatitis, constipation, diarrhea, and anorexia also occur.
- Skin: Extravasation of vinorelbine may cause local tissue injury and inflammation. Alopecia.
- Inappropriate secretion of antidiuretic hormone (SIADH).
- Neurotoxicity: Sensory neuropathy with numbness and paresthesias; dose related.
- Reproductive: Pregnancy category D. Breast feeding should be avoided.

Initiate antiemetic protocol:	Mildly emetogenic protocol.
Supportive drugs:	☐ pegfilgrastim (Neulasta) ☐ filgrastim (Neupogen)
	☐ epoetin alfa (Procrit) ☐ darbepoetin alfa (Aranesp)
Treatment schedule:	Chair time 4 hours on day 1 and 1 hour on day 8. Repeat cycle every 28 days until disease progression.
Estimated number of visits:	Three visits per cycle. Request three cycles worth of visits.

Dose Calculation by: 1. _____   2. _____

_____

Physician   Date

_____

Patient Name   ID Number

_____

Diagnosis   Ht   /   Wt   /   M^2

Vinorelbine + Doxorubicin

Baseline laboratory tests:	CBC: Chemistry panel and CA 27-29
Baseline procedures or tests:	MUGA scan
Initiate IV:	0.9% sodium chloride
Premedicate:	5-HT$_3$ and dexamethasone 10–20 mg in 100 cc of NS.
Administer:	**Vinorelbine** _____ mg (25 mg/m^2) IV on days 1 and 8

- **Vesicant**
- Available in 1- or 5-mL single-use vials at a concentration of 10 mg/mL.
- Further dilute in syringe or IV bag to concentration of 1.5–3.0 mg/mL.
- Reconstituted solution is stable for 24 hours refrigerated.

Doxorubicin _____ mg (50 mg/m^2) IV on day 1

- **Potent vesicant**
- Available as a 2-mg/mL solution.
- Doxorubicin will form a precipitate if it is mixed with heparin or 5-FU.

Major Side Effects

- Hypersensitivity Reaction: Presents as dyspnea and bronchospasm with vinorelbine.
- Bone Marrow Depression: WBC and platelet nadir 10–14 days after drug dose, with recovery from days 15–21. Myelosuppression may be severe but is less severe with weekly dosing.
- GI Toxicities: Nausea and vomiting are moderate to severe. Stomatitis is mild to moderate. Constipation, diarrhea, and anorexia also occur.
- Cardiac: Acutely, pericarditis-myocarditis syndrome may occur. With high cumulative doses > 550 mg/m^2 of doxorubicin, cardiomyopathy may occur. Increased risk of cardiotoxicity when doxorubicin is given with trastuzumab (Herceptin) or mitomycin.
- Neurotoxicity: Usually mild and occurs much less frequently than with other vinca alkaloids.
- Skin: Extravasation of vesicants causes severe tissue destruction. Hyperpigmentation, photosensitivity, and radiation recall occur. Alopecia likely.
- Reproductive: Pregnancy category D. Breast feeding should be avoided.

Initiate antiemetic protocol:	Moderately to highly emetogenic protocol.
Supportive drugs:	☐ pegfilgrastim (Neulasta) ☐ filgrastim (Neupogen)
	☐ epoetin alfa (Procrit) ☐ darbepoetin alfa (Aranesp)
Treatment schedule:	Chair time 1 hour on days 1 and 8. Repeat cycle every 21 days.
Estimated number of visits:	Three visits per cycle. Request four cycles worth of visits.

Dose Calculation by: 1. _____   2. _____

_____

Physician

Date

_____

Patient Name

ID Number

_____

Diagnosis

_____ / _____ / _____

Ht   Wt   M^2

Trastuzumab + Paclitaxel

Baseline laboratory tests:	CBC: Chemistry panel and CA 27-29
Baseline procedures or tests:	Her-2 testing of tumor using fluorescence in situ hybridization (FISH; preferred) or immunohistochemical (IHC) analysis, and MUGA scan
Initiate IV:	NS
Premedicate:	5-HT$_3$ and dexamethasone 10–20 mg in 100 cc of NS
	Diphenhydramine 25–50 mg and cimetidine 300 mg in 100 cc of NS

Administer:

Trastuzumab _____ mg (4 mg/kg) IV in 250 cc of NS over 90-minute loading dose, then

Trastuzumab _____ mg (2 mg/kg) IV in 250 cc of NS over 30 minutes weekly

Paclitaxel _____ mg (175 mg/m^2) IV over 3 hours on day 1

Repeat cycle every 21 days.

OR

Trastuzumab _____ mg (4 mg/kg) IV in 250 cc of NS over 90-minute loading dose, then

Trastuzumab _____ mg (2mg/kg) IV in 250 cc of NS over 30 minutes weekly

- Available as a lyophilized, sterile powder in 440-mg multiuse vials for IV use.
- Requires refrigeration. DO NOT FREEZE.
- Reconstitute with 20 mL of bacteriostatic water for injection, USP, containing 1.1% benzyl alcohol, which is supplied with each vial. DO NOT SHAKE.
- Reconstituted solution contains 21 mg/mL. Stable 28 days refrigerated.
- Further dilute desired dose in 250 cc of NS.

Paclitaxel _____ mg (80 mg/m^2) IV weekly

- Available in 6-mg/mL solution for IV use.
- Final concentration is $\leq$ 1.2 mg/mL.
- Stable for up to 27 hours at room temperature in 0.3–1.2 mg/mL solutions.
- **Use non-PVC containers and tubing with 0.22-micron inline filter for administration.**

Major Side Effects	• Infusion-related Symptoms: Fever, chills, urticaria, flushing, fatigue, headache, bronchospasm, dyspnea, angioedema, and hypotension. Usually mild to moderate and observed most commonly with initial dose of either drug. Symptoms usually resolve quickly when infusion is slowed or stopped. Premed as described.

- GI Toxicities: Nausea and vomiting, mucositis, and diarrhea—generally mild.
- Cardiotoxicity: Dyspnea, edema, and reduced left ventricular function seen with trastuzumab. Increased risk when used with paclitaxel.
- Pulmonary: Cough, dyspnea, pulmonary infiltrates, and/or pleural effusions.
- Myelosuppression: Leukopenia is dose-limiting toxicity. Use G-CSF support.
- Neurotoxicity: Dose-related sensory neuropathy with numbness and paresthesia. Can be dose limiting.
- Skin: Alopecia. Onycholysis seen in those receiving more than 6 courses of weekly paclitaxel.
- Reproductive: Pregnancy category D. Breast feeding should be avoided.

Initiate antiemetic protocol:	Mildly emetogenic protocol.
Supportive drugs:	☐ pegfilgrastim (Neulasta) ☐ filgrastim (Neupogen)
	☐ epoetin alfa (Procrit) ☐ darbepoetin alfa (Aranesp)
	☐ loperamide (Imodium) ☐ diphenoxylate/atropine sulfate (Lomotil)
Treatment schedule:	Chair time 5 hours on day 1 cycle 1 only, 4 hours day 1 subsequent cycles: 1 hour weeks 2 and 3. Repeat cycle every 21 days.
	OR
	Chair time 4 hours on day 1, 3 hours weekly thereafter. Repeat cycle every 4 weeks.
Estimated number of visits:	Three visits per cycle **OR** four visits per cycle. Request six cycles worth of treatments.

Dose Calculation by: 1. _____ 2. _____

_____
Physician

_____
Date

_____
Patient Name

_____
ID Number

_____
Diagnosis

_____ / _____ / _____
Ht   Wt   M²

Trastuzumab + Docetaxel

Baseline laboratory tests:	CBC: Chemistry panel and CA 27-29
Baseline procedures or tests:	Her-2 testing of tumor using FISH (preferred) or IHC, and MUGA scan
Initiate IV:	NS
Premedicate:	Dexamethasone 8 mg bid for 3 days, starting the day before treatment
	5-HT$_3$ and dexamethasone 10–20 mg in 100 cc of NS

Administer:

Trastuzumab _____ mg (4 mg/kg) IV in 250 cc of NS over 90-minute loading dose day 1 first cycle only, then

Trastuzumab _____ mg (2 mg/kg) IV in 250 cc of NS over 30 minutes on days 1, 8, and 15

Docetaxel _____ mg (35 mg/m^2) IV in 250 cc of NS over 1 hour on days 1, 8, and 15

The first cycle is administered weekly for 3 weeks, with 1 week rest.

For subsequent cycles:

Trastuzumab _____ mg (2 mg/kg) IV in 250 cc of NS over 30 minutes weekly

- Available as a lyophilized, sterile powder in 440-mg multiuse vials for IV use.
- Requires refrigeration. DO NOT FREEZE.
- Reconstitute with 20 mL of bacteriostatic water for injection, USP, containing 1.1% benzyl alcohol, which is supplied with each vial. DO NOT SHAKE.
- Reconstituted solution contains 21 mg/mL. Stable 28 days refrigerated.
- Further dilute desired dose in 250 cc of NS.

Docetaxel _____ mg (35 mg/m^2) IV in 250 cc of NS weekly

- Available in 20- or 80-mg packs with own diluent. Do not shake. Reconstituted vials stable at room temperature or refrigerated for 8 hours.
- Further dilute in 250 cc of D5W or NS.
- **Use non-PVC containers and tubing to administer.**

Major Side Effects

- Infusion-related Symptoms: Fever, chills, urticaria, flushing, fatigue, headache, bronchospasm, dyspnea, angioedema, and hypotension. Usually mild to moderate. Most common with initial dose of either drug. Symptoms usually resolve quickly when infusion is stopped. Premed with dexamethasone.
- GI Toxicities: Nausea and vomiting are mild to moderate. Mucositis and diarrhea can occur.
- Cardiotoxicity: Dyspnea, edema, and reduced left ventricular function seen with trastuzumab.
- Pulmonary: Cough, dyspnea, pulmonary infiltrates, and/or pleural effusions.
- Myelosuppression: Leukopenia is dose-limiting toxicity. Thrombocytopenia and anemia are also seen.
- Neurotoxicity: Dose-related sensory neuropathy with numbness and paresthesia.
- Fluid Balance: Fluid retention syndrome. Edema, pleural effusion, and ascites. Premedication with dexamethasone effective in preventing or minimizing fluid retention syndrome.
- Skin: Alopecia. Nail changes, rash, and dry, pruritic skin. Hand-foot syndrome has also been reported.
- Reproductive: Pregnancy category D. Breast feeding should be avoided.

Initiate antiemetic protocol:	Mildly emetogenic protocol.

Supportive drugs:

☐ pegfilgrastim (Neulasta) ☐ filgrastim (Neupogen)

☐ loperamide (Imodium) ☐ epoetin alfa (Procrit)

☐ darbepoetin alfa (Aranesp) ☐ diphenoxylate/atropine sulfate (Lomotil)

Treatment schedule:	Chair time 3 hours on day 1, 2 hours on days 8 and 15, and 2 hours weekly thereafter. Repeat cycle every 4 weeks.
Estimated number of visits:	Four visits per cycle. Request six cycles worth of treatments.

Dose Calculation by: 1. _____   2. _____

_____   _____
Physician   Date

_____   _____
Patient Name   ID Number

_____   _____/_____/_____
Diagnosis   Ht   Wt   M²

Gemcitabine + Paclitaxel

Baseline laboratory tests:	CBC: Chemistry panel, LFTs, and CA 27-29
Baseline procedures or tests:	N/A
Initiate IV:	0.9% sodium chloride
Premedicate:	5-HT$_3$ and dexamethasone 10–20 mg in 100 cc of NS
	Diphenhydramine 25–50 mg and cimetidine 300 mg in 100 cc of NS

Administer:

Gemcitabine _____ mg (1250 mg/m^2) IV on days 1 and 8

- Available in 1-g or 200-mg vials; reconstitute with 0.9% sodium chloride USP (5 cc for 200 mg, 25 cc for 1 g).
- Further dilute in 0.9% sodium chloride.
- Reconstituted solution is stable for 24 hours at room temperature.
- DO NOT refrigerate, because precipitate will form.

Paclitaxel _____ mg (175 mg/m^2) IV on day 1

- Available in solution as 6 mg/mL.
- Final concentration is < 1.2 mg/mL.
- Stable for up to 27 hours at room temperature in 0.3–1.2 mg/mL solutions.
- Use non-PVC containers and tubing with 0.22-micron inline filter for administration.

Major Side Effects

- Hypersensitivity Reaction: Occurs in 20%–40% of patients receiving paclitaxel. Characterized by generalized skin rash, flushing, erythema, hypotension, dyspnea, and/or bronchospasm. Usually occurs within the first 2–3 minutes of infusion and almost always within the first 10 minutes. Premedicate as described.
- Hematologic: Myelosuppression is dose limiting. G-CSF support recommended.
- Pulmonary: Mild dyspnea and drug induced pneumonitis.
- GI Symptoms: Mild-to-moderate nausea and vomiting, diarrhea, and mucositis.
- Neuropathy: Sensory neuropathy with numbness and paresthesias; dose related and dose limiting.
- Flulike Syndrome: Fever, malaise, chills, headache, and myalgias. Fever, in absence of infection 6–12 hours after treatment.
- Hepatic: Transient elevation of serum transaminase and bilirubin levels.
- Skin: Hand-foot syndrome. Rash and nail changes. Edema occurs in some patients. Alopecia is common, loss of total body hair likely.
- Reproductive: Pregnancy category D. Breast feeding should be avoided.

Initiate antiemetic protocol:	Mildly to moderately emetogenic protocol.
Supportive drugs:	☐ pegfilgrastim (Neulasta) ☐ filgrastim (Neupogen)
	☐ epoetin alfa (Procrit) ☐ darbepoetin alfa (Aranesp)
Treatment schedule:	Chair time 4 hours on day 1, 1 hour on day 8. Repeat cycle every 21 days until disease progression.
Estimated number of visits:	Three visits per cycle. Request three cycles worth of visits.

Dose Calculation by: 1. _____   2. _____

_____
Physician

_____
Date

_____
Patient Name

_____
ID Number

_____
Diagnosis

_____ / _____ / _____
Ht   Wt   M^2

Carboplatin + Paclitaxel

Baseline laboratory tests:	CBC: Chemistry (including Mg^{2+}) and CA 27-29
Baseline procedures or tests:	N/A
Initiate IV:	0.9% sodium chloride
Premedicate:	5-HT$_3$ and dexamethasone 10–20 mg in 100 cc of NS
	Diphenhydramine 25–50 mg and cimetidine 300 mg in 100 cc of NS

Administer:

Paclitaxel _____ mg (200 mg/m^2) IV over 3 hours on day 1

- Available in solution as 6 mg/mL.
- Final concentration is ≤ 1.2 mg/mL.
- Stable for up to 27 hours at room temperature in 0.3–1.2 mg/mL solutions.
- Use non-PVC containers and tubing with 0.22-micron inline filter to administer.

Carboplatin _____ mg (AUC 6) IV on day 1

- Available in solution as 10 mg/mL or as lyopholized powder.
- Reconstitute with sterile water for injection, 5% dextrose or 0.9% sodium.
- Reconstituted solution stable for 8 hours at room temperature.
- Do not use aluminum needles, because precipitate will form.
- Give carboplatin **after** paclitaxel to decrease toxicities.

Major Side Effects

- Hypersensitivity Reaction: Paclitaxel is usually seen with initial dose. Characterized by generalized skin rash, flushing, erythema, hypotension, dyspnea, and/or bronchospasm. Usually occurs within the first 2–3 minutes of infusion and almost always in the first 10 minutes. Premedicate as described. Increased risk of hypersensitivity reactions in patients receiving more than seven courses of carboplatin therapy.
- Bone Marrow Depression: Neutropenia, thrombocytopenia, and anemia are cumulative and dose related. Can be dose limiting. G-CSF support recommended.
- GI Toxicities: Moderate-to-severe nausea and vomiting may be acute or delayed. Mucositis and/or diarrhea seen in some patients.
- Hepatic: Transient elevations in serum transaminases, bilirubin and alkaline phosphatase.
- Renal: Nephrotoxicity less common than with cisplatin and rarely symptomatic.
- Electrolyte Imbalance: Decreases Mg^{2+}, K^+, Ca^{2+}, and Na^+.
- Neurotoxicity: Sensory neuropathy with numbness and paresthesias; dose related and can be dose limiting.
- Alopecia: Loss of total body hair occurs in nearly all patients.
- Reproductive: Pregnancy category D. Breast feeding should be avoided.

Initiate antiemetic protocol:	Moderately to highly emetogenic protocol.
Supportive drugs:	☐ pegfilgrastim (Neulasta) ☐ filgrastim (Neupogen)
	☐ epoetin alfa (Procrit) ☐ darbepoetin alfa (Aranesp)
Treatment schedule:	Chair time 5 hours on day 1. Repeat cycle every 21 days until disease progression.
Estimated number of visits:	Two visits per cycle. Request four cycles worth of visits.

Dose Calculation by: 1. _____ 2. _____

_____
Physician

_____
Date

_____
Patient Name

_____
ID Number

_____
Diagnosis

_____ / _____ / _____
Ht   Wt   M^2

Carboplatin + Docetaxel

Baseline laboratory tests:	CBC: Chemistry (including Mg^{2+}) and CA 27-29
Baseline procedures or tests:	N/A
Initiate IV:	0.9% sodium chloride
Premedicate:	Dexamethasone 8 mg PO bid for 3 days, starting the day before treatment
	5-HT_3 and dexamethasone 10–20 mg in 100 cc of NS on the day of treatment

Administer:

Docetaxel _____ mg ($75 mg/m^2$) IV on day 1

- Available in 20- or 80-mg doses; comes with own diluent. Do not shake.
- Reconstituted vials stable at room temperature or for 8 hours refrigerated.
- Further dilute in 250 cc of D5W or 0.9% sodium chloride.
- **Use non-PVC containers and tubings to administer.**

Carboplatin _____ mg (AUC 6) IV on day 1

- Available in solution as 10 mg/mL or as lyopholized powder.
- Reconstitute with sterile water for injection, 5% dextrose or 0.9% sodium.
- Reconstituted solution is stable for 8 hours at room temperature.
- Do not use aluminum needle, because precipitate will form.
- Available in powder or solution. Discard reconstituted powder after 8 hours.

Major Side Effects

- Hypersensitivity Reaction: Severe hypersensitivity reactions with docetaxel in 2%–3% of patients. Premedication with dexamethasone recommended. Carboplatin can cause rash, urticaria, erythema, and pruritus. Bronchospasm and hypotension are uncommon, but risk increases from 1% to 27% in patients receiving more than seven courses of carboplatin-based therapy.
- Bone Marrow Depression: Neutropenia, thrombocytopenia, and anemia are dose related and can be dose limiting.
- GI Toxicities: Moderate to severe nausea and vomiting within first 24 hours.
- Renal: Nephrotoxicity less common than with cisplatin and rarely symptomatic.
- Electrolyte Imbalance: Decreases Mg^{2+}, K^+, Ca^{2+}, and Na^+.
- Neuropathy: Neurologic dysfunction is infrequent, but there is increased risk in patients > 65 years of age or in those previously treated with cisplatin and receiving prolonged carboplatin treatment.
- Skin: Alopecia is common.
- Reproductive: Pregnancy category D. Breast feeding should be avoided.

Initiate antiemetic protocol:	Moderately to highly emetogenic protocol.
Supportive drugs:	☐ pegfilgrastim (Neulasta) ☐ filgrastim (Neupogen)
	☐ epoetin alfa (Procrit) ☐ darbepoetin alfa (Aranesp)
Treatment schedule:	Chair time 3 hours on day 1. Repeat cycle every 21 days until progression.
Estimated number of visits:	Two visits per cycle. Request six months worth.

Dose Calculation by: 1. _____   2. _____

_____
Physician

_____
Date

_____
Patient Name

_____
ID Number

_____
Diagnosis

_____/_____/_____
Ht   Wt M^2

Mitomycin + Vinblastine

Baseline laboratory tests:	CBC: Chemistry and CA 27-29
Baseline procedures or tests:	Central line placement
Initiate IV:	0.9% sodium chloride
Premedicate:	5-HT$_3$ and dexamethasone 10 in 100 cc of NS
Administer:	**Mitomycin** _____ mg (20 mg/m^2) IV bolus day 1

- Potent vesicant
- Dilute with sterile water to give a final concentration of 0.5 mg/mL.
- Reconstituted solution stable for 14 days refrigerated or 7 days at room temperature.

Vinblastine _____ mg (1.4–2 mg/m^2) IV continuous infusion days 1–5

- Vesicant
- Available in 10-mg vials for IV use.
- Solution containing 1 mg/mL should be prepared by adding 10 mL of bacteriostatic 0.9% sodium chloride preserved with benzyl alcohol.
- Also available in premixed solution to be stored in refrigerator.
- Reconstituted solution should be clear and free of particulate matter.

Major Side Effects

- Bone Marrow Depression: Dose limiting and cumulative toxicity, with leukopenia being more common than thrombocytopenia. Nadir counts are delayed at 4–6 weeks with mitomycin and at 4–6 days with vinblastine.
- GI Toxicities: Nausea and vomiting usually mild to moderate. Mucositis occurs. Constipation, abdominal pain, and paralytic ileus possible. Anorexia and fatigue common.
- Neurotoxicity: Occurs much less frequently than with vincristine. Presents with peripheral neuropathy (paresthesias, paralysis, loss of deep tendon reflexes, and constipation) and autonomic nervous system dysfunction (orthostatic hypotension, paralytic ileus, and urinary retention). Less commonly, cranial nerve paralysis, ataxia, cortical blindness, seizures, and coma may occur.
- CV Toxicities: Hypertension is most common cardiovascular side effect. Vascular events, such as stroke, myocardial infarction, and Raynaud's syndrome seen.
- Inappropriate secretion of antidiuretic hormone (SIADH).
- Hemolytic-uremic Syndrome: Hematocrit < 25%, platelets < 100 × 10^3/mm^3, and renal failure (serum creatinine >1.6 mg/dL). Rare event (< 2%).
- Pulmonary: Acute pulmonary edema, bronchospasm, acute respiratory distress, interstitial pulmonary infiltrates, and dyspnea have been reported on rare occasion.
- Skin: Mitomycin causes severe tissue necrosis if extravasated; vinblastine causes local skin damage if extravasated. Alopecia occurs frequently.
- Reproductive: Pregnancy category D. Breast feeding should be avoided.

Initiate antiemetic protocol:	Mildly to moderately emetogenic protocol.
Supportive drugs:	☐ pegfilgrastim (Neulasta) ☐ filgrastim (Neupogen)
	☐ epoetin alfa (Procrit) ☐ darbepoetin alfa (Aranesp)
Treatment schedule:	Chair time 1 hour on day. Repeat cycle every 6–8 weeks.
Estimated number of visits:	Six visits per treatment course.

Dose Calculation by: 1. _____   2. _____

_____
Physician

_____
Date

_____
Patient Name

_____
ID Number

_____
Diagnosis

_____ / _____ / _____
Ht   Wt   M^2

Single-Agent Regimens

Tamoxifen

Baseline laboratory tests:	CBC: Chemistry, LFTs, and CA 27-29
Baseline procedures or tests:	ER/PR testing
Initiate IV:	N/A
Premedicate:	Oral phenothiazine or 5-HT$_3$ if nausea occurs
Administer:	**Tamoxifen** 20 mg PO daily

- Available in 10- and 20-mg tablets.
- Monitor PT/INR closely in patients taking warfarin; increases PT/INR.

Major Side Effects
- GI Toxicities: Nausea and vomiting rarely observed.
- Tumor Flare: Usually occurs within the first 2 weeks of beginning of therapy. May observe increased bone pain, urinary retention, back pain with spinal cord compression and/or hypercalcemia.
- CV Toxicities: Deep vein thrombosis, pulmonary embolism, and superficial phlebitis are rare cardiovascular complications of tamoxifen therapy. Incidence of thromboembolic events may be increased when tamoxifen is given concomitantly with chemotherapy.
- Fluid/electrolyte Imbalance: Fluid retention and peripheral edema observed in about 30% of patients.
- Hormonal Effects: Menstrual irregularity, hot flashes, milk production in breasts, vaginal discharge, and bleeding. Usually not severe enough to discontinue therapy.
- Gynecological: Increased incidence of endometrial hyperplasia, polyps, and endometrial cancer.
- Sensory/perception Alteration: Headache, lethargy, and dizziness occur rarely. Visual disturbances, including cataract, retinopathy, and decreased visual acuity, have been described.
- Myelosuppression: Mild, transient leukopenia and thrombocytopenia occur rarely.
- Laboratory Values: Elevations in serum triglyceride levels.
- Reproductive: Pregnancy category D. Breast feeding should be avoided.

Initiate antiemetic protocol:	Mildly emetogenic protocol.
Treatment schedule:	No chair time. Daily dosing until disease progression.
Estimated number of visits:	One visit every 2–3 months. Request 12 months worth of visits.

Dose Calculation by: 1. _____   2. _____

_____
Physician

_____
Date

_____
Patient Name

_____
ID Number

_____
Diagnosis

_____ / _____ / _____
Ht   Wt   M^2

Toremifene Citrate (Fareston)

Baseline laboratory tests:	CBC: Chemistry, LFTs, and CA 27-29
Baseline procedures or tests:	ER/PR testing, eye exam.
Initiate IV:	N/A
Premedicate:	Oral phenothiazine or 5-HT$_3$ if nausea occurs
Administer:	Toremifene citrate 60 mg PO daily

- Available as toremifene citrate (88.5 mg of toremifene citrate is equivalent to 60 mg of toremifene) for oral use.
- Well absorbed after oral administration. Food does not interfere with absorption.
- Monitor PT/INR closely in patients taking warfarin.

Major Side Effects

- Tumor Flare: May cause flare reaction initially (bone and/or muscular pain, erythema, tumor pain, and transient increase in tumor size). Use with caution in the setting of brain and/or vertebral metastases.
- CV Toxicities: Toremifene is thrombogenic. Use with caution in patients with a prior history of thromboembolic events.
- GI Toxicities: Nausea, vomiting, and anorexia have occurred.
- Hormonal Effects: Menstrual irregularity, hot flashes, sweating, milk production in breasts, vaginal discharge and bleeding. Usually not severe enough to discontinue therapy.
- Myelosuppression: Mild, transient leukopenia and thrombocytopenia occur rarely.
- GU Toxicities: Increased risk of endometrial cancer associated with therapy.
- Ocular: Cataract formation and xerophthalmia. Baseline and biannual eye exams are recommended.
- Skin Toxicity: Rare. Presents as rash alopecia and peripheral edema.
- Reproductive: Pregnancy category D. Not known if excreted in breast milk.

Initiate antiemetic protocol:	Mildly emetogenic protocol.
Treatment schedule:	No chair time. Daily dosing until disease progression.
Estimated number of visits:	One visit every 2–3 months during treatment.

Dose Calculation by: 1. _____ 2. _____

_____

Physician

_____

Patient Name

_____

Diagnosis

_____

Date

_____

ID Number

_____/_____/_____

Ht   Wt   M^2

Exemestane (Aromasin)

Baseline laboratory tests:	CBC: Chemistry panel, LFTs, and CA 27-29
Baseline procedures or tests:	ER/PR testing
Initiate IV:	N/A
Premedicate:	Oral phenothiazine or 5-HT$_3$ if nausea occurs
Administer:	**Exemestane** 25 mg PO daily

- Available as a 25-mg tablet for oral use.
- Take once daily after a meal.

Major Side Effects

- Hot Flashes: Hot flashes, increased sweating, and pain reported.
- GI Toxicities: Mild-to-moderate nausea, increased appetite, and weight gain reported.
- CNS Toxicity: Depression and insomnia occurred in 13% and 11%, respectively. Headache and fatigue also seen.
- Reproductive: Pregnancy category D. Breast feeding should be avoided.

Initiate antiemetic protocol:	Mildly emetogenic protocol
Treatment schedule:	No chair time. Daily dosing until disease progression.
Estimated number of visits:	One visit every 2–3 months during treatment.

Dose Calculation by: 1. _____   2. _____

_____
Physician

_____
Patient Name

_____
Diagnosis

_____
Date

_____
ID Number

_____ / _____ / _____
Ht   Wt   M^2

Anastrozole (Arimidex)

Baseline laboratory tests:	CBC: Chemistry panel, LFTs, and CA 27-29
Baseline procedures or tests:	ER/PR testing
Initiate IV:	N/A
Premedicate:	Oral phenothiazine or 5-HT$_3$ if nausea occurs
Administer:	**Anastrozole** 1 mg PO daily

- Available as a 1-mg, white, film-coated tablet for oral use.
- Take orally with or without food, at approximately the same time daily.

Major Side Effects

- Hormonal: Hot flashes, and vaginal dryness may occur.
- CV Toxicities: Thrombophlebitis may occur but is uncommon. Mild swelling of arms or legs may occur.
- GI Toxicities: Mild nausea and vomiting. Mild constipation or diarrhea can also occur.
- Skin: Dry, scaling skin rash.
- Flulike Syndrome: Presents in the form of fever, malaise, and myalgias.
- Musculoskeletal: Arthralgias occur in 10%–15% of patients and involve hands, knees, hips, lower back, and shoulders. Early morning stiffness is usual presentation.
- CNS Toxicity: Headaches are mild and occur in about 13% of patients. Decreased energy and weakness are common.
- Reproductive: Pregnancy category D. Breast feeding should be avoided.

Initiate antiemetic protocol:	Mildly emetogenic protocol
Treatment schedule:	No chair time. Daily dosing until disease progression.
Estimated number of visits:	One visit every 2–3 months during treatment.

Dose Calculation by: 1. _____   2. _____

_____
Physician

_____
Date

_____
Patient Name

_____
ID Number

_____
Diagnosis

_____/ _____/ _____
Ht   Wt   M^2

Letrozole (Femara)

Baseline laboratory tests:	CBC: Chemistry panel, LFTs, and CA 27-29
Baseline procedures or tests:	ER/PR testing
Initiate IV:	N/A
Premedicate:	Oral phenothiazine or 5-HT$_3$ if nausea occurs
Administer:	**Letrozole** 2.5 mg PO daily

- Available as a 2.5-mg tablet for oral use
- Food does not interfere with oral absorption.

Major Side Effects

- Musculoskeletal: Most common side effects. Musculoskeletal pain (back, arms, legs) and arthralgias.
- Hormonal: Hot flashes occur in approximately 6% of patients.
- CV Toxicities: Thromboembolic events are rare and less common than with megestrol acetate. Chest pain reported in some patients.
- GI Toxicities: Mild nausea with vomiting and anorexia occurring less frequently. Mild constipation or diarrhea can also occur.
- Hepatic: Mild elevation in serum transaminase and serum bilirubin levels. Most often seen in patients with known metastatic disease in the liver.
- CNS Toxicity: Headaches and fatigue are mild.
- Reproductive: Pregnancy category D. Breast feeding should be avoided.

Initiate antiemetic protocol:	Mildly emetogenic protocol
Treatment schedule:	No chair time. Daily dosing until disease progression.
Estimated number of visits:	One visit every 2–3 months during treatment.

Dose Calculation by: 1. _____   2. _____

_____
Physician

_____
Date

_____
Patient Name

_____
ID Number

_____
Diagnosis

_____/ _____/ _____
Ht   Wt   M^2

Fulvestrant (Faslodex)

Baseline laboratory tests:	CBC: Chemistry panel, LFTs, and CA 27-29
Baseline procedures or tests:	ER/PR testing
Initiate IV:	N/A
Premedicate:	Oral phenothiazine or 5-HT$_3$ if nausea occurs
Administer:	**Fulvestrant** 250 mg IM on day 1

- Available as 250-mg/5mL and 125-mg/2.5mL prefilled syringes; concentration is 50 mg/mL.
- Unopened vials should be stored in the refrigerator.
- Drug can be left at room temperature for a short period before injection to increase patient comfort.
- Administer slowly by IM injection in one buttock (5 mL) or each buttock (2.5 mL) because drug is viscous.
- Use Z-track technique to prevent drug leakage into subcutaneous tissue.

Major Side Effects
- Musculoskeletal: Back and bone pain, arthralgias.
- Hormonal: Hot flashes occur in approximately 20% of patients.
- GI Toxicities: Mild nausea, vomiting, and anorexia. Abdominal pain, constipation, and/or diarrhea can also occur.
- CNS Toxicity: Mild headaches reported.
- Flulike Syndrome: Fever, malaise, and myalgias occur in 10% of patients.
- Skin: Injection site reactions with mild pain and inflammation that is usually transient. Occurs more frequently in 2.5-mL injections (28%) versus 5-mL injections (7%). Dry, scaling skin rash.
- Reproduction: Contraindicated in pregnancy and breastfeeding.

Initiate antiemetic protocol:	Mildly emetogenic protocol
Treatment schedule:	Monthly injection until disease progression.
Estimated number of visits:	One visit every month during treatment. Request 12 months worth of visits.

Dose Calculation by: 1. _____   2. _____

_____
Physician

_____
Patient Name

_____
Diagnosis

_____
Date

_____
ID Number

_____ / _____ / _____
Ht   Wt   M^2

Megestrol (Megace)

Baseline laboratory tests:	CBC: Chemistry, LFTs, and CA 27-29
Baseline procedures or tests:	ER/PR testing
Initiate IV:	N/A
Premedicate:	Oral phenothiazine or 5-HT$_3$ if nausea occurs
Administer:	**Megestrol** 40 mg PO qid

- Available in 20- and 40-mg tablets as well as a 40-mg/mL suspension

Major Side Effects

- GI Toxicities: Nausea and vomiting rarely observed. Increased appetite with accompanying weight gain.
- CV Toxicities: Use with caution in patients with a history of either thromboembolic or hypercoagulable disorders. Megestrol acetate has been associated with an increased incidence of thromboembolic events.
- Fluid/electrolyte Imbalance: Fluid retention.
- Endocrine: Hyperglycemia. Use with caution in patients with diabetes mellitus because megestrol may exacerbate this condition.
- Hepatic: Abnormal LFT results. Dose reduction recommended in patients with abnormal liver function.
- Hormonal: Breakthrough menstrual bleeding, hot flashes, sweating, and mood changes.
- Tumor flare.
- Reproduction: Pregnancy category D.

Initiate antiemetic protocol:	Mildly emetogenic protocol.
Treatment schedule:	No chair time. Daily dosing as tolerated or until disease progression.
Estimated number of visits:	Monthly during treatment.

Dose Calculation by: 1. _____   2. _____

_____
Physician

_____
Patient Name

_____
Diagnosis

_____
Date

_____
ID Number

_____/_____/_____
Ht   Wt   M^2

Trastuzumab (Herceptin Weekly Dosing)

Baseline laboratory tests:	CBC: Chemistry panel and CA 27-29
Baseline procedures or tests:	Her-2 testing of tumor using FISH (preferred) or IHC, and MUGA scan
Initiate IV:	NS
Premedicate:	No premedication recommended
Administer:	**Trastuzumab** _____ mg (4 mg/kg) IV in 250 cc of NS over 90-minute loading dose

Then

Trastuzumab _____ mg (2 mg/kg) IV in 250 cc of NS over 30 minutes weekly

- Available as a lyophilized, sterile powder in 440-mg multiuse vials for IV use.
- Require refrigeration. DO NOT FREEZE.
- Reconstitute with 20 mL of bacteriostatic water for injection, USP, containing 1.1% benzyl alcohol, which is supplied with each vial. DO NOT SHAKE.
- Reconstituted solution contains 22 mg/mL. Stable 28 days refrigerated.
- Further dilute desired dose in 250 cc of NS.

Major Side Effects

- Infusion-related Symptoms: Fever, chills, urticaria, flushing, fatigue, headache, bronchospasm, dyspnea, angioedema, and hypotension. Occurs in 40%–50% of patients. Usually mild to moderate in severity and observed most commonly with initial dose. Symptoms usually resolve quickly if infusion slowed or stopped.
- GI Toxicities: Nausea and vomiting, diarrhea—generally mild.
- Cardiotoxicity: Dyspnea, peripheral edema, and reduced left ventricular function. Significantly increased risk when used in combination with anthracycline/cyclophosphamide regimen. In most instances, cardiac dysfunction is readily reversible.
- Pulmonary: Toxicities in the form of increased cough, dyspnea, rhinitis, sinusitis, pulmonary infiltrates, and/or pleural effusions.
- Myelosuppression: Not significant. Increased risk and severity when trastuzumab is administered with chemotherapy.
- CNS Toxicities: Generalized pain, asthenia, and headache.
- Reproductive: Pregnancy category D. Breast feeding should be avoided.

Initiate antiemetic protocol:	Mildly emetogenic protocol.
Supportive drugs:	☐ pegfilgrastim (Neulasta) ☐ filgrastim (Neupogen) ☐ epoetin alfa (Procrit) ☐ darbepoetin alfa (Aranesp)
Treatment schedule:	Chair time 2 hours on day 1, 1 hour weekly thereafter.
	In the absence of disease progression, continue weekly maintenance dose of 2 mg/kg.
Estimated number of visits:	One visit per week. Request 6 month worth of visits.

Dose Calculation by: 1. _____ 2. _____

Physician _____   Date _____

Patient Name _____   ID Number _____

Diagnosis _____   Ht _____/ Wt _____/ M² _____

Trastuzumab (Herceptin Every 3 Weeks)

Baseline laboratory tests:	CBC: Chemistry panel and CEA
Baseline procedures or tests:	Her-2 testing of tumor using FISH (preferred) or IHC, and MUGA scan
Initiate IV:	NS
Premedicate:	No premedication recommended
Administer:	**Trastuzumab** _____ mg (8 mg/kg) IV in 250 cc of NS over 90-minute loading dose (if patient has been on weekly trastuzumab without a break the loading dose is not necessary. Start with the 6m/kg dose).

Then

Trastuzumab _____ mg (6 mg/kg) IV in 250 cc of NS over 30 minutes every three weeks.

- Available as a lyophilized, sterile powder in 440-mg multiuse vials for IV use.
- Require refrigeration. DO NOT FREEZE.
- Reconstitute with 20 mL of bacteriostatic water for injection, USP, containing 1.1% benzyl alcohol, which is supplied with each vial. DO NOT SHAKE.
- Reconstituted solution contains 22 mg/mL. Stable 28 days refrigerated.
- Further dilute desired dose in 250 cc of NS.

Major Side Effects

- Infusion-related Symptoms: Fever, chills, urticaria, flushing, fatigue, headache, bronchospasm, dyspnea, angioedema, and hypotension. Seen in 40%–50% of patients. Usually mild to moderate in severity and observed most commonly with initial dose. Symptoms usually resolve quickly if infusion is slowed or stopped.
- GI Toxicities: Nausea and vomiting, diarrhea—generally mild.
- Cardiotoxicity: Dyspnea, peripheral edema, and reduced left ventricular function. Significantly increased risk when used in combination with anthracycline/cyclophosphamide regimen. In most instances, cardiac dysfunction is readily reversible.
- Pulmonary: Toxicities seen in the form of increased cough, dyspnea, rhinitis, sinusitis, pulmonary infiltrates, and/or pleural effusions.
- Myelosuppression: Not significant. Increased risk and severity when trastuzumab is administered with chemotherapy.
- CNS Toxicities: Generalized pain, asthenia, and headache.
- Reproductive: Pregnancy category D. Breast feeding should be avoided.

Initiate antiemetic protocol:	Mildly emetogenic protocol.
Supportive drugs:	☐ pegfilgrastim (Neulasta) ☐ filgrastim (Neupogen) ☐ epoetin alfa (Procrit) ☐ darbepoetin alfa (Aranesp)
Treatment schedule:	Chair time 2 hours on day 1, 1 hour every 3 weeks thereafter. Repeat cycle every 3 weeks.
Estimated number of visits:	One visit every 3 weeks.

Dose Calculation by: 1. _____   2. _____

_____
Physician

_____
Date

_____
Patient Name

_____
ID Number

_____
Diagnosis

_____ / _____ / _____
Ht   Wt   M^2

Capecitabine (Xeloda)

Baseline laboratory tests:	CBC: Chemistry, bilirubin, LFTs, creatinine clearance, and CA 27-29
Baseline procedures or tests:	N/A
Initiate IV:	N/A
Premedicate:	Oral phenothiazine or 5-HT$_3$
Administer:	**Capecitabine** _____ mg (1250 mg/m^2) PO bid for 2 weeks followed by 1 week rest period.

- Dose may be decreased to 850–1000 mg/m^2 PO bid on days 1–14. This may reduce the risk of toxicity without compromising efficacy.
- Available in 150- and 500-mg tablets for oral use.
- Administer within 30 minutes of a meal with plenty of water.
- Monitor INRs closely in patients taking warfarin; may increase INR.

Major Side Effects

- Myelosuppression: Seen less frequently than with IV SFU. Leukopenia more common than thrombocytopenia.
- GI Toxicities: Nausea and vomiting, occurring in 30%–50% of patients, is usually mild to moderate. Diarrhea occurs in up to 40%, with 15% being grade 3–4. Stomatitis is common, 3% of which is severe.
- Skin: Hand-foot syndrome (palmar-plantar erythrodysesthesia) occurs in 15%–20% of patients. Characterized by tingling, numbness, pain, erythema, dryness, rash, swelling, increased pigmentation, and/or pruritus of the hands and feet. Less frequent in reduced doses.
- Ocular: Blepharitis, tear-duct stenosis, acute and chronic conjunctivitis.
- Hepatic: Elevations in serum bilirubin (20%–40%), alkaline phosphatase, and hepatic transaminases (aspartate transaminase, alanine transaminase) levels. Dose modifications may be required if hyperbilirubinemia occurs.
- Cardiac: Chest pain, EKG changes, and serum enzyme elevation occur rarely. Increased risk in patients with prior history of ischemic heart disease.
- Renal Insufficiency: Capecitabine is contraindicated in patients with baseline creatinine clearance < 30 mL/min. A dose reduction to 75% of capecitabine should be made with baseline creatinine clearance of 30–50 mL/min.
- Reproductive: Pregnancy category D. Breast feeding should be avoided.

Initiate antiemetic protocol:	Mildly to moderately emetogenic protocol.
Supportive drugs:	☐ pegfilgrastim (Neulasta) ☐ filgrastim (Neupogen)
	☐ epoetin alfa (Procrit) ☐ darbepoetin alfa (Aranesp)
	☐ loperamide (Imodium) ☐ diphenoxylate/atropine sulfate (Lomotil)
Treatment schedule:	No chair time. Repeat cycle every 21 days until disease progression.
Estimated number of visits:	One visit per cycle. Request six cycles worth of visits.

Dose Calculation by: 1. _____   2. _____

_____

Physician

_____

Patient Name

_____

Diagnosis

_____

Date

_____

ID Number

_____ / _____ / _____

Ht   Wt   M^2

Docetaxel

Baseline laboratory tests:	CBC: Chemistry and CA 27-29
Baseline procedures or tests:	None
Initiate IV:	0.9% sodium chloride
Premedicate:	Dexamethasone 8 mg bid for 3 days, starting the day before treatment
	Oral phenothiazine or 5-HT$_3$

Administer:

Docetaxel _____ mg (100 mg/m^2) IV on day 1

Repeat cycle every 21 days

OR

Docetaxel _____ mg (35–40 mg/m^2) IV weekly for 6 weeks

Repeat every 8 weeks

- Comes in 20- or 80-mg blister packs with own diluent. Do not shake. Reconstituted vials stable at room temperature or refrigerated for 8 hours.
- Further dilute in 250 cc of D5W or 0.9% sodium chloride.
- **Use non-PVC containers and tubing to administer.**

Major Side Effects

- Hypersensitivity Reactions: Severe hypersensitivity reactions with docetaxel in 2%–3% of patients. Premedication with dexamethasone recommended.
- Bone Marrow Depression: Neutropenia is dose-limiting with nadir at days 7–10 and recovery by day 14. Thrombocytopenia and anemia also occur.
- GI Toxicities: Nausea and vomiting are mild to moderate. Mucositis and diarrhea occur in 40% of patients.
- Neuropathy: Peripheral neuropathy may affect up to 49% of patients. Sensory alterations are paresthesias in a glove-and-stocking distribution, and numbness.
- Fluid Balance: Fluid retention syndrome. Symptoms include weight gain, peripheral and/or generalized edema, pleural effusion, and ascites. Occurs in about 50% of patients. Premedication with dexamethasone effective in preventing or minimizing occurrences.
- Skin: Alopecia occurs in 80% of patients. Nail changes, rash, and dry, pruritic skin seen. Hand-foot syndrome has also been reported.
- Reproductive: Pregnancy category D. Breast feeding should be avoided.

Initiate antiemetic protocol:	Mildly to moderately emetogenic protocol.
Supportive drugs:	☐ pegfilgrastim (Neulasta) ☐ filgrastim (Neupogen)
	☐ epoetin alfa (Procrit) ☐ darbepoetin alfa (Aranesp)

Treatment schedule:

Chair time 2 hours on day 1. Repeat cycle every 21 days.

OR

Chair time 2 hours on day 1 for 6 weeks. Repeat cycle every 8 weeks.

Estimated number of visits: Two visits per cycle OR six visits per cycle. Request three cycles worth of visits.

Dose Calculation by: 1. _____   2. _____

_____

Physician

_____

Patient Name

_____

Diagnosis

_____

Date

_____

ID Number

_____ / _____ / _____

Ht   Wt   M^2

Paclitaxel

Baseline laboratory tests:	CBC: Chemistry (including Mg^{2+}) and CA 27-29
Baseline procedures or tests:	N/A
Initiate IV:	0.9% sodium chloride
Premedicate:	5-HT$_3$ and dexamethasone 10–20 mg in 100 cc of NS
	Diphenhydramine 25–50 mg and cimetidine 300 mg in 100 cc of NS

Administer: **Paclitaxel** _____ mg (175 mg/m^2) IV over 3 hours on day 1

Repeat cycle every 21 days.

OR

Paclitaxel _____ mg (80–100 mg/m^2) IV weekly for 3 weeks

Repeat cycle every 4 weeks

- Available in solution as 6 mg/mL.
- Final concentration is $\leq$ 1.2 mg/mL.
- Stable for up to 27 hours at room temperature in 0.3–1.2 mg/mL solutions.
- **Use non-PVC containers and tubing with 0.22-micron inline filter for administration.**

Major Side Effects

- Hypersensitivity Reaction: Occurs in 20%–40% of patients. Characterized by generalized skin rash, flushing, erythema, hypotension, dyspnea, and/or bronchospasm. Usually occurs within the first 2–3 minutes of infusion and almost always within the first 10 minutes. Premedicate as described.
- Bone Marrow Depression: Dose-limiting neutropenia with nadir at days 8–10 and recovery by days 15–21. Decreased incidence of neutropenia with 3-hour schedule when compared with 24-hour schedule. G-CSF support recommended.
- Neurotoxicity: Sensory neuropathy with numbness and paresthesias; dose related. More frequent with longer infusions and at doses > 175 mg/m^2.
- Hepatic: Transient elevations in serum transaminases, bilirubin, and alkaline phosphatase.
- Skin: Onycholysis with weekly dosing. Alopecia total in nearly all patients on every 3 week schedule.
- Reproductive: Pregnancy category D. Breast feeding should be avoided.

Initiate antiemetic protocol: Mildly emetogenic protocol.

Supportive drugs:
☐ pegfilgrastim (Neulasta)   ☐ filgrastim (Neupogen)
☐ epoetin alfa (Procrit)   ☐ darbepoetin alfa (Aranesp)

Treatment schedule: Chair time 4 hours on day 1. Repeat every 21 days until disease progression

OR

Chair time 2 hours on day 1 for 3 weeks. Repeat cycle every 4 weeks until disease progression.

Estimated number of visits: Two visits per cycle. Request three cycles worth of visits **OR** three visits per cycle. Request three cycles worth of visits.

Dose Calculation by: 1. _____   2. _____

_____   _____
Physician   Date

_____   _____
Patient Name   ID Number

_____   _____/ _____/ _____
Diagnosis   Ht   Wt   M^2

Vinorelbine

Baseline laboratory tests:	CBC: Chemistry and CA 27-29
Baseline procedures or tests:	N/A
Initiate IV:	0.9% sodium chloride
Premedicate:	Oral phenothiazine or 5-HT$_3$
Administer:	**Vinorelbine** _____ mg (30 mg/m^2) IV on day 1

- **Vesicant**
- Available in 1- or 5-mL single-use vials at a concentration of 10 mg/mL.
- Further dilute in syringe or IV bag to concentration of 1.5–3.0 mg/mL.
- Reconstituted solution is stable for 24 hours refrigerated.

Major Side Effects

- Hypersensitivity Reaction: Presents as dyspnea and bronchospasm.
- Bone Marrow Depression: Leukopenia is dose-limiting toxicity. Nadir at 7–10 days. Severe thrombocytopenia and anemia are uncommon.
- GI Toxicities: Nausea and vomiting are mild in IV dosing (44% incidence). Stomatitis is mild to moderate (< 20% incidence). Constipation (35%), diarrhea (17%), and anorexia (< 20%) also seen.
- Hepatic: Use with caution in patients with abnormal liver function as toxicity may be significantly enhanced.
- Hormonal: SIADH.
- Skin: Extravasation of vinorelbine may cause local tissue injury and inflammation. Alopecia observed in 10%–15% of patients.
- Neurotoxicity: Usually mild in severity and occurs much less frequently than with other vinca alkaloids.
- Reproductive: Pregnancy category D. Breast feeding should be avoided.

Initiate antiemetic protocol:	Mildly emetogenic protocol.
Supportive drugs:	☐ pegfilgrastim (Neulasta) ☐ filgrastim (Neupogen)
	☐ epoetin alfa (Procrit) ☐ darbepoetin alfa (Aranesp)
Treatment schedule:	Chair time 1 hour on day 1. Repeat cycle weekly until disease progression.
Estimated number of visits:	One visit per cycle. Request 12 cycles worth of visits.

Dose Calculation by: 1. _____   2. _____

_____   _____
Physician   Date

_____   _____
Patient Name   ID Number

_____   _____/ _____/ _____
Diagnosis   Ht   Wt   M^2

Doxorubicin

Baseline laboratory tests:	CBC: Chemistry and CA 27-29
Baseline procedures or tests:	MUGA scan
Initiate IV:	0.9% sodium chloride
Premedicate:	5-HT$_3$ and dexamethasone 10–20 mg in 100 cc of NS.
Administer:	**Doxorubicin** _____ mg (20 mg/m^2) IV on day 1 weekly

- **Potent vesicant**
- Available as a 2-mg/mL solution.
- Doxorubicin will form a precipitate if it is mixed with heparin or 5-FU.

Major Side Effects

- Bone Marrow Depression: WBC and platelet nadir 10–14 days after drug dose, with recovery from days 15–21. Myelosuppression may be severe but is less severe with weekly dosing.
- GI Toxicities: Nausea and vomiting are moderate to severe and occur in 44% of patients. Stomatitis occurs in 10% of patients but is not dose limiting.
- Hepatic: Use with caution in patients with abnormal liver function. Dose reduction necessary in the presence of liver dysfunction.
- Cardiac: Acutely, pericarditis-myocarditis syndrome may occur. With high cumulative doses > 550 mg/m^2 cardiomyopathy may occur. Increased risk of cardiotoxicity when doxorubicin is given with trastuzumab (Herceptin) or mitomycin.
- Bladder Toxicities: Red-orange discoloration of urine; resolves by 24–48 hours.
- Skin: Extravasation of doxorubicin causes severe tissue destruction. Hyperpigmentation, photosensitivity, and radiation recall occur. Complete alopecia occurs with doses > 50 mg/m^2.
- Reproductive: Pregnancy category D. Breast feeding should be avoided.

Initiate antiemetic protocol:	Moderately to highly emetogenic protocol.
Supportive drugs:	☐ pegfilgrastim (Neulasta) ☐ filgrastim (Neupogen)
	☐ epoetin alfa (Procrit) ☐ darbepoetin alfa (Aranesp)
Treatment schedule:	Chair time 1 hour on day 1. Repeat cycle weekly until progression.
Estimated number of visits:	One visit per cycle. Request eight cycles worth of visits.

Dose Calculation by: 1. _____ 2. _____

_____

Physician

_____

Date

_____

Patient Name

_____

ID Number

_____

Diagnosis

_____ / _____ / _____

Ht   Wt   M^2

Gemcitabine

Baseline laboratory tests:	CBC: Chemistry panel, LFTs, and CA 27-29
Baseline procedures or tests:	N/A
Initiate IV:	0.9% sodium chloride
Premedicate:	Oral phenothiazine
	OR
	5-HT$_3$ and Dexamethasone 10 mg in 100 cc of NS

Administer: **Gemcitabine** _____ mg (725 mg/m^2) IV weekly for 3 weeks

- Available in 1-g or 200-mg vials, reconstitute with 0.9% sodium chloride USP (5 cc for 200 mg, 25 cc for 1 g). Further dilute in 0.9% sodium chloride.
- Reconstituted solution is stable 24 hours at room temperature. DO NOT refrigerate, because precipitate will form.

Major Side Effects

- Hematologic: Leukopenia (63%), thrombocytopenia (36%), and anemia (73%), with grade 3 and 4 thrombocytopenia more common in elderly patients. Myelosuppression is dose limiting. Nadir occurs in 10–14 days, with recovery at 21 days. Prolonged infusion time (> 60 minutes) is associated with higher toxicities.
- GI Symptoms: Mild-to-moderate nausea and vomiting (70%), diarrhea, and/or mucositis (15%–20%).
- Flulike Syndrome: Fever, malaise, chills, headache, and myalgias (20%). Fever in absence of infection 6–12 hours after treatment (40%).
- Pulmonary: Mild dyspnea and drug induced pneumonitis.
- Hepatic: Transient elevation of serum transaminase and bilirubin levels.
- Skin: Pruritic, maculopapular skin rash, usually involving trunk and extremities. Edema occurs in 30% of patients. Alopecia is rare.
- Reproductive: Pregnancy category D. Breast feeding should be avoided.

Initiate antiemetic protocol:	Mildly to moderately emetogenic protocol.
Supportive drugs:	☐ pegfilgrastim (Neulasta) ☐ filgrastim (Neupogen)
	☐ epoetin alfa (Procrit) ☐ darbepoetin alfa (Aranesp)
Treatment schedule:	Chair time 1 hour weekly for 3 weeks. Repeat cycle every 28 days.
Estimated number of visits:	Three visits per cycle. Request three cycles worth of visits.

Dose Calculation by: 1. _____   2. _____

_____

Physician

_____

Patient Name

_____

Diagnosis

_____

Date

_____

ID Number

_____ / _____ / _____

Ht   Wt   M^2

Liposomal Doxorubicin (Doxil)

Baseline laboratory tests:	CBC: Chemistry and CA 27-29
Baseline procedures or tests:	MUGA scan
Initiate IV:	0.9% sodium chloride
Premedicate:	5-HT$_3$ and dexamethasone 10–20 mg in 100 cc of NS.
Administer:	**Liposomal doxorubicin _____ mg (45–60 mg/m^2) IV on day 1**

- Available as a 2-mg/mL solution in 20- or 50-mg vials.
- Further dilute drug (doses up to 90 mg) in 250 cc of D5W
- Diluted drug may be stored for 24 hours refrigerated.

Major Side Effects

- Infusion Reaction: Flushing, dyspnea, facial swelling, headache, back pain, tightness in the chest and throat, and/or hypotension. Usually occurs during first treatment and occurs in 5%–10% of patients. Resolves quickly after infusion stopped.
- Bone Marrow Depression: Dose-limiting toxicity in the treatment of patients infected with the human immunodeficiency virus. Leukopenia occurs in 91% of patients, with anemia and thrombocytopenia being less common.
- GI Toxicities: Nausea and vomiting are usually mild to moderate. Stomatitis occurs in 7% of patients and diarrhea in 8%; both are usually mild.
- Cardiac: Acutely, pericarditis and/or myocarditis, electrocardiographic changes or arrhythmias. Not dose related. With high cumulative doses > 550 mg/m^2, cardiomyopathy may occur. Increased risk of cardiotoxicity when liposomal doxorubicin is given with trastuzumab (Herceptin) or mitomycin.
- GU Toxicity: Red-orange discoloration of urine.
- Skin: Skin toxicity manifested as hand-foot syndrome with skin rash, swelling, erythema, pain, and /or desquamation. Occurs in 3.4% of patients and is dose related. Hyperpigmentation of nails, skin rash, urticaria, and radiation recall occur. Alopecia occurs in 9% of patients with Kaposi's sarcoma.
- Reproductive: Pregnancy category D. Breast feeding should be avoided.

Initiate antiemetic protocol:	Mildly to moderately emetogenic protocol.
Supportive drugs:	☐ pegfilgrastim (Neulasta) ☐ filgrastim (Neupogen)
	☐ epoetin alfa (Procrit) ☐ darbepoetin alfa (Aranesp)
Treatment schedule:	Chair time 2 hours on day 1. Repeat cycle every 21–28 days.
Estimated number of visits:	Two visits per cycle. Request four cycles worth of visits.

Dose Calculation by: 1. _____   2. _____

_____   _____
Physician   Date

_____   _____
Patient Name   ID Number

_____   _____ / _____ / _____
Diagnosis   Ht   Wt   M^2

Paclitaxel Protein-bound Particles for Injectable Suspension (Abraxane)

Baseline laboratory tests:	CBC: Chemistry and CA 27-29
Baseline procedures or tests:	N/A
Initiate IV:	0.9% sodium chloride
Premedicate:	5-HT$_3$ in 100 cc of NS
Administer:	**Paclitaxel protein-bound particles for injectable suspension** _____ mg (260 mg/m^2) IV over 30 minutes every 3 weeks

OR

Paclitaxel protein-bound particles for injectable suspension _____ mg (100 mg/m^2) IV over 30 minutes weekly for 3 weeks

- Available as a lypholized powder in 100-mg single dose vial.
- Reconstitute with 20 mL 0.9% sodium chloride. Inject over 1 minute down the inside wall of the vial to prevent foaming. Allow vial to sit for a minimum of 5 minutes to ensure proper wetting of cake. Gently swirl vial for at least 2 minutes until complete dissolution of cake/powder occurs.
- Reconstituted solution contains 5 mg/mL paclitaxel. Solution should be milkly and homogenous without visible particulates.
- Inject dose into empty sterile PVC type IV bag.
- Use of non-PVC tubing not needed, use of in-line filter not recommended.
- Use reconstituted solution immediately, discard unused portion. May be stored in refrigerator for maximum of 8 hours if needed.

Major Side Effects

- Hypersensitivity Reactions: Mild symptoms reported in 1% of patients studied.
- Hematologic: Bone marrow suppression (primarily neutropenia) is dose dependent and dose limiting toxicity.
- Neurotoxicity: Sensory neuropathy occurs frequently and is a cumulative effect. If grade 3 sensory neuropathy develops, treatment should be withheld until resolution to grade 1 or 2 followed by a dose reduction. Symptoms improve in about 22 days.
- Ocular: Visual disturbances seen in 13%, 1% severe (keratitis and blurred vision).
- Respiratory: Dyspnea and cough reported in some cases. Rare reports of interstitial pneumonia, lung fibrosis, and radiation pneumonitis.
- Cardiovascular: ECG changes common usually asymptomatic.
- Musculoskeletal: Arthralgias/myalgias common.
- Gastrointestinal: Mild to moderate nausea, vomiting, and diarrhea. Mucositis occasionally reported.
- Skin: Alopecia.
- Reproduction: Pregnancy category D.

Initiate antiemetic protocol:	Mildly to moderately emetogenic protocol.
Supportive drugs:	☐ pegfilgrastim (Neulasta) ☐ filgrastim (Neupogen)
	☐ epoetin alfa (Procrit) ☐ darbepoetin alfa (Aranesp)
Treatment schedule:	Chair time 1 hour on day 1 for 3 weeks. Repeat cycle every 4 weeks **OR** chair time 1 hour on day 1. Repeat every 21 days until disease progression.
Estimated number of visits:	Three visits per cycle. Request three cycles worth of visits.

OR

Two visits per cycle. Request three cycles worth of visits.

Dose Calculation by: 1. _____   2. _____

_____   _____

Physician   Date

_____   _____

Patient Name   ID Number

_____   _____ / _____ / _____

Diagnosis   Ht   Wt M^2

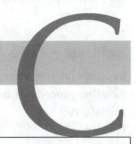
Paclitaxel: 200 mg/m^2 IV over 1 hour on day 1

Carboplatin: AUC of 6, IV on day 1

Etoposide: 50 mg alternating with 100 mg PO on days 1–10

Repeat cycle every 21 days.[85] Paclitaxel must be administered first before carboplatin

Etoposide: 100 mg/m^2 IV on days 1–5

Cisplatin: 100 mg/m^2 IV on day 1

Repeat cycle every 21 days.[86]

Cisplatin: 20 mg/m^2 IV on days 1–5

Etoposide: 100 mg/m^2 IV on days 1–5

Bleomycin: 30 units IV on days 1, 8, and 15

Repeat cycle every 21 days.[87]

Gemcitabine: 1000 mg/m^2 IV on days 1 and 8

Carboplatin: AUC 5, IV on day 1

Paclitaxel: 200 mg/m^2 IV on day 1

Repeat cycle every 21 days for four cycles.[88] This is to be followed by paclitaxel at 70 mg/m^2 IV every week for 6 weeks with a 2-week rest. Repeat for a total of three cycles.

Paclitaxel + Carboplatin + Etoposide (PCE)

Baseline laboratory tests:	CBC: Chemistry
Baseline procedures or tests:	N/A
Initiate IV:	0.9% sodium chloride
Premedicate:	5-HT$_3$ and dexamethasone 10–20 mg in 100 cc of NS on day 1
	Diphenhydramine 25–50 mg and cimetidine 300 mg in 100 cc of NS on day 1
	Oral phenothiazine or 5-HT$_3$ 30–60 minutes before etoposide on days 2–10

Administer:

Paclitaxel _____ mg (200 mg/m^2) IV over 1 hour on day 1

- Available in solution as 6 mg/mL.
- Final concentration is $\leq$ 1.2 mg/mL.
- Stable for up to 27 hours at room temperature in 0.3–1.2 mg/mL solutions.
- **Use non-PVC containers and tubing with 0.22-micron inline filter to administer.**

Carboplatin _____ mg (AUC 6) IV on day 1

- Available in solution as 10 mg/mL or as lyopholized powder.
- Reconstitute with sterile water for injection, 5% dextrose or 0.9% sodium chloride.
- Reconstituted solution stable for 8 hours at room temperature.
- Do not use aluminum needles, because precipitate will form.
- Give carboplatin **after** paclitaxel to decrease toxicities.

Etoposide 50 mg alternating with 100 mg PO days 1–10

- Oral capsules are available in 50- and 100-mg capsules and should be stored in the refrigerator.

Major Side Effects

- Hypersensitivity Reaction: Paclitaxel (30%–40%). Characterized by generalized skin rash, flushing, erythema, hypotension, dyspnea, and/or bronchospasm. Usually occurs within the first 2–3 minutes of infusion and almost always in the first 10 minutes. Premedicate as described. Increased risk of hypersensitivity reactions in patients receiving more than seven courses of carboplatin therapy.
- Bone Marrow Depression: Neutropenia, thrombocytopenia, and anemia are cumulative and dose related. Can be dose limiting. G-CSF support recommended.
- GI Toxicities: Moderate-to-severe nausea and vomiting may be acute or delayed. Oral dosing of etoposide has higher incidence of nausea/vomiting. Mucositis and/or diarrhea occur in 30%–40% of patients.
- Hepatic: Transient elevations in serum transaminases, bilirubin, and alkaline phosphatase.
- Renal: Nephrotoxicity less common than with cisplatin and rarely symptomatic.
- Electrolyte Imbalance: Decreases Mg^{2+}, K^+, Ca^{2+}, and Na^+.
- Neurotoxicity: Sensory neuropathy with numbness and paresthesias; dose related and can be dose limiting.
- Alopecia: Total loss of body hair occurs in nearly all patients.
- Reproductive: Pregnancy category D. Amenorrhea, azoospermia, impotence, and sterility.

Initiate antiemetic protocol:	Moderately to highly emetogenic protocol.
Supportive drugs:	☐ pegfilgrastim (Neulasta) ☐ filgrastim (Neupogen)
	☐ epoetin alfa (Procrit) ☐ darbepoetin alfa (Aranesp)
Treatment schedule:	Chair time 5 hours on day 1. Repeat cycle every 21 days until progression.
Estimated number of visits:	Two visits per cycle. Request four cycles worth of visits.

Dose Calculation by: 1. _____ 2. _____

_____

Physician   Date

_____   _____

Patient Name   ID Number

_____   _____/_____/_____

Diagnosis   Ht   Wt   M²

Etoposide + Cisplatin (EP)

Baseline laboratory tests:	CBC: Chemistry (including Mg^{2+})
Baseline procedures or tests:	N/A
Initiate IV:	0.9% sodium chloride
Premedicate:	$5\text{-}HT_3$ and dexamethasone 10–20 mg in 100 cc of NS
Administer:	**Etoposide** _____ mg ($100\ mg/m^2$) IV on days 1–5

- Available in 100-mg vials, when reconstituted with 5 or 10 mL of NS, D5W, or sterile water with benzyl alcohol makes a 20- or 10-mg/mL solution. Also available in solution as a 20-mg/mL concentration.
- May be further diluted in NS or D5W to a final concentration of 0.1 mg/mL.

Cisplatin _____ mg ($100\ mg/m^2$) IV on day 1

- Available in solution as 1 mg/mL.
- Do not use aluminum needles, because precipitate will form.
- Stable for 96 hours when protected from light and only 6 hours when not protected from light.
- Further dilute solution with 250 cc or more of NS.

Major Side Effects

- Hypersensitivity Reaction: Etoposide, bronchospasm, with or without fever, chills. Hypotension may occur during rapid infusion. Anaphylaxis may occur, but is rare. Cisplatin: facial edema, wheezing, bronchospasm, and hypotension.
- Bone Marrow Depression: Myelosuppression can be a dose-limiting toxicity.
- GI Toxicities: Moderate to severe nausea and vomiting. May be acute (first 24 hours) or delayed (> 24 hours). Mucositis and diarrhea are rare. Metallic taste and anorexia.
- Renal: Nephrotoxicity is dose related with cisplatin and presents at 10–20 days.
- Electrolyte Imbalance: Decreases Mg^{2+}, K^+, Ca^{2+}, Na^+, and P.
- Inappropriate secretion of antidiuretic hormone (SIADH).
- Neurotoxicity: Dose-limiting toxicity, usually in the form of peripheral sensory neuropathy. Paresthesias and numbness in a classic "stocking glove" pattern.
- Ototoxicity: High-frequency hearing loss and tinnitus.
- Secondary Malignancies: Increased risk with etoposide (especially with AML).
- Skin: Alopecia
- Reproductive: Azoospermia, impotence, and sterility. Pregnancy category D. Breast feeding should be avoided.

Initiate antiemetic protocol:	Moderately to highly emetogenic protocol.
Supportive drugs:	☐ pegfilgrastim (Neulasta) ☐ filgrastim (Neupogen)
	☐ epoetin alfa (Procrit) ☐ darbepoetin alfa (Aranesp)
Treatment schedule:	Chair time 3 hours on day 1, and 1 hour days 2–5. Repeat cycle every 21 days.
Estimated number of visits:	Six visits per cycle. Request three cycles worth of visits.

Dose Calculation by: 1. _____   2. _____

Physician _____   Date _____

Patient Name _____   ID Number _____

Diagnosis _____   _____ / _____ / _____

   Ht   Wt M^2

Cisplatin + Etoposide + Bleomycin (PEB)

Baseline laboratory tests:	CBC: Chemistry (including Mg^{2+})
Baseline procedures or tests:	Pulmonary function tests and chest x-ray studies at baseline and before each cycle of therapy.
Initiate IV:	0.9% sodium chloride
Premedicate:	5-HT_3 and dexamethasone 10–20 mg in 100 cc of NS
	Acetaminophen 30 minutes before bleomycin
Administer:	**Cisplatin** _____ mg (20 mg/m^2) IV on days 1–5

- Available in solution as 1 mg/mL.
- Do not use aluminum needles, because precipitate will form.
- Further dilute solution with 250 cc or more of NS.
- Stable for 96 hours when protected from light and only 6 hours when not protected from light.

Etoposide _____ mg (100 mg/m^2) IV on days 1–5

- Available in 100-mg vials; when reconstituted with 5 or 10 mL of NS, D5W, or sterile water with benzyl alcohol makes a 20- or 10-mg/mL solution. Also available in solution as a 20-mg/mL concentration.
- May be further diluted in NS or D5W to a final concentration of 0.1 mg/mL.

Bleomycin 30 units IV on days 1, 8, and 15

- A test dose of 2 units is recommended before the first dose to detect hypersensitivity
- Available as a powder in 15- or 30-unit sizes. Dilute powder in 0.9% sodium chloride or sterile water to maximum concentration 3 μ/mL.
- Reconstituted solution is stable for 24 hours at room temperature and 35 days if refrigerated and protected from light.

Major Side Effects

- Hypersensitivity Reaction: With bleomycin, fever and chills observed in up to 25% of patients. True anaphylactoid reactions are rare. With etoposide, bronchospasm, with or without fever, chills. Hypotension may occur during rapid infusion. Anaphylaxis may occur, but is rare. Cisplatin causes facial edema, wheezing, bronchospasm, and hypotension.
- Bone Marrow Depression: Myelosuppression can be a dose-limiting toxicity.
- GI Toxicities: Moderate-to-severe nausea and vomiting. May be acute (first 24 hours) or delayed (> 24 hours). Mucositis and diarrhea are rare. Metallic taste and anorexia.
- Pulmonary Toxicities: Pulmonary toxicity is dose limiting in bleomycin. Usually presents as pneumonitis with cough, dyspnea, dry inspiratory crackles, and infiltrates on CXR.
- Renal: Nephrotoxicity is dose related with cisplatin, presents at 10–20 days.
- Electrolyte Imbalance: Decreases Mg^{2+}, K^+, Ca^{2+}, Na^+, and P.
- Inappropriate secretion of antidiuretic hormone (SIADH).
- Neurotoxicity: Dose-limiting toxicity, usually in the form of peripheral sensory neuropathy. Paresthesias and numbness in a classic "stocking glove" pattern.
- Ototoxicity: High-frequency hearing loss and tinnitus.
- Secondary Malignancies: Increased risk with etoposide (especially AML).
- Skin: Alopecia
- Reproductive: Azoospermia, impotence, and sterility. Pregnancy category D. Breast feeding should be avoided.

Initiate antiemetic protocol:	Moderately to highly emetogenic protocol.
Supportive drugs:	☐ pegfilgrastim (Neulasta) ☐ filgrastim (Neupogen) ☐ epoetin alfa (Procrit) ☐ darbepoetin alfa (Aranesp)
Treatment schedule:	Chair time 4 hours on day 1, 1 hour days 2–5, 8, and 15. Repeat cycle every 21 days.
Estimated number of visits:	Seven visits per cycle. Request three cycles worth of visits.

Dose Calculation by: 1. _____   2. _____

_____   _____
Physician   Date

_____   _____
Patient Name   ID Number

_____   _____/_____/_____
Diagnosis   Ht   Wt M^2

Gemcitabine + Carboplatin + Paclitaxel (GCP)

Baseline laboratory tests:	CBC: Chemistry panel (including Mg^{2+}, LFTs)
Baseline procedures or tests:	N/A
Initiate IV:	0.9% sodium chloride
Premedicate:	5-HT$_3$ and dexamethasone 10–20 mg in 100 cc of NS
	Diphenhydramine 25–50 mg and cimetidine 300 mg in 100 cc of NS

Administer:

Carboplatin _____ mg (AUC 5) IV on day 1

- Available in solution as 10 mg/mL or as lyopholized powder.
- Reconstitute with sterile water for injection, 5% dextrose or 0.9% sodium chloride.
- Reconstituted solution stable for 8 hours at room temperature.
- Do not use aluminum needles, because precipitate will form.
- Give carboplatin **after** paclitaxel to decrease toxicities.

Gemcitabine _____ mg (1000 mg/m^2) IV on days 1 and 8

- Available in 1-g or 200-mg vials, reconstitute with 0.9% sodium chloride (5 cc for 200 mg and 25 cc for 1 g). Further dilute in 0.9% sodium chloride.
- Reconstituted solution is stable for 24 hours at room temperature.
- DO NOT refrigerate, because precipitate will form.

Paclitaxel _____ mg (200 mg/m^2) IV over 3 hours on day 1

Repeat cycle every 21 days for four cycles. Followed by:

Premedicate:

5-HT$_3$ and dexamethasone 10–20 mg in 100 cc of NS

Diphenhydramine 25–50 mg and cimetidine 300 mg in 100 cc of NS

Administer:

Paclitaxel _____ mg (70 mg/m^2) IV weekly for 6 weeks with a 2-week rest.

- Available in solution as 6 mg/mL.
- Final concentration is $\leq$ 1.2 mg/mL.
- Stable for up to 27 hours at room temperature in 0.3–1.2 mg/mL solutions.
- **Use non-PVC containers and tubing with 0.22-micron inline filter to administer.**

Repeat for a total of three cycles.

Major Side Effects

- Hypersensitivity Reaction: Paclitaxel (30%–40%). Characterized by generalized skin rash, flushing, erythema, hypotension, dyspnea, and/or bronchospasm. Usually occurs within the first 2–3 minutes of infusion and almost always in the first 10 minutes. Premedicate as described. Increased risk of hypersensitivity reactions in patients receiving more than seven courses of carboplatin therapy.
- Bone Marrow Depression: Neutropenia, thrombocytopenia, and anemia are cumulative and dose related. Can be dose limiting. G-CSF recommended.
- GI Toxicities: Moderate to severe nausea and vomiting, acute or delayed. Mucositis and diarrhea. Elevation of serum transaminase and bilirubin levels.
- Flulike Syndrome: Fever, malaise, chills, headache, and myalgias. Fever in absence of infection 6–12 hours after treatment.
- Hepatic: Transient elevations of serum transaminases and bilirubin.
- Renal: Nephrotoxicity less common than with cisplatin and rarely symptomatic.
- Electrolyte Imbalance: Decreases Mg^{2+}, K^+, Ca^{2+}, Na^+, and P.
- Inappropriate secretion of antidiuretic hormone (SIADH).
- Neurotoxicity: Sensory neuropathy with numbness and paresthesias dose related or can be dose limiting.
- Skin: Pruritic, maculopapular skin rash, usually involving trunk and extremities. Edema occurs in 30% of patients. Alopecia.
- Reproductive: Amenorrhea, azoospermia, impotence, and sterility. Pregnancy category D. Breast feeding should be avoided.

Initiate antiemetic protocol: Moderately to highly emetogenic protocol.

Supportive drugs: ☐ pegfilgrastim (Neulasta) ☐ filgrastim (Neupogen)
☐ epoetin alfa (Procrit) ☐ darbepoetin alfa (Aranesp)

Treatment schedule: Chair time 3 hours on day 1, and 1 hour on day 8. Repeat cycle every 21 days for four cycles. **Then** 2 hours weekly for 6 weeks. Repeat every 8 weeks for three cycles.

Estimated number of visits: Three visits per cycle; 12 visits first course. Then, 18 visits last course of treatment.

Dose Calculation by: 1. _____ 2. _____

_____
Physician   Date

_____
Patient Name   ID Number

_____
Diagnosis   Ht / Wt / M²

CARCINOID TUMORS

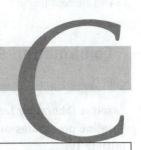

Combination Regimens

5-Fluorouracil + Streptozocin 134

5-Fluorouracil: 400 mg/m^2/day IV on days 1–5
Streptozocin: 500 mg/m^2/day IV on days 1–5
Repeat cycle every 6 weeks.[1,89]

Doxorubicin + Streptozocin 135

Doxorubicin: 50 mg/m^2 IV on days 1 and 22
Streptozocin: 500 mg/m^2/day IV on days 1–5
Repeat cycle every 6 weeks.[1,89]

Cisplatin + Etoposide 136

Cisplatin: 45 mg/m^2/day IV continuous infusion on days 2 and 3
Etoposide: 130 mg/m^2/day IV continuous infusion on days 1–3
Repeat cycle every 21 days.[1,90]

Single-Agent Regimens

Octreotide; Sandostatin LAR 137

Octreotide: 150–250 µg SC tid or
Sandostatin LAR: 20–40 mg IM every 4 weeks
Continue until disease progression[1,91–93]

Combination Regimens

5-Fluorouracil + Streptozocin

Baseline laboratory tests:	CBC: Chemistry and CA 19-9, creatinine clearance
Baseline procedures or tests:	N/A
Initiate IV:	0.9% sodium chloride
Premedicate:	5-HT$_3$ and dexamethasone 10–20 mg in 100 cc of normal saline (NS)
Administer:	**Fluorouracil** _____ mg (400 mg/m^2/day) IV on days 1–5

- Available 10 mg/mL. No dilution required. Can be further diluted with 0.9% sodium chloride or 5% dextrose and water (D5W).

Streptozocin _____ mg (500 mg/m^2) IV over 1 hour on days 1–5 omit if CrC < 60 mL/min

- 1 gm vial, reconstitute with sterile water or 0.9% sodium chloride
- Reconstituted solution is stable for 48 hours at room temperature, and 96 hours refrigerated.
- Irritant; avoid contact with skin and extravasation
- Administer with 1–2 L of hydration to avoid renal toxicity.

Major Side Effects

- Renal: Renal toxicity is dose limiting. Renal dysfunction occurs in 60% of patients receiving streptozocin. Usually transient proteinuria and azotemia, but may progress to permanent renal failure.
- Bone Marrow Depression: Myelosuppression occurs in about 9%–20% of patients with nadir at 7–14 days. Occasionally, severe leucopenia and thrombocytopenia occur. Mild anemia may occur.
- Gastrointestinal (GI) Toxicities: Nausea and vomiting occur in up to 90% of patients beginning 1–4 hours after administration. May worsen during 5-consecutive-day therapy.
- Skin: Hyperpigmentation, photosensitivity, and nail changes may occur. Hand-foot syndrome can be dose limiting.
- Blood Glucose Levels: Hypoglycemia (20%) or hyperglycemia may occur.
- Ocular: Photophobia, increased lacrimation, conjunctivitis, and blurred vision.

Initiate antiemetic protocol:	Moderately to highly emetogenic protocol.
Supportive drugs:	☐ pegfilgrastim (Neulasta) ☐ filgrastim (Neupogen) ☐ epoetin alfa (Procrit) ☐ darbepoetin alfa (Aranesp)
Treatment schedule:	Chair time 2 hours on days 1–5. Repeat cycle every 6 weeks as tolerated.
Estimated number of visits:	Five visits per treatment cycle. Request six cycles for complete treatment.

Dose Calculation by: 1. _____   2. _____

_____

Physician

_____

Patient Name

_____

Diagnosis

_____

Date

_____

ID Number

_____ / _____ / _____
Ht   Wt   M^2

Doxorubicin + Streptozocin

Baseline laboratory tests:	CBC: Chemistry, creatinine clearance
Baseline procedures or tests:	MUGA scan
Initiate IV:	0.9% sodium chloride
Premedicate:	5-HT$_3$ and dexamethasone 10–20 mg in 100 cc of NS.
Administer:	**Doxorubicin** _____ mg (50 mg/m^2) IV push on days 1 and 22

- Potent vesicant
- Available as a 2-mg/mL solution.
- Doxorubicin will form a precipitate if it is mixed with heparin or 5-FU.

Streptozocin _____ mg (500 mg/m^2/day) IV days 1–5 omit if CrC < 60 mL/min

- 1-g vial; reconstitute with sterile water or NS.
- Reconstituted solution is stable for 48 hours at room temperature, and 96 hours refrigerated.
- Irritant: Avoid contact with skin or extravasation.
- Administer with 1–2 L of hydration to avoid renal toxicity.

Major Side Effects

- Bone Marrow Depression: White blood cell (WBC) and platelet nadir 10–14 days after drug dose, with recovery from days 15–21. Myelosuppression may be severe.
- Renal: Renal toxicity is dose limiting. Renal dysfunction occurs in 60% of patients receiving streptozocin. Usually transient proteinuria and azotemia, but may progress to permanent renal failure.
- GI Toxicities: Nausea and vomiting is moderate to severe with doxorubicin. May worsen during 5-consecutive-day therapy of streptozocin. Stomatitis occurs in 10% of patients but is not dose limiting.
- Cardiac: Acutely, pericarditis-myocarditis syndrome may occur. With high cumulative doses < 450 mg/m^2, cardiomyopathy may occur.
- Skin: Extravasation of doxorubicin causes severe tissue destruction; irritation of tissue if streptozocin is extravasated. Hyperpigmentation, photosensitivity, and radiation recall occur. Complete alopecia occurs with doxorubicin doses < 50 mg/m^2.
- Blood Glucose Levels: Hypoglycemia (20%) or hyperglycemia may occur.
- Reproduction: Doxorubicin is teratogenic, mutagenic, and carcinogenic.

Initiate antiemetic protocol:	Moderately to highly emetogenic protocol.
Supportive drugs:	☐ pegfilgrastim (Neulasta) ☐ filgrastim (Neupogen)
	☐ epoetin alfa (Procrit) ☐ darbepoetin alfa (Aranesp)
Treatment schedule:	Chair time 2 hours on days 1–5, and 1 hour on day 22. Repeat cycle every 6 weeks.
Estimated number of visits:	One visit per cycle. Request four cycles for complete treatment.

Dose Calculation by: 1. _____   2. _____

_____
Physician

_____
Date

_____
Patient Name

_____
ID Number

_____
Diagnosis

_____ / _____ / _____
Ht   Wt   M^2

Cisplatin + Etoposide

Baseline laboratory tests:	CBC: Chemistry (including Mg^{2+})
Baseline procedures or tests:	Central line placement
Initiate IV:	0.9% sodium chloride
Premedicate:	5-HT$_3$ and dexamethasone 10–20 mg in 100 cc of NS
Administer:	**Etoposide** _____mg (130 mg/m^2/day) IV continuous infusion on days 1–3

- Stable for 96 hours at concentration 0.2 mg/mL.
- Available in 100-mg vials, when reconstituted with 5 or 10 mL of NS, D5W, or sterile water with benzyl alcohol, makes a 20- or 10-mg/mL solution. Also available in solution as a 20-mg/mL concentration.
- May be further diluted in NS or D5W to a final concentration of 0.1 mg/mL.

Cisplatin _____mg (45 mg/m^2/day) IV continuous infusion on days 2 and 3

- Stable for 96 hours when protected from light and only 6 hours if not protected from light.
- Do not use aluminum needles, as precipitate will form.
- Available in solution as 1 mg/mL.
- Further dilute solution with 250 cc or more of NS.

Major Side Effects

- Allergic Reaction: Bronchospasm, with or without fever, chills. Hypotension may occur during rapid infusion of etoposide. Anaphylaxis may occur but is rare.
- Bone Marrow Depression: Myelosuppression can be a dose-limiting toxicity.
- GI Toxicities: Moderate-to-severe nausea and vomiting. May be acute (first 24 hours) or delayed (> 24 hours). Mucositis and diarrhea are rare.
- Renal: Nephrotoxicity is dose related and with cisplatin presents at 10–20 days.
- Electrolyte Imbalance: Decreases Mg^{2+}, K, Ca^{2+}, Na, and P.
- Neurotoxicity: Dose-limiting toxicity, usually in the form of peripheral sensory neuropathy. Paresthesias and numbness in a classic "stocking glove" pattern.
- Ototoxicity: High-frequency hearing loss and tinnitus.
- Skin: Alopecia
- Reproduction: Drugs are mutagenic and teratogenic.

Initiate antiemetic protocol:	Moderately to highly emetogenic protocol.
Supportive drugs:	☐ pegfilgrastim (Neulasta) ☐ filgrastim (Neupogen)
	☐ epoetin alfa (Procrit) ☐ darbepoetin alfa (Aranesp)
Treatment schedule:	Chair time 1 hour on days 1–3. Discontinue pump day 4. Repeat cycle every 21 days.
Estimated number of visits:	Four visits per cycle. Request three cycles worth of visits. May require extra days for hydration.

Dose Calculation by: 1. _____   2. _____

_____

Physician

_____

Date

_____

Patient Name

_____

ID Number

_____

Diagnosis

_____/ _____/ _____

Ht   Wt   M^2

Single-Agent Regimens

Octreotide or Sandostatin LAR Depot (Octreotide acetate injectable suspension)

Baseline laboratory tests:	CBC: Chemistry, liver function tests (LFTs), thyroid function, 5–HIAA (urinary 5-hydroxyindole acetic acid) GH and IGF–1
Baseline procedures or tests:	CAT scan, PET scan
Initiate IV:	N/A
Premedicate:	None required

Administer: **Octreotide** 150–250 μg SC tid

- Available in 1- or 5-mL multidose vials. 50 mcg → 5000 mcg/mL.
- Patient may develop pain, stinging, tingling, or burning sensation at injection site, with redness and swelling.
- May change to long-acting depot if condition is already controlled on immediate-release preparation, or in a new patient, after response is assessed after 2 weeks of immediate-release dosing.

Or Administer: **Sandostatin** LAR 20–30 mg IM in gluteal muscle once per month

- Available in 10-, 20-, or 30-mg single dose kits.
- Closely follow mixing instructions, change the needle after mixing, administer immediately after changing the needle.
- Must be given deep IM in gluteal muscle, never given IV or SC.
- Patients should receive an initial trial of octreotide acetate subcutaneously to develop tolerability before starting Sandostatin LAR.
- Starting dose of 20 mg deep IM monthly for 3 months.
- Dose adjustment after 3 months based on the following criteria
  - GH < 2.5 ng/ml, IGF–1 normal and clinical symptoms controlled: maintain Sandostatin LAR at 20 mg every 4 weeks.
  - GH > 2.5 ng/ml, IGF–1 elevated and clinical symptoms uncontrolled: increase Sandostatin LAR to 30 mg every 4 weeks.
  - GH < 1 ng/ml, IGF–1 normal and clinical symptoms controlled: reduce Sandostatin LAR at 20 mg every 4 weeks.
  - Patients whose GH, IGF-1 and symptoms are not adequately controlled at a dose of 30 mg may increase to 40 mg every 4 weeks. Doses higher than 40 mg are not recommended.

Major Side Effects

- Nutrition: Transient hypoglycemia or hyperglycemia due to altered balance between hormones regulating serum glucose (insulin, glucagons, growth hormone); occurs rarely.
- Hypothyroidism has been reported. Baseline and periodic assessment of thyroid function is recommended.
- GI Toxicities: Nausea, vomiting, diarrhea, flatulence, and abdominal pain or discomfort occur in 27%–38% of patients.
- Other: Rarely, a patient may experience lightheadedness, dizziness, fatigue, pedal edema, headache, flushing of the face, weakness.
- Pain at injection site with Sandostatin LAR depot.

Initiate antiemetic protocol:	Mildly emetogenic protocol prn.
Supportive drugs:	☐ loperamide (Imodium) ☐ diphenoxylate/atropine sulfate (Lomotil)
Treatment schedule:	No chair time. Self administration of injections TID as tolerated. For patients receiving Sandostatin LAR: every 4-week appointments for injection
Estimated number of visits:	Monthly during treatment.

Dose Calculation by: 1. _____ 2. _____

_____

Physician _____ Date _____

_____

Patient Name _____ ID Number _____

_____

Diagnosis _____ Ht _____ / Wt _____ / M² _____

CERVICAL CANCER

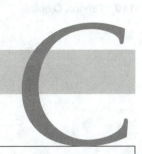

Combination Regimens

Radiation therapy: 1.8 to 2 Gy per fraction (total dose, 45 Gy)
Cisplatin: 40 mg/m^2 IV weekly (maximal dose, 70 mg/wk)
Cisplatin is given 4 hours before radiation therapy on weeks 1–6.[1,94]

Paclitaxel: 135 mg/m^2 IV over 24 hours on day 1
Cisplatin: 75 mg/m^2 IV on day 2
Repeat cycle every 21 days.[1,95]

Cisplatin: 50 mg/m^2 IV on day 1
Topotecan: 0.75 mg/m^2/day IV on days 1–3
Repeat cycle every 21 days.[1,95]

Bleomycin: 30 U IV over 24 hours on day 1
Ifosfamide: 5000 mg/m^2 IV over 24 hours on day 2
Mesna: 6000 mg/m^2 IV over 36 hours on day 2
Cisplatin: 50 mg/m^2 IV on day 2
Repeat cycle every 21 days.[1,96]

Bleomycin: 30 U IV on day 1
Ifosfamide: 2000 mg/m^2 IV on days 1–3
Mesna: 400 mg/m^2 IV, 15 minutes before ifosfamide dose,
then 400 mg/m^2 IV at 4 and 8 hours after ifosfamide
Carboplatin: 200 mg/m^2 IV on day 1
Repeat cycle every 21 days.[1,97]

Cisplatin: 75 mg/m^2 IV on day 1
5-Fluorouracil: 1000 mg/m^2 IV continuous infusion on days 2–5
Repeat cycle every 21 days.[1,98]

Cisplatin + Vinorelbine 150

Cisplatin: 80 mg/m^2 IV on day 1
Vinorelbine: 25 mg/m^2 IV on days 1 and 8
Repeat cycle every 21 days.[1,99]

Cisplatin + Irinotecan 151

Cisplatin: 60 mg/m^2 IV on day 1
Irinotecan: 60 mg/m^2 IV on days 1, 8, and 15
Repeat cycle every 28 days.[1,100]

MOBP 152

Mitomycin: 10 mg/m^2 IV on day 1
Vincristine: 0.5 mg/m^2 IV on days 1 and 4
Bleomycin: 30 U/day IV continuous infusion on days 1–4
Cisplatin: 50 mg/m^2 IV on days 1 and 22
Repeat cycle every 6 weeks.[1,101]

Single-Agent Regimens

Cisplatin 154

Cisplatin: 50–100 mg/m^2 IV on day 1
Repeat cycle every 21 days.[1,102]

Docetaxel 155

Docetaxel: 100 mg/m^2 IV on day 1
Repeat cycle every 21 days.[1,103]

Paclitaxel 156

Paclitaxel: 175 mg/m^2 IV over 3 hours on day 1
Repeat cycle every 21 days.[1,104]

Irinotecan 157

Irinotecan: 125 mg/m^2 IV weekly for 4 weeks
Repeat cycle every 6 weeks.[1,105]

Vinorelbine 158

Vinorelbine: 30 mg/m^2 IV weekly

Repeat cycle every week up to 12 cycles, to be followed by surgery or radiation therapy.[1,106]

Topotecan 159

Topotecan: 1.5 mg/m^2/day on days 1–5

Repeat cycle every 21 days.[1,107]

Combination Regimens

Cisplatin + Radiation Therapy

Baseline laboratory tests:	CBC: Chemistry panel (including Mg^{2+})
Baseline procedures or tests:	N/A
Initiate IV:	0.9% sodium chloride
Premedicate:	5-HT$_3$ and dexamethasone 10–20 mg in 100 cc of NS before cisplatin therapy
Administer:	**Radiation therapy:** 1.8 to 2 Gy per fraction (total dose, 45 Gy)

Cisplatin _____ mg (40 mg/m^2) IV weekly (maximal dose is 70 mg/wk)

- Available in 100-mg vials, 1 mg/mL
- Do not use aluminum needles, because precipitate will form.
- Further dilute solution with 250–1000 cc NS.
- Stable for 24 hours at room temperature.

Cisplatin is given 4 hours before radiation therapy on weeks 1–6.

Major Side Effects	- Bone Marrow Toxicity: WBCs, platelets, and red blood cells equally affected at lower doses.
	- GI Toxicities: Moderate-to-severe nausea and vomiting may be acute or delayed. Diarrhea can be severe.
	- Renal: Nephrotoxicity is dose related and with cisplatin presents at 10–20 days. Vigorous hydration before and after treatment required.
	- Electrolyte Imbalance: Decreases Mg^{2+}, K, Ca^{2+}, Na, and P.
	- Skin: Local tissue irritation progressing to desquamation can occur in radiation field. Do not use oil-based lotions or creams in radiation field. Alopecia.
	- Neurotoxicity: Peripheral sensory neuropathy; increased risk with cumulative doses.
	- Ototoxicity: High-frequency hearing loss and tinnitus.
Initiate antiemetic protocol:	Moderately emetogenic protocol.
Supportive drugs:	☐ pegfilgrastim (Neulasta) ☐ filgrastim (Neupogen)
	☐ epoetin alfa (Procrit) ☐ darbepoetin alfa (Aranesp)
Treatment schedule:	Chair time: 1–4 hours weekly for 6 weeks
Estimated number of visits:	Six visits per treatment course. May need more visits if patient needs hydration for nausea and vomiting.

Dose Calculation by: 1. _____ 2. _____

Physician	Date
Patient Name	ID Number
Diagnosis	Ht _____ / Wt _____ / M^2 _____

Paclitaxel + Cisplatin

Baseline laboratory tests:	CBC: Chemistry (including Mg^{2+})
Baseline procedures or tests:	Central line placement
Initiate IV:	0.9% sodium chloride
Premedicate:	5-HT$_3$ and dexamethasone 10–20 mg in 100 cc of NS (days 1 and 2)
	Diphenhydramine 25–50 mg and cimetidine 300 mg in 100 cc of NS (day 1 only)

Administer:

Paclitaxel _____mg (135 mg/m^2) IV over 24 hours on day 1

- Available in 30- and 300-mg vials 6m/mL and 100-mg vial 16.7 mg/mL.
- Further dilute in NS or D5W for final concentration < 1.2 mg/ml.
- **Use non-PVC containers and tubing with 0.22-micron inline filter for administration.**
- Stable for up to 27 hours at room temperature in 0.3–1.2 mg/mL solutions.

Cisplatin _____mg (75 mg/m^2) IV on day 2

- Available in 1-mg/mL concentrations.
- Further dilute solution with 250 cc or more of NS.
- Do not use aluminum needles, because precipitate will form.
- Stable for 96 hours when protected from light and only 6 hours when not protected from light.

Major Side Effects

- Hypersensitivity Reaction: Occurs in 20%–40% of patients. Characterized by generalized skin rash, flushing, erythema, hypotension, dyspnea, and/or bronchospasm. Usually occurs within the first 2–3 minutes of infusion and almost always within the first 10 minutes. Premedicate as described.
- Bone Marrow Depression: Neutropenia, thrombocytopenia, and anemia are cumulative and dose related. Can be dose limiting. G-CSF support recommended.
- GI Toxicities: Moderate-to-severe nausea and vomiting may be acute or delayed.
- Renal: Nephrotoxicity is dose related and with cisplatin presents at 10–20 days.
- Electrolyte Imbalance: Decreases Mg^{2+}, K, Ca^{2+}, Na, and P.
- Neurotoxicity: Sensory neuropathy with numbness and paresthesias; dose related.
- Alopecia: Total loss of body hair occurs in nearly all patients.

Initiate antiemetic protocol:	Moderately to highly emetogenic protocol.
Supportive drugs:	☐ pegfilgrastim (Neulasta) ☐ filgrastim (Neupogen)
	☐ epoetin alfa (Procrit) ☐ darbepoetin alfa (Aranesp)
Treatment schedule:	Chair time 1 hour on day 1, and 3 hours on day 2. Repeat every 21 days as tolerated or until disease progression.
Estimated number of visits:	Three visits per cycle. Request three cycles worth of visits.

Dose Calculation by: 1. _____ 2. _____

_____
Physician

_____
Date

_____
Patient Name

_____
ID Number

_____
Diagnosis

_____ / _____ / _____
Ht   Wt   M^2

Cisplatin + Topotecan

Baseline laboratory tests:	CBC: Chemistry (including Mg^{2+})
Baseline procedures or tests:	N/A
Initiate IV:	0.9% sodium chloride
Premedicate:	5-HT_3 and dexamethasone 10–20 mg in 100 cc of NS
Administer:	**Cisplatin** _____mg (50 mg/m^2) IV over 1–3 hours on day 1

- Do not use aluminum needles, because precipitate will form.
- Available in solution as 1 mg/mL.
- Further dilute solution with 250 cc or more of NS.
- Stable for 96 hours when protected from light and only 6 hours when not protected from light.

Topotecan _____mg (0.75 mg/m^2/day) IV on days 1–3

- Available as a 4-mg vial.
- Reconstitute vial with 4 mL of sterile water for injection.
- Further dilute in NS or D5W.
- Use immediately.

Major Side Effects

- Bone Marrow Depression: Myelosuppression can be severe, dose-limiting toxicity. May need dose reductions for severe neutropenia.
- GI Toxicities: Moderate-to-severe nausea and vomiting. May be acute (first 24 hours) or delayed (> 24 hours). Diarrhea or constipation possible. Abdominal pain not unusual.
- Hepatic Toxicities: Evidence of increased drug toxicity in patients with low protein and hepatic dysfunction. Dose reductions may be necessary.
- Renal: Nephrotoxicity is dose related and with cisplatin presents at 10–20 days. Use with caution in patients with abnormal renal function. Dose reduction is necessary in this setting.
- Electrolyte Imbalance: Decreases Mg^{2+}, K, Ca^{2+}, Na, and P.
- Neurotoxicity: Dose-limiting toxicity, usually in the form of peripheral sensory neuropathy. Paresthesias and numbness in a classic "stocking glove" pattern.
- Ototoxicity: High-frequency hearing loss and tinnitus.
- Skin: Alopecia.
- Reproduction: Cisplatin is mutagenic and probably teratogenic.

Initiate antiemetic protocol:	Moderately to highly emetogenic protocol.
Supportive drugs:	☐ pegfilgrastim (Neulasta) ☐ filgrastim (Neupogen)
	☐ epoetin alfa (Procrit) ☐ darbepoetin alfa (Aranesp)
Treatment schedule:	Chair time 3 hours on day 1, and 1 hour on days 2 and 3. Repeat cycle every 21 days. CBC weekly.
Estimated number of visits:	Four visits per cycle. Request six cycles worth of visits.

Dose Calculation by: 1. _____ 2. _____

_____
Physician

_____
Patient Name

_____
Diagnosis

_____
Date

_____
ID Number

_____/ _____/ _____
Ht   Wt   M^2

Bleomycin + Ifosfamide + Mesna + Cisplatin (BIP)

Baseline laboratory tests:	CBC: Chemistry (including Mg^{2+})
Baseline procedures or tests:	Central line placement, pulmonary function tests (PFTs), chest x-ray study (CXR)
Initiate IV:	0.9% sodium chloride
Premedicate:	Acetaminophen 325–500 mg^2 PO before bleomycin
	5-HT_3 and dexamethasone 10–20 mg in 100 cc of NS

Administer:

Bleomycin 30 units IV over 24 hours on day 1

- Test dose of 2 units SC or IM before first dose.
- Stable at room temperature for 24 hours and 35 days if refrigerated and protected from light. Maximum concentration 3 μ/mL.
- Available powder in 15- or 30-unit doses.
- Reconstitute powder with 0.9% sodium chloride or sterile water 3–10 mls.
- Do not reconstitute with dextrose-containing solutions.

Ifosfamide _____mg (5000 mg/m^2) IV over 24 hours on day 2

- Reconstitute powder with sterile water for injection; discard unused portion after 8 hours. 50 mg/mL final concentration.
- May further dilute in D5W or 0.9% sodium chloride.

Mesna _____mg (6000 mg/m^2) IV over 36 hours on day 2

- Diluted solution is stable for 24 hours at room temperature.

Cisplatin _____mg (50 mg/m^2) IV infusion on day 2

- Available in 100-mL vials. 1-mg/1-mL concentration.
- Stable for 96 hours when protected from light and only 6 hours when not protected from light.
- Do not use aluminum needles, because precipitate will form.
- Further dilute solution with 250–1000 cc or more of NS.

Major Side Effects

- Hypersensitivity Reaction: Fever and chills in 25% of patients. True anaphylactoid reactions are rare; more common in lymphoma patients.
- Bone Marrow Depression: Myelosuppression cumulative and dose limiting.
- GI Toxicities: Moderate-to-severe nausea and vomiting may be acute or delayed. Mucositis and/or diarrhea occurs in 30%–40% of patients.
- Pulmonary Toxicities: Pneumonitis seen in 10% of patients with cough, rales, dyspnea, and infiltrates on CXR. May progress to irreversible pulmonary fibrosis in 1% of patients.
- Renal: Nephrotoxicity and/or hemorrhagic cystitis may be dose limiting.
- Electrolyte Imbalance: Decreases Mg^{2+}, K, Ca^{2+}, Na, and P.
- Neurotoxicity: Sensory neuropathy with numbness and paresthesias.
- CNS: Somnolence, confusion, depressive psychosis, or hallucinations. Incidence may be higher in patients with decreased renal function.
- Skin: Erythema, rash, striae, hyperpigmentation, vesiculation, hyperkeratosis, nail changes, skin peeling, macular rash, and urticaria. Alopecia.
- Reproduction: Do not use in pregnancy. Mutagenic, teratogenic, and carcinogenic.

Initiate antiemetic protocol:	Moderately to highly emetogenic protocol.
Supportive drugs:	☐ pegfilgrastim (Neulasta) ☐ filgrastim (Neupogen)
	☐ epoetin alfa (Procrit) ☐ darbepoetin alfa (Aranesp)
Treatment schedule:	Chair time 1 hour on day 1, and 3 hours on day 2. Repeat cycle every 21 days.
Estimated number of visits:	Three visits per cycle. Request three cycles worth of visits.

Dose Calculation by: 1. _____ 2. _____

_____   _____
Physician   Date

_____   _____
Patient Name   ID Number

_____   _____ / _____ / _____
Diagnosis   Ht   Wt   M²

Bleomycin + Ifosfamide + Mesna + Carboplatin (BIC)

Baseline laboratory tests:	CBC: Chemistry (including Mg^{2+})
Baseline procedures or tests:	Pulmonary Function Tests (PFTs), CXR
Initiate IV:	0.9% sodium chloride
Premedicate:	Acetaminophen 325–500 mg^2 PO before bleomycin
	5-HT_3 and dexamethasone 10–20 mg in 100 cc of NS
Administer:	**Bleomycin** 30 units IV over 10 minutes on day 1

- Test dose of 2 units SC or IM before first dose.
- Stable at room temperature for 24 hours and 35 days if refrigerated and protected from light. Maximum concentration 3 μ/mL.
- Available powder in 15- or 30-unit doses.
- Reconstitute powder with 0.9% sodium chloride or sterile water.
- Do not reconstitute with dextrose-containing solutions.

Ifosfamide _____mg (2000 mg/m^2) IV on days 1–3

- Reconstitute powder with sterile water for injection; discard unused portion after 8 hours.
- May further dilute in D5W or 0.9% sodium chloride.

Mesna _____mg (400 mg/m^2) IV 15 minutes before and 4 and 8 hours after ifosfamide.

- Diluted solution is stable for 24 hours at room temperature. Refrigerate and use reconstituted solution within 6 hours.

Carboplatin _____mg (200 mg/m^2) IV infusion over 30–60 minutes on day 1

- Available as powder in 50-, 150-, and 450-mg vial or as solution. 10 mg/mL
- Reconstitute powder with sterile water, D5W, or NS for injection.
- Reconstituted solution stable at room temperature for 8 hours.

Major Side Effects	

- Hypersensitivity Reaction: Fever and chills in 25% of patients. True anaphylactic reactions with bleomycin are rare; more common in lymphoma patients. Increased risk of reaction with carboplatin after $\geq$ 7 doses are received.
- Bone Marrow Depression: Myelosuppression cumulative and dose limiting.
- GI Toxicities: Moderate-to-severe nausea and vomiting may be acute or delayed. Mild diarrhea may occur.
- Pulmonary Toxicities: Pneumonitis seen in 10% of patients with cough, rales, dyspnea, and infiltrates on CXR. May progress to irreversible pulmonary fibrosis in 1% of patients. Increased incidence in patients > 70 and with cumulative doses > 400 units.
- Renal: Nephrotoxicity and/or hemorrhagic cystitis possible.
- Electrolyte Imbalance: Decreases Mg^{2+}, K, Ca^{2+}, and Na.
- Neurotoxicity: Sensory neuropathy with numbness and SIADH paresthesias (< 10%)
- CNS: Somnolence, confusion, depressive psychosis, or hallucinations. Incidence may be higher in patients with decreased renal function.
- Skin: Erythema, rash, striae, hyperpigmentation, vesiculation, hyperkeratosis, nail changes, skin peeling, macular rash, urticaria. Alopecia.
- Reproduction: Do not use in pregnancy. Mutagenic, teratogenic, and carcinogenic.

Initiate antiemetic protocol:	Moderately to highly emetogenic protocol.
Supportive drugs:	☐ pegfilgrastim (Neulasta) ☐ filgrastim (Neupogen)
	☐ epoetin alfa (Procrit) ☐ darbepoetin alfa (Aranesp)
Treatment schedule:	Chair time 4 hours on day 1, and 3 hours on days 2 and 3. Repeat cycle every 21 days.
Estimated number of visits:	Three visits per cycle. Request three cycles worth of visits.

Dose Calculation by: 1. _____   2. _____

Physician _____   Date _____

Patient Name _____   ID Number _____

Diagnosis _____   _____/_____/_____
                                           Ht   Wt   M^2

Cisplatin + 5-Fluorouracil

Baseline laboratory tests:	CBC: Chemistry (including Mg^{2+})
Baseline procedures or tests:	Central line placement
Initiate IV:	0.9% sodium chloride
Premedicate:	5-HT$_3$ and dexamethasone 10–20 mg in 100 cc of NS
Administer:	**Cisplatin** _____ mg (75 mg/m^2) IV infusion on day 1

- Stable for 96 hours when protected from light and only 6 hours when not protected from light.
- Do not use aluminum needles, because precipitate will form.
- Further dilute solution with 250–1000 cc of NS.

5-Fluorouracil _____ mg (1000 mg/m^2) IV continuous infusion days 2–5

- No dilution required.
- May be further diluted with NS or D5W.

Major Side Effects

- Bone Marrow Depression: Neutropenia, thrombocytopenia, and anemia are dose related.
- GI Toxicities: Moderate to severe nausea and vomiting may be acute or delayed. Mucositis and diarrhea can be severe and dose limiting.
- Renal: Nephrotoxicity is dose related and with cisplatin presents at 10–20 days.
- Electrolyte Imbalance: Decreases Mg^{2+}, K, Ca^{2+}, Na, and P.
- Skin: Hyperpigmentation, photosensitivity, and nail changes may occur. Hand-foot syndrome can be dose limiting.
- Ocular: Photophobia, increased lacrimation, conjunctivitis, and blurred vision.

Initiate antiemetic protocol:	Moderately to highly emetogenic protocol.
Supportive drugs:	☐ pegfilgrastim (Neulasta) ☐ filgrastim (Neupogen)
	☐ epoetin alfa (Procrit) ☐ darbepoetin alfa (Aranesp)
Treatment schedule:	Chair time 3 hours on day 1, and 1 hour on day 2. Repeat cycle every 21 days.
Estimated number of visits:	Two visits per cycle. Ask for three cycles worth of visits.

Dose Calculation by: 1. _____   2. _____

_____
Physician

_____
Patient Name

_____
Diagnosis

_____
Date

_____
ID Number

_____ / _____ / _____
Ht   Wt   M^2

Cisplatin + Vinorelbine

Baseline laboratory tests:	CBC: Chemistry (including Mg^{2+})
Baseline procedures or tests:	N/A
Initiate IV:	0.9% sodium chloride
Premedicate:	5-HT$_3$ and dexamethasone 10–20 mg in 100 cc of NS
Administer:	**Cisplatin** _____mg (80 mg/m^2) IV on day 1

- Stable for 96 hours when protected from light and only 6 hours when not protected from light.
- Do not use aluminum needles, because precipitate will form.
- Available as 1-mg/mL solution.
- Further dilute in 250–1000 cc 0.9% sodium chloride.

Vinorelbine _____mg (25 mg/m^2) IV on days 1 and 8

- **Vesicant**
- Available in 1- or 5-mL single-use vials at a concentration of 10 mg/mL.
- Further dilute in syringe or IV bag to concentration of 1.5–3.0 mg/mL.
- Infuse over 6–10 minutes into sidearm port of freely flowing IV infusion, either peripherally or via central line. Use port CLOSEST TO THE IV BAG, not to the patient.
- Flush vein with at least 75–125 mL of IV fluid after drug infusion.
- Reconstituted solution is stable for 24 hours refrigerated.

Major Side Effects

- Bone Marrow Depression: Neutropenia, thrombocytopenia, and anemia are dose related and can be dose limiting.
- GI Toxicities: Moderate-to-severe nausea and vomiting may be acute or delayed. Constipation, diarrhea, stomatitis, and anorexia may be seen.
- Renal: Nephrotoxicity is dose related and with cisplatin presents at 10–20 days.
- Electrolyte Imbalance: Decreases Mg^{2+}, K, Ca^{2+}, Na, and P.
- Skin: Extravasation of vinorelbine may cause local tissue injury and inflammation. Alopecia likely.
- Musculoskeletal: Jaw pain, myalgia, and arthralgia.
- Respiratory: Dyspnea and hypersensitivity reaction.
- Neurotoxicity: Usually mild paresthesia and hypesthesia in severity and occurs much less frequently than with other vinca alkaloids.

Initiate antiemetic protocol:	Moderately to highly emetogenic protocol.
Supportive drugs:	☐ pegfilgrastim (Neulasta) ☐ filgrastim (Neupogen)
	☐ epoetin alfa (Procrit) ☐ darbepoetin alfa (Aranesp)
Treatment schedule:	Chair time 3 hours on day 1, and 1 hour on day 8. Repeat cycle every 21 days.
Estimated number of visits:	Three visits per cycle. Request three cycles worth of visits.

Dose Calculation by: 1. _____   2. _____

_____
Physician

_____
Date

_____
Patient Name

_____
ID Number

_____
Diagnosis

_____ / _____ / _____
Ht   Wt   M^2

Cisplatin + Irinotecan

Baseline laboratory tests:	CBC: Chemistry (including Mg^{2+})
Baseline procedures or tests:	N/A
Initiate IV:	0.9% sodium chloride
Premedicate:	5-HT$_3$ and dexamethasone 10–20 mg in 100 cc of NS
Administer:	**Cisplatin** _____ mg (60 mg/m^2) IV over 1–3 hours on day 1

- Stable for 96 hours when protected from light and only 6 hours when not protected from light.
- Do not use aluminum needles, because precipitate will form.
- Available in solution as 1 mg/mL.
- Further dilute solution with 250–1000 cc NS.

Irinotecan _____ mg (60 mg/m^2) IV on days 1, 8, and 15

- Available in 2- and 5-ml vials (20 mg/ml).
- Store at room temperature and protect from light.
- Dilute and mix drug in D5W (preferred) or NS, final concentration 0.12–2.8 mg/mL.
- Diluted drug is stable 24 hours at room temperature or, if diluted in D5W, stable for 48 hours if refrigerated and protected form light.

Major Side Effects

- Bone Marrow Depression: Myelosuppression can be severe, dose-limiting toxicity. May need dose reductions for severe neutropenia.
- GI Toxicities: Moderate-to-severe nausea and vomiting. May be acute (first 24 hours) or delayed (> 24 hours). Diarrhea or constipation possible. Abdominal pain not unusual. Early diarrhea, most likely a cholinergic reaction, can be managed with atropine before administration of irinotecan. Late diarrhea observed in 22% of patients, can be severe, and should be treated aggressively. Consider lomotil, immodium, tincture of opium, and hydration.
- Hepatic Toxicities: Evidence of increased drug toxicity in patients with low protein and hepatic dysfunction. Dose reductions may be necessary.
- Renal: Nephrotoxicity is dose related and with cisplatin presents at 10–20 days. Use with caution in patients with abnormal renal function. Dose reduction is necessary in this setting.
- Electrolyte Imbalance: Decreases Mg^{2+}, K, Ca^{2+}, Na, and P.
- Neurotoxicity: Dose-limiting toxicity, usually in the form of peripheral sensory neuropathy. Paresthesias and numbness in a classic "stocking glove" pattern.
- Ototoxicity: High-frequency hearing loss and tinnitus.
- Skin: Alopecia
- Reproduction: Cisplatin is mutagenic and probably teratogenic.

Initiate antiemetic protocol:	Moderately to highly emetogenic protocol.
Supportive drugs:	☐ pegfilgrastim (Neulasta) ☐ filgrastim (Neupogen)
	☐ epoetin alfa (Procrit) ☐ darbepoetin alfa (Aranesp)
Treatment schedule:	Chair time 4 hours on day 1, and 2 hours on days 2 and 3. Repeat cycle every 28 days.
Estimated number of visits:	Four visits per cycle. Request six cycles worth of visits.

Dose Calculation by: 1. _____   2. _____

_____
Physician

_____
Patient Name

_____
Diagnosis

_____
Date

_____
ID Number

_____/_____/_____
Ht   Wt   M^2

Mitomycin + Vincristine + Bleomycin + Cisplatin (MOBP)

Baseline laboratory tests:	CBC: Chemistry (including Mg^{2+})
Baseline procedures or tests:	PFTs and CXR baseline and before each cycle of therapy.
Initiate IV:	0.9% sodium chloride
Premedicate:	5-HT$_3$ and dexamethasone 10–20 mg in 100 cc of NS
	Acetaminophen 30 minutes before bleomycin

Administer:

Mitomycin _____ mg (10 mg/m^2) IV push or infusion through side arm of running infusion on day 1

- **Potent vesicant**
- Available in 5-, 20-, and 40-mg vials. Dilute with sterile water to 0.5 mg/mL.
- Reconstituted solution is stable for 12 days refrigerated or 7 days at room temperature.

Vincristine _____ mg (1 mg/m^2) IV push on days 1, 8, 22, and 29. **Total dose should not exceed 2 mg**.

- **Vesicant**
- Available in 1-, 2-, and 5-mg vials (1 mg/mL).
- Refrigerate until use.

Bleomycin 10 units IV on days 1, 8, and 15, and 22

- A test dose of 2 units is recommended before the first dose to detect hypersensitivity.
- Available as a powder in 15- or 30-unit sizes. Dilute powder in 0.9% sodium chloride or sterile water, 3–10 mL.
- Reconstituted solution is stable for 24 hours at room temperature.

Cisplatin _____ mg (50 mg/m^2) IV on days 1 and 22

- Stable for 96 hours when protected from light and only 6 hours when not protected from light.
- Do not use aluminum needles, because precipitate will form.
- Further dilute solution with 250–1000 cc of NS.

Major Side Effects

- Allergic Reaction: Bleomycin—fever and chills observed in up to 25% of patients. True anaphylactic reactions are rare except in patients with lymphoma.
- Bone Marrow Depression: Myelosuppression can be a dose-limiting toxicity.
- GI Toxicities: Moderate-to-severe nausea and vomiting, acute or delayed. Mucositis is common. Constipation, abdominal pain, and paralytic ileus may occur with vincristine.
- Pulmonary Toxicities: Interstitial pneumonitis with bleomycin and mitomycin. Characterized by cough, dyspnea, pneumonia, pulmonary infiltrates on CXR.
- Renal: Nephrotoxicity secondary to cisplatin. Hemolytic-uremic syndrome, creatinine > 1.6, Hct < 25%, and platelet count < $100 \times 10^3/mm^3$ occurs with mitomycin.
- Electrolyte Imbalance: Decreases Mg^{2+}, K, Ca^{2+}, Na, and P.
- Neurotoxicity: Peripheral sensory neuropathy. Dose-limiting toxicity.
- Skin: Tissue necrosis if vesicants extravasated. Alopecia, skin rash, and fever.
- Reproduction: Drugs are mutagenic and teratogenic.

Initiate antiemetic protocol:	Moderately to highly emetogenic protocol.
Supportive drugs:	☐ pegfilgrastim (Neulasta) ☐ filgrastim (Neupogen)
	☐ epoetin alfa (Procrit) ☐ darbepoetin alfa (Aranesp)
Treatment schedule:	Chair time 3 hours on day 1, 1 hour on days 8 and 15, and 3 hours on day 22. Repeat cycle every 6 weeks.
Estimated number of visits:	Four visits per cycle. Request three cycles worth of visits.

Dose Calculation by: 1. _____   2. _____

_____   _____
Physician   Date

_____   _____
Patient Name   ID Number

_____   _____/_____/_____
Diagnosis   Ht   Wt   M²

Single-Agent Regimens

Cisplatin

Baseline labs:	CBC: Chemistry (including Mg^{++})
Baseline procedures of tests:	N/A
Initiate IV:	0.9% sodium chloride
Premedicate:	$5HT_3$ and dexamethasone 10–20 mg in 100 cc normal saline
Administer:	**Cisplatin** _____ mg (50–100 mg/m^2) IV over 1–3 hours on day 1

- Stable for 96 hours when protected from light and only 6 hours when not protected from light.
- Do not use aluminum needles, as precipitate will form.
- Available in solution as 1 mg/ml.
- Further dilute solution with 250 cc or more normal saline.

Major Side Effects

- Bone Marrow Depression: Myelosuppression can be severe, dose-limiting toxicity. May need dose reductions for severe neutropenia.
- GI Toxicities: Nausea and vomiting moderate to severe. May be acute (first 24 hours) or delayed (> 24 hours). Diarrhea or constipation possible. Abdominal pain not unusual.
- Hepatic Toxicities: Evidence of increased drug toxicity in patients with low protein and hepatic dysfunction. Dose reductions may be necessary.
- Renal: Nephrotoxicity is dose related with cisplatin, presents at 10–20 days. Use with caution in patients with abnormal renal function. Dose reduction is necessary in this setting.
- Electrolyte Imbalance: Decreases Mg^{2+}, K, Ca^{2+}, Na, and P.
- Neurotoxicity: Dose-limiting toxicity, usually in the form of peripheral sensory neuropathy. Paresthesias and numbness in a classic "stocking-glove" pattern.
- Ototoxicity: High-frequency hearing loss and tinnitus.
- Skin: Alopecia.
- Reproduction: Cisplatin is mutagenic and probably teratogenic.

Initiate antiemetic protocol:	Moderately to highly emetogenic protocol.
Supportive drugs:	☐ pegfilgrastim (Neulasta) ☐ filgrastim (Neupogen)
	☐ epoetin alfa (Procrit) ☐ darbepoetin alfa (Aranesp)
Treatment schedule:	Chair time 3 hours day 1. Repeat cycle every 21 days.
Estimated number of visits:	Two visits per cycle, request six cycles worth of visits.

Dose Calculation by: 1. _____ 2. _____

_____
Physician

_____
Date

_____
Patient Name

_____
ID Number

_____
Diagnosis

_____ / _____ / _____
Ht   Wt   M^2

Docetaxel

Baseline laboratory tests:	CBC: Chemistry (including Mg^{2+}) and CEA
Baseline procedures or tests:	Central line placement
Initiate IV:	0.9% sodium chloride
Premedicate:	Dexamethasone 8 mg bid for 3 days, starting the day before treatment or
	$5HT_3$ and dexamethasone 10–20 mg in 100 cc NS
Administer:	**Docetaxel** _____ mg (100 mg/m²) IV on day 1

- Comes in 20- or 80-mg blister packs with own diluent. Do not shake. Reconstituted vials stable at room temperature or refrigerated for 8 hours.
- Further dilute in 250 cc D5W or 0.9% sodium chloride, final concentration 0.3–0.74 mg/mL.
- Use non-PVC containers and tubing to administer.
- Use within 24 hours of preparation.

Major Side Effects

- Hypersensitivity Reactions: Severe hypersensitivity reactions with docetaxel characterized by hypotension, bronchospasm, generalized rash and erythema, chest tightness, back pain, dyspnea, dry fever, or chills in 2%–3% of patients. Premedication with dexamethasone recommended.
- Bone Marrow Depression: Neutropenia is dose limiting, with nadir at days 7–10 and recovery by day 14. Thrombocytopenia and anemia also occur.
- GI Toxicities: Nausea and vomiting is mild to moderate. Mucositis and diarrhea occur in 40% of patients.
- Neuropathy: Peripheral neuropathy may affect up to 49% of patients. Sensory alterations are paresthesias in a "glove and stocking" distribution and numbness.
- Fluid Balance: Fluid retention syndrome. Symptoms include weight gain, peripheral and/or generalized edema, pleural effusion, and ascites. Occurs in about 50% of patients. Premedication with dexamethasone effective in preventing or minimizing occurrences.
- Skin: Alopecia occurs in 80% of patients. Nail changes, rash, dry and pruritic skin occurs. Hand-foot syndrome has also been reported.

Initiate antiemetic protocol:	Mildly to moderately emetogenic protocol.
Supportive drugs:	☐ pegfilgrastim (Neulasta) ☐ filgrastim (Neupogen)
	☐ epoetin alfa (Procrit) ☐ darbepoetin alfa (Aranesp)
Treatment schedule:	Chair time 2 hours on day 1. Repeat cycle every 21 days.
Estimated number of visits:	Two visits per cycle. Request three cycles worth of visits.

Dose Calculation by: 1. _____ 2. _____

_____
Physician

_____
Patient Name

_____
Diagnosis

_____
Date

_____
ID Number

_____ / _____ / _____
Ht   Wt   M²

Paclitaxel

Baseline laboratory tests:	CBC: Chemistry (including Mg^{2+}) and CEA
Baseline procedures of tests:	N/A
Initiate IV:	0.9% sodium chloride
Premedicate:	$5HT_3$ and dexamethasone 10–20 mg in 100 cc NS
	Diphenhydramine 25–50 mg and cimetidine 300 mg in 100 cc NS
Administer:	Paclitaxel _____mg (175 mg/m^2) IV over 3 hours day 1

- Available in 30- and 300-mg vials 6 m/mL and 100-mg vial 16.7 mg/mL.
- Further dilute in NS or D5W for final concentration < 1.2 mg/ml.
- **Use non-PVC containers and tubing with 0.22 micron inline filter for administration.**

Major Side Effects

- Hypersensitivy Reaction: Occurs in 20%–40% of patients. Characterized by generalized skin rash, flushing, erythema, hypotension, dyspneas, and/or bronchospasm. Usually occurs within the first 2–3 minutes of infusion and almost always within the first 10 minutes. Premedicate as described.
- Bone Marrow Depression: Dose-limiting neutropenia with nadir at day 8–10 and recovery by day 15–21. Decreased incidence of neutropenia with 3-hour schedule when compared to 24-hour schedule. G-CSF support recommended.
- Neurotoxicity: Sensory neuropathy with numbness and paresthesias, dose related. More frequent with longer infusions and at doses < 175 mg/m^2.
- Musculoskeletal: Arthralgias and myalgias up to 1 week after treatment.
- Alopecia: Loss of total body hair occurs in nearly all patients.

Initiate antiemetic protocol:	Mildly emetogenic protocol.
Supportive drugs:	☐ pegfilgrastim (Neulasta) ☐ filgrastim (Neupogen)
	☐ epoetin alfa (Procrit) ☐ darbepoetin alfa (Aranesp)
Treatment schedule:	Chair time 4–5 hours day 1. Repeat every 21 days as tolerated or until progression.
Estimated number of visits:	Two visits per cycle. Request three cycles worth of visits.

Dose Calculation by: 1. _____ 2. _____

_____

Physician   Date

_____

Patient Name   ID Number

_____   _____/_____/_____

Diagnosis   Ht   Wt   M^2

Irinotecan (weekly)

Baseline laboratory tests:	CBC: Chemistry panel and CEA
Baseline procedures or tests:	N/A
Initiate IV:	D5W 100 cc
Premedicate:	5HT$_3$ and dexamethasone 20 mg in 100 cc of D5W
	Atropine 0.25–1.0 mg IV unless contraindicated

Administer: **Irinotecan**_____mg (125 mg/m^2) IV in 500 cc of D5W over 90 minutes

- Available in 2- and 5-ml vials (20 mg/ml).
- Store at room temperature and protect from light.
- Dilute and mix drug in D5W (preferred) or NS. 0.12–2.8 mg/mL.
- Diluted drug is stable for 24 hours at room temperature or, if diluted in D5W, is stable for 48 hours if refrigerated and protected from light.

Major Side Effects

- GI Toxicities: Early diarrhea, most likely a cholinergic effect, can be managed with atropine before therapy. Late diarrhea observed in 22% of patients can be severe and should be treated aggressively. Consider Lomotil, Imodium, tincture of opium, and hydration. Nausea and vomiting occurs in 35%–60% of patients, with 17% experiencing grade 3–4 nausea and 13% experiencing grade 3–4 vomiting.
- Bone Marrow Depression: Dose-limiting, grade 3–4 neutropenia in 17%. Nadir in 6–9 days.
- Alopecia: Mild.

Initiate antiemetic protocol: Moderately to highly emetogenic protocol.

Supportive drugs:

- ☐ pegfilgrastim (Neulasta)
- ☐ filgrastim (Neupogen)
- ☐ epoetin alfa (Procrit)
- ☐ darbepoetin alfa (Aranesp)
- ☐ loperamide (Imodium)
- ☐ diphenoxylate/atropine sulfate (Lomotil)

Treatment schedule: Chair time 3 hours weekly × 4 weeks. May need additional days for hydration if patient has diarrhea. Repeat cycle every 6 weeks.

Estimated number of visits: Four visits per cycle. Request three cycles worth of visits.

Dose Calculation by: 1. _____ 2. _____

_____
Physician

_____
Date

_____
Patient Name

_____
ID Number

_____
Diagnosis

_____/ _____/ _____
Ht   Wt   M^2

Vinorelbine

Baseline laboratory tests:	CBC: Chemistry
Baseline procedures or tests:	N/A
Initiate IV:	0.9% sodium chloride
Premedicate:	Oral phenothiazine or 5-HT$_3$
Administer:	**Vinorelbine** _____ mg (30 mg/m^2) IV weekly

- **Vesicant**
- Available in 1- or 5-mL single-use vials at a concentration of 10 mg/mL.
- Further dilute in syringe or IV bag to concentration of 1.5–3.0 mg/mL.
- Infuse over 6–10 minutes into sidearm port of freely flowing IV infusion, either peripherally or via central line. Use port CLOSEST TO THE IV BAG, not to the patient.
- Flush vein with at least 75–125 mL of IV fluid after drug infusion.
- Reconstituted solution is stable for 24 hours refrigerated.

Major Side Effects

- Bone Marrow Depression: Leukopenia is dose-limiting toxicity. Nadir at 7–10 days. Severe thrombocytopenia and anemia are uncommon.
- GI Toxicities: Nausea and vomiting are mild in IV dosing with an incidence of 44%. Stomatitis is mild to moderate (< 20% incidence). Constipation (35%), diarrhea (17%), and anorexia (< 20%) also occur.
- Hormonal: Syndrome of inappropriate secretion of antidiuretic hormone.
- Skin: Extravasation of vinorelbine may cause local tissue injury and inflammation. Alopecia observed in 10%–15% of patients.
- Neurotoxicity: Usually mild and occurs much less frequently than with other vinca alkaloids.

Initiate antiemetic protocol:	Mildly emetogenic protocol.
Supportive drugs:	☐ pegfilgrastim (Neulasta) ☐ filgrastim (Neupogen)
	☐ epoetin alfa (Procrit) ☐ darbepoetin alfa (Aranesp)
Treatment schedule:	Chair time 1 hour weekly. Repeat cycle weekly up to 12 cycles, to be followed by surgery or radiation therapy.
Estimated number of visits:	One per week up to 12 weeks. Request 12 cycles worth of visits.

Dose Calculation by: 1. _____ 2. _____

Physician _____

Date _____

Patient Name _____

ID Number _____

Diagnosis _____

Ht _____ / Wt _____ / M^2 _____

Topotecan

Baseline laboratory tests:	CBC: Chemistry panel
Baseline procedures or tests:	N/A
Initiate IV:	0.9% sodium chloride
Premedicate:	5-HT$_3$ and dexamethasone 10 mg in 100 cc of NS
Administer:	**Topotecan** _____mg (1.5 mg/m^2/day) IV days 1–5

- Available as a 4-mg vial.
- Reconstitute vial with 4 mL of sterile water for injection.
- Further dilute in 0.9% sodium chloride or D5W.
- Use immediately.

Major Side Effects

- Hematologic: Severe grade 4 myelosuppression occurs during the first course of therapy in 60% of patients. Dose-limiting toxicity. Typical nadir occurs at days 7–10 with full recovery by days 21–28. If severe neutropenia occurs, reduce dose by 0.25 mg/m^2 for subsequent doses or may use granulocyte colony stimulating factor (G-CSF) to prevent neutropenia 24 hours after last day of topotecan.
- GI Toxicities: Nausea and vomiting, mild to moderate and dose related. Occurs in 60%–80% of patients. Diarrhea occurs in 42% of patients, and constipation occurs in 39%. Abdominal pain may occur in 33% of patients.
- Hepatic Toxicity: Evidence of increased drug toxicity in patients with low protein and hepatic dysfunction. Dose reductions may be necessary.
- Renal: Use with caution in patients with abnormal renal function. Dose reduction is necessary in this setting. Microscopic hematuria occurs in 10% of patients.
- Skin: Alopecia.

Initiate antiemetic protocol:	Mildly to moderately emetogenic protocol.
Supportive drugs:	☐ pegfilgrastim (Neulasta) ☐ filgrastim (Neupogen)
	☐ epoetin alfa (Procrit) ☐ darbepoetin alfa (Aranesp)
Treatment schedule:	Chair time 1 hour on days 1–5. Repeat every 21 days until disease progression.
Estimated number of visits:	Three visits per course. Request three courses.

Dose Calculation by: 1. _____   2. _____

_____   _____
Physician   Date

_____   _____
Patient Name   ID Number

_____   _____/ _____/ _____
Diagnosis   Ht   Wt   M^2

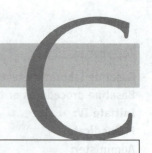

NEOADJUVANT COMBINED MODALITY THERAPY FOR RECTAL CANCER
Combination Regimens

5-Fluorouracil: 1000 mg/m^2/day IV continuous infusion on days 1–5

Repeat infusional 5-FU on weeks 1 and 5.

Radiation therapy: 180 cGy/day for 5 days per week (total dose, 5040 cGy)

Followed by surgical resection and then adjuvant chemotherapy with 5-FU at 500 mg/m^2 IV for 5 days every 28 days for a total of 4 cycles.[108]

Capecitabine: 825 mg/m^2 PO bid throughout the entire course of radiation therapy or

900–1000 mg/m^2 PO bid on days 1–5 of each week of radiation therapy

Radiation therapy: 180 cGy/day for 5 days per week (total dose, 5040 cGy)

Followed by surgical resection and then adjuvant chemotherapy with 5-FU or 5-FU/LV for a total of 4 cycles.[109]

NEOADJUVANT COMBINED MODALITY THERAPY FOR RECTAL CANCER
Combination Regimens

5-Fluorouracil + Radiation Therapy (German AIO Regimen)

Baseline laboratory tests:	CBC: Chemistry and CEA
Baseline procedures or tests:	Central line placement
Initiate IV:	0.9% sodium chloride
Premedicate:	Oral phenothiazine or 5-HT$_3$

Administer: **Fluorouracil** _____mg (1000 mg/m^2/day) IV continuous infusion Monday–Friday (days 1–5). Repeat infusional 5-FU on weeks 1 and 5.

- No dilution required. Concentration 50 mg/mL.
- Can be further diluted with 0.9% sodium chloride or D5W.

Radiation 180 cGy/day for 5 days per week (total dose 5040 cGy)

Followed by surgical resection and then adjuvant chemotherapy with 5-FU at 500 mg/m^2/day IV for 5 days every 28 days for a total of 4 cycles.

Major Side Effects

- Bone Marrow Depression: Nadir 10–14 days. Neutropenia, thrombocytopenia are dose related. Can be dose limiting for daily × 5 or weekly regimens.
- GI Toxicities: Nausea and vomiting occur in 30%–50% of patients but are usually mild. Mucositis and diarrhea can be severe and dose limiting.
- Skin: Local tissue irritation progressing to desquamation can occur. Do not use oil-based lotions or creams in radiation field. Hyperpigmentation, photosensitivity, and nail changes may occur. Hand-foot syndrome can be dose limiting.
- Ocular: Photophobia, increased lacrimation, conjunctivitis, and blurred vision.

Initiate antiemetic protocol: Mildly emetogenic protocol.

Supportive drugs:

☐ pegfilgrastim (Neulasta) ☐ filgrastim (Neupogen)

☐ epoetin alfa (Procrit) ☐ darbepoetin alfa (Aranesp)

☐ loperamide (Imodium) ☐ diphenoxylate/atropine sulfate (Lomotil)

Treatment schedule: Chair time 1 hour 2 days per week, weeks 1 and 5.

During adjuvant therapy, 2 visits per week every 28 days for 4 cycles.

Estimated number of visits: 12 to 14 visits per treatment course.

Dose Calculation by: 1. _____ 2. _____

_____

Physician

_____

Patient Name

_____

Diagnosis

_____

Date

_____

ID Number

_____/_____/_____

Ht   Wt   M^2

Capecitabine + Radiation Therapy

Baseline laboratory tests:	CBC: Chemistry, bilirubin, LFTs, CEA, and creatinine clearance
Baseline procedures or tests:	N/A
Initiate IV:	N/A
Premedicate:	Oral phenothiazine or 5-HT$_3$
Administer:	**Capecitabine** _____mg (825 mg/m^2/day) PO daily throughout the entire course of radiation therapy

OR

Capecitabine _____mg (900–1000 mg/m^2) PO bid Monday–Friday of each week of radiation therapy.

- Administer within 30 minutes of a meal with plenty of water.
- Monitor INRs closely in patients taking warfarin; may increase INR.
- Stop therapy at first sign of hand-foot syndrome or diarrhea.
- Available in 150 mg and 500 mg tablets.

Radiation: **Radiation 35 cGy (palliative) over 14 fractions (3 weeks)**

OR

Radiation 45–50.4 cGy (definitive) over 20 fractions (5 weeks)

Followed by surgical resection and then adjuvant chemotherapy with 5-FU or 5-FU/LV for a total of 4 cycles.

Major Side Effects

- GI Toxicities: Nausea and vomiting, in 30%–50% of patients, is usually mild to moderate. Diarrhea occurs in up to 40%, with 15% being grade 3–4. Stomatitis is common, 3% of which is severe.
- Skin: Local tissue irritation progressing to desquamation in radiation field. Do not use oil-based lotions or creams in radiation field. Hand-foot syndrome (palmar-plantar erythrodysesthesia) occurs in 15%–20% of patients. Characterized by tingling, numbness, pain, erythema, dryness, rash, swelling, increased pigmentation, and/or pruritus of the hands and feet.
- Renal Insufficiency: Xeloda contraindicated in patients with creatinine clearance < 30 mL/min, with creatinine clearance of 30–50 mL/min at baseline a dose reduction to 75% of capecitabine should be made.
- Ocular: Blepharitis, tear-duct stenosis, acute and chronic conjunctivitis.
- Hepatic: Elevations in serum bilirubin (20%–40%), alkaline phosphatase, and hepatic transaminase (SGOT, SGPT) levels. Dose modifications may be required if hyperbilirubinemia occurs.

Initiate antiemetic protocol:	Mildly to moderately emetogenic protocol.
Supportive drugs:	☐ pegfilgrastim (Neulasta) ☐ filgrastim (Neupogen)
	☐ loperamide (Imodium) ☐ epoetin alfa (Procrit)
	☐ darbepoetin alfa (Aranesp) ☐ diphenoxylate/atropine sulfate (Lomotil)
Treatment schedule:	Daily during radiation therapy
Estimated number of visits:	One visit per week for 3 or 5 weeks.

Dose Calculation by: 1. _____   2. _____

_____
Physician

_____
Date

_____
Patient Name

_____
ID Number

_____
Diagnosis

_____/_____/_____
Ht   Wt   M^2

ADJUVANT THERAPY

5-Fluorouracil: 425 mg/m^2 IV on days 1–5

Leucovorin: 20 mg/m^2 IV on days 1–5, administered before 5-Fluorouracil

Repeat cycle every 4–5 weeks for a total of six cycles.[111]

5-Fluorouracil: 500 mg/m^2 IV weekly for 6 weeks

Leucovorin: 500 mg/m^2 IV over 2 hours weekly for 6 weeks, administered
   before 5-Fluorouracil

Repeat cycle every 8 weeks for a total of four cycles (32 weeks total).[112]

5-Fluorouracil: 500 mg/m^2 IV weekly for 6 weeks

Leucovorin: 20 mg/m^2 IV weekly for 6 weeks, administered before
   5-Fluorouracil

Repeat cycle every 8 weeks for a total of four or six cycles (32 or 48 weeks
   total).[113]

Oxaliplatin: 85 mg/m^2 IV on day 1

5-Fluorouracil: 400 mg/m^2 IV bolus, followed by 600 mg/m^2 IV continuous infusion for 22 hours on days 1 and 2

Leucovorin: 200 mg/m^2 IV on days 1 and 2 as a 2-hour infusion before
   5-Fluorouracil

Repeat cycle every 2 weeks for a total of 12 cycles.[114]

Capecitabine: 1250 mg/m^2 PO bid on days 1–14

Repeat cycle every 21 days for a total of 8 cycles.[115] Dose may be decreased to 850–1000 mg/m^2 PO bid on days 1–14 to reduce the risk of
   toxicity without compromising clinical efficacy.

Adjuvant Therapy

5-Fluorouracil + Leucovorin (Mayo Clinic Regimen)

Baseline laboratory tests:	CBC: Chemistry and CEA
Baseline procedures or tests:	N/A
Initiate IV:	0.9% sodium chloride
Premedicate:	Oral phenothiazine or 5-HT$_3$
Administer:	**Leucovorin** _____ mg (20 mg/m^2/day) IV bolus on days 1–5

- Available in solution or powder. Reconstitute solution with sterile water. May further dilute with 0.9% sodium chloride or D5W.
- Do not mix in same solution with 5-FU, because a precipitate will form.

5-Fluorouracil _____ mg (425 mg/m^2/day) IV bolus 1 hour after start of leucovorin, days 1–5.

- 50 mg/mL, no dilution required. Can be further diluted with 0.9% sodium chloride or D5W.

Major Side Effects

- Bone Marrow Depression: Nadir 10–14 days. Neutropenia, thrombocytopenia are dose related. Can be dose limiting for daily × 5 or weekly regimens.
- GI Toxicities: Nausea and vomiting occur in 30%–50% of patients but is usually mild. Mucositis and diarrhea can be severe and dose limiting.
- Skin: Alopecia is more common in the 5-day course and results in diffuse thinning of hair. Hyperpigmentation, photosensitivity, and nail changes may occur. Hand-foot syndrome characterized by tingling, numbness, erythema, dryness, rash, swelling, or increased pigmentation of hands and/or feet can be dose limiting.
- Ocular: Photophobia, increased lacrimation, conjunctivitis, and blurred vision.
- Reproductive: Pregnancy category D. Breast feeding should be avoided.

Initiate antiemetic protocol:	Mildly emetogenic protocol.
Supportive drugs:	☐ pegfilgrastim (Neulasta) ☐ filgrastim (Neupogen)
	☐ epoetin alfa (Procrit) ☐ darbepoetin alfa (Aranesp)
	☐ loperamide (Imodium) ☐ diphenoxylate/atropine sulfate (Lomotil)
Treatment schedule:	Chair time 1 hour, days 1–5. Nadir at day 14. Repeat cycle every 28 days for 6 cycles.
Estimated number of visits:	Five days per cycle, 30 per treatment course.

Dose Calculation by: 1. _____   2. _____

_____
Physician

_____
Date

_____
Patient Name

_____
ID Number

_____
Diagnosis

_____ / _____ / _____
Ht   Wt   M^2

5-Fluorouracil + Leucovorin (Weekly Schedule/High Dose)

Baseline laboratory tests:	CBC: Chemistry and CEA
Baseline procedures or tests:	N/A
Initiate IV:	0.9% sodium chloride
Premedicate:	Oral phenothiazine or 5-HT$_3$
Administer:	**Leucovorin** _____mg (500 mg/m^2) IV over 2 hours, weekly for 6 weeks

- Available in solution or powder. Reconstitute solution with sterile water. May further dilute with 0.9% sodium chloride or D5W.
- Do not mix in same solution with 5-FU, because a precipitate will form.

5-Fluorouracil_____mg (500 mg/m^2) IV weekly for 6 weeks

- No dilution required. Can be further diluted with 0.9% sodium chloride or D5W.

Major Side Effects

- Bone Marrow Depression: Nadir 10–14 days. Neutropenia, thrombocytopenia are dose related. Can be dose limiting for daily × 5 or weekly regimens.
- GI Toxicities: Nausea and vomiting occur in 30%–50% of patients but are usually mild. Mucositis and diarrhea can be severe and dose limiting.
- Skin: Alopecia is more common in the 5-day course and results in diffuse thinning of hair. Hyperpigmentation, photosensitivity, and nail changes may occur. Hand-foot syndrome characterized by tingling, numbness, erythema, dryness, rash, pruritis, swelling, or increased pigmentation of hands and/or feet can be dose limiting.
- Ocular: Photophobia, increased lacrimation, conjunctivitis, and blurred vision.
- Reproductive: Pregnancy category D. Breast feeding should be avoided.

Initiate antiemetic protocol:	Mildly emetogenic protocol.
Supportive drugs:	☐ pegfilgrastim (Neulasta) ☐ filgrastim (Neupogen)
	☐ epoetin alfa (Procrit) ☐ darbepoetin alfa (Aranesp)
	☐ loperamide (Imodium) ☐ diphenoxylate/atropine sulfate (Lomotil)
Treatment schedule:	Chair time 1 hour weekly for 6 weeks. Nadir drawn between days 10 and 14. Repeat every 8 weeks for four cycles.
Estimated number of visits:	Twelve visits per cycle, 24 per course.

Dose Calculation by: 1. _____   2. _____

_____
Physician

_____
Date

_____
Patient Name

_____
ID Number

_____
Diagnosis

_____ / _____ / _____
Ht   Wt   M^2

5-Fluorouracil + Leucovorin (Weekly Schedule/Low Dose)

Baseline laboratory tests:	CBC: Chemistry and CEA
Baseline procedures or tests:	N/A
Initiate IV:	0.9% sodium chloride
Premedicate:	Oral phenothiazine or 5-HT$_3$
Administer:	**5-Fluorouracil** _____ mg (500 mg/m^2) IV weekly for 6 weeks

- No dilution required. Can be further diluted with 0.9% sodium chloride or D5W.

Leucovorin _____ mg (20 mg/m^2) IV weekly for 6 weeks, administer before 5-Fluorouracil

- Available in solution or powder. Reconstitute solution with sterile water. May further dilute with 0.9% sodium chloride or D5W.
- Do not mix in same solution with 5-FU, because a precipitate will form.

Major Side Effects
- Bone Marrow Depression: Nadir 10–14 days. Neutropenia, thrombocytopenia are dose related. Can be dose limiting for daily × 5 or weekly regimens.
- GI Toxicities: Nausea and vomiting occur in 30%–50% of patients but are usually mild. Mucositis and diarrhea can be severe and dose limiting.
- Skin: Alopecia is more common in the 5-day course and results in diffuse thinning of hair. Hyperpigmentation, photosensitivity, and nail changes may occur. Hand-foot syndrome characterized by tingling, numbness, erythema, dryness, rash, swelling, or increased pigmentation of hands and/or feet can be dose limiting.
- Ocular: Photophobia, increased lacrimation, conjunctivitis, and blurred vision.
- Reproductive: Pregnancy category D. Breast feeding should be avoided.

Initiate antiemetic protocol:	Mildly emetogenic protocol.
Supportive drugs:	☐ pegfilgrastim (Neulasta) ☐ filgrastim (Neupogen)
	☐ epoetin alfa (Procrit) ☐ darbepoetin alfa (Aranesp)
	☐ loperamide (Imodium) ☐ diphenoxylate/atropine sulfate (Lomotil)
Treatment schedule:	Chair time 1 hour weekly for 6 weeks. Repeat every 8 weeks for 6 cycles.
Estimated number of visits:	Twelve per cycle. Nadir drawn between day 10–14, 36 per course.

Dose Calculation by: 1. _____   2. _____

_____

Physician

_____

Patient Name

_____

Diagnosis

Date

ID Number

_____ / _____ / _____
Ht   Wt   M^2

Oxaliplatin + 5-Fluorouracil + Leucovorin (FOLFOX 4)

Baseline laboratory tests:	CBC: Chemistry panel and CEA
Baseline procedures or tests:	Central line required for continuous infusion
Initiate IV:	D5W
Premedicate:	$5HT_3$ and dexamethasone 20 mg in 100 cc of D5W
Administer:	**DAY 1: Oxaliplatin** _____ mg (85 mg/m^2) IV in 250–500 cc of D5W over 2 hours

Classified as an irritant, but extravasations have resulted in induration and formation of nodule lasting 9 months or more.

Available in 50- and 100-mg vials. Concentration is 5 mg/ml.

Do not use chloride containing solutions or aluminum needles.

Leucovorin _____ mg (200 mg/m^2) IV in 250–500 cc of D5W over 2 hours (oxaliplatin and leucovorin are infused concurrently, in separate bags through a Y-site over 2 hours).

• Available in solution or powder. Reconstitute powder with sterile water.

• Do not mix in same solution with 5-FU, as a precipitate will form.

5-Fluorouracil _____ mg (400 mg/m^2) IV bolus over 2–4 minutes, then

5-Fluorouacil _____ mg (600 mg/m^2) IV continuous infusion over 22 hours

DAY 2: Leucovorin _____ mg (200 mg/m^2) IV in 250–500 cc D5W

5-Fluorouracil _____ mg (400 mg/m^2) IV bolus over 2–4 minutes, then

5-Fluorouracil _____ mg (600 mg/m^2) IV continuous infusion over 22 hours

DAY 3: Discontinue pump

Major Side Effects

• Acute Neurotoxicities: Are temporary and can occur within hours of or up to 14 days after oxaliplatin. Often precipitated by exposure to cold and characterized by dysesthesias, transient paresthesias or hypothesias of hands, feet, perioral area, and throat. Pharyngolaryngeal dysesthesia (**sensation** of discomfort or tightness in the back of the throat and inability to breathe), is most frightening to patients.

• Peripheral Neuropathy: Affects about 48% of patients, usually with a cumulative dose of 800 mg/m^2. Symptoms include paresthesias, dysesthesias, hypoesthesias in a "stocking and glove" distribution, and altered proprioception (knowing where body parts are in relation to the whole).

• GI Toxicities: Nausea and vomiting occur in 65% of patients; can be severe. Diarrhea occurs in 80%–90% of patients.

• Bone Marrow Depression: Mild leukopenia, mild-to-moderate thrombocytopenia, and anemia are common.

• Anaphylactic/anaphylactoid reactions to eloxatin have been reported. Delayed hypersensitivity: May occur after 10–12 cycles. Symptoms range from mild symptoms, i.e., rash, urticaria, erythema, pruritus, or emesis to anaphylaxis / severe hypersensitivity characterized by dyspnea, angioedema bronchospasm, and hypotension. These reactions occur within minutes of administration and should be managed with appropriate supportive therapy. Drug-related deaths associated with platinum compounds from this reaction have been reported.

Initiate antiemetic protocol:	Moderately to highly emetogenic protocol.
Supportive drugs:	☐ pegfilgrastim (Neulasta) ☐ filgrastim (Neupogen)
	☐ epoetin alfa (Procrit) ☐ darbepoetin alfa (Aranesp)
	☐ loperamide (Imodium) ☐ diphenoxylate/atropine sulfate (Lomotil)
Treatment schedule:	Chair time 3 hours on days 1 and 2, and 15 minutes on day 3. Repeat every 14 days for 12 cycles.
Estimated number of visits:	36 visits (6 per month for 6 months)

Dose Calculation by: 1. _____   2. _____

Physician _____   Date _____

Patient Name _____   ID Number _____

Diagnosis _____   Ht _____ / Wt _____ / M² _____

Capecitabine (Xeloda)

Baseline laboratory tests:	CBC: Chemistry, bilirubin, LFTs, CEA and creatinine clearance
Baseline procedures or tests:	N/A
Initiate IV:	N/A
Premedicate:	Oral phenothiazine or 5-HT$_3$

Administer: **Capecitabine** _____ mg (1250 mg/m^2/day) PO bid on days 1–14

- Dose may be decreased to 850–1000 mg/m^2 PO bid on days 1–14. This may reduce the risk of toxicity without compromising efficacy.
- Available in 150 mg and 500 mg tablets.
- Administer within 30 minutes of a meal with plenty of water.
- Monitor INRs closely in patients taking warfarin; may increase INR.
- Stop therapy at first signs of hand-foot syndrome or diarrhea.

Major Side Effects

- GI Toxicities: Nausea and vomiting, in 30%–50% of patients, is usually mild to moderate. Diarrhea occurs in up to 40%, with 15% being grade 3–4. Stomatitis is common, 3% of which is severe.
- Renal Insufficiency: Xeloda contraindicated in patients with creatinine clearance < 30 mL/min, with creatinine clearance of 30–50 mL/min at baseline a dose reduction to 75% of capecitabine should be made.
- Skin: Hand-foot syndrome (palmar-plantar erythrodysesthesia) seen in 15%–20% of patients. Characterized by tingling, numbness, pain, erythema, dryness, rash, swelling, increased pigmentation, and/or pruritus of the hands and feet. Less frequent in reduced doses.
- Ocular: Blepharitis, tear-duct stenosis, acute and chronic conjunctivitis.
- Hepatic: Elevations in serum bilirubin (20%–40%), alkaline phosphatase, and hepatic transaminase (SGOT, SGPT) levels. Dose modifications may be required if hyperbilirubinemia occurs.
- Reproductive: Pregnancy category D. Breast feeding should be avoided.

Initiate antiemetic protocol: Mildly to moderately emetogenic protocol.

Supportive drugs:

☐ pegfilgrastim (Neulasta)   ☐ filgrastim (Neupogen)

☐ epoetin alfa (Procrit)   ☐ darbepoetin alfa (Aranesp)

☐ loperamide (Imodium)   ☐ diphenoxylate/atropine sulfate (Lomotil)

Treatment schedule: No chair time. Repeat cycle every 21 days for a total of 8 cycles. Dose may be decreased to 850–1000 mg/m^2 PO bid on days 1–14 to reduce the risk of toxicity without compromising clinical efficacy.

Dose Calculation by: 1. _____   2. _____

Physician _____   Date _____

Patient Name _____   ID Number _____

Diagnosis _____   _____/ _____/ _____

Ht   Wt   M^2

COLORECTAL CANCER

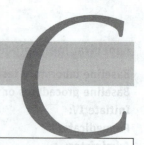

METASTATIC DISEASE
Combination Regimens

Irinotecan: 125 mg/m^2 IV over 90 minutes weekly for 4 weeks

5-Fluorouracil: 500 mg/m^2 IV weekly for 4 weeks

Leucovorin: 20 mg/m^2 IV weekly for 4 weeks

Repeat cycle every 6 weeks.[1,115]

Irinotecan: 125 mg/m^2 IV over 90 minutes weekly for 4 weeks

5-Fluorouracil: 500 mg/m^2 IV weekly for 4 weeks

Leucovorin: 20 mg/m^2 IV weekly for 4 weeks

Bevacizumab: 5 mg/kg IV every 2 weeks

Repeat cycle every 6 weeks.[1,116]

Irinotecan: 125 mg/m^2 IV over 90 minutes weekly for 2 weeks

5-Fluorouracil: 500 mg/m^2 IV weekly for 2 weeks

Leucovorin: 20 mg/m^2 IV weekly for 2 weeks

Repeat cycle every 3 weeks.[1,117]

Irinotecan: 180 mg/m^2 IV on day 1

5-Fluorouracil: 400 mg/m^2 IV bolus, followed by 600 mg/m^2 IV continuous infusion for 22 hours on days 1 and 2

Leucovorin: 200 mg/m^2 IV on days 1 and 2 as a 2-hour infusion before 5-Fluorouracil

Repeat cycle every 2 weeks.[1,118]

IFL FOLFIRI Regimen **181**

Irinotecan: 180 mg/m^2 IV on day 1

5-Fluorouracil: 400 mg/m^2 IV bolus on day 1, followed by 2400 mg/m^2 IV continuous infusion for 46 hours

Leucovorin: 200 mg/m^2 IV on day 1 as a 2-hour infusion before 5-Fluorouracil

Repeat cycle every 2 weeks.[1,119]

Oxaliplatin + 5-Fluorouracil + Leucovorin (FOLFOX4) **183**

Oxaliplatin: 85 mg/m^2 IV on day 1

5-Fluorouracil: 400 mg/m^2 IV bolus, followed by 600 mg/m^2 IV continuous infusion for 22 hours on days 1 and 2

Leucovorin: 200 mg/m^2 IV on days 1 and 2 as a 2-hour infusion before 5-Fluorouracil

Repeat cycle every 2 weeks.[1,120]

Oxaliplatin + 5-Fluorouracil + Leucovorin (FOLFOX6) **185**

Oxaliplatin: 100 mg/m^2 IV on day 1

5-Fluorouracil: 400 mg/m^2 IV bolus on day 1, followed by 2400 mg/m^2 IV continuous infusion for 46 hours

Leucovorin: 400 mg/m^2 IV on day 1 as a 2-hour infusion before 5-Fluorouracil

Repeat cycle every 2 weeks.[1,121]

Oxaliplatin + 5-Fluorouracil + Leucovorin (FOLFOX7) **187**

Oxaliplatin: 130 mg/m^2 IV on day 1

5-Fluorouracil: 2400 mg/m^2 IV continuous infusion on days 1 and 2 for 46 hours

Leucovorin: 400 mg/m^2 IV on day 1 as a 2-hour infusion before 5-Fluorouracil

Repeat cycle every 2 weeks.[1,122]

Cetuximab + Irinotecan 189

Cetuximab: 400 mg/m^2 IV loading dose day 1, then 250 mg/m^2 IV weekly
Irinotecan: 350 mg/m^2 IV on day 1
Repeat cycle every 21 days.[1,123]

Capecitabine + Oxaliplatin (XELOX) 191

Capecitabine: 1000 mg/m^2 PO bid on days 1–14
Oxaliplatin: 130 mg/m^2 IV on day 1
Repeat cycle every 21 days.[1,124]

Capecitabine + Irinotecan (XELIRI) 193

Capecitabine: 1000 mg/m^2 PO bid on days 1–14
Irinotecan: 250 mg/m^2 IV on day 1 or irinotecan 80 mg/m^2 days 1 and 8
Repeat cycle every 21 days.[1,125]

Oxaliplatin + Irinotecan (IROX Regimen) 194

Oxaliplatin: 85 mg/m^2 IV on day 1
Irinotecan: 200 mg/m^2 IV on day 1
Repeat cycle every 3 weeks.[1, 126]

5-Fluorouracil + Leucovorin (Mayo Clinic Regimen) 196

5-Fluorouracil: 425 mg/m^2 IV on days 1–5
Leucovorin: 20 mg/m^2 IV on days 1–5, administered before 5-Fluorouracil
Repeat cycle every 4–5 weeks.[1,127]

5-Fluorouracil + Leucovorin (Roswell Park Schedule, Hgh Dose) 197

5-Fluorouracil: 500 mg/m^2 IV weekly for 6 weeks
Leucovorin: 500 mg/m^2 IV weekly for 6 weeks, administered before
  5-Fluorouracil
Repeat cycle every 8 weeks.[1,128]

5-Fluorouracil + Leucovorin + Bevacizumab **198**

5-Fluorouracil: 500 mg/m^2 IV weekly for 6 weeks

Leucovorin: 500 mg/m^2 IV weekly for 6 weeks, administered before 5-Fluorouracil

Bevacizumab: 5 mg/kg IV every 2 weeks

Repeat cycle every 8 weeks.[1,129]

5-Fluorouracil + Leucovorin (German Schedule, Low Dose) **200**

5-Fluorouracil: 600 mg/m^2 IV weekly for 6 weeks

Leucovorin: 20 mg/m^2 IV weekly for 6 weeks, administered before 5-Fluorouracil

Repeat cycle every 8 weeks following a 2-week rest period.[1,130]

5-Fluorouracil + Leucovorin (de Gramont Regimen) **201**

5-Fluorouracil: 400 mg/m^2 IV and then 600 mg/m^2 IV for 22 hours on days 1 and 2

Leucovorin: 200 mg/m^2 IV on days 1 and 2 as a 2-hour infusion before 5-Fluorouracil

Repeat cycle every 2 weeks.[1,131]

FOLFOX4 + Bevacizumab **202**

Oxaliplatin: 85 mg/m^2 IV on day 1

5-Fluorouracil: 400 mg/m^2 IV bolus, followed by 600 mg/m^2 IV continuous infusion on days 1 and 2

Leucovorin: 200 mg/m^2 IV on days 1 and 2 as a 2-hour infusion before 5-Fluorouracil

Bevacizumab: 10 mg/kg IV every 2 weeks

Repeat cycle every 2 weeks.[1,132]

Capecitabine + Oxaliplatin (XELOX) + Bevacizumab...**204**

Capecitabine: 850 mg/m^2 PO bid on days 1–14

Oxaliplatin: 130 mg/m^2 IV on day 1

Bevacizumab: 7.5 mg/kg every 3 weeks

Repeat cycle every 21 days.[1,133]

Trimetrexate + 5-Fluorouracil + Leucovorin **206**

Trimetrexate: 110 mg/m^2 IV on day 1

Leucovorin: 200 mg/m^2 IV on day 2, 24 hours after trimetrexate dose

5-Fluorouracil: 500 mg/m^2 IV on day 2, immediately after leucovorin

Leucovorin: 15 mg PO every 6 hours for 7 doses, starting 6 hours after 5-Fluorouracil

Repeat on a weekly schedule for 6 weeks every 8 weeks.[1,134]

Hepatic Artery Infusion (HAI)

Floxuridine **207**

Floxuridine: 0.3 mg/kg/day HAI on days 1–14
Dexamethasone: 20 mg HAI on days 1–14
Heparin: 50,000 U HAI on days 1–14
Repeat cycle every 14 days.[1,135]

Single-Agent Regimens

Capecitabine (Xeloda) **208**

Capecitabine: 1250 mg/m^2 PO bid on days 1–14
Repeat cycle every 21 days.[1,136]
Dose may be decreased to 850–1000 mg/m^2 PO bid on days 1–14.
This dose reduction may reduce the risk of toxicity without compromising clinical efficacy.

Irinotecan (CPT-11/Weekly Schedule) **209**

CPT-11: 125 mg/m^2 IV over 90 minutes weekly for 4 weeks
Repeat cycle every 6 weeks.[1,137]
OR
CPT-11: 125 mg/m^2 IV over 90 minutes weekly for 2 weeks
Repeat cycle every 3 weeks.
OR
CPT-11: 175 mg/m^2 IV on days 1 and 10
Repeat cycle every 3 weeks.[1,138]

Irinotecan (CPT-11/Monthly Schedule) **210**

CPT-11: 350 mg/m^2 IV on day 1
Repeat cycle every 3 weeks.[1,139]

Cetuximab **211**

Cetuximab: 400 mg/m^2 IV loading dose, then 250 mg/m^2
 IV weekly
Repeat cycle on a weekly basis.[1,140]

5-Fluorouracil (Continuous Infusion) **213**

5-Fluorouracil: 2600 mg/m^2 IV over 24 hours weekly
Repeat cycle weekly for 4 weeks.[1,141]
OR
5-Fluorouracil: 1000 mg/m^2/day IV continuous infusion on days 1–4
Repeat cycle every 21–28 days.[1,142]

Combination Regimen

Irinotecan + 5-Fluorouracil + Leucovorin (IFL-Saltz Regimen)

Baseline laboratory tests:	CBC: Chemistry panel and CEA
Baseline procedures or tests:	None
Initiate IV:	NS or D5W
Premedicate:	5-HT$_3$ and dexamethasone 20 mg in 100 cc of NS or D5W
	Atropine 0.25–1.0 mg IV unless contraindicated

Administer:

Irinotecan_____mg (125 mg/m^2) IV in 500 cc of D5W over 90 minutes weekly for 4 weeks

- Available in 2- and 5-mL vials (20 mg/mL).
- Store at room temperature; protect from light.
- Dilute and mix drug in 250–500 cc of D5W (preferred) or NS.
- Diluted drug is stable 24 hours at room temperature, if diluted in D5W, and is stable for 48 hours if refrigerated and protected from light.

Leucovorin_____mg (20 mg/m^2) IV push weekly for 4 weeks

- Available in solution or powder. Reconstitute powder with sterile water. May further dilute with NS or D5W.
- Do not mix in same solution with 5-FU, because precipitate will form. 160 mg/min maximum rate. (Flush IV/port with NS before starting the 5-FU)

5-Fluorouracil_____mg (500 mg/m^2) IV push weekly for 4 weeks

- No dilution required. Concentration 50 mg/mL.
- Can be further diluted with NS or D5W.

Major Side Effects

- GI Toxicities: Acute diarrhea, most likely a cholinergic effect, can be managed with atropine before or during therapy. Symptoms include diarrhea, sweating, and abdominal cramping during or after drug administration. Late diarrhea observed in 44% of patients, can be severe, and should be treated aggressively. Dose-limiting toxicity. Nausea and vomiting in 35%–60% of those treated, with 17% experiencing grade 3–4 nausea and 13% experiencing grade 3–4 vomiting.
- Bone Marrow Depression: Dose-limiting, grade 3–4 neutropenia in 29%. Nadir in 7–10 days. CBC weekly.
- Pulmonary Toxicities: Occurs in up to 22% of patients, ranging from transient dyspnea to pulmonary infiltrates, fever, and cough.
- Alopecia: Mild.
- Reproductive: Pregnancy category D. Breast feeding should be avoided.

Initiate antiemetic protocol:	Moderately to highly emetogenic protocol. Initiate antidiarrheal protocol.

Supportive drugs:

☐ pegfilgrastim (Neulasta)   ☐ filgrastim (Neupogen)

☐ epoetin alfa (Procrit)   ☐ darbepoetin alfa (Aranesp)

Initiate antidiarrheal protocol: ☐ loperamide (Imodium)   ☐ diphenoxylate/atropine sulfate (Lomotil)

Treatment schedule: Chair time 3 hours every week for 4 weeks. Repeat cycle every 6 weeks.

Estimated number of visits: Five visits per cycle. Request six cycles worth of visits.

Dose Calculation by: 1. _____   2. _____

_____

Physician

_____

Date

_____

Patient Name

_____

ID Number

_____   _____/ _____/ _____

Diagnosis   Ht   Wt   M^2

Irinotecan + 5-Fluorouracil + Leucovorin (IFL-Saltz Regimen) + Bevacizumab (BV)

Baseline laboratory tests: CBC: Chemistry panel, CEA, urine test for protein baseline and periodically throughout treatment cycles

Baseline procedures or tests: None

Initiate IV: NS or D5W

Premedicate: 5-HT$_3$ and dexamethasone 20 mg in 100 cc of NS or D5W

Atropine 0.25–1.0 mg IV unless contraindicated

Acetaminophen 1000 mg

Cimetidine 300 mg and diphenhydramine 25–50 mg in 100 cc of NS

- Premedication only necessary with prior infusion reaction with Bevacizumab

Administer: Irinotecan_____mg (125 mg/m^2) IV in 500 cc of D5W over 90 minutes weekly for 4 weeks

- Available in 100-mg/5-mL single-use vials or 20 mg/mL, 2 mL vial.
- Store at room temperature; protect from light.
- Dilute and mix drug in 250–500 cc of D5W (preferred) or NS.
- Diluted drug is stable 24 hours at room temperature, if diluted in D5W, and is stable for 48 hours if refrigerated and protected from light.

Leucovorin_____mg (20 mg/m^2) IV push weekly for 4 weeks

- Available in solution or powder. Reconstitute powder with sterile water. May further dilute with NS or D5W.
- Do not mix in same solution with 5-FU, because precipitate will form. (Flush IV/port with NS before starting the 5-FU)

5-Fluorouracil _____mg (500 mg/m^2) IV push weekly for 4 weeks

- No dilution required. Concentration 50 mg/mL
- Can be further diluted with NS or D5W.

Bevacizumab _____mg (5 mg/kg) IV every 2 weeks

- Single-use vial (10 mg/mL); use within 8 hours of opening.
- Further dilute in NS (100–150 cc).
- Initial infusion over 90 minutes; if well tolerated, give second dose over 60 minutes, and if well tolerated, subsequent doses over 30 minutes.
- **DO NOT** administer perioperatively—may inhibit wound healing.

Major Side Effects

- Infusion reaction with bevacizumab: Characterized by fever, rigors, or chills. If reaction occurs: stop infusion, and keep main line open. May require meperidine, antihistamines, or dexamethasone for rigors, as prescribed by physician. Symptoms usually last about 20 minutes. May resume infusion 30 minutes after symptoms resolve.
- Cardiovascular: Hypertension (11%) in the form of hypertensive crisis or hypertension not controlled by current antihypertensive medications may require discontinuation of the drug (bevacizumab).
- Hemostasis: Thrombotic events (19%), bleeding (3.1%), or thrombocytopenia may occur.
- Renal: Nephrotic syndrome and proteinuria may occur. Check for presence of protein in urine. Dipstick or urinalyses to detect proteinuria. 24-hour urine for 4+ protein or use the protein-to-creatinine (UPC) ratio to monitor. (For UPC obtain a random urine protein and a random urine creatinine. Divide the urine protein by the urine creatinine to obtain the ratio. A ratio of <0.1 mg/dl is normal. UPC >2.5 suggests presence of nephritic range proteinuria. The clinical significance or increased proteinuria has not been determined.
- GI Toxicities: Acute diarrhea, most likely a cholinergic effect, can be managed with atropine before or during therapy. Symptoms include diarrhea, sweating, and abdominal cramping during or after drug administration. Late diarrhea observed in 44% of patients, can be severe, and should be treated aggressively. Dose-limiting toxicity. Nausea and vomiting in 35%–60% of those treated, with 17% experiencing grade 3–4 nausea and

13% experiencing grade 3–4 vomiting. Gastrointestinal perforation was observed in 2% of patients.

- Bone Marrow Depression: Dose-limiting, grade 3–4 neutropenia in 29%. Nadir in 7–10 days. CBC weekly.
- Pulmonary Toxicities: Occurs in up to 22% of patients, ranging from transient dyspnea to pulmonary infiltrates, fever, and cough.
- Alopecia: Mild.
- Reproductive: Pregnancy category D. Breast feeding should be avoided.

Initiate antiemetic protocol: Moderately to highly emetogenic protocol. Initiate antidiarrheal protocol.

Supportive drugs: ☐ pegfilgrastim (Neulasta)   ☐ filgrastim (Neupogen)

☐ epoetin alfa (Procrit)   ☐ darbepoetin alfa (Aranesp)

Initiate antidiarrheal protocol: ☐ loperamide (Imodium)   ☐ diphenoxylate/atropine sulfate (Lomotil)

Treatment schedule: Chair time 4 hours every week for 4 weeks. Repeat cycle every 6 weeks. CBC weekly.

Estimated number of visits: Five visits per cycle. Request six cycles worth of visits.

Dose Calculation by: 1. _____   2. _____

_____

Physician   Date

_____

Patient Name   ID Number

_____ / _____ / _____

Diagnosis   Ht   Wt   M²

Irinotecan + 5-Fluorouracil + Leucovorin (Modified IFL-Saltz Regimen)

Baseline laboratory tests:	CBC: Chemistry panel, CEA
Baseline procedures or tests:	None
Initiate IV:	NS or D5W
Premedicate:	5-HT$_3$ and dexamethasone 20 mg in 100 cc of NS or D5W
	Atropine 0.25–1.0 mg IV unless contraindicated

Administer:

Irinotecan_____mg (125 mg/m^2) IV in 500 cc of D5W over 90 minutes weekly for 2 weeks

- Available in 100-mg/5-mL single-use vials or 20 mg/mL, 2 mL vial.
- Store at room temperature; protect from light.
- Dilute and mix drug in 250–500 cc of D5W (preferred) or NS.
- Diluted drug is stable 24 hours at room temperature, if diluted in D5W, and is stable for 48 hours if refrigerated and protected from light.

Leucovorin_____mg (20 mg/m^2) IV push weekly for 2 weeks

- Available in solution or powder. Reconstitute powder with sterile water. May further dilute with NS or D5W. 160 mg/min maximum rate.
- Do not mix in same solution with 5-FU, because precipitate will form. (Flush IV/port with NS before starting the 5-FU)

5-Fluorouracil _____mg (500 mg/m^2) IV push weekly for 2 weeks

- No dilution required. Concentration 50 mg/mL.
- Can be further diluted with NS or D5W.

Major Side Effects

- GI Toxicities: Acute diarrhea, most likely a cholinergic effect, can be managed with atropine before or during therapy. Symptoms include diarrhea, sweating, and abdominal cramping during or after drug administration. Late diarrhea observed in 44% of patients, can be severe, and should be treated aggressively. Dose-limiting toxicity. Nausea and vomiting in 35%–60% of those treated, with 17% experiencing grade 3–4 nausea and 13% experiencing grade 3–4 vomiting.
- Bone Marrow Depression: Dose-limiting, grade 3–4 neutropenia in 29%. Nadir in 7–10 days. CBC weekly.
- Pulmonary Toxicities: Occur in up to 22% of patients, ranging from transient dyspnea to pulmonary infiltrates, fever, and cough.
- Alopecia: Mild.
- Reproductive: Pregnancy category D. Breast feeding should be avoided.

Initiate antiemetic protocol:	Moderately to highly emetogenic protocol. Initiate antidiarrheal protocol.
Supportive drugs:	☐ pegfilgrastim (Neulasta) ☐ filgrastim (Neupogen)
	☐ epoetin alfa (Procrit) ☐ darbepoetin alfa (Aranesp)
Initiate antidiarrheal protocol:	☐ loperamide (Imodium) ☐ diphenoxylate/atropine sulfate (Lomotil)
Treatment schedule:	Chair time 3 hours every week for 2 weeks. Repeat cycle every 3 weeks.
Estimated number of visits:	Two visits per cycle. Request six cycles worth of visits.

Dose Calculation by: 1. _____   2. _____

_____
Physician

_____
Date

_____
Patient Name

_____
ID Number

_____
Diagnosis

_____/_____/_____
Ht   Wt   M^2

IFL-Douillard Regimen

Baseline laboratory tests:	CBC: Chemistry panel and CEA
Baseline procedures or tests:	Central line required for continuous infusion
Initiate IV:	D5W
Premedicate:	5HT$_3$ and dexamethasone 20 mg in 100 cc of D5W
	Atropine 0.25–1.0 mg IV unless contraindicated
Administer:	DAY 1: **Irinotecan** _____mg (180 mg/m^2) IV in 250–500 cc of D5W

- Available in 2- and 5-ml vials (20 mg/ml).
- Store at room temperature and protect from light.
- Dilute and mix drug in D5W (preferred) or NS.
- Diluted drug is stable for 24 hours at room temperature or, if diluted in D5W, is stable for 48 hours if refrigerated and protected from light.

Leucovorin _____mg (200 mg/m^2) IV in 250–500 cc of D5W

- Available in solution or powder. Reconstitute powder with sterile water. May further dilute with NS or D5W.
- Do not mix in same solution with 5-FU, because precipitate will form. Irinotecan and leucovorin are infused concurrently, in separate bags through a Y-site over 2 hours. (Flush IV/port with NS before starting the 5-FU)

Then

5-Fluorouracil _____mg (400 mg/m^2) IV bolus over 2–4 min

- No dilution required. Concentration 50 mg/mL.
- Can be further diluted with 0.9% sodium chloride or D5W.

Then

5-Fluorouracil _____mg (600 mg/m^2) IV continuous infusion over 22 hours

DAY 2: **Leucovorin** _____mg (200 mg/m^2) IV in 250–500 cc of NS or D5W

5-Fluorouracil _____mg (400 mg/m^2) IV bolus over 2–4 minutes, then

5-Fluorouracil _____mg (600 mg/m^2) IV continuous infusion over 22 hours

DAY 3: Discontinue pump.

Major Side Effects	

- GI Toxicities: Early diarrhea, most likely a cholinergic effect, can be managed with atropine before therapy. Late diarrhea observed in 44% of patients, can be severe, and should be treated aggressively. Nausea and vomiting in 35%–60% of those treated, with 17% experiencing grade 3–4 nausea and 13% experiencing grade 3–4 vomiting.
- Skin: Hand-foot syndrome (palmar-plantar erythrodysesthesia) occurs in 15%–20% of patients. Characterized by tingling, numbness, pain, erythema, dryness, rash, swelling, increased pigmentation, and/or pruritus of the hands and feet. Less frequent in reduced doses.
- Ocular: Blepharitis, tear-duct stenosis, acute and chronic conjunctivitis.
- Bone Marrow Depression: Dose-limiting, grade 3–4 neutropenia in 29%. Nadir in 7–10 days. CBC weekly.
- Alopecia: Mild.
- Reproductive: Pregnancy category D. Breast feeding should be avoided.

Initiate antiemetic protocol:	Moderately to highly emetogenic protocol.
Supportive drugs:	☐ pegfilgrastim (Neulasta) ☐ filgrastim (Neupogen)
	☐ epoetin alfa (Procrit) ☐ darbepoetin alfa (Aranesp)
Initiate antidiarrheal protocol:	☐ loperamide (Imodium) ☐ diphenoxylate/atropine sulfate (Lomotil)
Treatment schedule:	Chair time 3 hours on days 1 and 2, and 15 minutes day 3. Repeat every 2 weeks until disease progression.
Estimated number of visits:	Six visits per month. Request three months worth. CBC weekly.

Dose Calculation by: 1. _____ 2. _____

_____

Physician   Date

_____

Patient Name   ID Number

_____   _____/_____/_____

Diagnosis   Ht   Wt   M²

IFL FOLFIRI Regimen

Baseline laboratory tests:	CBC: Chemistry panel and CEA
Baseline procedures or tests:	Central line required for continuous infusion
Initiate IV:	D5W
Premedicate:	$5HT_3$ and dexamethasone 20 mg in 100 cc of D5W
	Atropine 0.25–1.0 mg IV unless contraindicated

Administer:

DAY 1: Irinotecan _____ mg (180 mg/m^2) IV in 250–500-cc of D5W over 90 minutes

- Available in 2- and 5-ml vials (20 mg/ml).
- Store at room temperature and protect from light.
- Dilute and mix drug in D5W (preferred) or NS.
- Diluted drug is stable for 24 hours at room temperature or, if diluted in D5W, is stable for 48 hours if refrigerated and protected from light.

Leucovorin _____ mg (200 mg/m^2) IV in 250–500 cc of D5W over 2 hours. Infuse during irinotecan therapy. Prior to 5-FU infusion.

- Available in solution or powder. Reconstitute solution with sterile water. May further dilute with NS or D5W.
- Do not mix in same solution with 5-FU, because precipitate will form. (Flush IV/port with NS before starting the 5-FU)

5-Fluorouracil _____ mg (400 mg/m^2) IV bolus over 2–4 minutes

- No dilution required. Concentration 50 mg/mL.
- Can be further diluted with 0.9% sodium chloride or D5W.

Then

5-Fluorouacil _____ mg (2.4 g/m^2) IV continuous infusion over 46 hours

DAY 3: Discontinue pump.

Major Side Effects

- GI Toxicities: Early diarrhea, most likely a cholinergic effect, can be managed with atropine before therapy. Late diarrhea observed in 44% of patients, can be severe, and should be treated aggressively. Nausea and vomiting in 35%–60% of those treated, with 17% experiencing grade 3–4 nausea and 13% experiencing grade 3–4 vomiting.
- Bone Marrow Depression: Dose-limiting, grade 3–4 neutropenia in 29%. Nadir in 7–10 days.
- Skin: Hand-foot syndrome (palmar-plantar erythrodysesthesia) occurs in 15%–20% of patients. Characterized by tingling, numbness, pain, erythema, dryness, rash, swelling, increased pigmentation, and/or pruritus of the hands and feet. Less frequent in reduced doses.
- Ocular: Blepharitis, tear-duct stenosis, acute and chronic conjunctivitis.
- Reproductive: Pregnancy category D. Breast feeding should be avoided.
- Alopecia: Mild.
- Reproductive: Pregnancy category D. Breast feeding should be avoided.

Initiate antiemetic protocol:	Highly to moderately emetogenic protocol.

Supportive drugs:

☐ pegfilgrastim (Neulasta)	☐ filgrastim (Neupogen)
☐ epoetin alfa (Procrit)	☐ darbepoetin alfa (Aranesp)

Initiate antidiarrheal protocol:	☐ loperamide (Imodium) ☐ diphenoxylate/atropine sulfate (Lomotil)
Treatment schedule:	Chair time three hours on day 1 and 15 minutes on day 3. Repeat every 2 weeks.
Estimated number of visits:	Two visits per cycle. Request three months worth of visits.

Dose Calculation by: 1. _____   2. _____

_____
Physician

_____
Patient Name

_____
Diagnosis

Date _____

ID Number _____

Ht _____ / Wt _____ / M^2 _____

FOLFOX4

Baseline laboratory tests:	CBC: Chemistry panel and CEA
Baseline procedures or tests:	Central line required for continuous infusion
Initiate IV:	D5W
Premedicate:	Palonosetron (Aloxi) and dexamethasone 20 mg in 100 cc of D5W
Administer:	**DAY 1: Oxaliplatin** _____mg (85 mg/m^2) IV in 250–500 cc of D5W over 2 hours

Classified as an irritant, but extravasations have resulted in induration and formation of nodule lasting 9 months or more.

Available in 50- and 100-mg vials. Concentration is 5 mg/ml.

Do not use chloride containing solutions or aluminum needles.

Leucovorin _____mg (200 mg/m^2) IV in 250–500-cc of D5W over 2 hours

- Available in solution or powder. Reconstitute solution with sterile water. May further dilute with NS or D5W.

- Do not mix in same solution with 5-FU, because precipitate will form. (Oxaliplatin and leucovorin are infused concurrently, in separate bags through a Y-site over 2 hours).

- **DO NOT USE** sodium chloride-containing solutions or aluminum needles. (Flush IV/port with NS before starting the 5-FU)

5-Fluorouracil _____mg (400 mg/m^2) IV bolus over 2–4 minutes

- No dilution required. Concentration 50 mg/mL.

- Can be further diluted with 0.9% sodium chloride or D5W.

Then

5-Fluorouacil _____mg (600 mg/m^2) IV continuous infusion over 22 hours

DAY 2: Leucovorin _____mg (200 mg/m^2) IV in 250–500 cc of NS or D5W

5-Fluorouracil _____mg (400 mg/m^2) IV bolus over 2–4 minutes, then

5-Fluorouracil _____mg (600 mg/m^2) IV continuous infusion over 22 hours

DAY 3: Discontinue pump.

Major Side Effects

- Acute Neurotoxicities: Are temporary and can occur within hours of or up to 14 days after oxaliplatin. Often precipitated by exposure to cold and characterized by dysesthesias, transient paresthesias or hypothesias of hands, feet, perioral area, and throat. Pharyngolaryngeal dysesthesia (**sensation** of discomfort or tightness in the back of the throat and inability to breathe) is most frightening to patients.

- Peripheral Neuropathy: Affects about 48% of patients, usually with a cumulative dose of 800 mg/m^2. Symptoms include paresthesias, dysesthesias, hypoesthesias in a stocking and glove distribution, and altered proprioception (knowing where body parts are in relation to the whole).

- GI Toxicities: Nausea and vomiting in 65% of patients; can be severe. Diarrhea in 80%–90% of patients.

- Bone Marrow Depression: Mild leukopenia, mild-to-moderate thrombocytopenia, and anemia are common.

- Anaphylactic/anaphylactoid reactions to eloxatin have been reported. Delayed hypersensitivity: Symptoms range from mild symptoms, i.e., rash, urticaria, erythema, pruritus, or emesis to anaphylaxis/severe hypersensitivity characterized by dyspnea, angioedema bronchospasm, and hypotension. These reactions occur within minutes of administration and should be managed with appropriate supportive therapy. Drug-related deaths associated with platinum compounds from this reaction have been reported.

- Reproductive: Pregnancy category D. Breast feeding should be avoided.

Initiate antiemetic protocol:	Highly to moderately emetogenic protocol.

Supportive drugs:

☐ pegfilgrastim (Neulasta)	☐ filgrastim (Neupogen)
☐ epoetin alfa (Procrit)	☐ darbepoetin alfa (Aranesp)

Initiate antidiarrheal protocol:

☐ loperamide (Imodium)	☐ diphenoxylate/atropine sulfate (Lomotil)

Treatment schedule: Chair time 3 hours on days 1 and 2, and 15 minutes on day 3. Repeat every 2 weeks for 12 cycles.

Estimated number of visits: 36 visits (six per month for six months or until disease progression)

Dose Calculation by: 1. _____   2. _____

_____   _____
Physician   Date

_____   _____
Patient Name   ID Number

_____ / _____ / _____
Diagnosis   Ht   Wt   M²

FOLFOX6

Baseline laboratory tests:	CBC: Chemistry panel and CEA
Baseline procedures or tests:	Central line required for continuous infusion
Initiate IV:	D5W
Premedicate:	$5HT_3$ and dexamethasone 10–20 mg in 100 cc of D5W
Administer:	**DAY 1: Oxaliplatin** _____ mg (100 mg/m^2) IV in 250–500 cc of D5W

Classified as an irritant, but extravasations have resulted in induration and formation of nodule lasting 9 months or more.

Available in 50- and 100-mg vials. Concentration is 5 mg/ml.

Do not use chloride containing solutions or aluminum needles.

Leucovorin _____ mg (400 mg/m^2) IV in 250–500 cc of D5W

- Available in solution or powder. Reconstitute solution with sterile water. May further dilute with NS or D5W.
- Do not mix in same solution with 5-FU, because precipitate will form. Oxaliplatin and leucovorin are infused concurrently, in separate bags through a Y-site over 2 hours on day 1 only.
- **DO NOT USE** chloride-containing solutions or aluminum needles. (Flush IV/port with NS before starting the 5-FU)

5-Fluorouacil _____ mg (400 mg/m^2) IV bolus on day 1 only

- No dilution required. Concentration 50 mg/mL.
- Can be further diluted with 0.9% sodium chloride or D5W.

5-Fluorouacil _____ mg (2400–3000 mg/m^2) IV continuous infusion over 46 hours

DAY 3: Discontinue pump.

Major Side Effects	

- Acute Neurotoxicities: Are temporary and can occur within hours of or up to 14 days after oxaliplatin. Often precipitated by exposure to cold and characterized by dysesthesias, transient paresthesias or hypothesias of hands, feet, perioral area, and throat. Pharyngolaryngeal dysesthesia (**sensation** of discomfort or tightness in the back of the throat and inability to breathe) is most frightening to patients.
- Peripheral Neuropathy: Affects about 48% of patients, usually with a cumulative dose of 800 mg/m^2. Symptoms include paresthesias, dysesthesias, hypoesthesias in a "stocking and glove" distribution, and altered proprioception (knowing where body parts are in relation to the whole).
- GI Toxicities: Nausea and vomiting in 65% of patients; can be severe. Diarrhea in 80%–90% of patients.
- Bone Marrow Depression: Mild leukopenia, mild-to-moderate thrombocytopenia, and anemia are common.
- Anaphylactic/anaphylactoid reactions to eloxatin have been reported. Delayed hypersensitivity: Symptoms range from mild symptoms, i.e., rash, urticaria, erythema, pruritus, or emesis to anaphylaxis/severe hypersensitivity characterized by dyspnea, angioedema bronchospasm, and hypotension. These reactions occur within minutes of administration and should be managed with appropriate supportive therapy. Drug-related deaths associated with platinum compounds from this reaction have been reported.
- Reproductive: Pregnancy category D. Breast feeding should be avoided.

Initiate antiemetic protocol:	Highly to moderately emetogenic protocol.	
Supportive drugs:	☐ pegfilgrastim (Neulasta)	☐ filgrastim (Neupogen)
	☐ epoetin alfa (Procrit)	☐ darbepoetin alfa (Aranesp)
Initiate antidiarrheal protocol:	☐ loperamide (Imodium)	☐ diphenoxylate/atropine sulfate (Lomotil)
Treatment schedule:	Chair time three hours on day 1, and 30 minutes on day 3. Repeat every 14 days until disease progression.	
Estimated number of visits:	Four visits per month. Request 3 months worth of visits.	

Dose Calculation by: 1. _____ 2. _____

_____

Physician   Date

_____

Patient Name   ID Number

_____ / _____ / _____

Diagnosis   Ht   Wt M^2

FOLFOX7

Baseline laboratory tests:	CBC: Chemistry panel and CEA
Baseline procedures or tests:	Central line required for continuous infusion
Initiate IV:	D5W
Premedicate:	$5HT_3$ and dexamethasone 20 mg in 100 cc of D5W
Administer:	**DAY 1: Oxaliplatin** _____ mg (130 mg/m^2) IV in 250–500 cc of D5W

Classified as an irritant, but extravasations have resulted in induration and formation of nodule lasting 9 months or more.

Available in 50- and 100-mg vials. Concentration is 5 mg/ml.

Do not use chloride containing solutions or aluminum needles.

Leucovorin _____ mg (400 mg/m^2) IV in 250–500 cc of D5W

- Available in solution or powder. Reconstitute powder with sterile water. May further dilute with NS or D5W.
- Do not mix in same solution with 5-FU, because precipitate will form. Oxaliplatin and leucovorin are infused concurrently, in separate bags through a Y-site over 2 hours on day 1 only.
- **DO NOT USE** chloride-containing solutions or aluminum needles. Flush IV/port with NS before starting 5-FU

5-Fluorouracil _____ mg (2.4 g/m^2) IV continuous infusion on days 1 and 2 over 46 hours

DAY 3: Discontinue pump.

- No dilution required. Concentration 50 mg/mL.
- Can be further diluted with 0.9% sodium chloride or D5W.

Major Side Effects	• Acute Neurotoxicities: Are temporary and can occur within hours of or up to 14 days after oxaliplatin. Often precipitated by exposure to cold and characterized by dysesthesias, transient paresthesias or hypothesias of hands, feet, perioral area, and throat. Pharyngolaryngeal dysesthesia (**sensation** of discomfort or tightness in the back of the throat and inability to breathe) is most frightening to patients.

- Peripheral Neuropathy: Affects about 48% of patients, usually with a cumulative dose of 800 mg/m^2. Symptoms include paresthesias, dysesthesias, hypoesthesias in a "stocking and glove" distribution, and altered proprioception (knowing where body parts are in relation to the whole).
- GI Toxicities: Nausea and vomiting in 65% of patients; can be severe. Diarrhea in 80%–90% of patients.
- Bone Marrow Depression: Mild leukopenia, mild-to-moderate thrombocytopenia, and anemia are common.
- Anaphylactic/anaphylactoid reactions to eloxatin have been reported. Delayed hypersensitivity: Symptoms range from mild symptoms, i.e., rash, urticaria, erythema, pruritus, or emesis to anaphylaxis/severe hypersensitivity characterized by dyspnea, angioedema bronchospasm, and hypotension. These reactions occur within minutes of administration and should be managed with appropriate supportive therapy. Drug-related deaths associated with platinum compounds from this reaction have been reported.
- Reproductive: Pregnancy category D. Breast feeding should be avoided.

Initiate antiemetic protocol:	Moderately to highly emetogenic protocol.
Supportive drugs:	☐ pegfilgrastim (Neulasta) ☐ filgrastim (Neupogen)
	☐ epoetin alfa (Procrit) ☐ darbepoetin alfa (Aranesp)
Initiate antidiarrheal protocol:	☐ loperamide (Imodium) ☐ diphenoxylate/atropine sulfate (Lomotil)
Treatment schedule:	Chair time 3 hours on day 1, and 30 minutes on day 3. Repeat every 14 days until disease progression.
Estimated number of visits:	Four visits per month; request 3 months worth of visits

Dose Calculation by: 1. _____   2. _____

_____   _____
Physician   Date

_____   _____
Patient Name   ID Number

_____   _____/_____/_____   _____
Diagnosis   Ht   Wt   M²

Cetuximab + Irinotecan

Baseline laboratory tests:	CBC: Chemistry and CEA monitor electrolytes
Baseline procedures or tests:	EGFR expression using immunohistochemistry
Initiate IV:	NS
Premedicate:	Diphenhydramine 50 mg in 100 cc of NS
Administer:	**Cetuximab** _____mg (400 mg/m^2) IV over 2 hours week 1 only

Cetuximab _____mg (250 mg/m^2) IV over 1 hour weekly as maintenance dose. Followed by 1 hour observation for infusion reactions.

- Maximum infusion rate 5 mL/min.
- **Administer through low-protein-binding 0.22-micron in-line filter.**
- Place cetuximab in sterile evacuated container, prime tubing with drug, and then piggy-back into main line infusion of NS.
- Do not shake or dilute.
- Supplied in 100-mg/50-mL vials; discard 8 hours after opening if kept at room temperature, 12 hours if refrigerated.
- Dose reductions for skin reactions from package insert:

Severe Acneform Rash	ERBITUX	Outcome	ERBITUX Dose Modification
1st occurrence	Delay infusion 1 to 2 weeks	Improvement No Improvement	Continue at 250 mg/m^2 Discontinue ERBITUX
2nd occurrence	Delay infusion 1 to 2 weeks	Improvement No Improvement	Reduce dose to 200 mg/m^2 Discontinue ERBITUX
3rd occurrence	Delay infusion 1 to 2 weeks	Improvement No Improvement	Reduce dose to 150 mg/m2 Discontinue ERBITUX
4th occurrence	Discontine ERBITUX		

Initiate IV:	D5W
Premedicate:	5-HT$_3$ and dexamethasone 20 mg in 100 cc of D5W
	Atropine 0.25–1.0 mg IV unless contraindicated
Administer:	**Irinotecan** _____mg (175 mg/m^2) IV in 500 cc of D5W on day 1 and every 3 weeks

- Available in 2- and 5-mL vials (20 mg/mL).
- Store at room temperature and protect from light.
- Dilute and mix drug in D5W (preferred) or NS.
- Diluted drug is stable for 24 hours at room temperature or, if diluted in D5W, is stable for 48 hours if refrigerated and protected from light.

Major Side Effects

- Infusion Reaction: Seen with eribitux. Severe allergic reactions (3%–4%) with symptoms including rapid onset of airway obstruction (bronchospasm, stirdor, hoarseness), dyspnea, fever, chills, rash, itching, and/or hypotension require that treatment be stopped immediately and NOT started again. For mild or moderate (grade 1–2) infusion reactions (19%), infusion rate should be permanently reduced by 50%.
- Skin: Acneform rash (90%) can be severe and require dose modification (8%). Paronychial inflammation, especially in thumbs and great toes (14%). May be treated with topical antibiotic cream or oral antibiotics.
- Hypomagnesemia may occur in 50% of patients. Grade 3–4 in 10%–15% of patients. Electrolyte replacement may be necessary. Closely monitor magnesium, potassium, and calcium levels.
- GI Toxicities with Irinotecan: Early diarrhea, most likely a cholinergic effect, can be managed with atropine before therapy. Late diarrhea observed in 22% of patients, can be severe, and should be treated aggressively. Nausea and vomiting in 35%–72% of patients, with 17% experiencing grade 3–4 nausea and 13% experiencing grade 3–4 vomiting.
- Bone Marrow Depression: Dose-limiting, grade 3–4 neutropenia in 17%. Nadir in 6–9 days.

- Alopecia: Mild.
- Cardiopulmonary Toxicity: Interstitial Pneumonitis with non-cardiogenic pulmonary edema in < 0.5%. Onset between 4–11th doses. Monitor pulmonary symptoms; if interstitial lung disease develops, erbitux should be discontinued. Cardiopulmonary arrest/and or sudden death occurred in 2% of patients. Closely monitor electrolyes including serum magnesium, potassium, and calcium.
- Reproductive: Pregnancy category D. Breast feeding should be avoided.

Initiate antiemetic protocol: Mildly to moderately emetogenic protocol

Supportive drugs:

☐ epoetin alfa (Procrit)   ☐ darbepoetin alfa (Aranesp)

☐ oprelvekin (Neumega)   ☐ filgrastim (Neupogen)

☐ pegfilgrastim (Neulasta)   ☐ Other _____

Treatment schedule: Chair time 4 hours for first treatment with cetuximab and irinotecan, 1 hour for week cetuximab, 3 hours for all other courses. Repeat cycle every 21 days.

Estimated number of visits: Four visits per month. Request three months worth of visits.

Dose Calculation by: 1. _____   2. _____

_____   _____

Physician   Date

_____   _____

Patient Name   ID Number

_____   _____/_____/_____

Diagnosis   Ht   Wt   M²

XELOX (Capox)

Baseline laboratory tests:	CBC: Chemistry, bilirubin, LFTs, CEA, and creatinine clearance
Baseline procedures or tests:	N/A
Initiate IV:	D5W
Premedicate:	5-HT$_3$ and dexamethasone 10–20 mg in 100 cc of D5W
Administer:	**Oxaliplatin** _____mg (130 mg/m^2) IV in 250 cc of 5W over 2 hours on day 1

- Do not mix with chloride-containing solutions or use aluminum needles.
- Reconstitute with 10–40 mL of sterile water or D5W
- Further dilute in D5W. Stable for 24 hours at room temperature.

Capecitabine _____mg (1000 mg/m^2) PO bid on days 1–14

- Available in 150- or 500-mg tablets for oral use.
- Administer within 30 minutes of a meal with plenty of water.
- Monitor international normalized ratios (INRs) closely in patients taking warfarin; may increase INR.

Major Side Effects

- Acute Neurotoxicities: Are temporary and can occur within hours of or up to 14 days after oxaliplatin. Often precipitated by exposure to cold and characterized by dysesthesias, transient paresthesias or hypothesias of hands, feet, perioral area, and throat. Pharyngolaryngeal dysesthesia (**sensation** of discomfort or tightness in the back of the throat and inability to breathe) is most frightening to patients.
- Peripheral Neuropathy: Affects about 48% of patients, usually with a cumulative dose of 800 mg/m^2. Symptoms include paresthesias, dysesthesias, hypoesthesias in a stocking and glove distribution, and altered proprioception (knowing where body parts are in relation to the whole).
- GI Toxicities: Nausea and vomiting in 50%–65% of patients; can be severe. Diarrhea occurs in up to 40% with 15% being grade 3–4. Stomatitis is common, 3% of which is severe.
- Skin: Hand-foot syndrome (palmar-plantar erythrodysesthesia) occurs in 15%–20% of patients. Characterized by tingling, numbness, pain, erythema, dryness, rash, swelling, increased pigmentation, and/or pruritus of the hands and feet. Less frequent in reduced doses.
- Ocular: Blepharitis, tear-duct stenosis, acute and chronic conjunctivitis.
- Hepatic: Elevations in serum bilirubin (20%–40%), alkaline phosphatase, and hepatic transaminases (aspartate transaminase [SGOT], alanine transaminase [SGPT]). Dose modifications may be required if hyperbilirubinemia occurs.
- Renal Insufficiency: Xeloda contraindicated in patients with creatinine clearance < 30 mL/min, with creatinine clearance of 30–50 mL/min at baseline a dose reduction to 75% of capecitabine should be made.
- Bone Marrow Toxicity: Grade 3–4 neutropenia (15%), thrombocytopenia (4%)
- Anaphylactic/anaphylactoid reactions to eloxatin have been reported. Delayed hypersensitivity: Symptoms range from mild symptoms, i.e., rash, urticaria, erythema, pruritus, or emesis to anaphylaxis / severe hypersensitivity characterized by dyspnea, angioedema bronchospasm, and hypotension. These reactions occur within minutes of administration and should be managed with appropriate supportive therapy. Drug-related deaths associated with platinum compounds from this reaction have been reported.
- Reproductive: Pregnancy category D. Breast feeding should be avoided.

Initiate antiemetic protocol:	Highly to moderately emetogenic protocol.

Supportive drugs:

☐ pegfilgrastim (Neulasta)	☐ filgrastim (Neupogen)
☐ loperamide (Imodium)	☐ epoetin alfa (Procrit)

Initiate antidiarrheal protocol:	☐ darbepoetin alfa (Aranesp)	☐ diphenoxylate/atropine sulfate (Lomotil)
Treatment schedule:	Chair time 3 hours. Repeat cycle every 21 days until disease progression.	
Estimated number of visits:	One visit per cycle. Request three cycles worth.	

Dose Calculation by: 1. _____ 2. _____

_____

Physician   Date

_____

Patient Name   ID Number

_____/_____/_____

Diagnosis   Ht   Wt   M²

Capecitabine + Irinotecan (XELIRI)

Baseline laboratory tests:	CBC: Chemistry, bilirubin, LFTs, CEA, and creatinine clearance
Baseline procedures or tests:	N/A
Initiate IV:	NS or D5W
Premedicate:	5-HT$_3$ and dexamethasone 10–20 mg in 100 cc of NS or D5W
	Atropine 0.25–1.0 mg IV unless contraindicated.

Administer:

Capecitabine _____mg (1000 mg/m^2) PO bid days 1–14
- Available in 150- and 500-mg tablets.
- Administer within 30 minutes of a meal with plenty of water.
- Monitor INRs closely in patients taking warfarin; may increase INR.

Irinotecan _____mg (200–250 mg/m^2) IV in 250–500 cc of D5W over 90 minutes on day 1

OR

Irinotecan _____mg (80 mg/m^2) IV in 250 cc of D5W over 90 minutes on days 1 and 8
- Available in 2- and 5-ml vials (20 mg/ml).
- Store at room temperature and protect from light.
- Dilute and mix drug in D5W (preferred) or NS.
- Diluted drug is stable for 24 hours at room temperature or, if diluted in D5W, is stable for 48 hours if refrigerated and protected from light.

Major Side Effects
- GI Toxicities: Nausea and vomiting in 30%–50% of patients, 12% grade 3–4. Diarrhea is common, with 20% being grade 3–4. Stomatitis, 3% of which is severe.
- Skin: Hand-foot syndrome (palmar-plantar erythrodysesthesia) occurs in 15%–20% of patients. Characterized by tingling, numbness, pain, erythema, dryness, rash, swelling, increased pigmentation, and/or pruritus of the hands and feet. Less frequent in reduced doses. Grade 3–4 (6%) with XELIRI.
- Bone Marrow Toxicity: Grade 3–4 neutropenia, 25%.
- Renal Insufficiency: Xeloda contraindicated in patients with creatinine clearance < 30 mL/min, with creatinine clearance of 30–50 mL/min at baseline a dose reduction to 75% of capecitabine should be made.
- Ocular: Blepharitis, tear-duct stenosis, acute and chronic conjunctivitis.
- Hepatic: Elevations in serum bilirubin (20%–40%), alkaline phosphatase, and hepatic transaminase (SGOT, SGPT) levels. Dose modifications may be required if hyperbilirubinemia occurs.
- Reproductive: Pregnancy category D. Breast feeding should be avoided.

Initiate antiemetic protocol:	Moderately to highly emetogenic protocol.
Supportive drugs:	☐ pegfilgrastim (Neulasta) ☐ filgrastim (Neupogen)
	☐ loperamide (Imodium) ☐ epoetin alfa (Procrit)
Initiate antidiarrheal protocol:	☐ darbepoetin alfa (Aranesp) ☐ diphenoxylate/atropine sulfate (Lomotil)
Treatment schedule:	Chair time 2 hours. Repeat cycle every 21 days as tolerated or until disease progression.
Estimated number of visits:	One visit per cycle. Request three cycles.

Dose Calculation by: 1. _____   2. _____

_____

Physician   Date

_____

Patient Name   ID Number

_____   _____/_____/_____

Diagnosis   Ht   Wt   M^2

Oxaliplatin + Irinotecan (IROX Regimen)

Baseline laboratory tests:	CBC: Chemistry panel and CEA
Baseline procedures or tests:	N/A
Initiate IV:	D5W
Premedicate:	5-HT$_3$ and dexamethasone 20 mg in 100 cc of D5W
Administer:	**Oxaliplatin** _____ mg (85 mg/m^2) IV in 250–500 cc of D5W on day 1

- Available in 50- and 100-mg vials for IV use.
- Dilute with 10–40 mL with sterile water or D5W.
- Further dilute in a solution of 250 or 500 cc of D5W.
- Do not administer drug undiluted.
- **NEVER** use NS or saline-containing solutions.
- Reconstituted solution is stable for 24 hours at room temperature.

Irinotecan _____ mg (200 mg/m^2) IV in 500 cc of D5W day 1

- Available in 100-mg vials, 20 mg/mL.
- Store at room temperature and protect from light.
- Dilute and mix drug in D5W (preferred) or NS.
- Diluted drug is stable for 24 hours at room temperature or, if diluted in D5W, is stable for 48 hours if refrigerated and protected from light.

Major Side Effects

- Acute Neurotoxicities: Are temporary and can occur within hours of or up to 14 days after oxaliplatin. Often precipitated by exposure to cold and characterized by dysesthesias, transient paresthesias or hypothesias of hands, feet, perioral area, and throat. Pharyngolaryngeal dysesthesia (**sensation** of discomfort or tightness in the back of the throat and inability to breathe) is most frightening to patients.
- Peripheral Neuropathy: Affects about 48% of patients, usually with a cumulative dose of 800 mg/m^2. Symptoms include paresthesias, dysesthesias, hypoesthesias in a stocking and glove distribution, and altered proprioception (knowing where body parts are in relation to the whole).
- GI Toxicities: Nausea and vomiting; can be severe. Diarrhea can be dose limiting. Early diarrhea, most likely a cholinergic effect, can be managed with atropine before therapy. Late diarrhea can be severe and should be treated aggressively.
- Bone Marrow Depression: Myelosuppression, dose-limiting neutropenia. CBC weekly.
- Renal: Renal toxicity is uncommon.
- Ototoxicity: Rare in contrast to cisplatin.
- Anaphylactic/anaphylactoid reactions to eloxatin have been reported. Delayed hypersensitivity: Symptoms range from mild symptoms, i.e., rash, urticaria, erythema, pruritus, or emesis to anaphylaxis / severe hypersensitivity characterized by dyspnea, angioedema bronchospasm, and hypotension. These reactions occur within minutes of administration and should be managed with appropriate supportive therapy. Drug-related deaths associated with platinum compounds from this reaction have been reported.
- Reproductive: Pregnancy category D. Breast feeding should be avoided.

Initiate antiemetic protocol:	Highly to moderately emetogenic protocol.
Supportive drugs:	☐ pegfilgrastim (Neulasta) ☐ filgrastim (Neupogen)
	☐ epoetin alfa (Procrit) ☐ darbepoetin alfa (Aranesp)
Initiate antidiarrheal protocol:	☐ loperamide (Imodium) ☐ diphenoxylate/atropine sulfate (Lomotil)
Treatment schedule:	Chair time 4 hours on day 1. Repeat cycle every 3 weeks until disease progression.
Estimated number of visits:	Weekly visits. Request four cycles worth of visits.

Dose Calculation by: 1. _____   2. _____

_____

Physician   Date

_____   _____

Patient Name   ID Number

_____   _____/_____/_____   _____

Diagnosis   Ht   Wt   M²

5-Fluorouracil + Leucovorin (Mayo Clinic Regimen)

Baseline laboratory tests:	CBC: Chemistry and CEA
Baseline procedures or tests:	N/A
Initiate IV:	0.9% sodium chloride
Premedicate:	Oral phenothiazine or 5-HT$_3$ and 10–20 mg of dexamethasone if necessary
Administer:	**5-Fluorouracil** _____ mg (425 mg/m^2/day) IV on days 1–5

- No dilution required. Concentration 50 mg/mL.
- Can be further diluted with 0.9% sodium chloride or D5W.

Leucovorin _____ mg (20 mg/m^2/day) IV on days 1–5, administered before 5-FU

- Available in solution or powder. Reconstitute solution with sterile water. May further dilute with 0.9% sodium chloride or D5W.
- Do not mix in same solution with 5-FU, because a precipitate will form.

Major Side Effects

- Bone Marrow Depression: Nadir 10–14 days. Neutropenia, thrombocytopenia are dose related. Can be dose limiting for daily × 5 or weekly regimens.
- GI Toxicities: Nausea and vomiting occur in 30%–50% of patients but are usually mild. Mucositis and diarrhea can be severe and dose limiting.
- Skin: Alopecia is more common in the 5-day course and results in diffuse thinning of hair. Hyperpigmentation, photosensitivity, and nail changes may occur. Hand-foot syndrome can be dose limiting.
- Ocular: Photophobia, increased lacrimation, conjunctivitis, and blurred vision.
- Reproductive: Pregnancy category D. Breast feeding should be avoided.

Initiate antiemetic protocol:	Mildly to moderately emetogenic protocol.
Supportive drugs:	☐ pegfilgrastim (Neulasta) ☐ filgrastim (Neupogen)
	☐ epoetin alfa (Procrit) ☐ darbepoetin alfa (Aranesp)
Initiate antidiarrheal protocol:	☐ loperamide (Imodium) ☐ diphenoxylate/atropine sulfate (Lomotil)
Treatment schedule:	Chair time 1 hour on days 1–5. Repeat cycle every 4–5 weeks.
Estimated number of visits:	6 days per cycle. Request four cycles worth of visits.

Dose Calculation by: 1. _____   2. _____

Physician _____   Date _____

Patient Name _____   ID Number _____

Diagnosis _____   _____/ Ht   _____/ Wt   _____ M^2

5-Fluorouracil + Leucovorin (Roswell Park Cancer Institute Regimen/High Dose)

Baseline laboratory tests:	CBC: Chemistry and CEA
Baseline procedures or tests:	N/A
Initiate IV:	0.9% sodium chloride
Premedicate:	Oral phenothiazine or 5-HT$_3$ and 10–20 mg of dexamethasone if necessary
Administer:	**5-Fluorouracil**_____mg (500 mg/m^2) IV bolus 1 hour after start of leucovorin weekly for 6 weeks

- No dilution required. Concentration 50 mg/mL.
- Can be further diluted with 0.9% sodium chloride or D5W.

Leucovorin _____mg (500 mg/m^2) IV over 2 hours, weekly for 6 weeks

- Available in solution or powder. Reconstitute solution with sterile water. May further dilute with 0.9% sodium chloride or D5W.
- Do not mix in same solution with 5-FU, because a precipitate will form.

Major Side Effects

- Bone Marrow Depression: Nadir 10–14 days. Neutropenia, thrombocytopenia are dose related. Can be dose limiting for daily × 5 or weekly regimens.
- GI Toxicities: Nausea and vomiting occur in 30%–50% of patients but are usually mild. Mucositis and diarrhea can be severe and dose limiting.
- Skin: Alopecia is more common in the 5-day course and results in diffuse thinning of hair. Hyperpigmentation, photosensitivity, and nail changes may occur. Hand-foot syndrome can be dose limiting.
- Ocular: Photophobia, increased lacrimation, conjunctivitis, and blurred vision.
- Reproductive: Pregnancy category D. Breast feeding should be avoided.

Initiate antiemetic protocol:	Mildly emetogenic protocol.
Supportive drugs:	☐ pegfilgrastim (Neulasta) ☐ filgrastim (Neupogen)
	☐ epoetin alfa (Procrit) ☐ darbepoetin alfa (Aranesp)
Initiate antidiarrheal protocol:	☐ loperamide (Imodium) ☐ diphenoxylate/atropine sulfate (Lomotil)
Treatment schedule:	Chair time 1 hour weekly for 6 weeks. Repeat every 6 weeks for four cycles.
Estimated number of visits:	Six visits per cycle, 24 per course.

Dose Calculation by: 1. _____   2. _____

_____

Physician

_____

Patient Name

_____/_____/_____

Diagnosis

Date _____

ID Number _____

Ht _____   Wt _____   M^2 _____

5-Fluorouracil + Leucovorin + Bevacizumab

Baseline laboratory tests:	CBC: Chemistry and CEA and urine test for protein baseline and periodically throughout treatment cycles
Initiate IV:	0.9% sodium chloride
Premedicate:	Oral phenothiazine or 5-HT$_3$ and 10–20 mg of dexamethasone if necessary
Administer:	**Leucovorin** _____ mg (500 mg/m^2) IV over 2 hours, weekly for 6 weeks

- Available in solution or powder. Reconstitute solution with sterile water. May further dilute with 0.9% sodium chloride or D5W.
- Do not mix in same solution with 5-FU, because a precipitate will form.

5-Fluorouracil _____ mg (500 mg/m^2) IV weekly for 6 weeks

- No dilution required. Can be further diluted with 0.9% sodium chloride or D5W.

Administer:	**Bevacizumab** _____ mg (5 mg/kg) IV every 2 weeks

- Single-use vial (10 mg/mL); use within 8 hours of opening.
- Further dilute in NS (100–150 cc).
- Initial infusion over 90 minutes; if well tolerated, give second dose over 60 minutes, and if well tolerated, subsequent doses over 30 minutes.
- **DO NOT** administer perioperatively—may inhibit wound healing.

Major Side Effects

- Infusion reaction with bevacizumab: Characterized by fever, rigors, or chills. If reaction occurs: stop infusion, and keep main line open. May require meperidine, antihistamines, or dexamethasone for rigors, as prescribed by physician. Symptoms usually last about 20 minutes. May resume infusion 30 minutes after symptoms resolve.
- Cardiovascular: Hypertension (11%) in the form of hypertensive crisis or hypertension not controlled by current antihypertensive medications may require discontinuation of the drug (bevacizumab).
- Hemostasis: Thrombotic events (19%), bleeding (3.1%), or thrombocytopenia may occur.
- Renal: Nephrotic syndrome and proteinuria may occur. Check for presence of protein in urine. Dipstick or urinalyses to detect proteinuria. 24-hour urine for 4+ protein or use the protein-to-creatinine (UPC) ratio to monitor. (For UPC obtain a random urine protein and a random urine creatinine. Divide the urine protein by the urine creatinine to obtain the ratio. A ratio of < 0.1 mg/dl is normal. UPC > 2.5 suggests presence of nephritic range proteinuria. The clinical significance or increased proteinuria has not been determined.
- Bone Marrow Depression: Nadir 10–14 days. Neutropenia, thrombocytopenia are dose related. Can be dose limiting for daily × 5 or weekly regimens.
- GI Toxicities: Nausea and vomiting occur in 30%–50% of patients but are usually mild. Mucositis and diarrhea can be severe and dose limiting.
- Skin: Alopecia is more common in the 5-day course and results in diffuse thinning of hair. Hyperpigmentation, photosensitivity, and nail changes may occur. Hand-foot syndrome can be dose limiting.
- Ocular: Photophobia, increased lacrimation, conjunctivitis, and blurred vision.
- Reproductive: Pregnancy category D. Breast feeding should be avoided.

Initiate antiemetic protocol:	Mildly emetogenic protocol.	
Supportive drugs:	☐ pegfilgrastim (Neulasta)	☐ filgrastim (Neupogen)
	☐ epoetin alfa (Procrit)	☐ darbepoetin alfa (Aranesp)
Initiate antidiarrheal protocol:	☐ loperamide (Imodium)	☐ diphenoxylate/atropine sulfate (Lomotil)
Treatment schedule:	Chair time 1 hour weekly for 6 weeks. Nadir drawn between days 10 and 14. Repeat every 8 weeks for four cycles.	
Estimated number of visits:	Six visits per cycle, 24 visits per course.	

Dose Calculation by: 1. _____   2. _____

_____

Physician   Date

_____

Patient Name   ID Number

_____   ____ / ____ / ____

Diagnosis   Ht   Wt   M^2

5-Fluorouracil + Leucovorin (German Schedule/Low Dose)

Baseline laboratory tests:	CBC: Chemistry and CEA
Baseline procedures or tests:	N/A
Initiate IV:	0.9% sodium chloride
Premedicate:	Oral phenothiazine or 5-HT$_3$ and 10–20 mg of dexamethasone if necessary
Administer:	**5-Fluorouracil** _____ mg (600 mg/m^2) IV weekly for 6 weeks

- No dilution required. Concentration 50 mg/mL.
- Can be further diluted with 0.9% sodium chloride or D5W.

Leucovorin _____ mg (20 mg/m^2) IV weekly for 6 weeks; administer before 5-Fluorouracil

- Available in solution or powder. Reconstitute powder with sterile water. May further dilute with 0.9% sodium chloride or D5W.
- Do not mix in same solution with 5-FU, because a precipitate will form.

Major Side Effects

- Bone Marrow Depression: Nadir at day 10–14. Neutropenia, thrombocytopenia are dose related. Can be dose limiting for daily × 5 or weekly regimens.
- GI Toxicities: Nausea and vomiting occur in 30%–50% of patients but are usually mild. Mucositis and diarrhea can be severe and dose limiting.
- Skin: Alopecia is more common in the 5-day course and results in diffuse thinning of hair. Hyperpigmentation, photosensitivity, and nail changes may occur. Hand-foot syndrome can be dose limiting.
- Ocular: Photophobia, increased lacrimation, conjunctivitis, and blurred vision.
- Reproductive: Pregnancy category D. Breast feeding should be avoided.

Initiate antiemetic protocol:	Mildly emetogenic protocol.

Supportive drugs:

☐ pegfilgrastim (Neulasta)　　　　☐ filgrastim (Neupogen)

☐ epoetin alfa (Procrit)　　　　☐ darbepoetin alfa (Aranesp)

Initiate antidiarrheal protocol:　☐ loperamide (Imodium)　　☐ diphenoxylate/atropine sulfate (Lomotil)

Treatment schedule:	Chair time 1 hour weekly for 6 weeks. Repeat cycle every 8 weeks.
Estimated number of visits:	Twelve visits per cycle. Nadir drawn between days 10–14. Request four cycles worth of visits.

Dose Calculation by:　1. _____　2. _____

_____　　　　_____
Physician　　　　　　　　　　　　Date

_____　　　　_____
Patient Name　　　　　　　　　　ID Number

_____　　_____/_____/_____
Diagnosis　　　　　　　　　　Ht　　　　　　Wt　　　　　　M^2

Dose Calculation by: 1. _____   2. _____

_____

Physician   Date

_____

Patient Name   ID Number

_____   _____/_____/_____

Diagnosis   Ht   Wt   M²

5-Fluorouracil + Leucovorin (German Schedule/Low Dose)

Baseline laboratory tests:	CBC: Chemistry and CEA
Baseline procedures or tests:	N/A
Initiate IV:	0.9% sodium chloride
Premedicate:	Oral phenothiazine or 5-HT$_3$ and 10–20 mg of dexamethasone if necessary
Administer:	**5-Fluorouracil** _____ mg (600 mg/m^2) IV weekly for 6 weeks

- No dilution required. Concentration 50 mg/mL.
- Can be further diluted with 0.9% sodium chloride or D5W.

Leucovorin _____ mg (20 mg/m^2) IV weekly for 6 weeks; administer before 5-Fluorouracil

- Available in solution or powder. Reconstitute powder with sterile water. May further dilute with 0.9% sodium chloride or D5W.
- Do not mix in same solution with 5-FU, because a precipitate will form.

Major Side Effects

- Bone Marrow Depression: Nadir at day 10–14. Neutropenia, thrombocytopenia are dose related. Can be dose limiting for daily × 5 or weekly regimens.
- GI Toxicities: Nausea and vomiting occur in 30%–50% of patients but are usually mild. Mucositis and diarrhea can be severe and dose limiting.
- Skin: Alopecia is more common in the 5-day course and results in diffuse thinning of hair. Hyperpigmentation, photosensitivity, and nail changes may occur. Hand-foot syndrome can be dose limiting.
- Ocular: Photophobia, increased lacrimation, conjunctivitis, and blurred vision.
- Reproductive: Pregnancy category D. Breast feeding should be avoided.

Initiate antiemetic protocol:	Mildly emetogenic protocol.

Supportive drugs:	☐ pegfilgrastim (Neulasta)	☐ filgrastim (Neupogen)
	☐ epoetin alfa (Procrit)	☐ darbepoetin alfa (Aranesp)
Initiate antidiarrheal protocol:	☐ loperamide (Imodium)	☐ diphenoxylate/atropine sulfate (Lomotil)

Treatment schedule:	Chair time 1 hour weekly for 6 weeks. Repeat cycle every 8 weeks.
Estimated number of visits:	Twelve visits per cycle. Nadir drawn between days 10–14. Request four cycles worth of visits.

Dose Calculation by: 1. _____   2. _____

Physician

Date

Patient Name

ID Number

Diagnosis

Ht _____ / Wt _____ / M^2 _____

5-Fluorouracil (de Gramont Regimen)

Baseline laboratory tests:	CBC: Chemistry and CEA
Baseline procedures or tests:	Central line placement
Initiate IV:	0.9% sodium chloride
Premedicate:	Oral phenothiazine or 5-HT$_3$ and 10–20 mg dexamethasone if necessary
Administer:	**DAYS 1 & 2: 5-Fluorouracil** _____ mg (400 mg/m^2) IV bolus, **then**

5-Fluorouracil _____ mg (600 mg/m^2) IV over 22 hours days 1 and 2

- No dilution required. Concentration 50 mg/mL.
- Can be further diluted with 0.9% sodium chloride or D5W.

Leucovorin _____ mg (200 mg/m^2) IV over 2 hours before 5-FU days 1 and 2

- Available in solution or powder. Reconstitute powder with sterile water. May further dilute with NS or D5W.
- Do not mix in same solution with 5-FU, because precipitate will form.

DAY 3: Discontinue pump.

Major Side Effects

- Bone Marrow Depression: Nadir 10–14 days. Neutropenia, thrombocytopenia are dose related. Can be dose limiting for daily × 5 or weekly regimens.
- GI Toxicities: Nausea and vomiting occur in 30%–50% of patients but are usually mild. Mucositis and diarrhea can be severe and dose limiting.
- Skin: Alopecia is more common in the 5-day course and results in diffuse thinning of hair. Hyperpigmentation, photosensitivity, and nail changes may occur. Hand-foot syndrome can be dose limiting.
- Ocular: Photophobia, increased lacrimation, conjunctivitis, and blurred vision.
- Reproductive: Pregnancy category D. Breast feeding should be avoided.

Initiate antiemetic protocol:	Mildly emetogenic protocol.
Supportive drugs:	☐ pegfilgrastim (Neulasta) ☐ filgrastim (Neupogen)
	☐ epoetin alfa (Procrit) ☐ darbepoetin alfa (Aranesp)
Initiate antidiarrheal protocol:	☐ loperamide (Imodium) ☐ diphenoxylate/atropine sulfate (Lomotil)
Treatment schedule:	Chair time 3 hours on days 1 and 2, and 15 minutes day 3. Repeat cycle every 2 weeks.
Estimated number of visits:	Two visits per cycle. Request three to four cycles worth of visits.

Dose Calculation by: 1. _____   2. _____

_____   _____
Physician   Date

_____   _____
Patient Name   ID Number

_____   _____/_____/_____
Diagnosis   Ht   Wt   M^2

FOLFOX4 + Bevacizumab

Baseline laboratory tests:	CBC: Chemistry panel, and urine test for protein baseline and periodically throughout treatment cycles.
Baseline procedures or tests:	Central line required for continuous infusion
Initiate IV:	D5W
Premedicate:	5 HT$_3$ and dexamethasone 20 mg in 100 cc of D5W
Administer:	

Day 1: Bevacizumab _____mg (10 mg/kg) IV every 2 weeks

- Single-use vial (10 mg/mL); use within 8 hours of opening
- Further dilute in NS (100–150 cc).
- Initial infusion over 90 minutes; if well tolerated, give second dose over 60 minutes, and if well tolerated, subsequent doses over 30 minutes.
- **DO NOT** administer perioperatively—may inhibit wound healing.

DAY 1: Oxaliplatin _____mg (85 mg/m^2) IV in 250–500 cc of D5W over 2 hours

Classified as an irritant, but extravasations have resulted in induration and formation of nodule lasting 9 months or more.

- Available in 50- and 100-mg vials. Concentration is 5 mg/ml.
- Do not use chloride containing solutions or aluminum needles.

Leucovorin_____mg (200 mg/m^2) IV in 250–500 cc of D5W over 2 hours

- Available in solution or powder. Reconstitute solution with sterile water. May further dilute with NS or D5W.
- Do not mix in same solution with 5-FU, because precipitate will form.

(Oxaliplatin and leucovorin are infused concurrently, in separate bags through a Y-site over 2 hours). **DO NOT USE** sodium chloride–containing solutions or aluminum needles.

5-Fluorouracil _____mg (400 mg/m2) IV bolus over 2–4 minutes,

- No dilution required. Concentration 50 mg/mL.
- Can be further diluted with 0.9% sodium chloride or D5W.

then

5-Fluorouracil _____mg (600 mg/m^2) IV continuous infusion over 22 hours

DAY 2: Leucovorin _____mg (200 mg/m^2) IV in 250–500 cc of NS or D5W

5-Fluorouracil _____mg (400 mg/m^2) IV bolus over 2–4 minutes, then

5-Fluorouracil ____mg (600 mg/m^2) IV continuous infusion over 22 hours

DAY 3: Discontinue pump.

Major Side Effects

- Anaphylactic/anaphylactoid reactions to eloxatin have been reported. Delayed hypersensitivity: Symptoms range from mild symptoms, i.e., rash, urticaria, erythema, pruritus, or emesis to anaphylaxis / severe hypersensitivity characterized by dyspnea, angioedema bronchospasm, and hypotension. These reactions occur within minutes of administration and should be managed with appropriate supportive therapy. Drug-related deaths associated with platinum compounds from this reaction have been reported.

- Infusion Reaction with bevacizumab: Characterized by fever, rigors, or chills. If reaction occurs: stop infusion, and keep main line open. May require meperidine, antihistamines, or dexamethasone for rigors, as prescribed by physician. Symptoms usually last about 20 minutes. May resume infusion 30 minutes after symptoms resolve.

- Cardiovascular: Hypertension (11%) in the form of hypertensive crisis or hypertension not controlled by current antihypertensive medications may require discontinuation of the drug (bevacizumab).

- Hemostasis: Thrombotic events (19%), bleeding (3.1%), or thrombocytopenia may occur.

- Renal: Nephrotic syndrome and proteinuria may occur. Check for presence of protein in urine. Dipstick or urinalyses to detect proteinuria. 24-hour urine for 4+ protein or use the protein-to-creatinine (UPC) ratio to monitor. (For UPC obtain a random urine protein and a random urine creatinine.) Divide the urine protein by the urine creatinine to obtain the ratio. A ratio of < 0.1 mg/dl is normal. UPC < 2.5 suggests presence of nephritic range proteinuria. The clinical significance or increased proteinuria has not been determined.

- Acute Neurotoxicities: Are temporary and can occur within hours of or up to 14 days after oxaliplatin. Often precipitated by exposure to cold and characterized by dysesthesias, transient paresthesias or hypothesias of hands, feet, perioral area, and throat. Pharyngolaryngeal dysesthesia (**sensation** of discomfort or tightness in the back of the throat and inability to breathe) is most frightening to patients.

- Peripheral Neuropathy: Affects about 48% of patients, usually with a cumulative dose of 800 mg/m^2. Symptoms include paresthesias, dysesthesias, hypoesthesias in a stocking and glove distribution, and altered proprioception (knowing where body parts are in relation to the whole).

- GI Toxicities: Nausea and vomiting in 65% of patients; can be severe. Diarrhea in 80%–90% of patients.

- Bone Marrow Depression: Mild leukopenia, mild-to-moderate thrombocytopenia, and anemia are common.

- Reproductive: Pregnancy category D. Breast feeding should be avoided.

Initiate antiemetic protocol:	Highly to mildly emetogenic protocol.	
Supportive drugs:	☐ pegfilgrastim (Neulasta)	☐ filgrastim (Neupogen)
	☐ epoetin alfa (Procrit)	☐ darbepoetin alfa (Aranesp)
Initiate antidiarrheal protocol:	☐ loperamide (Imodium)	☐ diphenoxylate/atropine sulfate (Lomotil)
Treatment schedule:	Chair time 4–5 hours on days 1, 3 hours on day 2, and 15 minutes on day 3. Repeat every 2 weeks for 12 cycles.	
Estimated number of visits:	36 visits (6 per month for 6 months or until disease progression)	

Dose Calculation by: 1. _____ 2. _____

_____

Physician   Date

_____

Patient Name   ID Number

_____   _____/_____/_____

Diagnosis   Ht   Wt   M^2

Capecitabine + Oxaliplatin (XELOX) + Bevacizumab

Baseline laboratory tests:	CBC: Chemistry, bilirubin, LFTs, CEA, creatinine clearance, and urine test for protein baseline and periodically throughout treatment cycles.
Initiate IV:	D5W
Premedicate:	5-HT$_3$ and dexamethasone 10–20 mg in 100 cc of D5W
Administer:	**Bevacizumab** _____ mg (7.5 mg/kg) IV every 2 weeks

- Single-use vial (10 mg/mL); use within 8 hours of opening.
- Further dilute in NS (100–150 cc).
- Initial infusion over 90 minutes; if well tolerated, give second dose over 60 minutes, and if well tolerated, subsequent doses over 30 minutes.
- **DO NOT** administer perioperatively—may inhibit wound healing.

Oxaliplatin _____ mg (130 mg/m^2) IV in 250 cc of D5W over 2 hours on day 1

- Available in 50- and 100-mg vials. Concentration is 5 mg/mL.
- Do not mix with chloride-containing solutions or use aluminum needles.
- Reconstitute with 10–40 mL of sterile water or D5W.
- Further dilute in D5W. Stable for 24 hours at room temperature.

Capecitabine _____ mg (850 mg/m^2) PO bid on days 1–14

- Available in 150- or 500-mg tablets for oral use.
- Administer within 30 minutes of a meal with plenty of water.
- Monitor international normalized ratios (INRs) closely in patients taking warfarin; may increase INR.

Major Side Effects

- Infusion Reaction with bevacizumab: Characterized by fever, rigors, or chills. If reaction occurs: stop infusion, and keep main line open. May require meperidine, antihistamines, or dexamethasone for rigors, as prescribed by physician. Symptoms usually last about 20 minutes. May resume infusion 30 minutes after symptoms resolve.

- Anaphylactic/anaphylactoid reactions to eloxatin have been reported. Delayed hypersensitivity: May occur after 10–12 cycles. Symptoms range from mild symptoms, i.e., rash, urticaria, erythema, pruritus, or emesis to anaphylaxis / severe hypersensitivity characterized by dyspnea, angioedema bronchospasm, and hypotension. These reactions occur within minutes of administration and should be managed with appropriate supportive therapy. Drug-related deaths associated with platinum compounds from this reaction have been reported.

- Cardiovascular: Hypertension (11%) in the form of hypertensive crisis or hypertension not controlled by current antihypertensive medications may require discontinuation of the drug (bevacizumab).

- Hemostasis: Thrombotic events (19%), bleeding (3.1%), or thrombocytopenia may occur.

- Renal Insufficiency: Xeloda contraindicated in patients with creatinine clearance < 30 mL/min, with creatinine clearance of 30–50 mL/min at baseline a dose reduction to 75% of capecitabine should be made.

- Renal: Nephrotic syndrome and proteinuria may occur. Check for presence of protein in urine. Dipstick or urinalyses to detect proteinuria. 24-hour urine for 4+ protein or use the protein-to-creatinine (UPC) ratio to monitor. (For UPC obtain a random urine protein and a random urine creatinine.) Divide the urine protein by the urine creatinine to obtain the ratio. A ratio of < 0.1 mg/dl is normal. UPC < 2.5 suggests presence of nephritic range proteinuria. The clinical significance or increased proteinuria has not been determined.

- Acute neurotoxicities: Are temporary and can occur within hours of or up to 14 days after oxaliplatin. Often precipitated by exposure to cold and characterized by dysesthesias, transient paresthesias or hypothesias of hands, feet, perioral area, and throat. Pharyngolaryngeal dysesthesia (**sensation** of discomfort or tightness in the back of the throat and inability to breathe) is most frightening to patients.

- Peripheral Neuropathy: Affects about 48% of patients, usually with a cumulative dose of 800 mg/m². Symptoms include paresthesias, dysesthesias, hypoesthesias in a stocking and glove distribution, and altered proprioception (knowing where body parts are in relation to the whole).
- GI Toxicities: Nausea and vomiting in 50%–65% of patients; can be severe. Diarrhea occurs in up to 40%, with 15% being grade 3–4. Stomatitis is common, 3% of which is severe.
- Skin: Hand-foot syndrome (palmar-plantar erythrodysesthesia) occurs in 15%–20% of patients. Characterized by tingling, numbness, pain, erythema, dryness, rash, swelling, increased pigmentation, and/or pruritus of the hands and feet. Less frequent in reduced doses.
- Ocular: Blepharitis, tear-duct stenosis, acute and chronic conjunctivitis.
- Hepatic: Elevations in serum bilirubin (20%–40%), alkaline phosphatase, and hepatic transaminases (aspartate transaminase [SGOT], alanine transaminase [SGPT]). Dose modifications may be required if hyperbilirubinemia occurs.
- Bone Marrow Toxicity: Grade 3–4 neutropenia (15%), thrombocytopenia (4%).
- Anaphylactic/anaphylactoid reactions to eloxatin have been reported. Delayed hypersensitivity: Symptoms range from mild symptoms, i.e., rash, urticaria, erythema, pruritus, or emesis to anaphylaxis/severe hypersensitivity characterized by dyspnea, angioedema bronchospasm, and hypotension. These reactions occur within minutes of administration and should be managed with appropriate supportive therapy. Drug-related deaths associated with platinum compounds from this reaction have been reported.
- Reproductive: Pregnancy category D. Breast feeding should be avoided.

Initiate antiemetic protocol: Highly to moderately emetogenic protocol.

Supportive drugs:
☐ pegfilgrastim (Neulasta)   ☐ filgrastim (Neupogen)
☐ loperamide (Imodium)   ☐ epoetin alfa (Procrit)

Initiate antidiarrheal protocol: ☐ darbepoetin alfa (Aranesp)   ☐ diphenoxylate/atropine sulfate (Lomotil)

Treatment schedule: Chair time 4–5 hours first cycle, then 3 hours for other courses. Repeat cycle every 21 days until disease progression.

Estimated number of visits: One visit per cycle. Request three cycles worth.

Dose Calculation by: 1. _____   2. _____

_____   _____
Physician   Date

_____   _____
Patient Name   ID Number

_____   _____/_____/_____
Diagnosis   Ht   Wt   M²

Trimetrexate + 5-Fluorouracil + Leucovorin

Baseline laboratory tests:	CBC: Chemistry and CEA
Baseline procedures or tests:	N/A
Initiate IV:	0.9% sodium chloride
Premedicate:	Oral phenothiazine or 5-HT$_3$ and 10–20 mg of dexamethasone if necessary
Administer:	**Trimetrexate** _____ mg (110 mg/m^2) IV in 250 cc of D5W on day 1

- Available as a lyophilized powder in 5- or 30-mL multidose vials for IV use.
- Reconstitute with 2 mL of D5W or sterile water.
- Filter with a 0.22-micron filter before further dilution. Inspect for cloudiness or precipitate.
- Further dilute in D5W to a final concentration of 0.25–2.0 mg/mL.
- Stable for 24 hours at room temperature or refrigerated.
- Incompatible with chloride solutions, because precipitate forms immediately, and leucovorin.

5-Fluorouracil _____ mg (500 mg/m^2) IV on day 2, immediately after leucovorin

- No dilution required. Concentration 50 mg/mL.
- Can be further diluted with 0.9% sodium chloride or D5W.

Leucovorin _____ mg (200 mg/m^2) IV on day 2; administer before 5-Fluorouracil

- Available in solution or powder. Reconstitute solution with sterile water. May further dilute with 0.9% sodium chloride or D5W.
- Do not mix in same solution with 5-FU, because a precipitate will form.

Leucovorin 15 mg PO every 6 hours for seven doses, starting 6 hours after 5-Fluorouracil

Major Side Effects	

- Bone Marrow Depression: Leukopenia is dose-limiting toxicity.
- GI Toxicities: Nausea and vomiting occur in 30%–50% of patients but are usually mild. Mucositis and diarrhea can be severe and dose limiting.
- Hepatic Toxicities: Transient elevation in serum transaminase levels. Clinically asymptomatic.
- Pulmonary: Dyspnea may occur and can be severe.
- Skin: Hyperpigmentation, photosensitivity, and nail changes may occur. Hand-foot syndrome can be dose limiting. Alopecia likely.
- Ocular: Photophobia, increased lacrimation, conjunctivitis, and blurred vision.
- Reproductive: Pregnancy category D. Breast feeding should be avoided.

Initiate antiemetic protocol:	Mildly to moderately emetogenic protocol.

Supportive drugs:
- ☐ pegfilgrastim (Neulasta)
- ☐ epoetin alfa (Procrit)
- ☐ filgrastim (Neupogen)
- ☐ darbepoetin alfa (Aranesp)

Initiate antidiarrheal protocol:
- ☐ loperamide (Imodium)
- ☐ diphenoxylate/atropine sulfate (Lomotil)

Treatment schedule:	Chair time 1 hour weekly for 6 weeks. Repeat cycle every 8 weeks.
Estimated number of visits:	Six visits per cycle. Request four cycles worth of visits.

Dose Calculation by: 1. _____   2. _____

_____
Physician

_____
Date

_____
Patient Name

_____
ID Number

_____
Diagnosis

_____/_____/_____
Ht   Wt   M^2

Hepatic Artery Infusion

Floxuridine

Baseline laboratory tests:	CBC: Chemistry panel, LFTs, and CEA
Baseline procedures or tests:	Hepatic artery line for arterial infusion.
Initiate IV:	N/A
Premedicate:	Oral phenothiazine or 5-HT$_3$ if nausea occurs

H_2 antagonist antihistamine (i.e., ranitidine 150 mg PO bid) administered concurrently during intra-arterial infusion to prevent development of peptic ulcer disease.

Administer:

Floxuridine _____ (0.3 mg/kg/day) HAI days 1–14

- Available as a 500-mg vial of lyophilized powder for intra-arterial use.
- Dilute with 5 mL of sterile water and then further dilute with NS or D5W.
- Reconstituted solution is stable for up to 2 weeks under refrigeration.

Dexamethasone 20 mg HAI on days 1–14

Heparin 50,000 units HAI on days 1–14

Major Side Effects

- GI Toxicities: Nausea and vomiting occur infrequently and are mild. Anorexia is common, as is mild mucositis. Gastritis may occur, with abdominal cramping and pain. Duodenal ulcers may occur, be painless, and lead to gastric outlet obstruction and vomiting.
- Hepatic: Chemical hepatitis may be severe, with increased alkaline phosphatase, liver transaminase, and bilirubin levels. Sclerosing cholangitis is a rare event.
- Intra-arterial Catheter Problems: Leakage, arterial ischemia or aneurysm, bleeding at catheter site, catheter occlusion, thrombosis or embolism of artery, vessel perforation or dislodged catheter, infection, and biliary sclerosis.
- Skin: Hand-foot syndrome. Erythema, dermatitis, pruritus, or rash may occur.
- Neurotoxicity: Manifested by somnolence, confusion, seizures, cerebellar ataxia, vertigo, nystagmus, depression, hemiplegia, hiccups, and lethargy. Blurred vision, and rarely encephalopathy.
- Bone Marrow Suppression: Myelosuppression occurs rarely. Nadir day 9–14.
- Cardiac Toxicity: Symptoms of chest pain, electrocardiographic changes, and serum enzyme elevation occur rarely. Increased risk in patients with prior history of ischemic heart disease.
- Ocular: Blepharitis, tear-duct stenosis, acute and chronic conjunctivitis.
- Miscellaneous: Fever malaise, catheter infections.

Initiate antiemetic protocol:	Mildly emetogenic protocol.

Supportive drugs:

☐ pegfilgrastim (Neulasta)   ☐ filgrastim (Neupogen)

☐ epoetin alfa (Procrit)   ☐ darbepoetin alfa (Aranesp)

Initiate antidiarrheal protocol:	☐ loperamide (Imodium) ☐ diphenoxylate/atropine sulfate (Lomotil)
Treatment schedule:	Chair time 1 hour on days 1–14. Repeat cycle every 14 days until disease progression.
Estimated number of visits:	14 visits per cycle. Ask for three to four cycles worth of visits. May require hospitalization for all or part of treatment.

Dose Calculation by: 1. _____   2. _____

_____   _____
Physician   Date

_____   _____
Patient Name   ID Number

_____ / _____ / _____
Diagnosis   Ht   Wt   M^2

Single-Agent Regimens

Capecitabine (Xeloda)

Baseline laboratory tests:	CBC: Chemistry, bilirubin, LFTs, CEA, and creatinine clearance
Baseline procedures or tests:	N/A
Initiate IV:	N/A
Premedicate:	Oral phenothiazine or 5-HT$_3$
Administer:	**Capecitabine** _____ mg (1250 mg/m^2/day) PO bid on days 1–14

- Dose may be decreased to 850–1000 mg/m^2 PO bid on days 1–14. This may reduce the risk of toxicity without compromising efficacy.
- Administer within 30 minutes of a meal with plenty of water.
- Monitor INRs closely in patients taking warfarin; may increase INR.
- Stop therapy at first signs of hand-foot syndrome or diarrhea.

Major Side Effects

- GI Toxicities: Nausea and vomiting, in 30%–50% of patients, is usually mild to moderate. Diarrhea occurs in up to 40%, with 15% being grade 3–4. Stomatitis is common, 3% of which is severe.
- Bone Marrow Suppression: Less than 5-FU.
- Renal Insufficiency: Contraindicated in patients with creatinine clearance < 30 mL/min, CrCl 30–50 mL/min at baseline should have dose reduction to 75% of total dose.
- Skin: Hand-foot syndrome (palmar-plantar erythrodysesthesia) seen in 15%–20% of patients. Characterized by tingling, numbness, pain, erythema, dryness, rash, swelling, increased pigmentation, and/or pruritus of the hands and feet. Less frequent in reduced doses.
- Ocular: Blepharitis, tear-duct stenosis, acute and chronic conjunctivitis.
- Hepatic: Elevations in serum bilirubin (20%–40%), alkaline phosphatase, and hepatic transaminase (SGOT, SGPT) levels. Dose modifications may be required if hyperbilirubinemia occurs.
- Reproductive: Pregnancy category D. Breast feeding should be avoided.

Initiate antiemetic protocol:	Mildly to moderately emetogenic protocol.
Supportive drugs:	☐ pegfilgrastim (Neulasta) ☐ filgrastim (Neupogen)
	☐ darbepoetin alfa (Aranesp) ☐ diphenoxylate/atropine sulfate (Lomotil)
Initiate diarrheal protocol:	☐ loperamide (Imodium) ☐ epoetin alfa (Procrit)
Treatment schedule:	No chair time. Repeat cycle every 21 days.
Estimated number of visits:	One to two visits per cycle. Request six cycles worth of visits.

Dose Calculation by: 1. _____ 2. _____

_____
Physician

_____
Date

_____
Patient Name

_____
ID Number

_____
Diagnosis

_____ / _____ / _____
Ht   Wt   M^2

Irinotecan (CPT-11/Weekly Schedule)

Baseline laboratory tests:	CBC: Chemistry panel and CEA
Baseline procedures or tests:	N/A
Initiate IV:	D5W
Premedicate:	5-HT$_3$ and dexamethasone 20 mg in 100 cc of D5W
	Atropine 0.25–1.0 mg IV unless contraindicated

Administer:

Irinotecan _____ mg (125 mg/m^2) IV in 500 cc of D5W over 90 minutes weekly for 4 weeks, repeat every 6 weeks

OR

Irinotecan _____ mg (125 mg/m^2) IV in 500 cc of D5W over 90 minutes weekly for 2 weeks, repeat every 3 weeks

OR

Irinotecan _____ mg (175 mg/m^2) IV in 500 cc of D5W on days 1 and 10 every 3 weeks

- Available in 100-mg vials.
- Store at room temperature and protect from light.
- Dilute and mix drug in D5W (preferred) or NS.
- Diluted drug is stable for 24 hours at room temperature or, if diluted in D5W, is stable for 48 hours if refrigerated and protected from light.

Major Side Effects

- GI Toxicities: Early diarrhea, most likely a cholinergic effect, can be managed with atropine before therapy. Late diarrhea observed in 22% of patients, can be severe, and should be treated aggressively. Nausea and vomiting in 35%–60% of patients, with 17% experiencing grade 3–4 nausea and 13% experiencing grade 3–4 vomiting.
- Bone Marrow Depression: Dose-limiting, grade 3–4 neutropenia in 17%. Nadir in 6–9 days. Monitor CBC weekly.
- Alopecia: Mild.
- Reproductive: Pregnancy category D. Breast feeding should be avoided.

Initiate antiemetic protocol:	Moderately to highly emetogenic protocol.

Supportive drugs:

☐ pegfilgrastim (Neulasta) ☐ filgrastim (Neupogen)

☐ epoetin alfa (Procrit) ☐ darbepoetin alfa (Aranesp)

Initiate antidiarrheal protocol:

☐ loperamide (Imodium) ☐ diphenoxylate/atropine sulfate (Lomotil)

Treatment schedule:	Chair time 2 hours weekly for 4 weeks. Repeat cycle every 6 weeks until disease progression.
Estimated number of visits:	Weekly for 4 weeks. Request 6 cycles worth of visits.

Dose Calculation by: 1. _____ 2. _____

_____   _____

Physician   Date

_____   _____

Patient Name   ID Number

_____   _____/_____/_____

Diagnosis   Ht   Wt   M^2

Irinotecan (CPT-11/Monthly Schedule)

Baseline laboratory tests:	CBC: Chemistry panel and CEA
Baseline procedures or tests:	N/A
Initiate IV:	D5W
Premedicate:	5-HT$_3$ and dexamethasone 20 mg in 100 cc of D5W
	Atropine 0.25–1.0 mg IV unless contraindicated
Administer:	**Irinotecan**_____mg (350 mg/m^2) IV on day 1 repeat every 3 weeks

- Store at room temperature; protect from light.
- Dilute and mix drug in D5W (preferred) or NS.
- Diluted drug is stable for 24 hours at room temperature; if diluted in D5W, is stable for 48 hours if refrigerated and protected from light.

Major Side Effects	

- GI Toxicities: Early diarrhea, most likely a cholinergic effect, can be managed with atropine before therapy. Late diarrhea observed in 22% of patients, can be severe, and should be treated aggressively. Nausea and vomiting in 35%–60% of patients, with 17% experiencing grade 3–4 nausea and 13% experiencing grade 3–4 vomiting.
- Bone Marrow Depression: Dose-limiting, grade 3–4 neutropenia in 17%. Nadir in 6–9 days.
- Alopecia: Mild.

Initiate antiemetic protocol:	Moderately to highly emetogenic protocol.
Supportive drugs:	☐ pegfilgrastim (Neulasta) ☐ filgrastim (Neupogen)
	☐ epoetin alfa (Procrit) ☐ darbepoetin alfa (Aranesp)
Initiate antidiarrheal protocol:	☐ loperamide (Imodium) ☐ diphenoxylate/atropine sulfate (Lomotil)
Treatment schedule:	Chair time 2 hours on day 1. Repeat cycle every 3 weeks as tolerated or until disease progression.
Estimated number of visits:	One visit per cycle. Request four cycles worth of visits.

Dose Calculation by: 1. _____   2. _____

Physician _____   Date _____

Patient Name _____   ID Number _____

Diagnosis _____   Ht _____ / Wt _____ / M^2 _____

Cetuximab (Erbitux)

Baseline laboratory tests:	CBC: Chemistry and CEA, monitor electrolytes
Baseline procedures or tests:	EGFR expression using immunohistochemistry
Initiate IV:	NS
Premedicate:	Diphenhydramine 50 mg in 100 cc of NS
Administer:	**Cetuximab** _____mg (400 mg/m^2) IV over 2 hours week 1 only

Cetuximab _____mg (250 mg/m^2) IV over 1 hour weekly as maintenance dose. Followed by 1 hour observation for infusion reactions.

- Maximum infusion rate 5 mL/min.
- **Administer through low-protein-binding 0.22-micron in-line filter.**
- Place cetuximab in sterile evacuated container, prime tubing with drug, and then piggyback into main line infusion of NS.
- Do not shake or dilute.
- Supplied in 100-mg/50-mL vials; discard 8 hours after opening if kept at room temperature, 12 hours if refrigerated.
- Dose reductions for skin reactions from package insert:

Severe Acneform Rash	ERBITUX	Outcome	ERBITUX Dose Modification
1st occurrence	Delay infusion 1 to 2 weeks	Improvement No Improvement	Continue at 250 mg/m^2 Discontinue ERBITUX
2nd occurrence	Delay infusion 1 to 2 weeks	Improvement No Improvement	Reduce dose to 200 mg/m^2 Discontinue ERBITUX
3rd occurrence	Delay infusion 1 to 2 weeks	Improvement No Improvement	Reduce dose to 150 mg/m2 Discontinue ERBITUX
4th occurrence	Discontine ERBITUX		

Major Side Effects

- Infusion Reaction: Severe allergic reactions (3%–4%) with symptoms including rapid onset of airway obstruction (bronchospasm, stirdor, hoarseness), dyspnea, fever, chills, rash, itching, and/or hypotension require that treatment be stopped immediately and NOT started again. For mild or moderate (grade 1–2) infusion reactions (19%), infusion rate should be permanently reduced by 50%.
- Skin: Acneform rash (90%) can be severe and require dose modification (8%). Paronychial inflammation, especially in thumbs and great toes (14%). May be treated with topical antibiotic cream or oral antibiotics.
- Hypomagnesemia may occur in 50% of patients. Grade 3–4 in 10%–15% of patients. Electrolyte replacement may be necessary. Closely monitor magnesium, potassium, and calcium levels.
- GI Symptoms: Nausea and vomiting, 25% in monotherapy and 72% in combination with irinotecan.
- Pulmonary Toxicity: Interstitial pneumonitis with non-cardiogenic pulmonary edema in < 0.5%. Onset between 4–11th doses. Monitor pulmonary symptoms; if interstitial lung disease develops, erbitux should be discontinued.
- Reproductive: Pregnancy category D. Breast feeding should be avoided.

Initiate antiemetic protocol:	Mildly to moderately emetogenic protocol
Supportive drugs:	☐ epoetin alfa (Procrit) ☐ darbepoetin alfa (Aranesp)
	☐ oprelvekin (Neumega) ☐ filgrastim (Neupogen)
	☐ pegfilgrastim (Neulasta) ☐ Other _____
Treatment schedule:	Chair time 2 hours. Repeat cycle every 3–4 weeks.
Treatment schedule:	Chair time 2–3 hours includes premeds, drug infusion, and 1-hour observation time. Repeat weekly as tolerated or until disease progression.
Estimated number of visits:	Four visits per month. Request three months worth of visits.

Dose Calculation by: 1. _____   2. _____

_____   _____
Physician   Date

_____   _____
Patient Name   ID Number

_____   _____ / _____ / _____
Diagnosis   Ht   Wt   M²

5-Fluorouracil (Continuous Infusion)

Baseline laboratory tests:	CBC: Chemistry and CEA
Baseline procedures or tests:	Central line placement
Initiate IV:	0.9% sodium chloride only if administering IV antiemetics
Premedicate:	Oral phenothiazine or 5-HT$_3$

Administer:

Fluorouracil _____ mg (2600 mg/m^2) IV over 24 hours weekly for 4 weeks

OR

Fluorouracil _____ mg (1000 mg/m^2/day) IV continuous infusion on days 1–4

- No dilution required. Concentration 50 mg/mL.
- Can be further diluted with 0.9% sodium chloride or D5W.

Major Side Effects

- Bone Marrow Depression: Nadir 10–14 days. Neutropenia, thrombocytopenia are dose related. Can be dose limiting for daily × 5 or weekly regimens.
- GI Toxicities: Nausea and vomiting occur in 30%–50% of patients but are usually mild. Mucositis and diarrhea can be severe and dose limiting.
- Skin: Alopecia is more common in the 5-day course and results in diffuse thinning of hair. Hyperpigmentation, photosensitivity, and nail changes may occur. Hand-foot syndrome can be dose limiting.
- Ocular: Photophobia, increased lacrimation, conjunctivitis, and blurred vision.
- Reproductive: Pregnancy category D. Breast feeding should be avoided.

Initiate antiemetic protocol: Mildly emetogenic protocol.

Supportive drugs:

☐ pegfilgrastim (Neulasta)   ☐ filgrastim (Neupogen)

☐ epoetin alfa (Procrit)   ☐ darbepoetin alfa (Aranesp)

Initiate antidiarrheal protocol: ☐ loperamide (Imodium)   ☐ diphenoxylate/atropine sulfate (Lomotil)

Treatment schedule: Chair time 1 hour weekly for 4 weeks. Repeat cycle every 21–28 days.

Estimated number of visits: Four visits per cycle. Request four cycles worth of visits.

Dose Calculation by: 1. _____   2. _____

_____

Physician   Date

_____

Patient Name   ID Number

_____

Diagnosis   Ht _____ / Wt _____ / M^2 _____

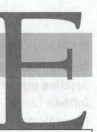

Combination Regimens

Paclitaxel: 175 mg/m^2 IV over 3 hours on day 1
Carboplatin: area under the curve (AUC) 5–7, IV on day 1
Repeat cycle every 28 days.[1,143]

Doxorubicin: 60 mg/m^2 IV on day 1
Cyclophosphamide: 500 mg/m^2 IV on day 1
Repeat cycle every 21 days.[1,144]

Doxorubicin: 50 mg/m^2 IV on day 1
Cisplatin: 50 mg/m^2 IV on day 1
Repeat cycle every 21 days.[1,145]

Doxorubicin: 50 mg/m^2 IV on day 1
Paclitaxel: 150 mg/m^2 IV on day 1
Repeat cycle every 21 days.[1,146]

Cisplatin: 50 mg/m^2 IV on day 1
Doxorubicin: 45 mg/m^2 IV on day 1
Paclitaxel: 160 mg/m^2 IV over 3 hours on day 2
Filgrastim: 5 µg/kg SC on days 3–12
Repeat cycle every 21 days.[1,147]

Cyclophosphamide: 500 mg/m^2 IV on day 1
Doxorubicin: 50 mg/m^2 IV on day 1
Cisplatin: 50 mg/m^2 IV on day 1
Repeat cycle every 21 days.[1,148]

Single-Agent Regimens

Doxorubicin **224**

Doxorubicin: 60 mg/m^2 IV on day 1
Repeat cycle every 21 days.[1,149]

Megestrol **225**

Megestrol: 160 mg PO daily
Repeat on a daily basis.[1,150]

Paclitaxel **226**

Paclitaxel: 200 mg/m^2 IV over 3 hours on day 1
Repeat cycle every 21 days.[1,151]
Reduce dose to 175 mg/m^2 IV for patients with prior pelvic radiation
  therapy.

Topotecan **227**

Topotecan: 1.0 mg/m^2/day IV on days 1–5
Repeat cycle every 21 days.[1,152]
Reduce dose to 0.8 mg/m^2/day IV on days 1–3 in patients with prior radia-
  tion therapy.

Medroxyprogesterone **228**

Medroxyprogesterone: 200 mg PO daily
Repeat on a daily basis.[1,153]

Combination Regimens

Paclitaxel and Carboplatin

Baseline laboratory tests:	CBC: Chemistry
Baseline procedures or tests:	N/A
Initiate IV:	0.9% sodium chloride
Premedicate:	5-HT$_3$ and dexamethasone 10–20 mg in 100 cc of NS
	Diphenhydramine 25–50 mg and cimetidine 300 mg in 100 cc of NS

Administer:

Paclitaxel _____ mg (175 mg/m^2) IV over 3 hours on day 1

- Stable for up to 27 hours at room temperature, 0.3–1.2 mg/mL solutions.
- Final concentration is ≤ 1.2 mg/mL
- Available in 50-, 100-, and 200-mg vials; 1 mg/mL
- **Use non-PVC containers and tubing with 0.22-micron inline filter to administer.**

Carboplatin _____ mg (AUC 5–7) IV on day 1

- Use within 24 hours of reconstitution or preparation.
- Available in 50-, 150-, and 450-mg lyophilized powder; mix with sterile water, D5W or NS for concentration of 10 mg/ml; stable for 8 hours after mixing.
- Also available in 50-, 150-, 450- and 600-mg aqueous solution 10 mg/mL multidose vial; multidose vials stable for 14 days with multiple needle sticks; once diluted stable for 8 hours.
- Do not use aluminum needles, because precipitate will form.
- Give carboplatin after paclitaxel to decrease toxicities

Major Side Effects

- Hypersensitivity Reaction: Paclitaxel (30%–40%). Premedicate as described. Characterized by generalized rash, flushing, back pain, erythema, hypotension, dyspnea, and/or bronchospasm. Increased risk of hypersensitivity reactions in patients receiving more than seven courses of carboplatin therapy.
- Bone Marrow Depression: Neutropenia, thrombocytopenia, and anemia are cumulative and dose related. Can be dose limiting. G-CSF support recommended.
- GI Toxicities: Moderate-to-severe nausea and vomiting may be acute or delayed. Mucositis and/or diarrhea occurs in 30%–40% of patients.
- Renal: Nephrotoxicity less common than with cisplatin and rarely symptomatic.
- Electrolyte Imbalance: Decreases Mg^{2+}, K, Ca^{2+}, Na, and P.
- Neurotoxicity: Sensory neuropathy with numbness and paresthesias; dose related.
- Alopecia: Loss of total body hair occurs in nearly all patients.
- Reproductive: Pregnancy category D. Breast feeding should be avoided.

Initiate antiemetic protocol:	Moderately to severely emetogenic protocol.
Supportive drugs:	☐ pegfilgrastim (Neulasta) ☐ filgrastim (Neupogen)
	☐ epoetin alfa (Procrit) ☐ darbepoetin alfa (Aranesp)
Treatment schedule:	Chair time 5 hours on day 1. Repeat cycle every 28 days until disease progression.
Estimated number of visits:	One visit per cycle. Request three cycles worth of visits.

Dose Calculation by: 1. _____   2. _____

_____

Physician

_____

Patient Name

_____

Diagnosis

_____

Date

_____

ID Number

_____ / _____ / _____

Ht   Wt   M^2

Doxorubicin + Cyclophosphamide (AC)

Baseline laboratory tests:	CBC: Chemistry and LFTs
Baseline procedures or tests:	MUGA scan
Initiate IV:	0.9% sodium chloride
Premedicate:	5-HT$_3$ and dexamethasone 20 mg in 100 cc of NS.
Administer:	**Doxorubicin** _____mg (60 mg/m^2) IV on day 1

- Potent vesicant
- Available as a 2-mg/mL solution.
- Doxorubicin will form a precipitate if it is mixed with heparin or 5-FU.

Cyclophosphamide _____mg (500 mg/m^2) IV on day 1

- Available in 100-, 200-, 500-, 1000-, and 2000-mg vials
- Dilute with sterile water to make final concentration 20 mg/mL; shake well to ensure that solution is completely dissolved.
- Reconstituted solution stable for 24 hours at room temperature, and for 6 days refrigerated.

Major Side Effects

- Bone Marrow Depression: Leukopenia, thrombocytopenia, and anemia all occur; may be severe.
- GI Toxicities: Nausea and vomiting is moderate to severe and can be acute or delayed. Stomatitis and diarrhea occurs in 10% of patients but is not dose limiting.
- Cardiac: Acutely, pericarditis-myocarditis syndrome may occur. With high cumulative doses < 450 mg/m^2, cardiomyopathy may occur. Cyclophosphamide may increase the risk of doxorubicin-induced cardiotoxicity.
- Hepatic: Use with caution in patients with abnormal liver function. Dose reduction is required in the presence of liver dysfunction.
- Bladder Toxicities: Hemorrhagic cystitis, dysuria, and urinary frequency. Usually preventable with adequate hydration.
- GU: Red-orange discoloration of urine; resolves in 24–48 hours.
- Skin: Extravasation of doxorubicin causes severe tissue destruction. Hyperpigmentation, photosensitivity, and radiation recall occur. Complete alopecia.
- Reproduction: Drugs are teratogenic and mutagenic.

Initiate antiemetic protocol:	Moderately to severely emetogenic protocol.
Supportive drugs:	☐ pegfilgrastim (Neulasta)　　☐ filgrastim (Neupogen)
	☐ epoetin alfa (Procrit)　　☐ darbepoetin alfa (Aranesp)
Treatment schedule:	Chair time 2 hours on day 1. Repeat cycle every 21 days.
Estimated number of visits:	Two visits per cycle. Request four cycles worth of visits.

Dose Calculation by:　　1. _____　　2. _____

_____

Physician

_____

Date

_____

Patient Name

_____

ID Number

_____

Diagnosis

_____ / _____ / _____
Ht　　　　　Wt　　　　　M^2

Doxorubicin + Cisplatin (AP)

Baseline laboratory tests:	CBC: Chemistry (including Mg^{2+})
Baseline procedures or tests:	MUGA scan
Initiate IV:	0.9% sodium chloride
Premedicate:	5-HT$_3$ and dexamethasone 20 mg in 100 cc of NS.
Administer:	**Doxorubicin** _____mg (50 mg/m^2) IV push on day 1

- Potent vesicant
- Available as a 2-mg/mL solution.
- Doxorubicin will form a precipitate if it is mixed with heparin or 5-FU.

Cisplatin _____mg (50 mg/m^2) IV over 1–2 hours on day 1

- Do not use aluminum needles, because precipitate will form.
- Stable for 96 hours when protected from light and only 6 hours when not protected from light.
- Available in solution as 1 mg/mL.
- Further dilute solution with 250 cc or more NS (1–2 liters).

Major Side Effects

- Bone Marrow Depression: Leukopenia, thrombocytopenia, and anemia all seen, may be severe.
- GI Toxicities: Nausea and vomiting is moderate to severe and can be acute or delayed. Stomatitis occurs in 10% of patients but is not dose limiting.
- Cardiac: Acutely, pericarditis-myocarditis syndrome may occur. With high cumulative doses > 550 mg/m^2, cardiomyopathy may occur. Risk of cardiotoxicity increased when doxorubicin is given with trastuzumab (Herceptin) or mitomycin.
- Renal: Nephrotoxicity is dose related with cisplatin and presents at 10–20 days.
- Electrolyte Imbalance: Decreases Mg^{2+}, K, Ca^{2+}, Na, and P.
- Skin: Extravasation of doxorubicin causes severe tissue destruction. Hyperpigmentation, photosensitivity, and radiation recall occur. Complete alopecia occurs with doses > 50 mg/m^2.
- Neurotoxicity: Dose-limiting toxicity, usually in the form of peripheral sensory neuropathy. Paresthesias and numbness in a classic "stocking glove" pattern.
- Ototoxicity: High-frequency hearing loss and tinnitus with cisplatin.
- Reproduction: Drugs are teratogenic and mutagenic.

Initiate antiemetic protocol:	Moderately to severely emetogenic protocol.
Supportive drugs:	☐ pegfilgrastim (Neulasta) ☐ filgrastim (Neupogen)
	☐ epoetin alfa (Procrit) ☐ darbepoetin alfa (Aranesp)
Treatment schedule:	Chair time 3 hours on day 1. Repeat cycle every 21 days.
Estimated number of visits:	Two visits per cycle. Request four cycles worth of visits.

Dose Calculation by: 1. _____   2. _____

_____
Physician

_____
Date

_____
Patient Name

_____
ID Number

_____
Diagnosis

_____ / _____ / _____
Ht   Wt   M^2

Doxorubicin + Paclitaxel (AT)

Baseline laboratory tests:	CBC: Chemistry (including Mg^{2+})
Baseline procedures or tests:	Central line placement for continuous infusion and MUGA scan
Initiate IV:	0.9% sodium chloride
Premedicate:	5-HT$_3$ and dexamethasone 10–20 mg in 100 cc of NS
	Diphenhydramine 25–50 mg and cimetidine 300 mg in 100 cc of NS

Administer:

Doxorubicin _____ mg (50 mg/m^2) IV on day 1

- **Potent vesicant**
- Available as a 2-mg/mL solution
- Doxorubicin will form precipitate if it is mixed with heparin or 5-FU.

Paclitaxel _____ mg (150 mg/m^2) IV on day 1

- Stable for up to 27 hours at room temperature, 0.3–1.2 mg/mL solutions.
- Available in 30- and 300-mg vials 6 mg/mL and 100-mg vial 16.7 mg/mL.
- Futher dilute in NS or D5W for final concentration < 1.2 mg/ml.
- **Use non-PVC containers and tubing with 0.22-micron inline filter for administration.**

Major Side Effects

- Hypersensitivity Reaction: Occurs in 20%–40% of patients. Characterized by generalized skin rash, flushing, erythema, hypotension, dyspnea, back pain, and/or bronchospasm. Usually occurs within the first 2–3 minutes of infusion and almost always within the first 10 minutes. Premedicate as described–.
- Bone Marrow Depression: Dose-limiting neutropenia. Use G-CSF support.
- GI Toxicities: Nausea and vomiting is moderate to severe. Stomatitis can occur but is not dose limiting.
- GU: Red-orange discoloration of urine; resolves in 24–48 hours.
- Cardiac: Acutely, pericarditis-myocarditis syndrome may occur. With high cumulative doses < 450 mg/m^2, cardiomyopathy may occur. Cyclophosphamide may increase the risk of doxorubicin-induced cardiotoxicity.
- Neurotoxicity: Sensory neuropathy with numbness/paresthesias; dose related.
- Skin: Extravasation of doxorubicin causes severe tissue destruction. Hyperpigmentation, photosensitivity, and radiation recall occur. Alopecia.
- Reproduction: Teratogenic, mutagenic, and carcinogenic.

Initiate antiemetic protocol:	Moderately emetogenic protocol.
Supportive drugs:	☐ pegfilgrastim (Neulasta) ☐ filgrastim (Neupogen)
	☐ epoetin alfa (Procrit) ☐ darbepoetin alfa (Aranesp)
Treatment schedule:	Repeat every 21 days.
Estimated number of visits:	Chair time 4–5 hours every 3 weeks. Nadir day 10–14.

Dose Calculation by: 1. _____   2. _____

Physician _____

Date _____

Patient Name _____

ID Number _____

Diagnosis _____

Ht _____ / Wt _____ / M^2 _____

Cisplatin + Doxorubicin + Paclitaxel

Baseline laboratory tests:	CBC: Chemistry (including Mg^{2+})
Baseline procedures or tests:	MUGA scan
Initiate IV:	0.9% sodium chloride
Premedicate:	5-HT$_3$ and dexamethasone 20 mg in 100 cc of NS.
Administer:	**Cisplatin** _____mg (50 mg/m^2) IV on day 1

- Do not use aluminum needles, because precipitate will form.
- Stable for 96 hours when protected from light and only 6 hours when not protected from light.
- Available in solution as 1 mg/mL.
- Further dilute solution with at least 250 cc or mm of NS

Doxorubicin _____mg (45 mg/m^2) IV push on day 1

- Potent vesicant
- Available as a 2-mg/mL solution.
- Doxorubicin will form a precipitate if mixed with heparin or 5-FU.

Paclitaxel _____mg (160 mg/m^2) IV over 3 hours on day 2

- Stable for up to 27 hours at room temperature, 0.3–1.2 mg/mL solutions.
- Available in 30- and 300-mg vials 6 mg/mL and 100-mg vial 16.7 mg/mL.
- Futher dilute in NS or D5W for final concentration < 1.2 mg/ml
- **Use non-PVC containers and tubing with 0.22-micron inline filter for administration.**

Major Side Effects

- Hypersensitivity Reaction: Occurs in 20%–40% of patients. Characterized by generalized skin rash, flushing, erythema, hypotension, dyspnea, back pain, and/or bronchospasm. Usually occurs within the first 2–3 minutes of infusion and almost always within the first 10 minutes. Premedicate as described.
- Bone Marrow Depression: Leukopenia, thrombocytopenia, and anemia all seen, may be severe. Dose-limiting neutropenia with nadir at days 8–10 and recovery by days 15–21. Decreased incidence of neutropenia with 3-hour schedule when compared with 24-hour schedule. G-CSF support recommended.
- Neurotoxicity: Sensory neuropathy. More frequent with longer infusions and at doses < 175 mg/m^2. Dose-limiting toxicity, usually in the form of peripheral sensory neuropathy in a classic "stocking glove" pattern.
- Ototoxicity: High-frequency hearing loss and tinnitus with cisplatin.
- GI Toxicities: Nausea and vomiting is moderate to severe and can be acute or delayed. Stomatitis occurs in 10% of patients but is not dose limiting.
- Cardiac: Acutely, pericarditis-myocarditis syndrome may occur. With high cumulative doses < 450 mg/m^2, cardiomyopathy may occur. Risk of cardiotoxicity increased when doxorubicin is given with trastuzumab (Herceptin) or mitomycin.
- Renal: Nephrotoxicity is dose related with cisplatin and presents at 10–20 days. Red-orange discoloration of urine; resolves by 24–48 hours.
- Electrolyte Imbalance: Decreases Mg^{2+}, K, Ca^{2+}, Na, and P.
- Skin: Extravasation of doxorubicin causes severe tissue destruction. Hyperpigmentation, photosensitivity, and radiation recall occur. Complete alopecia occurs with doses < 50 mg/m^2.
- Reproduction: Drugs are teratogenic and mutagenic.

Initiate antiemetic protocol:	Moderately to highly emetogenic protocol.
Supportive drugs:	☐ pegfilgrastim (Neulasta) ☐ filgrastim (Neupogen)
	☐ epoetin alfa (Procrit) ☐ darbepoetin alfa (Aranesp)
Treatment schedule:	Chair time 3 hours on day 1, 4 hours day 2. Repeat cycle every 21 days.
Estimated number of visits:	Two visits per cycle. Request four cycles worth of visits.

Dose Calculation by: 1. _____   2. _____

_____   _____
Physician   Date

_____   _____/_____/_____
Patient Name   ID Number

_____   _____ _____ _____
Diagnosis   Ht   Wt   M²

Cyclophosphamide + Doxorubicin + Cisplatin (CAP)

Baseline laboratory tests:	CBC: Chemistry (including Mg^{2+})
Baseline procedures or tests:	MUGA
Initiate IV:	0.9% sodium chloride
Premedicate:	5-HT_3 and dexamethasone 10–20 mg in 100 cc of NS
Administer:	**Cyclophosphamide** _____mg (500 mg/m^2) IV on day 1

- Available in 100-, 200-, 500-, 1000-, and 2000-mg vials.
- Dilute with sterile water to make final concentration 20 mg/mL; shake well to ensure that solution is completely dissolved.
- Further dilute with 250–1000 cc NS maximum concentration for IV infusion 20 mg/mL.
- Reconstituted solution is stable for 24 hours at room temperature and for 6 days refrigerated.

Doxorubicin _____mg (50 mg/m^2) IV on day 1

- **Potent vesicant**
- Available as a 2-mg/mL solution.
- Doxorubicin will form a precipitate if it is mixed with heparin or 5-FU.

Cisplatin _____mg (50 mg/m^2) IV over 1–3 hours on day 1

- Stable for 96 hours when protected from light and only 6 hours when not protected from light.
- Do not use aluminum needles, because precipitate will form.
- Available in solution as 1 mg/mL.
- Further dilute solution with 250 cc or more of NS.

Major Side Effects

- Bone Marrow Depression: Neutropenia, thrombocytopenia, and anemia occur equally in 25%–30% of patients. Leukopenia and thrombocytopenia are dose related.
- GI Toxicities: Moderate-to-severe nausea and vomiting. May be acute (first 24 hours) or delayed (> 24 hours). Mucositis may occur. Red-orange discoloration of urine; resolves in 24–48 hours. Adequately hydrate to decrease risk.
- GU: Nephrotoxicity is dose related and with cisplatin presents at 10–20 days. Bladder toxicity in the form of hemorrhagic cystitis, dysuria, and increased urinary frequency.
- Electrolyte Imbalance: Decreases Mg^{2+}, K, Ca^{2+}, Na, and P.
- Cardiac: Acutely, pericarditis-myocarditis syndrome may occur. With high cumulative doses < 450 mg/m^2, cardiomyopathy may occur. Cyclophosphamide may increase the risk of doxorubicin-induced cardiotoxicity.
- Neurotoxicity: Dose-limiting toxicity, usually in the form of peripheral sensory neuropathy. Paresthesias and numbness in a classic "stocking glove" pattern.
- Ototoxicity: High-frequency hearing loss and tinnitus.
- Skin: Extravasation of doxorubicin causes severe tissue damage. Hyperpigmentation, photosensitivity, and radiation recall occur. Alopecia.
- Reproduction: Drugs are mutagenic and teratogenic.

Initiate antiemetic protocol:	Moderately to severely emetogenic protocol.
Supportive drugs:	☐ pegfilgrastim (Neulasta)　　☐ filgrastim (Neupogen)
	☐ epoetin alfa (Procrit)　　☐ darbepoetin alfa (Aranesp)
Treatment schedule:	Chair time 3 hours on day 1. Repeat cycle every 21 days.
Estimated number of visits:	One visit per cycle. Request six cycles worth of visits.

Dose Calculation by: 1. _____   2. _____

_____   _____
Physician   Date

_____   _____
Patient Name   ID Number

_____   _____/_____/_____
Diagnosis   Ht   Wt   M^2

Single-Agent Regimens

Doxorubicin

Baseline laboratory tests:	CBC: Chemistry
Baseline procedures or tests:	MUGA scan
Initiate IV:	0.9% sodium chloride
Premedicate:	5-HT$_3$ and dexamethasone 10–20 mg in 100 cc of NS.
Administer:	**Doxorubicin** _____ mg (60 mg/m^2) IV on day 1

- Potent vesicant
- Available as a 2-mg/mL solution.
- Doxorubicin will form a precipitate if it is mixed with heparin or 5-FU.

Major Side Effects

- Bone Marrow Depression: WBC and platelet nadir 10–14 days after drug dose, with recovery from days 15–21. Myelosuppression may be severe but is less severe with weekly dosing.
- GI Toxicities: Nausea and vomiting are moderate to severe and occur in 44% of patients. Stomatitis occurs in 10% of patients but is not dose limiting.
- Cardiac: Acutely, pericarditis-myocarditis syndrome may occur. With high cumulative doses > 450 mg/m^2, cardiomyopathy may occur.
- Skin: Extravasation of doxorubicin causes severe tissue destruction. Hyperpigmentation, photosensitivity, and radiation recall occur. Complete alopecia occurs with doses > 50 mg/m^2.
- Gu: Red-orange discoloration of urine; resolves by 24–48 hours.
- Reproduction: Doxorubicin is teratogenic, mutagenic, and carcinogenic.

Initiate antiemetic protocol:	Moderately to severely emetogenic protocol.
Supportive drugs:	☐ pegfilgrastim (Neulasta) ☐ filgrastim (Neupogen)
	☐ epoetin alfa (Procrit) ☐ darbepoetin alfa (Aranesp)
Treatment schedule:	Chair time 1 hour on day 1. Repeat cycle every 21 days.
Estimated number of visits:	Two visits per cycle. Request four cycles worth of visits. Nadir days 15–21.

Dose Calculation by: 1. _____   2. _____

_____
Physician

_____
Patient Name

_____
Diagnosis

_____
Date

_____
ID Number

_____ / _____ / _____
Ht   Wt   M^2

Megestrol

Baseline laboratory tests:	CBC: Chemistry and LFTs
Baseline procedures or tests:	None
Initiate IV:	N/A
Premedicate:	Oral phenothiazine or 5-HT$_3$ if nausea occurs
Administer:	Megestrol 160 mg PO daily

Major Side Effects

- GI Toxicities: Nausea and vomiting rarely observed. Increased appetite with accompanying weight gain.
- CV Toxicities: Use with caution in patients with history of either thromboembolic or hypercoagulable disorders because megestrol acetate has been associated with an increased incidence of thromboembolic events.
- Fluid/electrolyte Imbalance: Fluid retention. Use with caution in patients with diabetes mellitus because megestrol may exacerbate this condition.
- Hepatic: Increased LFTs. Dose reduction recommended in patients with abnormal liver function.
- Gynecologic: Breakthrough menstrual bleeding.
- Reproduction: Pregnancy category D. Breast feeding should be avoided.

Initiate antiemetic protocol:	Mildly emetogenic protocol.
Supportive drugs:	☐ pegfilgrastim (Neulasta) ☐ filgrastim (Neupogen)
	☐ epoetin alfa (Procrit) ☐ darbepoetin alfa (Aranesp)
Treatment schedule:	No chair time. Daily PO dosing as tolerated or until disease progression.
Estimated number of visits:	Monthly during treatment.

Dose Calculation by: 1. _____   2. _____

_____

Physician

_____

Patient Name

_____

Diagnosis

_____

Date

_____

ID Number

_____/ _____/ _____

Ht   Wt   M^2

Paclitaxel

Baseline laboratory tests:	CBC: Chemistry (including Mg^{2+}) and CEA
Baseline procedures or tests:	N/A
Initiate IV:	0.9% sodium chloride
Premedicate:	5-HT_3 and dexamethasone 10–20 mg in 100 cc of NS
	Diphenhydramine 25–50 mg and cimetidine 300 mg in 100 cc of NS
Administer:	**Paclitaxel** _____ mg (200 mg/m^2) IV over 3 hours on day 1

- Stable for up to 27 hours at room temperature, 0.3–1.2 mg/mL solutions.
- Available in 30- and 300-mg vials 6 mg/mL and 100-mg vial 16.7 mg/mL.
- Futher dilute in NS or D5W for final concentration < 1.2 mg/ml.
- **Use non-PVC containers and tubing with 0.22-micron inline filter for administration.**

Major Side Effects

- Hypersensitivity reaction: Occurs in 20%–40% of patients. Characterized by generalized skin rash, flushing, erythema, hypotension, dyspnea, back pain, and/or bronchospasm. Usually occurs within the first 2–3 minutes of infusion and almost always within the first 10 minutes. Premedicate as described.
- Bone Marrow Depression: Dose-limiting neutropenia with nadir at days 8–10 and recovery by days 15–21. Decreased incidence of neutropenia with 3-hour schedule when compared with 24-hour schedule. G-CSF support recommended.
- Neurotoxicity: Sensory neuropathy with numbness and paresthesias; dose related. More frequent with longer infusions and at doses > 175 mg/m^2.
- Alopecia: Total loss of body hair occurs in nearly all patients.
- Reproductive: Pregnancy category D. Breast feeding should be avoided.

Initiate antiemetic protocol:	Mildly emetogenic protocol.
Supportive drugs:	☐ pegfilgrastim (Neulasta) ☐ filgrastim (Neupogen)
	☐ epoetin alfa (Procrit) ☐ darbepoetin alfa (Aranesp)
Treatment schedule:	Chair time 4 hours on day 1. Repeat every 21 days as tolerated or until disease progression.
Estimated number of visits:	Two visits per cycle. Request three cycles worth of visits. Nadir days 15–21.

Dose Calculation by: 1. _____   2. _____

_____   _____
Physician   Date

_____   _____
Patient Name   ID Number

_____   _____/_____/_____
Diagnosis   Ht   Wt   M^2

Topotecan

Baseline laboratory tests:	CBC: Chemistry panel, LFTs, and CA 19-9
Baseline procedures or tests:	N/A
Initiate IV:	0.9% sodium chloride
Premedicate:	5-HT$_3$ and dexamethasone 10 mg in 100 cc of NS
Administer:	**Topotecan** _____ mg (0.1 mg/m^2) IV on days 1–5

Reduce dose to _____ 0.8 mg/m^2 IV on days 1–3 in patients with prior radiation therapy

- Available as a 4-mg vial.
- Reconstitute vial with 4 mL of sterile water for injection.
- Further dilute in 0.9% sodium chloride or D5W.
- Use immediately.

Major Side Effects

- Hematologic: Severe grade 4 myelosuppression may occur during the first course of therapy in 60% of patients. Dose-limiting toxicity. Typical nadir occurs at days 7–10 with full recovery by days 21–28. If severe neutropenia occurs, reduce dose by 0.25 mg/m^2 for subsequent doses or may use G-CSF to prevent neutropenia 24 hours after last day of topotecan therapy.
- GI Toxicities: Nausea and vomiting, mild to moderate and dose related. Occur in 60%–80% of patients. Diarrhea occurs in 42% of patients, and constipation occurs in 39%. Abdominal pain may occur in 33% of patients.
- Hepatic Toxicity: Evidence of increased drug toxicity in patients with low protein and hepatic dysfunction. Dose reductions may be necessary.
- Renal: Use with caution in patients with abnormal renal function. Dose reduction is necessary in this setting. Microscopic hematuria occurs in 10% of patients.
- Skin: Alopecia.

Initiate antiemetic protocol:	Mildly to moderately emetogenic protocol.
Supportive drugs:	☐ pegfilgrastim (Neulasta) ☐ filgrastim (Neupogen)
	☐ epoetin alfa (Procrit) ☐ darbepoetin alfa (Aranesp)
Treatment schedule:	Chair time 1 hour on days 1–5. Repeat every 21 days until disease progression.
Estimated number of visits:	Three to six visits per course. Request three courses. Weekly CBC.

Dose Calculation by: 1. _____   2. _____

_____
Physician

_____
Date

_____
Patient Name

_____
ID Number

_____
Diagnosis

_____ / _____ / _____
Ht   Wt   M^2

Medroxyprogesterone

Baseline laboratory tests:	CBC: Chemistry, LFTs
Baseline procedures or tests:	None
Initiate IV:	N/A
Premedicate:	Oral phenothiazine or 5-HT$_3$ if nausea occurs
Administer:	Medroxyprogesterone 200 mg PO daily

Major Side Effects

- GI Toxicities: Nausea and vomiting rarely observed.
- Cardiovascular Toxicities: Use with caution in patients with a history of thromboembolic or hypercoagulable disorders.
- Fluid/electrolyte Imbalance: Fluid retention
- Hepatic: Increased LFTs.

Initiate antiemetic protocol:	Mildly emetogenic protocol.
Supportive drugs:	☐ pegfilgrastim (Neulasta) ☐ filgrastim (Neupogen)
	☐ epoetin alfa (Procrit) ☐ darbepoetin alfa (Aranesp)
Treatment schedule:	No chair time. Daily dosing as tolerated or until disease progression.
Estimated number of visits:	Monthly during treatment.

Dose Calculation by: 1. _____ 2. _____

Physician _____ Date _____

Patient Name _____ ID Number _____

Diagnosis _____ Ht _____ / Wt _____ / M^2 _____

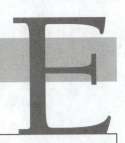

ESOPHAGEAL CANCER

Combination Regimens

5-FU + Cisplatin + Radiation Therapy (Herskovic Regimen) 231

5-Fluorouracil: 1000 mg/m²/day IV continuous infusion on days 1–4

Cisplatin: 75 mg/m² IV on day 1

Repeat on weeks 1, 5, 8, and 11.[1,154]

Radiation therapy: 200 cGy/day for 5 days per week (total dose, 3000 cGy), followed by a boost to the field of 2000 cGy.

5-FU + Cisplatin + Paclitaxel + Radiation Therapy (Hopkins/Yale Regimen) 232

Preoperative chemoradiation:

5-Fluorouracil 225 mg/m²/day IV continuous infusion on days 1–30

Cisplatin 20 mg/m²/day IV on days 1–5 and 26–30

Radiation therapy: 200 cGy/day to a total dose of 4400 cGy.
Followed by esophagectomy and then adjuvant chemotherapy in patients who had total gross removal of disease with negative margins.

Adjuvant chemotherapy:

Paclitaxel 135 mg/m² IV for 24 hours on day 1

Cisplatin 75 mg/m² IV on day 2

Chemotherapy is given concurrently with radiation therapy.

Adjuvant chemotherapy is given 8–12 weeks after esophagectomy, and each cycle is given every 21 days for a total of three cycles.[1,155]

Metastatic Disease

5-FU + Cisplatin 234

5-Fluorouracil: 1000 mg/m²/day IV continuous infusion on days 1–5

Cisplatin: 100 mg/m² IV on day 1

Repeat cycle on weeks 1, 5, 8, and 11.[1,156]

Irinotecan + Cisplatin 235

Irinotecan: 65 mg/m² IV weekly for 4 weeks

Cisplatin: 30 mg/m² IV weekly for 4 weeks

Repeat cycle every 6 weeks.[1,157]

Paclitaxel + Cisplatin..**236**

Paclitaxel: 200 mg/m^2 IV over 24 hours on day 1

Cisplatin: 75 mg/m^2 IV on day 2

Repeat cycle every 21 days.[1,158] G-CSF support is recommended.

5-FU + Cisplatin + Definitive Radiation Therapy **237**

5-FU 1000 mg/m^2 IV continuous infusion on days 1–4, 29–32, 50–53, and 71–74

Cisplatin 75 mg/m^2 IV on days 1, 29, 50, and 71

External-beam radiation therapy 50 cGy at 1.8 cGy per day, 5 days per week.[1,159]

Single-Agent Regimens

Paclitaxel **238**

Paclitaxel: 250 mg/m^2 IV over 24 hours on day 1

Repeat cycle every 21 days.[1,160] G-CSF support is recommended.

Combination Regimens

5-FU + Cisplatin + Radiation Therapy (Herskovic Regimen)

Baseline laboratory tests:	CBC: Chemistry (including Mg^{2+}) and CEA
Baseline procedures or tests:	Central line placement
Initiate IV:	0.9% sodium chloride
Premedicate:	$5\text{-}HT_3$ and dexamethasone 10–20 mg in 100 cc of NS
Administer:	**Fluorouracil** _____ mg (1000 mg/m²/day) IV continuous infusion on days 1–4

• No dilution required. Can be further diluted with 0.9% sodium chloride or D5W.

AND

Cisplatin _____ mg (75 mg/m²/day) IV on day 1

• Stable for 96 hours when protected from light and only 6 hours when not protected from light.

• Available in 1-mg/mL concentrations.

• Further dilute solution with 250 cc or more of NS.

• Do not use aluminum needles, because precipitate will form.

Repeat on weeks 1, 5, 8, and 11.

Radiation therapy 200 cGy/day, 5 days per week (total dose 3000 cGy), followed by a boost to the field of 2000 cGy

Major Side Effects

• Bone Marrow Depression: Neutropenia, thrombocytopenia, and anemia are cumulative and dose related. Can be dose limiting.

• GI Toxicities: Moderate-to-severe nausea and vomiting may be acute or delayed. Mucositis and diarrhea can be severe and dose limiting.

• Renal: Nephrotoxicity is dose related and with cisplatin presents at 10–20 days.

• Electrolyte Imbalance: Decreases Mg^{2+}, K, Ca^{2+}, Na, and P.

• Skin: Local tissue irritation progressing to desquamation can occur. Do not use oil-based lotions or creams in radiation field. Hyperpigmentation, photosensitivity, and nail changes may occur. Hand-foot syndrome can be dose limiting.

• Ocular: Photophobia, increased lacrimation, conjunctivitis, and blurred vision.

• Reproductive: Pregnancy category D. Breast feeding should be avoided.

Initiate antiemetic protocol:	Moderate to severely emetogenic protocol.
Supportive drugs:	☐ pegfilgrastim (Neulasta) ☐ filgrastim (Neupogen)
	☐ epoetin alfa (Procrit) ☐ darbepoetin alfa (Aranesp)
Treatment schedule:	Chair time 2 to 3 hours on day 1. Repeat at weeks 5, 8, and 11.
Estimated number of visits:	Four visits per treatment course. May require extra visits for hydration.

Dose Calculation by: 1. _____   2. _____

_____   _____
Physician   Date

_____   _____
Patient Name   ID Number

                                                          _____/_____/_____
Diagnosis   Ht   Wt   M²

5-FU + Cisplatin + Paclitaxel + Radiation Therapy (Hopkins/Yale Regimen)

Baseline laboratory tests:	CBC: Chemistry (including Mg^{2+}) and CEA
Baseline procedures or tests:	Central line placement
Initiate IV:	0.9% sodium chloride
Premedicate:	5-HT$_3$ and dexamethasone 10–20 mg in 100 cc of NS; followed by diphenhydramine 25–50 mg, and cimetidine 300 mg in 100 cc of NS (for paclitaxel only)
Administer:	Preoperative Chemoradiation

Fluorouracil _____ mg (225 mg/m^2/day) IV continuous infusion on days 1–30

- No dilution required. Can be further diluted with 0.9% sodium chloride or D5W.

AND

Cisplatin _____ mg (20 mg/m^2/day) IV on days 1–5 and 26–30

- Stable for 96 hours when protected from light and only 6 hours when not protected from light.
- Available in 1-mg/mL concentrations.
- Further dilute solution with 250 cc or more of NS.
- Do not use aluminum needles, because precipitate will form.

Radiation therapy 200 cGy/day to total dose of 4400 cGy, followed by esophagectomy and then adjuvant chemotherapy in patients who had total gross removal of disease with negative margins.

ADJUVANT CHEMOTHERAPY

Paclitaxel _____ mg (135 mg/m^2) IV for 24 hours on day 1

- Stable for up to 27 hours at room temperature, 0.3–1.2 mg/mL solutions.
- Available in 30- and 300-mg vials 6 mg/mL and 100-mg vial 16.7 mg/mL.
- Futher dilute in NS or D5W for final concentration < 1.2 mg/ml.
- **Use non-PVC containers and tubing with 0.22-micron inline filter for administration.**

Cisplatin _____ mg (75 mg/m^2) IV on day 2

Chemotherapy is given concurrently with radiation therapy. Adjuvant chemotherapy is given 8–12 weeks after esophagectomy. Repeat cycle every 21 days for three cycles.

Major Side Effects	- Hypersensitivity Reaction: Occurs in 20%–40% of patients. Characterized by generalized skin rash, flushing, erythema, hypotension, dyspnea, and/or bronchospasm. Usually occurs within the first 2–3 minutes of infusion and almost always within the first 10 minutes. Premedicate as described.
	- Bone Marrow Depression: Neutropenia, thrombocytopenia, and anemia are cumulative and dose related. Can be dose limiting.
	- GI Toxicities: Moderate-to-severe nausea and vomiting may be acute or delayed. Mucositis and diarrhea can be severe and dose limiting.
	- Renal: Nephrotoxicity is dose related and with cisplatin presents at 10–20 days. Provide adequate hydration to reduce risk.
	- Electrolyte Imbalance: Decreases Mg^{2+}, K, Ca^{2+}, Na, and P.
	- Skin: Local tissue irritation progressing to desquamation. Do not use oil-based lotions or creams in radiation field. Hand-foot syndrome can be dose limiting.
	- Neurotoxicity: Sensory neuropathy with numbness and paresthesias; dose related.
	- Alopecia: Loss of total body hair occurs in nearly all patients.
	- Reproductive: Pregnancy category D. Breast feeding should be avoided.
Initiate antiemetic protocol:	Moderate to severely emetogenic protocol.
Supportive drugs:	☐ pegfilgrastim (Neulasta) ☐ filgrastim (Neupogen) ☐ epoetin alfa (Procrit) ☐ darbepoetin alfa (Aranesp)
Treatment schedule:	Preoperative chemotherapy: Chair time 2 hours on days 1–5, 26–30 Adjuvant therapy: Chair time 1 hour on day 1, and 2 hours on day 2. Repeat every 3 weeks for six cycles.
Estimated number of visits:	Preoperative visits: 10 adjuvant therapy visits: two/cycle, six for total course

Dose Calculation by: 1. _____   2. _____

_____   _____
Physician   Date

_____   _____
Patient Name   ID Number

_____   _____/_____/_____
Diagnosis   Ht   Wt   M²

Metastatic Disease

5-FU + Cisplatin

Baseline laboratory tests:	CBC: Chemistry (including Mg^{2+}) and CEA
Baseline procedures or tests:	Central line placement
Initiate IV:	0.9% sodium chloride
Premedicate:	5-HT$_3$ and dexamethasone 10–20 mg in 100 cc of NS
Administer:	**Fluorouracil** _____mg (1000 mg/m^2/day) IV continuous infusion days 1–5

- No dilution required. Can be further diluted with 0.9% sodium chloride or D5W.

AND

Cisplatin _____mg (100 mg/m^2) IV on day 1

- Stable for 96 hours when protected from light and only 6 hours when not protected from light.
- Available in 1-mg/mL concentrations.
- Further dilute solution with 250 cc or more of NS.
- Do not use aluminum needles, because precipitate will form.

Repeat cycle on weeks 1, 5, 8, and 11.

Major Side Effects

- Bone Marrow Depression: Neutropenia, thrombocytopenia, and anemia are dose related. Can be dose limiting for daily × 5 or weekly regimens.
- GI Toxicities: Moderate-to-severe nausea and vomiting may be acute or delayed. Mucositis and diarrhea can be severe and dose limiting
- Renal: Nephrotoxicity is dose related and with cisplatin presents at 0–20 days. Provide adequate hydration to reduce risk.
- Electrolyte Imbalance: Decreases Mg^{2+}, K, Ca^{2+}, Na, and P.
- Skin: Hyperpigmentation, photosensitivity, and nail changes may occur. Hand-foot syndrome can be dose limiting.
- Ocular: Photophobia, increased lacrimation, conjunctivitis, and blurred vision.
- Reproductive: Pregnancy category D. Breast feeding should be avoided.

Initiate antiemetic protocol:	Moderate to severely emetogenic protocol.
Supportive drugs:	☐ pegfilgrastim (Neulasta) ☐ filgrastim (Neupogen)
	☐ epoetin alfa (Procrit) ☐ darbepoetin alfa (Aranesp)
Treatment schedule:	Chair time 3 hours on day 1. Repeat cycle on weeks 1, 5, 8, and 11.
Estimated number of visits:	Four per course. May require extra visits for hydration.

Dose Calculation by: 1. _____   2. _____

_____   _____

Physician   Date

_____   _____

Patient Name   ID Number

_____   _____/_____/_____

Diagnosis   Ht   Wt   M^2

Irinotecan + Cisplatin

Baseline laboratory tests:	CBC: Chemistry panel, CEA
Baseline procedures or tests:	N/A
Initiate IV:	D5W
Premedicate:	5HT$_3$ and dexamethasone 20 mg in 100 cc of D5W
	Atropine 0.25–1.0 mg IV unless contraindicated

Administer:

Irinotecan _____ mg (65 mg/m^2) IV in 500 cc of D5W over 90 minutes weekly for 4 weeks

- Available in 100-mg/5-mL single-use vials.
- Store at room temperature; protect from light.
- Dilute and mix drug in D5W (preferred) or NS.
- Diluted drug is stable 24 hours at room temperature; if diluted in D5W, it is stable for 48 hours if refrigerated and protected from light.

Cisplatin _____ mg (30 mg/m^2) IV weekly for 4 weeks

- Stable for 96 hours when protected from light and only 6 hours when not protected from light.
- Available in 1-mg/mL concentrations.
- Further dilute solution with 250 cc or more of NS.
- Do not use aluminum needles, because precipitate will form.

Major Side Effects

- GI Toxicities: Early diarrhea, most likely a cholinergic effect, can be managed with atropine before therapy. Late diarrhea observed in 22% of patients, can be severe, and should be treated aggressively. Nausea and vomiting in 35%–60% of patients, with 17% experiencing grade 3–4 nausea and 13% experiencing grade 3–4 vomiting.
- Bone Marrow Depression: Neutropenia can be dose limiting.
- Renal: Nephrotoxicity is dose related and with cisplatin presents at 10–20 days. Provide adequate hydration to reduce risk.
- Electrolyte Imbalance: Decreases in Mg^{2+}, K$^+$, Ca^{2+}, Na$^+$, and P.
- Alopecia: Mild.
- Reproductive: Pregnancy category D. Breast feeding should be avoided.

Initiate antiemetic protocol:	Highly to moderately emetogenic protocol.
Supportive drugs:	☐ pegfilgrastim (Neulasta) ☐ filgrastim (Neupogen)
	☐ epoetin alfa (Procrit) ☐ darbepoetin alfa (Aranesp)
	☐ loperamide (Imodium) ☐ diphenoxylate/atropine sulfate (Lomotil)
Treatment schedule:	Chair time 4 hours weekly for 4 weeks. Repeat cycle every 6 weeks as tolerated or until disease progression.
Estimated number of visits:	Four visits per cycle. Request three cycles worth of visits.

Dose Calculation by: 1. _____   2. _____

_____
Physician

_____
Date

_____
Patient Name

_____
ID Number

_____
Diagnosis

_____ / _____ / _____
Ht   Wt   M^2

Paclitaxel + Cisplatin

Baseline laboratory tests:	CBC: Chemistry (including Mg^{2+}) and CEA
Baseline procedures or tests:	Central line placement
Initiate IV:	0.9% sodium chloride
Premedicate:	5-HT$_3$ and dexamethasone 10–20 mg in 100 cc of NS (days 1 and 2)
	Diphenhydramine 25–50 mg and cimetidine 300 mg in 100 cc of NS (day 1 only)

Administer:

Paclitaxel _____mg (200 mg/m^2) IV over 24 hours on day 1

- Stable for up to 27 hours at room temperature, 0.3–1.2 mg/mL solutions.
- Available in 30- and 300-mg vials 6 mg/mL and 100-mg vial 16.7 mg/mL.
- Further dilute in NS or D5W for final concentration < 1.2 mg/ml.
- **Use non-PVC containers and tubing with 0.22-micron inline filter for administration.**

Cisplatin _____mg (75 mg/m^2) IV on day 2

- Stable for 96 hours when protected from light and only 6 hours when not protected from light.
- Available in 1-mg/mL concentrations.
- Further dilute solution with 250 cc or more of NS.
- Do not use aluminum needles, because precipitate will form.

Repeat cycle every 21 days.

Major Side Effects

- Hypersensitivity Reaction: Occurs in 20%–40% of patients. Characterized by generalized skin rash, flushing, erythema, hypotension, dyspnea, and/or bronchospasm. Usually occurs within the first 2–3 minutes of infusion and almost always within the first 10 minutes. Premedicate as described.
- Bone Marrow Depression: Neutropenia, thrombocytopenia, and anemia are cumulative and dose related. Can be dose limiting. G-CSF support recommended.
- GI Toxicities: Moderate-to-severe nausea and vomiting may be acute or delayed.
- Renal: Nephrotoxicity is dose related and with cisplatin presents at 10–20 days. Provide adequate hydration to reduce risk.
- Electrolyte Imbalance: Decreases Mg^{2+}, K, Ca^{2+}, Na, and P.
- Neurotoxicity: Sensory neuropathy with numbness and paresthesias; dose related.
- Alopecia: Total loss of body hair occurs in nearly all patients.
- Reproductive: Pregnancy category D. Breast feeding should be avoided.

Initiate antiemetic protocol:	Highly to severely emetogenic protocol.

Supportive drugs:

☐ pegfilgrastim (Neulasta)   ☐ filgrastim (Neupogen)

☐ epoetin alfa (Procrit)   ☐ darbepoetin alfa (Aranesp)

Treatment schedule:	Chair time 1 hour on day 1, and 3 hours on day 2. Repeat every 21 days as tolerated or until disease progression.
Estimated number of visits:	Three visits per cycle. Request three cycles worth of visits.

Dose Calculation by: 1. _____   2. _____

_____

Physician

_____

Patient Name

_____

Diagnosis

_____

Date

_____

ID Number

_____/_____/_____

Ht   Wt   M^2

5-FU + Cisplatin + Definitive Radiation Therapy

Baseline laboratory tests:	CBC: Chemistry (including Mg^{2+}) and CEA
Baseline procedures or tests:	Central line placement
Initiate IV:	0.9% sodium chloride
Premedicate:	5-HT$_3$ and dexamethasone 10–20 mg in 100 cc of NS
Administer:	**Fluorouracil** _____mg (1000 mg/m^2/day) IV continuous infusion on days 1–4, 29–32, 50–53, and 71–74

- No dilution required. Can be further diluted with 0.9% sodium chloride or D5W.

AND

Cisplatin _____mg (75 mg/m^2/day) IV on days 1, 29, 50, and 71

- Stable for 96 hours when protected from light and only 6 hours when not protected from light.
- Available in 1-mg/mL concentrations.
- Further dilute solution with 250 cc or more of NS.
- Do not use aluminum needles, because precipitate will form.

External-beam radiation therapy, 50.4 Gy at 1.8 Gy per day, 5 days per week

Major Side Effects

- Bone Marrow Depression: Neutropenia, thrombocytopenia, and anemia are cumulative and dose related. Can be dose limiting.
- GI Toxicities: Moderate-to-severe nausea and vomiting may be acute or delayed. Mucositis and diarrhea can be severe and dose limiting.
- Renal: Nephrotoxicity is dose related and with cisplatin presents at 10–20 days. Provide adequate hydration to reduce risk.
- Electrolyte Imbalance: Decreases Mg^{2+}, K, Ca^{2+}, Na, and P.
- Skin: Local tissue irritation progressing to desquamation can occur. Do not use oil-based lotions or creams in radiation field. Hyperpigmentation, photosensitivity, and nail changes may occur. Hand-foot syndrome can be dose limiting.
- Ocular: Photophobia, increased lacrimation, conjunctivitis, and blurred vision.
- Reproductive: Pregnancy category D. Breast feeding should be avoided.

Initiate antiemetic protocol:	Moderately to highly emetogenic protocol.
Supportive drugs:	☐ pegfilgrastim (Neulasta) ☐ filgrastim (Neupogen)
	☐ epoetin alfa (Procrit) ☐ darbepoetin alfa (Aranesp)
Treatment schedule:	Chair time 2 hours on days 1, 29, 50, and 71.
Estimated number of visits:	Four visits per treatment course. May require extra visits for hydration.

Dose Calculation by: 1. _____   2. _____

_____

Physician

_____

Date

_____

Patient Name

_____

ID Number

_____

Diagnosis

_____ / _____ / _____

Ht   Wt   M^2

Single-Agent Regimens

Paclitaxel

Baseline laboratory tests:	CBC: Chemistry (including Mg^{2+}) and CEA
Baseline procedures or tests:	Central line placement
Initiate IV:	0.9% sodium chloride
Premedicate:	5-HT$_3$ and dexamethasone 10–20 mg in 100 cc of NS
	Diphenhydramine 25–50 mg and cimetidine 300 mg in 100 cc of NS
Administer:	**Paclitaxel** _____mg (250 mg/m^2) IV over 24 hours on day 1

- Stable for up to 27 hours at room temperature, 0.3–1.2 mg/mL solutions.
- Available in 30- and 300-mg vials 6 mg/mL and 100-mg vial 16.7 mg/mL.
- Further dilute in NS or D5W for final concentration < 1.2 mg/ml.
- **Use non-PVC containers and tubing with 0.22-micron inline filter for administration.**

Major Side Effects

- Hypersensitivity Reaction: Occurs in 20%–40% of patients. Characterized by generalized skin rash, flushing, erythema, hypotension, dyspnea, back pain, and/or bronchospasm. Usually occurs within the first 2–3 minutes of infusion and almost always within the first 10 minutes. Premedicate as described–.
- Bone Marrow Depression: Dose-limiting neutropenia with nadir at days 8–10 and recovery by days 15–21. Decreased incidence of neutropenia with 3-hour schedule when compared with 24-hour schedule. G-CSF support recommended.
- Neurotoxicity: Sensory neuropathy with numbness and paresthesias, dose related. More frequent with longer infusions and at doses < 175 mg/m^2.
- Alopecia: Total loss of body hair occurs in nearly all patients.
- Reproductive: Pregnancy category D. Breast feeding should be avoided.

Initiate antiemetic protocol:	Mildly emetogenic protocol.
Supportive drugs:	☐ pegfilgrastim (Neulasta) ☐ filgrastim (Neupogen)
	☐ epoetin alfa (Procrit) ☐ darbepoetin alfa (Aranesp)
	☐ loperamide (Imodium) ☐ diphenoxylate/atropine sulfate (Lomotil)
Treatment schedule:	Chair time 1 hour. 1 hour for day 2 to discontinue pump. Repeat every every 21 days as tolerated or until disease progression.
Estimated number of visits:	Two visits per cycle. Request three cycles worth of visits.

Dose Calculation by: 1. _____   2. _____

_____

Physician

_____

Patient Name

_____

Diagnosis

_____

Date

_____

ID Number

_____ / _____ / _____

Ht   Wt   M^2

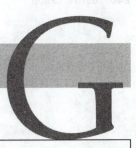

Adjuvant Therapy

One cycle of chemotherapy is administered as follows:

5-Fluorouracil: 425 mg/m^2 IV on days 1–5

Leucovorin: 20 mg/m^2 IV on days 1–5

Chemoradiotherapy is then started 28 days after the start of the initial cycle of chemotherapy as follows:

Radiation therapy: 180 cGy/day to a total dose of 4500 cGy, starting on day 28

5-Fluorouracil: 400 mg/m^2 IV on days 1–4 and days 23–25 of radiation therapy

Leucovorin: 20 mg/m^2 IV on days 1–4 and days 23–25 of radiation therapy

Chemoradiotherapy is followed by two cycles of chemotherapy that are given 1 month apart and include[1,161]:

5-Fluorouracil: 425 mg/m^2 IV on days 1–5

Leucovorin: 20 mg/m^2 IV on days 1–5

Combination Regimens

Docetaxel: 75 mg/m^2 IV on day 1

Cisplatin: 75 mg/m^2 IV over 1–3 hours on day 1

5-FU: 750 mg/m^2/day IV continuous infusion on days 1–5

Repeat cycle every 21 days.[1,162]

Cisplatin: 100 mg/m^2 IV over 1–3 hours on day 1

5-FU: 1000 mg/m^2/day IV continuous infusion on days 1–5

Repeat cycle every 28 days.[1,162]

Etoposide: 120 mg/m^2 IV on days 4–6

Doxorubicin: 20 mg/m^2 IV on days 1 and 7

Cisplatin: 40 mg/m^2 IV on days 2 and 8

Repeat cycle every 21–28 days.[1,163]

Epirubicin: 50 mg/m^2 IV on day 1

Cisplatin: 60 mg/m^2 IV on day 1

5-Fluorouracil: 200 mg/m^2/day IV continuous infusion for 21 weeks

Repeat cycle every 21 days.[1,164]

Etoposide: 120 mg/m^2 IV on days 1–3

Leucovorin: 300 mg/m^2 IV on days 1–3

5-Fluorouracil: 500 mg/m^2 IV on days 1–3

Repeat cycle every 21–28 days.[1,165]

Irinotecan: 70 mg/m^2 IV on days 1 and 15

Cisplatin: 80 mg/m^2 IV on day 1

Repeat cycle every 28 days.[1,166]

5-Fluorouracil: 600 mg/m^2 IV on days 1, 8, 29, and 36

Doxorubicin: 30 mg/m^2 IV on days 1 and 29

Mitomycin: 10 mg/m^2 IV on day 1

Repeat cycle every 8 weeks.[1,167]

5-Fluorouracil: 1500 mg/m^2 IV on day 1, starting 1 hour after methotrexate (MTX)

Leucovorin: 15 mg/m^2 PO every 6 hours for 12 doses, starting 24 hours
after MTX

Doxorubicin: 30 mg/m^2 IV on day 15

Methotrexate: 1500 mg/m^2 IV on day 1

Repeat cycle every 28 days.[1,168]

5-Fluorouracil: 300 mg/m^2 IV on days 1–5

Doxorubicin: 40 mg/m^2 IV on day 1

Cisplatin: 60 mg/m^2 IV on day 1

Repeat cycle every 5 weeks.[1,169]

Docetaxel + Cisplatin **255**

Docetaxel: 85 mg/m^2 IV on day 1
Cisplatin: 75 mg/m^2 IV on day 1
Repeat cycle every 21 days.[1,170]

Single-Agent Regimens

5-Fluorouracil **256**

5-Fluorouracil: 500 mg/m^2 IV on days 1–5
Repeat cycle every 28 days.[1,171]

Docetaxel **257**

Docetaxel: 100 mg/m^2 IV on day 1
Repeat cycle every 21 days.[1,172]
OR
Docetaxel: 36 mg/m^2 IV weekly for 6 weeks
Repeat cycle every 8 weeks.[1,172]

Adjuvant Therapy

5-FU + Leucovorin + 5-FU + Radiation Therapy

Baseline laboratory tests:	CBC: Chemistry and CEA
Baseline procedures or tests:	N/A
Initiate IV:	0.9% sodium chloride
Premedicate:	5-HT$_3$ and dexamethasone 10–20 mg in 100 cc of NS
Administer:	**Chemotherapy (one 28-day cycle):**

5-FU_____mg (425 mg/m^2/day) IV days 1–5

- 50 mg/mL, no dilution required. Can be further diluted with 0.9% sodium chloride or D5W.

Leucovorin_____mg (20 mg/m^2/day) IV days 1–5

- Available in solution or powder. Reconstitute powder with sterile water. May further dilute with 0.9% sodium chloride or D5W.
- Do not mix in same solution with 5-FU, because a precipitate will form.

Chemoradiotherapy (starts on day 28 after the start of the initial cycle of chemotherapy as follows):

Radiation therapy 180 cGy/day to a total dose of 4500 cGy

5-FU _____mg (400 mg/m^2/day) IV on days 1–4 and days 23–25 of radiation therapy

Leucovorin _____mg (20 mg/m^2/day) IV on days 1–4 and days 23–25 of radiation therapy

One-month recovery period

Chemotherapy (two-28 day cycles):

5-FU _____mg (425 mg/m^2/day) IV days 1–5

Leucovorin _____mg (20 mg/m^2/day) IV days 1–5

Major Side Effects	• Bone Marrow Depression: Neutropenia, thrombocytopenia, and anemia are cumulative and dose related. Can be dose limiting.
	• GI Toxicities: Mucositis and diarrhea can be severe and dose limiting.
	• Skin: Local tissue irritation progressing to desquamation can occur. Do not use oil-based lotions or creams in radiation field. Hyperpigmentation, photosensitivity, and nail changes may occur. Hand-foot syndrome can be dose limiting.
	• Ocular: Photophobia, increased lacrimation, conjunctivitis, and blurred vision.
	• Reproductive: Pregnancy category D. Breast feeding should be avoided.
Initiate antiemetic protocol:	Mildly emetogenic protocol.
Supportive drugs:	☐ pegfilgrastim (Neulasta) ☐ filgrastim (Neupogen)
	☐ epoetin alfa (Procrit) ☐ darbepoetin alfa (Aranesp)
	☐ loperamide (Imodium) ☐ diphenoxylate/atropine sulfate (Lomotil)
Treatment schedule:	Chemotherapy: 1 hour on day 1
	Chemoradiotherapy: 1 hour on day 1 week 1, 1 hour on day 4 week 5
	One month rest:
	then
	Chemotherapy: 1 hour on day 1 × 2
Estimated number of visits:	Four visits per treatment course (21 weeks' total therapy)
	Note: May need additional visits for IV hydration.

Dose Calculation by: 1. _____ 2. _____

_____   _____
Physician   Date

_____   _____
Patient Name   ID Number

_____   _____/_____/_____
Diagnosis   Ht   Wt   M²

Combination Regimens

Docetaxel + Cisplatin + 5-FU (DCF)

Baseline laboratory tests:	CBC: Chemistry (including Mg^{2+}) and CEA
Baseline procedures or tests:	Central line placement
Initiate IV:	0.9% sodium chloride
Premedicate:	5-HT$_3$ and dexamethasone 10–20 mg in 100 cc of NS
	Dexamethasone 8 mg bid for 3 days, starting the day before treatment
Administer:	**Docetaxel** _____ mg (75 mg/m^2) IV on day 1

- Comes in 20- or 80-mg blister packs with own diluent. Do not shake. Reconstituted vials stable at room temperature or refrigerated for 8 hours.
- Further dilute in 250 cc of D5W or 0.9% sodium chloride.
- Use non-PVC containers and tubing to administer.
- Use within 24 hours of preparation.

Cisplatin _____ mg (75 mg/m^2) IV over 1–3 hours on day 1

- Stable for 96 hours when protected from light and only 6 hours when not protected from light.
- Available in 1-mg/1-mL solution.
- Do not use aluminum needles, because precipitate will form.
- Further dilute in 250 cc or more of 0.9% sodium chloride.

Fluorouracil _____ mg (750 mg/m^2/day) IV continuous infusion on days 1–5

- 50-mg/10-mL concentration. No dilution required. Can be further diluted with 0.9% sodium chloride or D5W.

Major Side Effects	

- Hypersensitivity Reactions: Severe hypersensitivity reactions with docetaxel in 2%–3% of patients. Characterized by generalized skin rash, flushing, erythema, hypotension, dyspnea, and/or bronchospasm. Usually occurs within the first 2–3 minutes of infusion and almost always within the first 10 minutes. Premedicate as describe.
- Bone Marrow Depression: Neutropenia, thrombocytopenia, and anemia are dose related.
- GI Toxicities: Moderate-to-severe nausea and vomiting may be acute or delayed. Mucositis and diarrhea can be severe and dose limiting
- Renal: Nephrotoxicity is dose related and with cisplatin presents at 10–20 days. Provide adequate hydration to reduce risk.
- Neuropathy: Peripheral neuropathy may affect up to 49% of patients.
- Electrolyte Imbalance: Decreases Mg^{2+}, K, Ca^{2+}, Na, and P.
- Skin: Hyperpigmentation, photosensitivity, and nail changes may occur. Hand-foot syndrome can be dose limiting.
- Ocular: Photophobia, increased lacrimation, conjunctivitis, and blurred vision.
- Reproductive: Pregnancy category D. Breast feeding should be avoided.

Initiate antiemetic protocol:	Moderately to severely emetogenic protocol.	
Supportive drugs:	☐ pegfilgrastim (Neulasta)	☐ filgrastim (Neupogen)
	☐ epoetin alfa (Procrit)	☐ darbepoetin alfa (Aranesp)
Treatment schedule:	Chair time 4 hours on day 1. Repeat cycle every 21 days.	
Estimated number of visits:	One visit per cycle. Request three cycles worth of visits.	

Dose Calculation by: 1. _____   2. _____

_____

Physician

_____

Patient Name

_____

Diagnosis

_____

Date

_____

ID Number

_____/_____/_____

Ht   Wt   M^2

5-FU + Cisplatin (CF)

Baseline laboratory tests:	CBC: Chemistry (including Mg^{2+}) and CEA
Baseline procedures or tests:	Central line placement
Initiate IV:	0.9% sodium chloride
Premedicate:	5-HT_3 and dexamethasone 10–20 mg in 100 cc of NS
Administer:	**Cisplatin** _____mg (100 mg/m^2) IV over 1–3 hours on day 1

- Stable for 96 hours when protected from light and only 6 hours when not protected from light.
- Available in 1-m/1-mL solution.
- Do not use aluminum needles, because precipitate will form.
- Further dilute solution with 250 cc or more NS.

Fluorouracil _____mg (1000 mg/m^2/day) IV continuous infusion days 1–5

- 50-mg/10-ml solution. No dilution required. Can be further diluted with 0.9% sodium chloride or D5W.

Major Side Effects	• Bone Marrow Depression: Neutropenia, thrombocytopenia, and anemia are dose related.

- GI Toxicities: Moderate-to-severe nausea and vomiting may be acute or delayed. Mucositis and diarrhea can be severe and dose limiting.
- Renal: Nephrotoxicity is dose related and with cisplatin presents at 10–20 days. Provide adequate hydration to reduce risk.
- Electrolyte Imbalance: Decreases Mg^{2+}, K, Ca^{2+}, Na, and P.
- Skin: Hyperpigmentation, photosensitivity, and nail changes may occur. Hand-foot syndrome can be dose limiting.
- Ocular: Photophobia, increased lacrimation, conjunctivitis, and blurred vision.
- Reproductive: Pregnancy category D. Breast feeding should be avoided.

Initiate antiemetic protocol:	Moderately to severely emetogenic protocol.
Supportive drugs:	☐ pegfilgrastim (Neulasta) ☐ filgrastim (Neupogen)
	☐ epoetin alfa (Procrit) ☐ darbepoetin alfa (Aranesp)
	☐ loperamide (Imodium) ☐ diphenoxylate/atropine sulfate (Lomotil)
Treatment schedule:	Chair time 3 hours on day 1. Repeat cycle every 28 days.
Estimated number of visits:	Three visits per cycle. Request 6 months worth. May require extra visits for hydration.

Dose Calculation by: 1. _____   2. _____

_____

Physician   Date

_____

Patient Name   ID Number

_____/ _____/ _____

Diagnosis   Ht   Wt   M^2

Etoposide + Doxorubicin + Cisplatin (EAP)

Baseline laboratory tests:	CBC: Chemistry (including Mg^{2+}), LFTs, and CEA
Baseline procedures or tests:	MUGA scan
Initiate IV:	0.9% sodium chloride
Premedicate:	5-HT$_3$ and dexamethasone 10–20 mg in 100 cc of NS
Administer:	**Etoposide** _____ (120 mg/m^2) IV over 30–60 minutes on days 4–6

- Available in 20-mg/mL solution.
- May be further diluted with NS or D5W.
- Stability is dependent on final concentration. A concentration of 0.2 mg/mL is stable for 48 hours in a plastic container at room temperature or for 96 hours in a glass container at room temperature (under normal fluorescent light).

Doxorubicin _____ (20 mg/m^2) IV push on days 1 and 7

- **Potent vesicant**
- Available in 2-mg/mL solution; no need to further dilute.

Cisplatin _____ mg (40 mg/m^2) IV over 1–3 hours on days 2 and 8

- Stable for 96 hours when protected from light and only 6 hours when not protected from light.
- Available in 1-m/1-mL solution.
- Do not use aluminum needles, because precipitate will form.
- Further dilute solution with 250 cc or more of NS.

Major Side Effects

- Hypersensitivity reaction with etoposide: Characterized by generalized skin rash, flushing, erythema, hypotension, dyspnea, and/or bronchospasm. Usually occurs with rapid infusions. Always infuse over 30–60 minutes. Premedicate as described.
- Bone Marrow Depression: Neutropenia, thrombocytopenia, and anemia. Effects are dose related.
- GI Toxicities: Moderate-to-severe nausea and vomiting may be acute or delayed. Mucositis can occur.
- GU: Red-orange discoloration of urine; resolves in 24–48 hours.
- Renal: Nephrotoxicity is dose related and with cisplatin presents at 10–20 days. Provide adequate hydration to reduce risk.
- Electrolyte Imbalance: Decreases Mg^{2+}, K, Ca^{2+}, Na, and P.
- Skin: Tissue necrosis with extravasation. Hyperpigmentation, radiation recall, and nail changes are seen. Alopecia is dose dependent.
- Cardiovascular: Hypotension may occur with rapid infusion of etoposide. Cardiomyopathy may occur with high cumulative doses of doxorubicin.
- Reproduction: Etoposide and doxorubicin are mutagenic and teratogenic.

Initiate antiemetic protocol:	Moderately to highly emetogenic protocol.
Supportive drugs:	☐ pegfilgrastim (Neulasta) ☐ filgrastim (Neupogen)
	☐ epoetin alfa (Procrit) ☐ darbepoetin alfa (Aranesp)
Treatment schedule:	Chair time 1 hour on days 1, 4, 5, 6, and 7; 3 hours on days 2 and 8. Repeat cycle every 21–28 days.
Estimated number of visits:	Nine visits per cycle. Request three cycles worth. May require extra visits for hydration.

Dose Calculation by: 1. _____   2. _____

_____   _____
Physician   Date

_____   _____
Patient Name   ID Number

_____   _____/_____/_____
Diagnosis   Ht   Wt   M^2

Epirubicin + Cisplatin + Fluorouracil (ECF)

Baseline laboratory tests: CBC: Chemistry (including Mg^{2+}) and CEA

Baseline procedures or tests: Central line placement, MUGA scan

Initiate IV: 0.9% sodium chloride

Premedicate: 5-HT$_3$ and dexamethasone 10–20 mg in 100 cc of NS

Administer:

Epirubicin _____ mg (50 mg/m^2) IV on day 1

- **Vesicant**
- Available as a preservative-free solution (2 mg/mL).
- Use within 24 hours of preparation.

Cisplatin _____ mg (60 mg/m^2) IV over 1–3 hours on day 1

- Stable for 96 hours when protected from light and only 6 hours when not protected from light.
- Available in 1-mg/mL solutions.
- Do not use aluminum needles, because precipitate will form.
- Further dilute solution with 250 cc or more of NS.

Fluorouracil _____ mg (200 mg/m^2/day) IV continuous infusion for 21 days

- 50-mg/10-mL solution. No dilution required. Can be further diluted with 0.9% sodium chloride or D5W.

Major Side Effects

- Bone Marrow Depression: Neutropenia, thrombocytopenia, and anemia are dose related. Can be dose limiting.
- GI Toxicities: Moderate-to-severe nausea and vomiting may be acute or delayed. Mucositis and diarrhea can be severe and dose limiting
- Renal: Nephrotoxicity is dose related and with cisplatin presents at 10–20 days. Provide adequate hydration to reduce risk.
- Cardiovascular: Acute or delayed cardiotoxicities may be seen. Acute symptoms (sinus tachycardia and electrocardiographic abnormalities) are usually of no clinical significance. Delayed toxicities, such as decreased left ventricular ejection fraction and congestive heart failure, are clinically significant.
- Electrolyte Imbalance: Decreases Mg^{2+}, K, Ca^{2+}, Na, and P.
- Skin: Tissue necrosis if extravasation occurs. Hyperpigmentation, photosensitivity, radiation recall, and nail changes may occur. Hand-foot syndrome can be dose limiting. Alopecia is universal.
- Ocular: Photophobia, increased lacrimation, conjunctivitis, and blurred vision.
- Reproductive: Epirubicin is genotoxic, mutagenic, and carcinogenic.

Initiate antiemetic protocol: Moderately to highly emetogenic protocol.

Supportive drugs:
☐ pegfilgrastim (Neulasta)   ☐ filgrastim (Neupogen)
☐ epoetin alfa (Procrit)   ☐ darbepoetin alfa (Aranesp)
☐ loperamide (Imodium)   ☐ diphenoxylate/atropine sulfate (Lomotil)

Treatment schedule: Chair time 3 hours on day 1, and 1 hour on days 8 and 15. Repeat cycle every 21 days.

Estimated number of visits: Four visits per cycle. Request three cycles worth of visits.

Dose Calculation by: 1. _____ 2. _____

_____
Physician

_____
Date

_____
Patient Name

_____
ID Number

_____
Diagnosis

_____ / _____ / _____
Ht   Wt   M^2

Etoposide + Leucovorin + Fluorouracil (ELF)

Baseline laboratory tests: CBC: Chemistry and CEA
Baseline procedures or tests: N/A
Initiate IV: 0.9% sodium chloride
Premedicate: Oral phenothiazine or 5-HT$_3$
Administer:

Etoposide _____ mg (120 mg/m^2) IV on days 1–3
- Available in 20-mg/mL solution.
- May be further diluted in NS or D5W.
- Stability is dependant on final concentration. A concentration of 0.2 mg/mL is stable for 48 hours in a plastic container at room temperature or for 96 hours in a glass container at room temperature (under fluorescent light).

Leucovorin _____ mg (300 mg/m^2) IV on days 1–3
- Available in solution or powder. Reconstitute powder with sterile water. May further dilute with 0.9% sodium chloride or D5W.
- Do not mix in same solution with 5-FU, because a precipitate will form.

5-Fluorouracil _____ mg (500 mg/m^2) IV on days 1–3
- 50-mg/10-mL solution. No dilution required. Can be further diluted with 0.9% sodium chloride or D5W.

Major Side Effects
- Hypersensitivity reaction with etoposide: Characterized by generalized skin rash, flushing, erythema, hypotension, dyspnea, and/or bronchospasm. Usually occurs with rapid infusions. Always infuse over 30–60 minutes. Premedicate as described
- Bone Marrow Depression: Nadir 10–14 days. Neutropenia, thrombocytopenia are dose related. Can be dose limiting for daily × 5 or weekly regimens.
- GI Toxicities: Nausea and vomiting occur in 30%–50% of patients but are usually mild. Mucositis and diarrhea can be severe and dose limiting.
- Cardiovascular: Hypotension with rapid infusion of etoposide.
- Skin: Alopecia is dose dependent. Hyperpigmentation, photosensitivity, and nail changes may occur. Hand-foot syndrome can be dose limiting.
- Ocular: Photophobia, increased lacrimation, conjunctivitis, and blurred vision.
- Reproduction: Etoposide is teratogenic and mutagenic.

Initiate antiemetic protocol: Mildly emetogenic protocol.
Supportive drugs:
☐ pegfilgrastim (Neulasta)   ☐ filgrastim (Neupogen)
☐ epoetin alfa (Procrit)   ☐ darbepoetin alfa (Aranesp)
☐ loperamide (Imodium)   ☐ diphenoxylate/atropine sulfate (Lomotil)

Treatment schedule: Chair time 1 hour on days 1–3. Repeat every 21–28 days as tolerated.
Estimated number of visits: Four visits per cycle. Request three cycles worth of visits.

Dose Calculation by: 1. _____ 2. _____

Physician _____ Date _____

Patient Name _____ ID Number _____

Diagnosis _____ Ht _____ / Wt _____ / M^2 _____

Irinotecan + Cisplatin (IP)

Baseline laboratory tests:	CBC: Chemistry (including Mg^{2+})
Baseline procedures or tests:	N/A
Initiate IV:	0.9% sodium chloride
Premedicate:	5-HT$_3$ and dexamethasone 10–20 mg in 100 cc of NS
Administer:	

Irinotecan _____ mg (70 mg/m^2) IV on days 1 and 15

- Available in 2- and 5-ml vials (20 mg/ml).
- Store at room temperature and protect from light.
- Dilute and mix drug in D5W (preferred) or NS.
- Diluted drug is stable 24 hours at room temperature or, if diluted in D5W, stable for 48 hours if refrigerated and protected from light

Cisplatin _____ mg (80 mg/m^2) IV over 1–3 hours on day 1

- Stable for 96 hours when protected from light and only 6 hours when not protected from light.
- Do not use aluminum needles, because precipitate will form.
- Available in solution as 1 mg/mL.
- Further dilute solution with 250–1000 cc NS.

Major Side Effects

- Bone Marrow Depression: Myelosuppression can be severe, dose-limiting toxicity. May need dose reductions for severe neutropenia.
- GI Toxicities: Moderate-to-severe nausea and vomiting. May be acute (first 24 hours) or delayed (> 24 hours). Diarrhea or constipation possible. Abdominal pain not unusual. Early diarrhea, most likely a cholinergic reaction, can be managed with atropine before administration of irinotecan. Late diarrhea observed in 22% of patients, can be severe, and should be treated aggressively. Consider lomotil, immodium, tincture of opium, and hydration.
- Hepatic Toxicities: Evidence of increased drug toxicity in patients with low protein and hepatic dysfunction. Dose reductions may be necessary.
- Renal: Nephrotoxicity is dose related and with cisplatin presents at 10–20 days. Use with caution in patients with abnormal renal function. Dose reduction is necessary in this setting. Provide adequate hydration to reduce risk.
- Electrolyte Imbalance: Decreases Mg^{2+}, K, Ca^{2+}, Na, and P.
- Neurotoxicity: Dose-limiting toxicity, usually in the form of peripheral sensory neuropathy. Paresthesias and numbness in a classic "stocking glove" pattern.
- Ototoxicity: High-frequency hearing loss and tinnitus.
- Skin: Alopecia
- Reproduction: Cisplatin is mutagenic and probably teratogenic.

Initiate antiemetic protocol:	Moderately to highly emetogenic protocol.
Supportive drugs:	☐ pegfilgrastim (Neulasta) ☐ filgrastim (Neupogen)
	☐ epoetin alfa (Procrit) ☐ darbepoetin alfa (Aranesp)
Initiate antidiarrheal protocol:	☐ loperamide (Imodium) ☐ diphenoxylate/atropine sulfate (Lomotil)
Treatment schedule:	Chair time 4 hours on day 1, and 2 hours on days 2 and 3. Repeat cycle every 28 days.
Estimated number of visits:	Four visits per cycle. Request six cycles worth of visits.

Dose Calculation by: 1. _____   2. _____

_____
Physician

_____
Patient Name

_____
Diagnosis

_____
Date

_____
ID Number

_____ / _____ / _____
Ht   Wt   M^2

5-Fluorouracil + Doxorubicin + Mitomycin (FAM)

Baseline laboratory tests:	CBC: Chemistry and CA 19-9
Baseline procedures or tests:	MUGA scan
Initiate IV:	0.9% sodium chloride
Premedicate:	5-HT$_3$ and dexamethasone 10–20 mg in 100 cc of NS
Administer:	**Fluorouracil** _____ mg (600 mg/m^2/day) IV on days 1, 8, 29, and 36

- 50-mg/10-mL solution. No dilution required. Can be further diluted with 0.9% sodium chloride or D5W.

Doxorubicin _____ mg (30 mg/m^2) IV on days 1 and 29

- Potent vesicant
- Available in 2-mg/1-mL solution.
- Drug will form a precipitate if it is mixed with heparin or 5-FU.

Mitomycin _____ mg (10 mg/m^2) IV bolus on day 1

- Potent vesicant
- Available in 5-, 20-, and 40-mg vials. Dilute with sterile water to give a final concentration of 0.5 mg/mL. Reconstituted solution stable for 14 days refrigerated or 7 days at room temperature

Major Side Effects

- Bone Marrow Depression: Dose-limiting and cumulative toxicity, with leukopenia being more common than thrombocytopenia. Nadir counts are delayed at 4–6 weeks with mitomycin but occur at 10–14 days with doxorubicin.
- GI Toxicities: Nausea and vomiting in 50% of patients and are moderate to severe. Mucositis and diarrhea can be severe and dose limiting.
- GU: Red-orange discoloration of urine; resolves in 24–48 hours.
- Skin: Vesicants cause tissue necrosis if extravasated. Hyperpigmentation, photosensitivity, radiation recall, and nail changes may occur. Hand-foot syndrome can be dose limiting.
- Cardiac: Doxorubicin can cause cardiomyopathy with cumulative doses > 450 mg/m^2.
- Ocular: Photophobia, increased lacrimation, conjunctivitis, and blurred vision.
- Hemolytic-uremic syndrome: Hematocrit < 25%, platelets < 100×10^3/mm^3 and renal failure (serum creatinine > 1.6 mg/dL). Rare event (< 2%).
- Reproductive: Pregnancy category D. Breast feeding should be avoided.

Initiate antiemetic protocol:	Moderately to highly emetogenic protocol.
Supportive drugs:	☐ pegfilgrastim (Neulasta) ☐ filgrastim (Neupogen)
	☐ epoetin alfa (Procrit) ☐ darbepoetin alfa (Aranesp)
Initiate antidiarrheal protocol:	☐ loperamide (Imodium) ☐ diphenoxylate/atropine sulfate (Lomotil)
Treatment schedule:	Chair time 1 hour on days 1, 8, 29, and 36. Repeat every 56 day until disease progression.
Estimated number of visits:	Four visits per treatment course.

Dose Calculation by: 1. _____ 2. _____

_____

Physician

_____

Patient Name

_____

Diagnosis

_____

Date

_____

ID Number

_____ / _____ / _____

Ht Wt M^2

5-Fluorouracil + Doxorubicin + Methotrexate (FAMTX)

Baseline laboratory tests:	CBC: Chemistry and CA 19-9
Baseline procedures or tests:	MUGA scan
Initiate IV:	0.9% sodium chloride
Pre-/Posthydration:	1000 cc of 0.9% sodium chloride with two ampules of $NaHCO_3$
Premedicate:	5-HT$_3$ and dexamethasone 10–20 mg in 100 cc of NS
Administer:	**Fluorouracil** _____ mg (1500 mg/m^2) IV on day 1, starting 1 hour after MTX

- Available in 50-mg/20-mL solution. No dilution required. Can be further diluted with 0.9% sodium chloride or D5W.

Leucovorin _____ mg (15 mg/m^2) PO every 6 hours for 12 doses, starting 24 hours after MTX.

- Leucovorin rescue must be given on time, as ordered.
- Leucovorin should continue until MTX level is < 50 nM.

Doxorubicin _____ mg (30 mg/m^2) IV on day 15

- **Potent vesicant**
- Available in 2-mg/1-mL solution.
- Drug will form a precipitate if it is mixed with heparin or 5-FU.

Methotrexate _____ mg (1500 mg/m^2) IV over minimum of 3 hours on day 1

- Stable for 7 days at room temperature.
- Available in 25-mg/mL solutions. High doses cross the blood-brain barrier; reconstitute with preservative-free 0.9% sodium chloride.
- Urine should be alkalized before and after administration to prevent crystallization in the kidneys.

Major Side Effects	• Renal Toxicity: MTX may precipitate in renal tubules, causing acute renal tubular necrosis if urine pH greater than 7.0 is not maintained for 48–72 hours after administration.

- Bone Marrow Depression: Dose-limiting and cumulative toxicity with leukopenia being more common than thrombocytopenia.
- GI Toxicities: Moderate-to-severe nausea and vomiting and can begin during MTX infusion. Mucositis and diarrhea can be severe and dose limiting.
- GU: Red-orange discoloration in urine; resolves in 24–48 hours.
- Skin: Tissue necrosis if extravasated. Hyperpigmentation, photosensitivity, radiation recall, and nail changes may occur. Hand-foot syndrome can be dose limiting.
- Cardiac: Doxorubicin can cause cardiomyopathy at cumulative doses > 450 mg/m^2.
- Ocular: Photophobia, increased lacrimation, conjunctivitis, and blurred vision.
- Reproductive: Menstrual irregularities, abortion, and fetal deaths in women. Reversible oligospermia with testicular failure reported in men with high-dose therapy. Pregnancy category D. Breast feeding should be avoided.

Initiate antiemetic protocol:	Moderately to highly emetogenic protocol.
Supportive drugs:	☐ pegfilgrastim (Neulasta) ☐ filgrastim (Neupogen) ☐ epoetin alfa (Procrit) ☐ darbepoetin alfa (Aranesp)
Initiate antidiarrheal protocol:	☐ loperamide (Imodium) ☐ diphenoxylate/atropine sulfate (Lomotil)
Treatment schedule:	Chair time 8 hours on day 1, and 1 hour on day 15. Repeat cycle every 28 days.
Estimated number of visits:	Two visits per treatment course. Request three courses worth of treatments.

Dose Calculation by: 1. _____   2. _____

_____

Physician   Date

_____

Patient Name   ID Number

_____ / _____ / _____

Diagnosis   Ht   Wt   M²

Fluorouracil + Doxorubicin + Cisplatin (FAP)

Baseline laboratory tests:	CBC: Chemistry (including Mg^{2+}) and CEA
Baseline procedures or tests:	MUGA scan
Initiate IV:	0.9% sodium chloride
Premedicate:	5-HT_3 and dexamethasone 10–20 mg in 100 cc of NS
Administer:	**Fluorouracil** _____mg (300 mg/m^2) IV days 1–5

- 50-mg/10-mL solution. No dilution required. Can be further diluted with 0.9% sodium chloride or D5W.

Doxorubicin _____mg (40 mg/m^2) IV on day 1

- Potent vesicant
- Available in 2-mg/mL solution.
- Drug will form a precipitate if it is mixed with heparin or 5-FU.

Cisplatin _____mg (60 mg/m^2) IV over 1–3 hours on day 1

- Stable for 96 hours when protected from light and only 6 hours when not protected from light.
- Available in 1-mg/1-mL solution.
- Do not use aluminum needles, because precipitate will form.
- Further dilute solution with 250 cc or more NS.

Major Side Effects

- Bone Marrow Depression: Neutropenia, thrombocytopenia, and anemia are dose related.
- GI Toxicities: Moderate-to-severe nausea and vomiting may be acute or delayed. Mucositis and diarrhea can be severe and dose limiting.
- GU: Red-orange discoloration of urine; resolves in 24–48 hours.
- Cardiovascular: Doxorubicin can cause cardiomyopathy with cumulative doses > 450 mg/m^2.
- Renal: Nephrotoxicity is dose related and with cisplatin presents at 10–20 days. Provide adequate hydration to reduce risk.
- Electrolyte Imbalance: Decreases Mg^{2+}, K, Ca^{2+}, Na, and P.
- Skin: Tissue necrosis if extravasation occurs. Hyperpigmentation, radiation recall, photosensitivity, and nail changes may occur. Hand-foot syndrome can be dose limiting.
- Ocular: Photophobia, increased lacrimation, conjunctivitis, and blurred vision.
- Reproduction: Cisplatin and doxorubicin are mutagenic and teratogenic.

Initiate antiemetic protocol:	Moderately to highly emetogenic protocol.

Supportive drugs:

☐ pegfilgrastim (Neulasta)	☐ filgrastim (Neupogen)
☐ epoetin alfa (Procrit)	☐ darbepoetin alfa (Aranesp)

Initiate antidiarrheal protocol:

☐ loperamide (Imodium)	☐ diphenoxylate/atropine sulfate (Lomotil)

Treatment schedule:	Chair time 3 hours on day 1, and 1 hour on days 2–5. Repeat cycle every 5 weeks.
Estimated number of visits:	Five visits per cycle. Request three cycles worth of visits.

Dose Calculation by: 1. _____ 2. _____

_____
Physician

_____
Patient Name

_____
Diagnosis

_____
Date

_____
ID Number

_____/_____/_____
Ht   Wt   M^2

Docetaxel + Cisplatin

Baseline laboratory tests:	CBC: Chemistry (including Mg^{2+}) and CEA
Baseline procedures or tests:	Central line placement
Initiate IV:	0.9% sodium chloride
Premedicate:	Dexamethasone 8 mg PO bid for 3 days, starting the day before treatment. $5-HT_3$ and dexamethasone 10–20 mg in 100 cc of NS day of treatment

Administer:

Docetaxel _____mg (85 mg/m^2) IV on day 1

- Available in 20- or 80-mg doses; comes with own diluent. Do not shake.
- Reconstituted vials stable at room temperature or refrigerated for 8 hours.
- Further dilute in 250 cc of D5W or 0.9% sodium chloride.
- Use non-PVC containers and tubings to administer.
- Use within 24 hours of preparation.

Cisplatin _____mg (75 mg/m^2) IV over 1–3 hours on day 1

- Stable for 96 hours when protected from light and only 6 hours when not protected from light.
- Available in 1-mg/1-mL solution.
- Do not use aluminum needles, because precipitate will form.
- Further dilute solution with 250 cc or more of NS.

Major Side Effects

- Hypersensitivity Reaction: Occurs in 2%–3% of patients. Characterized by generalized skin rash, flushing, erythema, hypotension, dyspnea, and/or bronchospasm. Usually occurs within the first 2–3 minutes of infusion and almost always within the first 10 minutes. Premedicate as described.
- Bone Marrow Depression: Neutropenia, thrombocytopenia, and anemia are dose related and can be dose limiting.
- GI Toxicities: Moderate-to-severe nausea and vomiting may be acute or delayed.
- Renal: Nephrotoxicity is dose related and with cisplatin presents at 10–20 days. Provide adequate hydration to reduce risk.
- Electrolyte Imbalance: Decreases Mg^{2+}, K, Ca^{2+}, Na, and P.
- Neuropathy: Peripheral neuropathy may affect up to 49% of patients. Paresthesias in a "glove and stocking" distribution and numbness.
- Skin: Alopecia is common. Nail changes may occur.
- Reproductive: Pregnancy category D. Breast feeding should be avoided.

Initiate antiemetic protocol:	Moderately to severely emetogenic protocol.
Supportive drugs:	☐ pegfilgrastim (Neulasta) ☐ filgrastim (Neupogen)
	☐ epoetin alfa (Procrit) ☐ darbepoetin alfa (Aranesp)
Treatment schedule:	Chair time 4 hours on day 1. Repeat cycle every 21 days.
Estimated number of visits:	One visit per cycle. Request six months worth. May require extra visits for hydration.

Dose Calculation by: 1. _____   2. _____

_____
Physician

_____
Patient Name

_____
Diagnosis

_____
Date

_____
ID Number

_____/ _____/ _____
Ht   Wt   M^2

Single-Agent Regimens

5-Fluorouracil

Baseline laboratory tests:	CBC: Chemistry and CEA
Baseline procedures or tests:	N/A
Initiate IV:	0.9% sodium chloride
Premedicate:	Oral phenothiazine or 5-HT$_3$
Administer:	**5-Fluorouracil** _____ mg (500 mg/m^2/day) IV on days 1–5

- 50-mg/10-mL solution. No dilution required. Can be further diluted with 0.9% sodium chloride or D5W.

Major Side Effects

- Bone Marrow Depression: Nadir 10–14 days. Neutropenia, thrombocytopenia are dose related. Can be dose limiting for daily × 5 or weekly regimens.
- GI Toxicities: Nausea and vomiting occur in 30%–50% of patients but are usually mild. Mucositis and diarrhea can be severe and dose limiting.
- Skin: Alopecia is more common in the 5-day course and results in diffuse thinning of hair. Hyperpigmentation, photosensitivity, and nail changes may occur. Hand-foot syndrome can be dose limiting.
- Ocular: Photophobia, increased lacrimation, conjunctivitis, and blurred vision.
- Reproductive: Pregnancy category D. Breast feeding should be avoided.

Initiate antiemetic protocol:	Mildly emetogenic protocol.
Supportive drugs:	☐ pegfilgrastim (Neulasta) ☐ filgrastim (Neupogen)
	☐ epoetin alfa (Procrit) ☐ darbepoetin alfa (Aranesp)
	☐ loperamide (Imodium) ☐ diphenoxylate/atropine sulfate (Lomotil)
Treatment schedule:	Chair time 1 hour on days 1–5. Repeat cycle every 28 days.
Estimated number of visits:	Five days per cycle. Request six cycles worth of visits.

Dose Calculation by: 1. _____   2. _____

_____

Physician   Date

_____

Patient Name   ID Number

_____

Diagnosis   Ht _____ / Wt _____ / M^2 _____

Docetaxel

Baseline laboratory tests:	CBC: Chemistry (including Mg^{2+}) and CEA
Baseline procedures or tests:	Central line placement
Initiate IV:	0.9% sodium chloride
Premedicate:	Dexamethasone 8 mg bid for 3 days, starting the day before treatment
	Oral phenothiazine or 5-HT$_3$

Administer:

Docetaxel _____mg (100 mg/m^2) IV on day 1 repeat every 21 days

Or

Docetaxel _____mg (36 mg/m^2) IV weekly for 6 weeks; repeat every 8 weeks

- Comes in 20- or 80-mg blister packs with own diluent. Do not shake. Reconstituted vials stable at room temperature or if refrigerated for 8 hours.
- Further dilute in 250 cc D5W or 0.9% sodium chloride.
- Use non-PVC containers and tubing to administer.

Major Side Effects

- Hypersensitivity Reaction: Occurs in 2%–3% of patients. Characterized by generalized skin rash, flushing, erythema, hypotension, dyspnea, and/or bronchospasm. Usually occurs within the first 2–3 minutes of infusion and almost always within the first 10 minutes. Premedicate as described.
- Bone Marrow Depression: Neutropenia is dose limiting with nadir at days 7–10 and recovery by day 14. Thrombocytopenia and anemia also occur.
- GI Toxicities: Nausea and vomiting is mild to moderate. Mucositis and diarrhea occur in 40% of patients.
- Neuropathy: Peripheral neuropathy may affect up to 49% of patients. Sensory alterations are paresthesias in a "glove and stocking" distribution; numbness.
- Fluid Balance: Fluid retention syndrome. Symptoms include weight gain, peripheral and/or generalized edema, pleural effusion, and ascites. Occurs in about 50% of patients. Premedication with dexamethasone effective in preventing or minimizing occurrences.
- Skin: Alopecia occurs in 80% of patients. Nail changes, rash, and dry, pruritic skin seen. Hand-foot syndrome has also been reported.

Initiate antiemetic protocol:	Mildly to moderately emetogenic protocol.
Supportive drugs:	☐ pegfilgrastim (Neulasta) ☐ filgrastim (Neupogen)
	☐ epoetin alfa (Procrit) ☐ darbepoetin alfa (Aranesp)
Treatment schedule:	Chair time 2 hours on day 1. Repeat cycle every 21 days. OR weekly × 6 weeks, repeating every 8 weeks
Estimated number of visits:	Two visits per cycle; request three cycles worth of visits OR weekly for 6 weeks

Dose Calculation by: 1. _____   2. _____

_____   _____
Physician   Date

_____   _____
Patient Name   ID Number

_____   _____/_____/_____
Diagnosis   Ht   Wt   M^2

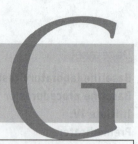

GASTROINTESTINAL STROMAL TUMOR (GIST)

Single-Agent Regimens

Imatinib: 400 mg/day PO

Continue treatment until disease progression.[1,173]

Increase dose to 600–800 mg/day if no response is seen.

Sutent: 50 mg PO once daily

4 weeks on schedule followed by 2 weeks off.[1,174]

Single-Agent Regimens

Imatinib (Gleevec)

Baseline laboratory tests:	CBC: Chemistry and LFTs
Baseline procedures or tests:	c-kit (CD117) expression
Initiate IV:	N/A
Premedicate:	Oral phenothiazine or 5-HT$_3$
Administer:	Start **imatinib** at 400–600 mg PO per day

- May increase dose to 600 or 800 mg PO per day if no response. 800 mg dose is given 400 mg bid.
- Available in 100- or 400-mg capsules.
- Taken with food and a large glass of water. Do NOT take with grapefruit juice.
- Monitor INRs closely in patients taking warfarin; inhibits metabolism of warfarin.

Major Side Effects

- GI Toxicities: Nausea 63%–75% and vomiting, 38%–55% of patients. Usually relieved when the drug is taken with food. Diarrhea observed in 54%; constipation in 13% of patients.
- Bone Marrow Suppression: Myelosuppression, neutropenia, and thrombocytopenia common and can be dose related. Median duration of Neutropenia 3–4 weeks. Dose should be held for ANC, 1.0×10^9/L and platelets $> 50 \times 10^9$/L. Resume dose at 400 mg; if recurrence decrease to 300 mg.
- Fluid/electrolyte Imbalance: Fluid retention is most common side effect, especially in the elderly, 77%–81%. Periorbital and lower-extremity edema primarily occur. However, pleural effusions, ascites, rapid weight gain, and pulmonary edema may develop. Hypokalemia reported in 2%–12% of patients.
- Muscle cramps, arthralgias, headache, fatigue, and abdominal pain affecting 25%–37% of patients.
- Rash may occur in 32%–36% of patients; treat with systemic antihistamine; topical or systemic corticosteroid.
- Laboratory Values: Mild, transient elevation in serum transaminase and bilirubin levels.
- Multiple drug interactions with CYP3A4 pathway:
- Drugs that increase Gleevec plasma levels: Erythomycin, ketoconazole, itraconazole, and clarithromycin.
- Drugs that decrease Gleevec plasma levels: Carbamazepine (tegretol), dexamethasone, phenobarbitol, rifampin, and St. John's Wort.
- Drugs whose plasma levels may be increased by Gleevec: Acetaminophen, cyclosporine, Dihydropyridine calcium channel blockers, HMG-CoA redcutase inhibitors (e.g., simvastatin), pimozide, triazolobenzodiazepines, and warfarin.
- Drugs whose plasma levels may be decreased by Gleevec: Warfarin.
- Reproduction: Drug is teratogenic.

Initiate antiemetic protocol:	Mildly to moderately emetogenic protocol.
Supportive drugs:	☐ loperamide (Imodium) ☐ diphenoxylate/atropine sulfate (Lomotil)
Treatment schedule:	Daily as tolerated until disease progression.
Estimated number of visits:	Monthly during treatment.

Dose Calculation by: 1. _____   2. _____

_____
Physician

_____
Date

_____
Patient Name

_____
ID Number

_____
Diagnosis

_____ / _____ / _____
Ht   Wt   M^2

Sutent: 50 mg PO once daily
4 weeks on schedule followed by 2 weeks off (Pfizer package insert)

Baseline laboratory tests:	CBC: Chemistry with P and LFT
Premedicate:	Oral phenothiazine or 5-HT$_3$
Administer:	**Sutent** 50 mg PO per day, 4 weeks on 2 weeks off.

- Available in 12.5-, 25-, and 50-mg capsules.
- May be taken with or without food.
- Dose modification: Increase or decrease by 12.5 mg based on individual safety and tolerance.

Major Side Effects

- Gastrointestinal: Diarrhea 81%, nausea and vomiting 49%–63%, stomatitis 58%, constipation 41%, and abdominal pain 57%.
- Cardiac: 15% of patients had decreases in Left Ventricular Ejection Fraction Dysfunction (LVEF). Monitor for signs and symptoms of Congestive Heart Failure (CHF). Patients with cardiac history should have a baseline LVEF.
- Hypertension: 15%, grade 3, 4%.
- Hemorrhagic Events: Epistaxis is the most common hemorrhagic event, bleeding from all sites 37%.
- Musculoskeletal: Arthalgia 24%, back pain 23%, and myalgias 28%
- Multiple Drug Interacations: CYP3A4 pathway.
- Reproduction: Drug is teratogenic.

Initiate antiemetic protocol:	Mildly to moderately emetogenic protocol.
Supportive drugs:	☐ loperamide (Imodium) ☐ diphenoxylate/atropine sulfate (Lomotil)
Treatment schedule:	Daily as tolerated until disease progression.
Estimated number of visits:	Monthly during treatment.

Dose Calculation by: 1. _____   2. _____

_____
Physician   Date

_____
Patient Name   ID Number

_____
Diagnosis   Ht _____ / Wt _____ / M^2 _____

HEAD AND NECK CANCER

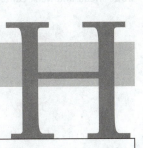

Combination Regimens

261

Cisplatin: 100 mg/m^2 IV on day 1

5-Fluorouracil: 1000 mg/m^2/day IV continuous infusion on days 1–5

Repeat cycle every 21–28 days.[1,180]

Cisplatin: 100 mg/m^2 IV on day 1

5-Fluorouracil: 800 mg/m^2/day IV continuous infusion on days 1–5

Leucovorin: 50 mg/m^2 PO every 6 hours on days 1–5

Repeat cycle every 21 days.[1,181]

Cisplatin: 100 mg/m^2 IV on day 1

5-Fluorouracil: 1000 mg/m^2/day IV continuous infusion on days 1–5

Radiation therapy: 6600–7600 cGy in 180- to 200-cGy fractions

Repeat cycle every 21–28 days for three cycles.[1,182]

Cisplatin: 100 mg/m^2 IV on days 1, 22, and 43

Radiation therapy: 7000 cGy in 200 cGy fractions

Administer cisplatin concurrently with radiation therapy.[183]

Cisplatin: 100 mg/m^2 IV on days 1, 22, and 43 during radiotherapy

Radiation therapy: Total dose of 7000 cGy in 180- to 200-cGy fractions

At the completion of chemoradiotherapy, chemotherapy is administered as
  follows:

Cisplatin: 80 mg/m^2 IV on day 1

5-Fluorouracil: 1000 mg/m^2/day IV continuous infusion on days 1–4

Repeat cycle every 28 days for a total of three cycles.[1,184]

Carboplatin: 300–400 mg/m^2 IV on day 1

5-Fluorouracil: 600 mg/m^2 IV on day 1

Repeat cycle every 21 days.[1,185]

Vinorelbine: 25 mg/m^2 IV on days 1 and 8

Cisplatin: 80 mg/m^2 IV on day 1

Repeat cycle every 21 days.[1,186]

Single-Agent Regimens

Docetaxel **280**

Docetaxel: 100 mg/m^2 IV over 1 hour on day 1
Repeat cycle every 21 days.[1,187]

Paclitaxel **281**

Paclitaxel: 250 mg/m^2 IV over 24 hours on day 1
Repeat cycle every 21 days.[1, 188]
OR
Paclitaxel: 137–175 mg/m^2 IV over 3 hours on day 1
Repeat cycle every 21 days.[1,188]

Methotrexate **282**

Methotrexate: 40 mg/m^2 IV or IM weekly
Repeat cycle every week.[1,189]

Vinorelbine **283**

Vinorelbine: 30 mg/m^2 IV weekly
Repeat cycle every week.[1,190]

Capecitabine (Xeloda) **284**

Capecitabine: 1000 mg/m^2/day PO BID on days 1–14.[1,191]

Combination Regimens

Paclitaxel + Ifosfamide + Mesna + Cisplatin (TIP)

Baseline laboratory tests:	CBC: Chemistry (including Mg^{2+})
Baseline procedures or tests:	N/A
Initiate IV:	0.9% sodium chloride
Premedicate:	5-HT_3 and dexamethasone 10–20 mg in 100 cc of normal saline (NS) (days 1–3)
	Diphenhydramine 25–50 mg and cimetidine 300 mg in 100 cc of NS (day 1 only)

Administer:

Paclitaxel _____ mg (175 mg/m²) IV over 3 hours on day 1

- Available in 50-, 100-, and 300-mg vials, 6 mg/ml or 100 mg/16.7 ml
- Further dilute in NS or D5W to a final concentration is ≤1.2 mg/mL.
- Diluted solution stable for 27 hours at room temperature.
- **Use non-PVC tubing and containers and a 0.22-micron inline filter to administer.**

Ifosfamide _____ mg (1000 mg/m²) IV over 2 hours on days 1–3

- Reconstitute powder with (20 ml for 1-gram or 60 mL for 3-gram vial) sterile water for injection.
- Chemically stable for 7 days, but discard after 8 hours due to lack of bacteriostatic preservative.
- May further dilute in D5W or NS.

Mesna _____ mg (400 mg/m²) IV before ifosfamide on day 1

Mesna _____ mg (200 mg/m²) IV 4 hours after ifosfamide on days 1–3

- Available in 100 mg/ml and 1000 mg vials.
- Diluted solution is stable for 24 hours at room temperature.
- Mesna tablets may be given orally in a dosage equal to 40% of the ifosfamide dose.

Cisplatin _____ mg (60 mg/m²) IV day 1

- Available in 100-mL vials. 1-mg/1-mL concentrations.
- Do not use aluminum needles, as precipitate will form.
- Further dilute solution with 250 cc or more NS.
- 100-mL vial stable for 28 days protected from light, 7 days under florescent light.

Major Side Effects

- Hypersensitivity Reaction: Paclitaxel and cisplatin, with anaphylaxis and severe hypersensitivity reactions in 2%–4%. Characterized by dyspnea, hypotension, andioedema, and generalized urticaria. May also see tachycardia, wheezing, and facial edema. Patients with mild reactions can be rechallenged after 24 hour corticosteroid prophylaxis. Patients with severe reactions should not be rechallenged. Monitor vitals signs every 15 minutes for the first hour. Premedicate as described.
- Bone Marrow Depression: Neutropenia, thrombocytopenia, and anemia are cumulative and dose related. Can be dose limiting. G-CSF support recommended. Give paclitaxel before cisplatin to decrease the severity of myelosuppression.
- Gastrointestinal Toxicities: Moderate to severe nausea and vomiting may be severe, acute, or delayed. Mucositis and/or diarrhea are seen in 30%–40% of patients.
- Renal: Nephrotoxicity may be dose-limiting toxicity. Preventable with adequate hydration. Mannitol or furosemide diuresis may be needed. Hemorrhagic cystitis possible.
- Electrolyte Imbalance: Decreases Mg^{2+}, K^+, Ca^{2+}, Na^+, and P.
- Neurotoxicity: Sensory neuropathy with numbness and paresthesias. Ototoxicity.
- Central Nervous System (CNS): Somulence, confusion, depressive psychosis, or hallucinations (12%).
- Alopecia: A total loss of body hair occurs in nearly all patients.
- Reproduction: Ifosfamide is mutagenic, teratogenic, and excreted in breast milk. Paclitaxel is embryotoxic. Cisplatin may result in Azoospermia, impotence, and sterility.

Initiate antiemetic protocol: Moderately to highly emetogenic protocol.

Supportive drugs: ☐ pegfilgrastim (Neulasta)   ☐ filgrastim (Neupogen)
                         ☐ epoetin alfa (Procrit)   ☐ darbepoetin alfa (Aranesp)

Treatment schedule: Chair time 7–8 hours on day 1 and 3 hours on days 2 and 3. Repeat cycle every 21–28 days.

Estimated number of visits: Three visits per cycle. Request three cycles worth of visits.

Dose Calculation by: 1. _____   2. _____

_____   _____
Physician   Date

_____   _____
Patient Name   ID Number

_____   _____/_____/_____ _____
Diagnosis   Ht   Wt   M²

Docetaxel + Cisplatin + 5-FU (TPF)

Baseline laboratory tests:	CBC: Chemistry (including Mg^{2+}) and carcinoembryonic antigen (CEA)
Baseline procedures or tests:	Central line placement
Initiate IV:	0.9% sodium chloride
Premedicate:	5-HT$_3$ and dexamethasone 20 mg in 100 cc of NS
	Dexamethasone 8-mg bid for 3 days, starting the day before treatment
Administer:	**Docetaxel** _____ mg (75 mg/m^2) IV on day 1

- Comes in 20- or 80-mg blister packs with own diluent. Do not shake. Final concentration 10-mg/mL.
- Reconstituted vials stable at room temperature or refrigerate for 8 hours.
- Further dilute in 250 cc of 5% dextrose or 0.9% sodium chloride. Thoroughly mix by manual rotation.
- Use non-PVC containers and tubing to administer.

Cisplatin _____ mg (75–100 mg/m^2) IV over 24 hours on day 1

- Available in 100-mL vials. 1-mg/1-mL concentrations.
- Do not use aluminum needles, as precipitate will form.
- Further dilute solution with 250 cc or more NS.
- 100-mL vial stable for 28 days protected from light, 7 days under florescent light.

Fluorouracil _____ mg (1000 mg/m^2/day) IV continuous infusion on days 1–4

- No dilution is required. Can be further diluted with NS or D5W.

Major Side Effects

- Hypersensitivity Reaction: Docetaxel and cisplatin, with anaphylaxis and severe hypersensitivity reactions in 2%–4%. Characterized by dyspnea, hypotension, andioedema, and generalized urticaria. May also see tachycardia, wheezing, and facial edema. Patients with mild reactions can be rechallenged after 24 hour corticosteroid prophylaxis. Patients with severe reactions should not be rechallenged. Monitor vitals signs every 15 minutes for the first hour. Premedicate as described.
- Bone Marrow Depression: Neutropenia, thrombocytopenia, and anemia are dose related. Can be dose limiting for daily × 5 or weekly regimens.
- Gastrointestinal Toxicities: Moderate to severe nausea and vomiting may be acute or delayed. Mucositis and diarrhea can be severe and dose limiting.
- Renal: Nephrotoxicity is dose related and with cisplatin presents at 10–20 days. May be dose-limiting toxicity. Preventable with adequate hydration. Mannitol or furosemide diuresis may be needed. Hemorrhagic cystitis possible.
- Fluid Retention Syndrome: Weight gain, peripheral and/or generalized edema, pleural effusion and/or ascites. Incidence increases with total dose > 400 mg/m^2. Occurs in 50% of patients. Premedicate as directed.
- Neurotoxicity: Dose limiting peripheral sensory neuropathy. Paresthesias and numbness in classic "stocking glove" pattern. Risk increases with cumulative doses. Loss of motor function, facial encephalopathy and seizures observed. Neurologic effects may be irreversible.
- Electrolyte Imbalance: Decreases magnesium, potassium, calcium, sodium, and phosphorus.
- Skin: Hyperpigmentation, photosensitivity, and nail changes may occur. Hand-foot syndrome (palmar-plantar erythrodysesthesia) characterized by tingling, numbness, pain, erythema, dryness, rash, swelling, increased pigmentation, and/or pruritus of the hands and feet. Less frequent in reduced doses, can be dose limiting.
- Ocular: Photophobia, increased lacrimation, conjunctivitis, and blurred vision.
- Reproduction: Pregnancy category D. Breast feeding should be avoided.
- Azoospermia, impotence, and sterility.

Initiate antiemetic protocol:	Moderately to highly emetogenic protocol.
Supportive drugs:	☐ pegfilgrastim (Neulasta) ☐ filgrastim (Neupogen)
	☐ epoetin alfa (Procrit) ☐ darbepoetin alfa (Aranesp)

Treatment schedule: Chair time 2 hours on day 1. Repeat cycle every 21 days.

Estimated number of visits: Three visits per cycle. Request three cycles worth of visits. Discontinue cisplatin pump on day 2 and fluorouracil pump on day 5.

Dose Calculation by: 1. _____   2. _____

_____

Physician   Date

_____

Patient Name   ID Number

_____ / _____ / _____

Diagnosis   Ht   Wt   M^2

Paclitaxel + Ifosfamide + Mesna + Carboplatin (TIC)

Baseline laboratory tests:	CBC: Chemistry (including BUN, creatinine, and Mg^{2+})
Baseline procedures or tests:	N/A
Initiate IV:	0.9% sodium chloride
Premedicate:	5-HT_3 and dexamethasone 10–20 mg in 100 cc of NS (days 1–3)
	Diphenhydramine 25–50 mg and cimetidine 300 mg in 100 cc of NS (day 1 only)

Administer:

Paclitaxel _____mg (175 mg/m^2) IV over 3 hours on day 1

- Available in 30-mg (6 m/mL), 100-mg (16.7 mg/mL), and 300-mg (6 mg/mL) vials.
- Further dilute in 250–500 cc NS or D5W. Final concentration is ≤1.2 mg/mL.
- **Use non-PVC tubing and containers and a 0.22-micron inline filter to administer.**

Ifosfamide _____mg (1000 mg/m^2) IV over 2 hours on days 1–3

- Reconstitute powder with sterile water for injection (20 ml for 1 gram or 60 mL for 3-gram vial) sterile water for injection.
- Chemically stable for 7 days, but discard after 8 hours due to lack of bacteriostatic preservative.
- May further dilute in D5W or NS, and discard the unused portion after 8 hours.

Mesna _____mg (400 mg/m^2) IV before ifosfamide

Mesna _____mg (200 mg/m^2) IV for 4 hours after ifosfamide on days 1–3

- Available in 100-mg/mL 1000-mg vials.
- May further dilute in 250–1000 cc NS or D5W.
- Diluted solution is stable for 24 hours at room temperature.
- Stable for 8 hours at room temperature.
- Refrigerate and use reconstituted solution within 6 hours.

Carboplatin _____mg (AUC 6) IV on day 1

- Available in 1-mg/mL solution. Do not use aluminum needles, as precipitate will form.
- Further dilute in 250–1000 cc 0.9% sodium chloride.
- Give after paclitaxel to decrease toxicity.

Major Side Effects

- Hypersensitivity Reaction: Paclitaxel and carboplatin, with anaphylaxis and severe hypersensitivity reactions in 2%–4%. Characterized by dyspnea, hypotension, andioedema, and generalized urticaria. May also see tachycardia, wheezing, and facial edema. Patients with mild reactions can be rechallenged after 24 hour corticosteroid prophylaxis. Patients with severe reactions should not be rechallenged. Monitor vitals signs every 15 minutes for the first hour. Premedicate as described. There is an increased risk of hypersensitivity reactions to carboplatin after more than seven doses.
- Bone Marrow Depression: Neutropenia, thrombocytopenia, and anemia are cumulative and dose related. Can be dose-limiting. G-CSF support recommended.
- Gastrointestinal Toxicities: Moderate to severe nausea and vomiting may be acute or delayed. Mucositis and/or diarrhea are seen in 30%–40% of patients.
- Renal: Nephrotoxicity may be dose-limiting toxicity. Preventable with adequate hydration. Hemorrhagic cystitis possible with symptoms of hematuria, dysuria, and urinary frequency
- Electrolyte Imbalance: Decreases Mg^{2+}, K^+, Ca^{2+}, Na^+, and P.
- Neurotoxicity: Dose limiting peripheral sensory neuropathy. Paresthesias and numbness in classic "stocking glove" pattern. Risk increases with cumulative doses. Loss of motor function, facial encephalopathy and seizures observed. Neurologic effects may be irreversible.
- CNS: Somulence, confusion, depressive psychosis, or hallucinations (12%).
- Alopecia: Total loss of body hair occurs in nearly all patients.
- Reproduction: Ifosfamide is mutagenic, teratogenic, and excreted in breast milk. Paclitaxel is embryotoxic.

Initiate antiemetic protocol: Moderately to highly emetogenic protocol.

Supportive Drugs: ☐ pegfilgrastim (Neulasta)   ☐ filgrastim (Neupogen)

☐ epoetin alfa (Procrit)   ☐ darbepoetin alfa (Aranesp)

Treatment schedule: Chair time 7 hours on day 1 and 4 hours on days 2 and 3. Repeat cycle every 21–28 days.

Estimated number of visits: Four visits per cycle. Request three cycles worth of visits.

Dose Calculation by: 1. _____   2. _____

_____

Physician   Date

_____

Patient Name   ID Number

_____ / _____ / _____

Diagnosis   Ht   Wt   M²

Paclitaxel and Carboplatin (Head and Neck CA)

Baseline laboratory tests:	CBC: Chemistry
Baseline procedures or tests:	N/A
Initiate IV:	0.9% sodium chloride
Premedicate:	5-HT$_3$ and dexamethasone 10–20 mg in 100 cc of NS
	Diphenhydramine 25–50 mg and cimetidine 300 mg in 100 cc of NS

Administer:

Paclitaxel _____ mg (175 mg/m^2) IV over 3 hours on day 1
- Available in 30-mg (6 mg/mL), 100-mg (16.7 mg/mL), and 300-mg (6-mg/mL) vials.
- Further dilute in 250–500 cc NS or D5W. Final concentration is ≤1.2 mg/mL.
- **Use non-PVC tubing and containers and a 0.22-micron inline filter for administration.**

Carboplatin _____ mg (AUC 6) IV day 1
- Available in 50-, 150-, and 450-mg lyophilized powder; dilute with sterile water. Also available in 50-mg and 150-mg, 10-mg/mLg/mL solution; 450-mg and 60-mg 10-mg/mL multidose vials stable for 15 days after first use.
- Do not use aluminum needles, as precipitate will form.
- Further dilute in 250–1000 cc 0.9% sodium chloride or D5W.
- Chemically stable for 24 hours, discard after 8 hours because of lack of bacteriostatic reservative.
- Give carboplatin **after** paclitaxel to decrease toxicities.

Major Side Effects

- Hypersensitivity Reaction: Paclitaxel and carboplatin, with anaphylaxis and severe hypersensitivity reactions in 2%–4%. Characterized by dyspnea, hypotension, andioedema, and generalized urticaria. May also see tachycardia, wheezing, and facial edema. Patients with mild reactions can be rechallenged after 24 hour corticosteroid prophylaxis. Patients with severe reactions should not be rechallenged. Monitor vitals signs every 15 minutes for the first hour. Premedicate as described. There is an increased risk of hypersensitivity reactions after 7–8 doses of carboplatin.
- Bone Marrow Depression: Neutropenia, thrombocytopenia, and anemia are cumulative and dose related. Can be dose limiting. G-CSF support recommended.
- Gastrointestinal Toxicities: Moderate to severe nausea and vomiting may be acute or delayed. Mucositis and/or diarrhea seen in 30%–40% of patients.
- Renal: Nephrotoxicity is less common than with cisplatin and is rarely symptomatic.
- Electrolyte Imbalance: Decreases Mg^{2+}, K$^+$, Ca^{2+}, Na$^+$, and P.
- Neurotoxicity: Dose limiting peripheral sensory neuropathy. Paresthesias and numbness in classic "stocking glove" pattern. Risk increases with cumulative doses. Loss of motor function, facial encephalopathy and seizures observed. Neurologic effects may be irreversible.
- Alopecia: Total loss of body hair occurs in nearly all patients.
- Reproduction: Pregnancy category D. Breast feeding should be avoided.

Initiate antiemetic protocol:	Moderately to highly emetogenic protocol.

Supportive drugs:

☐ pegfilgrastim (Neulasta) ☐ filgrastim (Neupogen)
☐ epoetin alfa (Procrit) ☐ darbepoetin alfa (Aranesp)

Treatment schedule:	Chair time 5 hours on day 1. Repeat the cycle every 21 days until progression.
Estimated number of visits:	Two visits per cycle. Request three cycles worth of visits.

Dose Calculation by: 1. _____   2. _____

_____

Physician   Date

_____   _____

Patient Name   ID Number

_____   ____/____/____

Diagnosis   Ht   Wt   M²

Paclitaxel and Cisplatin (Head and Neck CA)

Baseline laboratory tests: CBC: Chemistry (including Mg^{2+}) and CEA

Baseline procedures or tests: N/A

Initiate IV: 0.9% sodium chloride

Premedicate: 5-HT$_3$ and dexamethasone 10–20 mg in 100 cc of NS (days 1 and 2)

Diphenhydramine 25 to 50 mg and cimetidine 300 mg in 100 cc of NS (day 1 only)

Administer: **Paclitaxel** _____mg (175 mg/m^2) IV over 3 hours on day 1

- Available in 30-mg (6 mg/mL), 100-mg (16.7 mg/mL), and 300-mg (6-mg/mL) vials.
- Further dilute in NS or D5W to a final concentration of $\leq$1.2 mg/mL.
- Diluted solution stable for 27 hours at room temperature.
- **Use non-PVC containers and tubing with a 0.22-micron inline filter for administration.**

Cisplatin _____mg (75 mg/m^2) IV day 2

- Available in 100-mL vials. 1-mg/1-mL concentrations.
- Do not use aluminum needles, as precipitate will form.
- Further dilute solution with 250 cc or more NS.
- 100-mL vial stable for 28 days protected from light, 7 days under florescent light.

Major Side Effects

- Hypersensitivity Reaction: Anaphylaxis and severe hypersensitivity reactions in 2%–4% with Paciltaxel and cisplatin. Characterized by dyspnea, hypotension, andioedema, and generalized urticaria. May also see tachycardia, wheezing, and facial edema. Patients with mild reactions can be rechallenged after 24 hour corticosteroid prophylaxis. Patients with severe reactions should not be rechallenged. Monitor vitals signs every 15 minutes for the first hour. Premedicate as described.
- Bone Marrow Depression: Neutropenia, thrombocytopenia, and anemia are cumulative and dose related. Can be dose limiting. G-CSF support recommended.
- Gastrointestinal Toxicities: Moderate to severe nausea and vomiting may be acute or delayed. Mucositis and/or diarrhea are seen in 30%–40% of patients. Metallic taste to food and loss of appetite.
- Renal: Nephrotoxicity is dose related and with cisplatin presents at 10–20 days.
- Electrolyte Imbalance: Decreases Mg^{2+}, K^+, Ca^{2+}, Na^+, and P.
- Neurotoxicity: Dose limiting peripheral sensory neuropathy. Paresthesias and numbness in classic "stocking glove" pattern. Risk increases with cumulative doses. Loss of motor function, facial encephalopathy and seizures observed. Neurologic effects may be irreversible.
- Alopecia: A total loss of body hair occurs in nearly all patients.
- Reproduction: Pregnancy category D. Breast feeding should be avoided.

Initiate antiemetic protocol: Moderate to highly emetogenic protocol

Supportive drugs:

☐ pegfilgrastim (Neulasta)   ☐ filgrastim (Neupogen)

☐ epoetin alfa (Procrit)   ☐ darbepoetin alfa (Aranesp)

Treatment schedule: Chair time 4 hours on days 1 and 2. Repeat every 21 days until progression.

Estimated number of visits: Three visits per cycle. Request three cycles worth of visits.

Dose Calculation by: 1. _____   2. _____

_____

Physician

_____

Date

_____

Patient Name

_____

ID Number

_____

Diagnosis

_____/_____/_____

Ht   Wt   M^2

5-FU and Cisplatin (PF)

Baseline laboratory tests: CBC: Chemistry (including Mg^{2+}) and CEA

Baseline procedures or tests: Central line placement

Initiate IV: 0.9% sodium chloride

Premedicate: 5-HT_3 and dexamethasone 10–20 mg in 100 cc of NS

Administer: **Cisplatin** _____ mg (100 mg/m^2) IV on day 1

- Available in 100-mL vials. 1-mg/1-mL concentrations.
- Do not use aluminum needles, as precipitate will form.
- Further dilute solution with 250 cc or more NS.
- 100-mL vial stable for 28 days protected from light, 7 days under florescent light.

Fluorouracil _____ mg (1000 mg/m^2/day) IV continuous infusion on days 1–5.

- Available as 500 mg/10-mL.
- No dilution required. Can be further diluted with 0.9% sodium chloride or D5W.

Major Side Effects
- Hypersensitivity Reactions: Facial edema, wheezing, bronchospasm and hypotension. May occur with in minutes of administration of cisplatin.
- Bone Marrow Depression: Neutropenia, thrombocytopenia, and anemia are dose related. Can be dose limiting for 5-Fluorouracil daily × 5 or weekly regimens.
- Gastrointestinal Toxicities: Moderate to sever nausea and vomiting may be acute or delayed. Mucositis and diarrhea can be severe and dose limiting. Metallic taste of foods and loss of appetite.
- Renal: Nephrotoxicity is dose related and with cisplatin presents at 10–20 days.
- Electrolyte Imbalance: Decreases magnesium, potassium, calcium, sodium, and phosphorus.
- Neurotoxicity: Dose limiting peripheral sensory neuropathy. Paresthesias and numbness in classic "stocking glove" pattern. Risk increases with cumulative doses. Loss of motor function, facial encephalopathy and seizures observed. Neurologic effects may be irreversible.
- Skin: Hyperpigmentation, photosensitivity, and nail changes may occur. Hand-foot syndrome (palmar-plantar erythrodysesthesia) characterized by tingling, numbness, pain, erythema, dryness, rash, swelling, increased pigmentation, and/or pruritus of the hands and feet. Less frequent in reduced doses, can be dose limiting.
- Ocular: Photophobia, increased lacrimation, conjunctivitis, and blurred vision.
- Reproduction: Pregnancy category D. Breast feeding should be avoided.
- Azoospermia, impotence, and sterility.

Initiate antiemetic protocol: Moderately to highly emetogenic protocol.

Supportive drugs:
☐ pegfilgrastim (Neulasta) ☐ filgrastim (Neupogen)
☐ epoetin alfa (Procrit) ☐ darbepoetin alfa (Aranesp)

Treatment schedule: Chair time 3 hours on day 1. Repeat the cycle every 21 to 28 days.

Estimated number of visits: Three visits per cycle. Request three cycles worth of visits. May require extra visits for hydration; discontinuation of infusion pump and nadir.

Dose Calculation by: 1. _____ 2. _____

_____
Physician

_____
Date

_____
Patient Name

_____
ID Number

_____
Diagnosis

_____ / _____ / _____
Ht   Wt   M^2

Cisplatin + Fluorouracil + Leucovorin (PFL)

Baseline laboratory tests: CBC: Chemistry (including Mg^{2+}) and CEA

Baseline procedures or tests: Central line placement

Initiate IV: 0.9% sodium chloride

Premedicate: 5-HT_3 and dexamethasone 10–20 mg in 100 cc of NS

Administer:

Cisplatin _____ mg (100 mg/m^2) IV on day 1
- Available in 100-mL vials. 1-mg/1-mL concentrations.
- Do not use aluminum needles, as precipitate will form.
- Further dilute solution with 250 cc or more NS.
- 100-mL vial stable for 28 days protected from light, 7 days under florescent light.

Fluorouracil _____ mg (800 mg/m^2/day) IV continuous infusion days 1–5
- Available as 500 mg/10 mL.
- No dilution required. Can be further diluted with 0.9% sodium chloride or D5W.

Leucovorin _____ mg (50 mg/m^2) PO every 6 hours on days 1–5
- Available as 5- and 15-mg scored tablets for oral use. Protect from light and moisture.

Major Side Effects
- Hypersensitivity Reactions: Facial edema, wheezing, bronchospasm and hypotension. May occur within minutes of administration.
- Bone Marrow Depression: Neutropenia, thrombocytopenia, and anemia are dose related. Can be dose limiting for daily × 5 or weekly regimens.
- Gastrointestinal Toxicities: Moderate to severe nausea and vomiting may be acute or delayed. Mucositis and diarrhea can be severe and dose limiting.
- Renal: Nephrotoxicity is dose related and with cisplatin presents at 10–20 days.
- Electrolyte Imbalance: Decreases Mg^{2+}, K^+, Ca^{2+}, Na^+, and P.
- Neurotoxicity: Dose limiting peripheral sensory neuropathy. Paresthesias and numbness in classic "stocking glove" pattern. Risk increases with cumulative doses. Loss of motor function, facial encephalopathy and seizures observed. Neurologic effects may be irreversible.
- Skin: Hyperpigmentation, photosensitivity, and nail changes may occur. Hand-foot syndrome (palmar-plantar erythrodysesthesia) characterized by tingling, numbness, pain, erythema, dryness, rash, swelling, increased pigmentation, and/or pruritus of the hands and feet. Less frequent in reduced doses, can be dose limiting.
- Ocular: Photophobia, increased lacrimation, conjunctivitis, and blurred vision.
- Reproduction: Pregnancy category D. Breast feeding should be avoided.
- Azoospermia, impotence, and sterility.

Initiate antiemetic protocol: Moderately to highly emetogenic protocol.

Supportive drugs:
- ☐ pegfilgrastim (Neulasta)
- ☐ filgrastim (Neupogen)
- ☐ epoetin alfa (Procrit)
- ☐ darbepoetin alfa (Aranesp)

Treatment schedule: Chair time 3 hours on day 1. Repeat cycle every 21 days.

Estimated number of visits: Three visits per cycle. Request three cycles worth of visits. May require extra visits for hydration; discontinuation of pump and nadir.

Dose Calculation by: 1. _____ 2. _____

_____

Physician

_____

Patient Name

_____

Diagnosis

_____

Date

_____

ID Number

_____ / _____ / _____

Ht   Wt   M^2

Cisplatin + Fluorouracil + Radiation Therapy (PF-Larynx Preservation)

Baseline laboratory tests:	CBC: Chemistry (including Mg^{2+}) and CEA
Baseline procedures or tests:	Central line placement
Initiate IV:	0.9% sodium chloride
Premedicate:	5-HT$_3$ and dexamethasone 10–20 mg in 100 cc NS
Administer:	

Cisplatin _____ mg (100 mg/m²/day) IV day 1

- Available in 100-mL vials. 1-mg/1-mL concentrations.
- Do not use aluminum needles, as precipitate will form.
- Further dilute solution with 250 cc or more NS.
- 100-mL vial stable for 28 days protected from light, 7 days under florescent light.

Fluorouracil _____ mg (1000 mg/m²/day) IV continuous infusion on days 1–5

- Available as 500 mg/10 mL.
- No dilution required. Can be further diluted with 0.9% sodium chloride or D5W.

Radiation therapy: 6600–7600 cGy in 180- to 200-cGy fractions

Major Side Effects

- Hypersensitivity Reactions: Facial edema, wheezing, bronchospasm and hypotension. May occur within minutes of administration.
- Bone Marrow Depression: Neutropenia, thrombocytopenia, and anemia are cumulative and dose related. Can be dose limiting.
- Gastrointestinal Toxicities: Nausea and vomiting moderate to severe, may be acute or delayed. Mucositis and diarrhea can be severe and dose limiting.
- Renal: Nephrotoxicity is dose related and with cisplatin presents at 10–20 days.
- Neurotoxicity: Dose limiting peripheral sensory neuropathy. Paresthesias and numbness in classic "stocking glove" pattern. Risk increases with cumulative doses. Loss of motor function, facial encephalopathy and seizures observed. Neurologic effects may be irreversible.
- Electrolyte Imbalance: Decreases Mg^{2+}, K^+, Ca^{2+}, Na^+, and P.
- Skin: Local tissue irritation progressing to desquamation can occur. Do not use oil-based lotions or creams in radiation field. Hyperpigmentation, photosensitivity, and nail changes may occur. Hand-foot syndrome (palmar-plantar erythrodysesthesia) characterized by tingling, numbness, pain, erythema, dryness, rash, swelling, increased pigmentation, and/or pruritus of the hands and feet. Less frequent in reduced doses, can be dose limiting.
- Ocular: Photophobia, increased lacrimation, conjunctivitis, and blurred vision.
- Reproduction: Pregnancy category D. Breast feeding should be avoided.

Initiate antiemetic protocol:	Moderately to highly emetogenic protocol.
Supportive drugs:	☐ pegfilgrastim (Neulasta) ☐ filgrastim (Neupogen)
	☐ epoetin alfa (Procrit) ☐ darbepoetin alfa (Aranesp)
Treatment schedule:	Chair time 3 hours on day 1. Repeat the cycle every 21–28 days for three cycles.
Estimated number of visits:	Three visits per cycle, three visits for course. May require extra visits for hydration; discontinuation of infusion pump and nadir.

Dose Calculation by: 1. _____ 2. _____

Physician _____ Date _____

Patient Name _____ ID Number _____

Diagnosis _____ Ht _____ / Wt _____ / M²

Concurrent Chemo-Radiation Therapy for Laryngeal Preservation

Baseline laboratory tests:	CBC: Chemistry (including Mg^{2+})
Baseline procedures or tests:	Central line placement
Initiate IV:	0.9% sodium chloride
Premedicate:	5-HT$_3$ and dexamethasone 10–20 mg in 100 cc of NS
Administer:	Chemoradiotherapy:

Cisplatin _____mg (100 mg/m^2) IV on days 1, 22, and 43 during radiotherapy

- Available in 100-mL vials. 1-mg/1-mL concentrations.
- Do not use aluminum needles, as precipitate will form.
- Further dilute solution with 250 cc or more NS.
- 100-mL vial stable for 28 days protected from light, 7 days under florescent light.

Radiation therapy: Total dose of 7000 cGy in 200-cGy fractions

Administer cisplatin concurrently with radiation therapy

Major Side Effects

- Bone Marrow Depression: Neutropenia, thrombocytopenia, and anemia are cumulative and dose related. Can be dose limiting.
- Gastrointestinal Toxicities: Nausea and vomiting can be acute or delayed and are moderate to severe. Mucositis and diarrhea can be severe and dose limiting.
- Renal: Nephrotoxicity is dose related and with cisplatin presents at 10–20 days.
- Electrolyte Imbalance: Decreases in magnesium, potassium, calcium, sodium, and phosphorus are seen.
- Skin: Local tissue irritation progressing to desquamation can occur. Do not use oil-based lotions or creams in radiation field.
- Reproduction: Pregnancy category D. Breast feeding should be avoided.
- Azoospermia, impotence, and sterility.

Initiate antiemetic protocol:	Moderately to highly emetogenic protocol.
Supportive drugs:	☐ pegfilgrastim (Neulasta) ☐ filgrastim (Neupogen)
	☐ epoetin alfa (Procrit) ☐ darbepoetin alfa (Aranesp)
Treatment schedule:	Chair time 3 hours on days 1, 22, and 43 of radiotherapy.
Estimated number of visits:	Six to twelve visits per treatment course. May need additional visits for hydration; discontinuation of infusion pump and nadir.

Dose Calculation by: 1. _____   2. _____

_____

Physician

_____

Date

_____

Patient Name

_____

ID Number

_____

Diagnosis

_____/_____/_____

Ht   Wt   M^2

Chemoradiotherapy for Nasopharyngeal Cancer

Baseline laboratory tests:	CBC: Chemistry (including Mg^{2+})
Baseline procedures or tests:	Central line placement
Initiate IV:	0.9% sodium chloride
Premedicate:	5-HT$_3$ and dexamethasone 10–20 mg in 100 cc of NS
Administer:	**Chemoradiotherapy:**

Cisplatin _____ mg (100 mg/m^2) IV on days 1, 22, and 43 during radiotherapy

- Available in 100-mL vials. 1-mg/1-mL concentrations.
- Do not use aluminum needles, as precipitate will form.
- Further dilute solution with 250 cc or more NS.
- 100-mL vial stable for 28 days protected from light, 7 days under florescent light.

Radiation therapy: Total dose of 7000 cGy in 180- to 200-cGy fractions

At the completion of chemoradiotherapy, chemotherapy is administered as follows:

Chemotherapy: (three 28-day cycles)

Cisplatin _____ mg (80 mg/m^2) IV on day 1

Fluorouracil _____ mg (1000 mg/m^2/day) IV continuous infusion on days 1–4

- Available as 500 mg/10 mL.
- No dilution required. May further dilute in NS or D5W.

Major Side Effects

- Bone Marrow Depression: Neutropenia, thrombocytopenia, and anemia are cumulative and dose related. Can be dose limiting.
- Gastrointestinal Toxicities: Nausea and vomiting can be acute or delayed and are moderate to severe. Mucositis and diarrhea can be severe and dose limiting. Metallic taste to food and loss of appetite.
- Renal: Nephrotoxicity is dose related and with cisplatin presents at 10–20 days.
- Electrolyte Imbalance: Decreases in Mg^{2+}, K^+, Ca^{2+}, Na^+, and P.
- Skin: Local tissue irritation progressing to desquamation can occur. Do not use oil-based lotions or creams in radiation field.
- Skin Alterations: Hyperpigmentation, photosensitivity, and nail changes may occur. Hand-foot syndrome (palmar-plantar erythrodysesthesia) characterized by tingling, numbness, pain, erythema, dryness, rash, swelling, increased pigmentation, and/or pruritus of the hands and feet. Less frequent in reduced doses.
- Reproduction: Pregnancy category D. Breast feeding should be avoided.

Initiate antiemetic protocol:	Moderately to highly emetogenic protocol
Supportive drugs:	☐ pegfilgrastim (Neulasta) ☐ filgrastim (Neupogen)
	☐ epoetin alfa (Procrit) ☐ darbepoetin alfa (Aranesp)
Treatment schedule:	Chair time 3 hours on days 1, 22, and 43 of radiotherapy. Three hours on day 1 of chemotherapy.
Estimated number of visits:	Six to twelve visits per treatment course. May need additional visits for hydration; discontinuation of infusion pump and nadir.

Dose Calculation by: 1. _____ 2. _____

_____
Physician

_____
Date

_____
Patient Name

_____
ID Number

_____ / _____ / _____
Ht   Wt   M^2

_____
Diagnosis

Carboplatin and Fluorouracil (Head and Neck CA)

Baseline laboratory tests:	CBC: Chemistry (including Mg^{2+})
Baseline procedures or tests:	N/A
Initiate IV:	0.9% sodium chloride
Premedicate:	5-HT$_3$ and dexamethasone 10–20 mg in 100 cc of NS
Administer:	**Carboplatin** _____ mg (300–400 mg/m^2) IV on day 1

- Available in 50-, 150-, and 450-mg lyophilized powder; dilute with sterile water. Also available in 50 mg and 150 mg, 10 mg/mL solution; 450 mg and 600 mg 10 mg/mL multidose vials stable for 15 days after first use.
- Do not use aluminum needles, as precipitate will form.
- Further dilute in 250–1000 cc 0.9% sodium chloride.
- Chemically stable for 24 hours, discard after 8 hours because of lack of bacteriostatic preservative.

Fluorouracil _____ mg (600 mg/m^2/day) IV on day 1

- Available as 500 mg/10 mL.
- No dilution required. Can be further diluted with 0.9% sodium chloride or D5W.

Major Side Effects

- Hypersensitivity Reactions: Facial edema, wheezing, bronchospasm and hypotension. May occur within minutes of administration.
- Bone Marrow Depression: Neutropenia and thrombocytopenia are dose related and can be dose limiting. Anemia may occur with prolonged treatment.
- Gastrointestinal Toxicities: Moderate to severe nausea and vomiting may be acute or delayed. Mucositis and diarrhea can be severe and dose limiting.
- Renal: Nephrotoxicity is less common than with cisplatin and is rarely symptomatic.
- Electrolyte Imbalance: Decreases Mg^{2+}, K^+, Ca^{2+}, and Na^+.
- Skin: Hyperpigmentation, photosensitivity, and nail changes may occur. Hand-foot syndrome (palmar-plantar erythrodysesthesia) characterized by tingling, numbness, pain, erythema, dryness, rash, swelling, increased pigmentation, and/or pruritus of the hands and feet. Less frequent in reduced doses, can be dose limiting.
- Ocular: Photophobia, increased lacrimation, conjunctivitis, and blurred vision.
- Reproduction: Pregnancy category D. Breast feeding should be avoided.

Initiate antiemetic protocol:	Moderately to highly emetogenic protocol.
Supportive drugs:	☐ pegfilgrastim (Neulasta) ☐ filgrastim (Neupogen)
	☐ epoetin alfa (Procrit) ☐ darbepoetin alfa (Aranesp)
Treatment schedule:	Chair time 2 hours on day 1. Repeat the cycle every 21 days.
Estimated number of visits:	Two visits per course. Request three courses worth of visits.

Dose Calculation by: 1. _____   2. _____

_____   _____
Physician   Date

_____   _____
Patient Name   ID Number

_____   _____/_____/_____
Diagnosis   Ht   Wt   M^2

Vinorelbine and Cisplatin (VP)

Baseline laboratory tests:	CBC: Chemistry (including Mg^{2+})
Baseline procedures or tests:	Central line placement
Initiate IV:	0.9% sodium chloride
Premedicate:	5-HT$_3$ and dexamethasone 10–20 mg in 100 cc of NS
Administer:	**Vinorelbine** _____mg (25 mg/m^2) IV days 1 and 8

- **Vesicant**
- Available in 1- or 5-mL single-use vials at a concentration of 10 mg/mL.
- Further dilute in syringe or IV bag to concentration of 1.5–3.0 mg/mL. Infuse diluted drug IV over 6–10 minutes into sidearm port of freely flowing IV infusion, either peripherally or via central line. Use port CLOSEST to the IV bag, not to the patient, as vinorelbine causes venous irritation when infused. Central line for venous access is recommended.
- Flush with at least 75–125 mL of IV fluid after administration.
- Reconstituted solution is stable for 24 hours refrigerated.

Cisplatin _____mg (80 mg/m^2) IV day 1

- Available in 100-mL vials. 1-mg/1-mL concentrations.
- Do not use aluminum needles, as precipitate will form.
- Further dilute solution with 250 cc or more NS.
- 100-mL vial stable for 28 days protected from light, 7 days under florescent light.

Major Side Effects	- Bone Marrow Depression: Neutropenia, thrombocytopenia, and anemia are dose related and can be dose limiting.

- Gastrointestinal Toxicities: Moderate to severe nausea and vomiting may be acute or delayed. Constipation, diarrhea, stomatitis, and anorexia may be seen.
- Renal: Nephrotoxicity is dose related and with cisplatin presents at 10–20 days.
- Electrolyte Imbalance: Decreases Mg^{2+}, K^+, Ca^{2+}, Na^+, and P.
- Skin: Extravasation of vinorelbine may cause local tissue injury and inflammation. Alopecia likely.
- Neurotoxicity: Dose-limiting toxicity, usually in the form of peripheral sensory neuropathy. Paresthesias and numbness in a classic "stocking-glove" pattern, with numbness, tinglings, and sensory loss in arms and legs.
- Ototoxicity: High-frequency hearing loss and tinnitus.
- Reproduction: Pregnancy category D. Breast feeding should be avoided.
- Azoospermia, impotence, and sterility.

Initiate antiemetic protocol:	Moderately to highly emetogenic protocol.
Supportive drugs:	☐ pegfilgrastim (Neulasta) ☐ filgrastim (Neupogen)
	☐ epoetin alfa (Procrit) ☐ darbepoetin alfa (Aranesp)
Treatment schedule:	Chair time 3 hours on day 1 and 1 hour on day 8. Repeat the cycle every 21 days.
Estimated number of visits:	Three visits per cycle. Request three cycles worth of visits.

Dose Calculation by: 1. _____   2. _____

_____   _____

Physician   Date

_____   _____

Patient Name   ID Number

_____   _____/_____/_____

Diagnosis   Ht   Wt   M^2

Single-Agent Regimens

Docetaxel

Baseline laboratory tests:	CBC: Chemistry (including Mg^{2+}) and CEA
Baseline procedures or tests:	Central line placement
Initiate IV:	0.9% sodium chloride
Premedicate:	Dexamethasone 8-mg bid for 3 days, starting the day before treatment
	Oral phenothiazine or 5-HT$_3$ and dexamethasone 10–20 mg in 100 cc of NS
Administer:	**Docetaxe**l _____mg (100 mg/m^2) IV on day 1

- Comes in 20- or 80-mg blister packs with own diluent. Do not shake. Reconstituted vials stable at room temperature or refrigerated for 8 hours.
- Further dilute in 250-cc D5W or 0.9% NS.
- Use non-PVC containers and tubing to administer.

Major Side Effects

- Hypersensitivity Reaction: Anaphylaxis and severe hypersensitivity reactions seen less frequently than with paclitaxel. Characterized by dyspnea, hypotension, andioedema, and generalized urticaria. May also see tachycardia, wheezing, and facial edema. Patients with mild reactions can be rechallenged after 24 hour corticosteroid prophylaxis. Monitor vitals signs every 15 minutes for the first hour. Patients with severe reactions should not be rechallenged. Premedicate as described.
- Bone Marrow Depression: Neutropenia is dose limiting with nadir at days 7–10 and recovery by day 14. Thrombocytopenia and anemia are also seen.
- Gastrointestinal Toxicities: Nausea and vomiting are mild to moderate. Mucositis and diarrhea are seen in 40% of the patients.
- Neuropathy: Peripheral neuropathy may affect up to 49% of the patients. Sensory alterations are paresthesias in a glove-and-stocking distribution and numbness.
- Fluid Balance: Fluid retention syndrome. Symptoms include weight gain, peripheral and/or generalized edema, pleural effusion, and ascites. This is seen in about 50% of patients. Premedication with dexamethasone is effective in preventing or minimizing occurrences.
- Skin: Alopecia occurs in 56%–75% of patients. Maculopapular, violaceous/erythematous, and purtitic rash may occur, usually on the feet and/or hands but can be on arms, face, or thorax. Usually resolve prior to next treatment. Nail changes may occur in 11%–40% of patients and may include onycholysis (loss of nail). Hand-foot syndrome has also been reported.
- Reproduction: Pregnancy category D. Breast feeding should be avoided.

Initiate antiemetic protocol:	Mildly to moderately emetogenic protocol
Supportive drugs:	☐ pegfilgrastim (Neulasta) ☐ filgrastim (Neupogen)
	☐ epoetin alfa (Procrit) ☐ darbepoetin alfa (Aranesp)
Treatment schedule:	Chair time 2 hours on day 1. Repeat the cycle every 21 days.
Estimated number of visits:	Two visits per cycle. Request three cycles worth of visits.

Dose Calculation by: 1. _____   2. _____

_____   _____
Physician   Date

_____   _____
Patient Name   ID Number

_____   _____/ _____/ _____
Diagnosis   Ht   Wt   M^2

Paclitaxel

Baseline laboratory tests:	CBC: Chemistry
Baseline procedures or tests:	N/A
Initiate IV:	0.9% sodium chloride
Premedicate:	5-HT$_3$ and dexamethasone 10–20 mg in 100 cc of NS
	Diphenhydramine 25–50 mg and cimetidine 300 mg in 100 cc of NS

Administer:

Paclitaxel _____ mg (250 mg/m^2) IV over 24 hours on day 1

OR

Paclitaxel _____ mg (137–175 mg/m^2) IV over 3 hours on day 1

- Available in 30-mg (6 mg/mL), 100-mg (16.7 mg/mL), and 300-mg (6-mg/mL) vials.
- Further dilute in NS or D5W to a final concentration of ≤1.2 mg/mL.
- Diluted solution stable for 27 hours at room temperature.
- **Use non-PVC tubing and containers and a 0.22-micron inline filter for administration.**

Major Side Effects

- Hypersensitivity Reaction: With anaphylaxis and severe hypersensitivity reactions in 2%–4%. Characterized by dyspnea, hypotension, andioedema, and generalized urticaria. May also see tachycardia, wheezing, and facial edema. Usually happens within first 2–3 minutes of infusion. Patients with mild reactions can be rechallenged after 24 hour corticosteroid prophylaxis. Patients with severe reactions should not be rechallenged. Premedicate as described. Monitor vital signs every 15 minutes for first hour of infusion.
- Bone Marrow Depression: Dose-limiting neutropenia with nadir at days 8–10 and recovery by days 15–21. Decreased the incidence of neutropenia with a 3-hour schedule when compared with a 24-hour schedule. G-CSF support is recommended.
- Gastrointestinal Toxicity: Mild to moderate nausea and vomiting, usually brief in duration. Mucositis and/or diarrhea seen in 30%–40% of patients. Mucositis is more common with the 24-hour schedule.
- Neurotoxicity: Dose limiting peripheral sensory neuropathy. Paresthesias and numbness in classic "stocking glove" pattern. Risk increases with cumulative doses. Loss of motor function, facial encephalopathy and seizures observed. Neurologic effects may be irreversible.
- Alopecia: A total loss of body hair occurs in nearly all patients.
- Reproduction: Pregnancy category D. Breast feeding should be avoided.

Initiate antiemetic protocol:	Mildly to moderately emetogenic protocol.

Supportive drugs:

- ☐ pegfilgrastim (Neulasta)
- ☐ epoetin alfa (Procrit)
- ☐ filgrastim (Neupogen)
- ☐ darbepoetin alfa (Aranesp)

Treatment schedule:	Chair time 2 hours or 4 hours. Repeat every 21 days as tolerated.
Estimated number of visits:	Two visits per cycle. Request three cycles worth of visits.

Dose Calculation by: 1. _____   2. _____

_____
Physician

_____
Date

_____
Patient Name

_____
ID Number

_____
Diagnosis

_____ / _____ / _____
Ht   Wt   M^2

Methotrexate

Baseline laboratory tests: CBC: Chemistry

Baseline procedures or tests: N/A

Initiate IV: 0.9% sodium chloride

Premedicate: Oral phenothiazine or 5-HT$_3$

Administer: **Methotrexate** _____mg (40 mg/m^2) IV or IM weekly.

- Available in 50-, 100-, 200-, and 1000-mg single-use reconstituted vials.
- May dilute further in 0.9% sodium chloride.
- Reconstituted solution is stable for 24 hours at room temperature.

Major Side Effects

- Bone Marrow Depression: Dose-limiting toxicity, leukocyte nadir at 4–7 days, and recovery by day 14.
- Gastrointestinal Toxicities: Nausea and vomiting are mild. Mucositis can be dose limiting, typical onset 3–7 days after treatment.
- Renal: Acute renal failure, azotemia, urinary retention, and uric acid nephropathy have been observed. Methotrexate is insoluble in acid urine and may precipitate in renal tubules at higher doses.
- Pulmonary: Poorly defined pneumonitis characterized by fever, cough, and interstitial pulmonary infiltrates.
- Skin: Alopecia and dermatitis are uncommon. Pruritus, urticaria may occur. Photosensitivity, sunburn-like rash (1–5 days after treatment), and radiation recall seen.
- Reproduction: Menstrual irregularities, abortion, and fetal deaths reported.

Initiate antiemetic protocol: Moderately to highly emetogenic protocol.

Supportive drugs: ☐ pegfilgrastim (Neulasta)   ☐ filgrastim (Neupogen)
☐ epoetin alfa (Procrit)   ☐ darbepoetin alfa (Aranesp)

Treatment schedule: Chair time 1 hour weekly if given IV. If IM schedule injection only or teach patient self injection. Repeat the cycle every week.

Estimated number of visits: One visit per week. Request 12 weeks worth of visits.

Dose Calculation by: 1. _____   2. _____

Physician _____   Date _____

Patient Name _____   ID Number _____

Diagnosis _____   Ht _____/ Wt _____/ M^2 _____

Vinorelbine

Baseline laboratory tests:	CBC: Chemistry
Baseline procedures or tests:	Central line placement
Initiate IV:	0.9% sodium chloride
Premedicate:	5-HT$_3$
Administer:	**Vinorelbine** _____ mg (30 mg/m^2) IV weekly

- **Vesicant**
- Available in 1- or 5-mL single-use vials at a concentration of 10 mg/mL.
- Further dilute in syringe or IV bag to concentration of 1.5–3.0 mg/mL. Infuse diluted drug IV over 6–10 minutes into sidearm port of freely flowing IV infusion, either peripherally or via central line. Use port CLOSEST to the IV bag, not to the patient, as vinorelbine causes venous irritation when infused.
- Flush with at least 75–125 mL of IV fluid after administration.
- Reconstituted solution is stable for 24 hours refrigerated.

Major Side Effects

- Bone Marrow Depression: Leukopenia is a dose-limiting toxicity. Nadir at 7–10 days. Severe thrombocytopenia and anemia are uncommon.
- Gastrointestinal Toxicities: Nausea and vomiting are moderate with an incidence of 44%. Mild to moderate stomatitis has a < 20% incidence. Constipation (35%), diarrhea (17%), and anorexia (< 20%) are also seen.
- Hormonal: Syndrome of inappropriate secretion of antidiuretic hormone.
- Skin: Extravasation of vinorelbine may cause local tissue injury and inflammation. Alopecia observed in 10%–15% of patients.
- Neurotoxicity: Usually mild in severity and occurs much less frequently than with other vinca alkaloids.
- Reproduction: Pregnancy category D. Breast feeding should be avoided.

Initiate antiemetic protocol:	Moderately emetogenic protocol.
Supportive drugs:	☐ pegfilgrastim (Neulasta) ☐ filgrastim (Neupogen)
	☐ epoetin alfa (Procrit) ☐ darbepoetin alfa (Aranesp)
Treatment schedule:	Chair time 1 hour weekly. Repeat the cycle every week.
Estimated number of visits:	One visit per cycle. Request 12 cycles worth of visits.

Dose Calculation by: 1. _____   2. _____

_____
Physician

_____
Patient Name

_____
Diagnosis

_____
Date

_____
ID Number

_____ / _____ / _____
Ht   Wt   M^2

Capecitabine (Xeloda)

Baseline laboratory tests:	CBC: Chemistry, bilirubin, and LFTs
Baseline procedures or tests:	N/A
Initiate IV:	N/A
Premedicate:	Oral phenothiazine or 5-HT$_3$
Administer:	**Capecitabine** _____ mg (1000 mg/m^2/day) PO bid on days 1–14

- Available in 150- and 500-mg tablets. Do not break tablets in half. Do not give Maalox 30 minutes before or 2 hour after administration. Administer within 30 minutes after a meal with plenty of water.
- Monitor INRs closely in patients on warfarin, may increase INR.
- Dose may be reduced to 825–900 mg/m^2 PO bid on days 1–14 to decrease the risk of toxicity without compromising clinical efficacy.
- Patient should be instructed to stop Xeloda at the first sign of hand-and-foot syndrome, or with stomatitis, or diarrhea uncontrolled by antidiarrheal protocol.

Major Side Effects

- Gastrointestinal Toxicities: Nausea and vomiting occur in 15%–53% of patients and are usually mild to moderate. Diarrhea is seen in up to 40% with 15% being grades 3–4. Stomatitis is common, 3% of which is severe.
- Skin: Hand-foot syndrome (palmar-plantar erythrodysesthesia) is seen in 15%–20% of patients. Characterized by tingling, numbness, pain, erythema, dryness, rash, swelling, increased pigmentation, and/or pruritus of the hands and feet. This is less frequent in reduced doses.
- Ocular: Blepharitis, tear-duct stenosis, and acute and chronic conjunctivitis.
- Hepatic: Elevations in serum bilirubin (20%–40%), alkaline phosphatase, and hepatic transaminases. Dose modifications may be required if hyperbilirubinemia occurs or if patient has hepatic metastasis, which may require a 25% dose reduction.
- Renal Insufficiency: Capecitabine is contraindicated in patients with baseline creatinine clearance < 30 mL/min. A dose reduction to 75% of capecitabine should be made with baseline creatinine clearance of 30–50 mL/min.
- Reproduction: Pregnancy category D. Breast feeding should be avoided.

Initiate antiemetic protocol:	Mildly to moderately emetogenic protocol.
Supportive drugs:	☐ pegfilgrastim (Neulasta) ☐ filgrastim (Neupogen)
	☐ epoetin alfa (Procrit) ☐ darbepoetin alfa (Aranesp)
	☐ diphenoxylate/ ☐ loperamide (Imodium) atropine sulfate (Lomotil)
Treatment schedule:	14 days on 7 days off per cycle. Repeat as tolerated until progression.
Estimated number of visits:	One visit per cycle. Repeat cycle every 3 weeks.

Dose Calculation by: 1. _____ 2. _____

_____
Physician

_____
Date

_____
Patient Name

_____
ID Number

_____
Diagnosis

_____/_____/_____
Ht   Wt   M^2

HEPATOCELLULAR CANCER

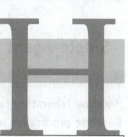

Single Agent Regimens

Doxorubicin: 20–30 mg/m^2 IV weekly
Repeat cycle every week.[1,192]

Cisplatin: 80 mg/m^2 IV on day 1
Repeat cycle every 28 days.[1,193]

Capecitabine: 1000 mg/m^2 PO bid on days 1–14
Repeat cycle every 21 days.[1,194]

Dose may be reduced to 825–900 mg/m^2. PO bid on days 1–14. This dose reduction may decrease the risk of toxicity without compromising clinical efficacy.

Single-Agent Regimens

Doxorubicin

Baseline laboratory tests:	CBC: Chemistry
Baseline procedures or tests:	Multigated angiogram (MUGA) scan/consider central line placement
Initiate IV:	0.9% sodium chloride
Premedicate:	5-HT$_3$ and dexamethasone 10–20 mg in 100 cc of NS
Administer:	**Doxorubicin** _____mg (20–30 mg/m^2) IV weekly

- **Potent vesicant**
- Available as a 2-mg/mL solution.
- Doxorubicin will form a precipitate if mixed with heparin or 5-FU.
- Should be given IV push through the side port of a free-flowing IV.

Major Side Effects

- Bone Marrow Depression: White blood cell (WBC) and platelet nadir 10–14 days after drug dose, with recovery from days 15–21. Myelosuppression may be severe but is less severe with weekly dosing.
- Gastrointestinal Toxicities: Nausea and vomiting are moderate to severe and occur in 44% of the patients. Stomatitis occurs in 10% of the patients but is not dose limiting.
- GU: Red-orange discoloration of urine for up to 48 hours.
- Cardiac: Acutely, pericarditis-myocarditis syndrome may occur. With high cumulative doses of > 550 mg/m^2, cardiomyopathy may occur. There is an increased risk of cardiotoxicity when doxorubicin is given with Herceptin or mitomycin C.
- Skin: Extravasation of doxorubicin causes severe tissue destruction. Hyperpigmentation, photosensitivity, and radiation recall occur. Complete alopecia occurs with doses of more than 50 mg/m^2.
- Reproduction: Doxorubicin is teratogenic, mutagenic, and carcinogenic.

Initiate antiemetic protocol:	Moderately to highly emetogenic protocol.
Supportive drugs:	☐ pegfilgrastim (Neulasta) ☐ filgrastim (Neupogen)
	☐ epoetin alfa (Procrit) ☐ darbepoetin alfa (Aranesp)
Treatment schedule:	Chair time 1 hour on day 1. Repeat the cycle every 7 days until progression.
Estimated number of visits:	One visit per week. Request eight weeks worth of visits.

Dose Calculation by: 1. _____   2. _____

_____
Physician

_____
Date

_____
Patient Name

_____
ID Number

_____
Diagnosis

_____ / _____ / _____
Ht   Wt   M^2

Cisplatin

Baseline laboratory tests:	CBC: Chemistry (including Mg^{2+}) and CEA
Baseline procedures or tests:	N/A
Initiate IV:	0.9% sodium chloride
Premedicate:	5-HT$_3$ and dexamethasone 10–20 mg in 100 cc of NS
Administer:	**Cisplatin** _____ mg (80 per m^2) IV over 1–3 hours on day 1

- Available in 100-mL vials. 1-mg/1-mL concentrations.
- Do not use aluminum needles, as precipitate will form.
- Further dilute solution with 250 cc or more NS.
- 100-mL vial stable for 28 days protected from light, 7 days under florescent light.

Major Side Effects

- Bone Marrow Depression: Neutropenia, thrombocytopenia, and anemia occur equally in 25%–30% of patients. Leukopenia and thrombocytopenia are dose related.
- Gastrointestinal Toxicities: Moderate to severe nausea and vomiting. May be acute (first 24 hours) or delayed (> 24 hours). Metallic taste of foods and loss of appetite.
- Renal: Nephrotoxicity is dose related, with cisplatin presents at 10–20 days.
- Electrolyte Imbalance: Decreases magnesium, potassium, calcium, sodium, and phosphorus.
- Neurotoxicity: Dose limiting peripheral sensory neuropathy. Paresthesias and numbness in classic "stocking glove" pattern. Risk increases with cumulative doses. Loss of motor function, facial encephalopathy and seizures observed. Neurologic effects may be irreversible.
- Ototoxicity: High-frequency hearing loss and tinnitus.
- Skin: Alopecia.
- Reproduction: Cisplatin is mutagenic and probably teratogenic. Azoospermia, impotence, and sterility.

Initiate antiemetic protocol:	Moderately to highly emetogenic protocol.
Supportive drugs:	☐ pegfilgrastim (Neulasta) ☐ filgrastim (Neupogen)
	☐ epoetin alfa (Procrit) ☐ darbepoetin alfa (Aranesp)
Treatment schedule:	Chair time 3 hours on day 1. Repeat cycle every 28 days.
Estimated number of visits:	Two visits per cycle. Request six cycles worth of visits.

Dose Calculation by: 1. _____ 2. _____

_____

Physician

Date _____

_____

Patient Name

ID Number _____

_____

Diagnosis

_____ / _____ / _____

Ht   Wt M^2

Capecitabine (Xeloda)

Baseline laboratory tests:	CBC: Chemistry, bilirubin, LFTs, and CEA
Baseline procedures or tests:	N/A
Initiate IV:	N/A
Premedicate:	Oral phenothiazine or 5-HT$_3$
Administer:	**Capecitabine** _____mg (1000 mg/m^2/day) PO BID, days 1–14, followed by 7 days of rest.

- Administer within 30 minutes after a meal with plenty of water.
- Available in 150- and 500-mg tablets. Do not break tablets in half. Do not give Maalox 30 minutes before or 2 hours after administration.
- Monitor INRs closely in patients on warfarin, may increase INR.
- Patient should be instructed to stop Xeloda at the first sign of hand-and-foot syndrome, or with stomatitis, or diarrhea uncontrolled by antidiarrheal protocol.

Major Side Effects

- Gastrointestinal Toxicities: Nausea and vomiting, 30%–50% of patients, are usually mild to moderate. Diarrhea is seen in up to 40%, with 15% being grades 3–4. Stomatitis is common, 3% of which is severe.
- Skin: Hand-foot syndrome (palmar-plantar erythrodysesthesia) seen in 15%–20% of patients. Characterized by tingling, numbness, pain, erythema, dryness, rash, swelling, increased pigmentation, and/or pruritus of the hands and feet. Less frequent in reduced doses.
- Ocular: Blepharitis, tear-duct stenosis, and acute and chronic conjunctivitis.
- Hepatic: Elevations in serum bilirubin (20%–40%), alkaline phosphatase, and hepatic transaminases. Dose modifications may be required if hyperbilirubinemia occurs or if patient has hepatic metastasis, which may require a 25% dose reduction.
- Renal: Patients with mild to moderate renal impairment should start with a 25% dose reduction.
- Renal Insufficiency: Capecitabine is contraindicated in patients with baseline creatinine clearance < 30 mL/min. A dose reduction to 75% of capecitabine should be made with baseline creatinine clearance of 30–50 mL/min.
- Reproduction: Pregnancy category D. Breast feeding should be avoided.

Initiate antiemetic protocol:	Mildly to moderately emetogenic protocol.
Supportive drugs:	☐ pegfilgrastim (Neulasta) ☐ filgrastim (Neupogen)
	☐ epoetin alfa (Procrit) ☐ darbepoetin alfa (Aranesp)
	☐ diphenoxylate/ ☐ loperamide (Imodium)
	atropine sulfate (Lomotil)
Treatment schedule:	14 days on followed by 7 days off per cycle. Repeat cycle every 3 weeks as tolerated until progression.
Estimated number of visits:	One visit per cycle. Request three to six cycles of visits.

Dose Calculation by: 1. _____ 2. _____

_____

Physician   Date

_____

Patient Name   ID Number

_____

Diagnosis   Ht _____ / Wt _____ / M^2

KAPOSI'S SARCOMA

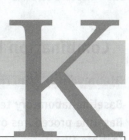

Combination Regimens

Bleomycin: 10 U/m^2 IV on days 1 and 15
Vincristine: 1.4 mg/m^2 IV on days 1 and 15 (maximum, 2 mg)
Repeat cycle every 2 weeks.[1,195]

Doxorubicin: 40 mg/m^2 IV on day 1
Bleomycin: 15 U/m^2 IV on days 1 and 15
Vinblastine: 6 mg/m^2 IV on day 1
Repeat cycle every 28 days.[1,196]

Single-Agent Regimens

DaunoXome: 40 mg/m^2 IV on day 1
Repeat cycle every 14 days.[1,197]

Doxil: 20 mg/m 2 IV on day 1
Repeat cycle every 21 days.[1,198]

Paclitaxel: 135 mg/m^2 IV over 3 hours on day 1
Repeat cycle every 21 days.[1,199]
OR
Paclitaxel: 100 mg/m^2 IV on day 1
Repeat cycle every 2 weeks.[1,200]

Interferon α-2a: 36 million IU/m^2 SC or IM, daily for 8–12 weeks[1,201]
Interferon α-2b: 30 million IU/m^2 SC or IM, 3 times weekly[1,202]

Combination Regimens

Bleomycin + Vincristine (BV)

Baseline laboratory tests:	CBC: Chemistry
Baseline procedures or tests:	Pulmonary function tests (PFTs) and chest x-ray (CXR)
Initiate IV:	0.9% sodium chloride
Premedicate:	Tylenol or Tylenol ES 2 tablets orally 30 minutes before treatment and every 6 hours after oral 5-HT$_3$ if prior nausea exhibited (phenothiazines enhance activity of bleomycin)

Administer:

Bleomycin _____ units (10 U/m^2) IV on days 1 and 15

- A test dose of 2 U is recommended before the first dose to detect hypersensitivity.
- Available as a powder in 15- or 30-unit sizes. Dilute powder in NS or sterile water 1–5 cc for the 15-unit vial and 2–10 cc for the 30-unit vial. Should NOT be diluted in D5W.
- Stable for 24 hours when diluted with NS.
- Given IV push or further diluted in NS and infused or pushed over at least 10 minutes.

Vincristine _____ mg (1.4 mg/m^2) IV on days 1 and 15.

Maximum dose of 2 mg.

- **Vesicant**
- Available in 1-, 2-, and 5-mg vials at a concentration of 1 mg/mL.
- Given IV push through side port of free-flowing IV of NS or D5W.

Major Side Effects

- Hypersensitivity Reaction: Fever and chills observed in up to 25% of patients. True anaphylactoid reactions are rare but more common in patients with lymphoma (1%).
- Pulmonary: Pulmonary toxicity is dose limiting in bleomycin.
- Bone Marrow Depression: Myelosuppression is mild.
- Gastrointestinal Toxicities: Nausea with or without vomiting may occur but is usually mild. Constipation, abdominal pain, and paralytic ileus are common. A prophylactic bowel regimen for constipation is recommended.
- Skin: Extravasation of vincristine may cause local tissue injury, inflammation, and necrosis. Phlebitis at the IV site may occur. Alopecia is common. Skin changes with or without rash and nail changes or loss have been seen.
- Neurotoxicity: Peripheral neuropathies occur as a result of toxicity to nerve fibers. Symptoms include absent deep tendon reflexes, numbness, weakness, myalgias, cramping, and late severe motor difficulties. Impotence may result in secondary to nerve damage.
- Reproduction: Bleomycin is teratogenic and mutagenic.

Initiate antiemetic protocol:	Mildly emetogenic protocol.
Supportive drugs:	☐ pegfilgrastim (Neulasta) ☐ filgrastim (Neupogen) ☐ epoetin alfa (Procrit) ☐ darbepoetin alfa (Aranesp)
Treatment schedule:	Chair time 1 hour on days 1 and 15. Repeat cycle every 2 weeks.
Estimated number of visits:	Two visits per cycle. Request six cycles worth of visits.

Dose Calculation by: 1. _____ 2. _____

_____ _____
Physician   Date

_____ _____
Patient Name   ID Number

_____ _____/_____/_____
Diagnosis   Ht   Wt   M^2

Doxorubicin + Bleomycin + Vinblastine (ABV)

Baseline laboratory tests:	CBC: Chemistry
Baseline procedures or tests:	MUGA scan PFTs and CXR baseline; PFTs and CXR
Initiate IV:	0.9% sodium chloride
Premedicate:	Tylenol or Tylenol ES 2 tablets orally 30 minutes before treatment and every 6 hours after
	5-HT$_3$ and dexamethasone 10–20 mg in 100 cc of NS over 30 minutes (phenothiazines enhance activity of bleomycin)

Administer:

Doxorubicin _____ mg (40 mg/m^2) IV day 1

- Potent vesicant
- Available as a 2-mg/mL solution. Given IV push through side port of free-flowing IV of NS or D5W.
- Doxorubicin will form a precipitate if mixed with heparin or 5-FU.
- Given IV push through the side port of a free-lowing IV.

Bleomycin _____ units (15 U/m^2) IV on days 1 and 15

- A test dose of 2 U is recommended before the first dose to detect hypersensitivity.
- Available as a powder in 15- or 30-unit sizes. Dilute powder in 0.9% sodium chloride or sterile water: 1–5 cc for the 15-unit vial and 2–10 cc for the 30-unit vial. Should NOT be diluted in D5W.
- Stable for 24 hours when diluted with NS.
- Given IV push over at least 10 minutes or further diluted and NS infused or pushed over at least 10 minutes.

Vinblastine _____ mg (6 mg/m^2) IV on day 1

- Vesicant
- Available in 10-mg vials at a concentration of 1 mg/mL.
- Given IV push through side port of free-flowing IV of NS or D5W.

Major Side Effects

- Hypersensitivity Reaction: Fever and chills observed in up to 25% of patients. True anaphylactoid reactions are rare but more common in patients with lymphoma (1%).
- Pulmonary: Pulmonary toxicity is dose limiting in bleomycin.
- Bone Marrow Depression: Myelosuppression may be severe with WBC and platelet nadir at 10–14 days and recovery on days 15–21.
- Gastrointestinal Toxicities: Nausea and vomiting are moderate to severe and occur in 44% of patients. Stomatitis occurs in 10% of patients but is not dose limiting. Constipation, abdominal pain, and paralytic ileus are common. A prophylactic bowel regimen for constipation is recommended.
- GU: Red-orange discoloration of urine for up to 48 hours after doxorubicin.
- Cardiotoxicity: Acutely, myocarditis or subsequent cardiomyopathy can occur.
- Skin: Extravasation of doxorubicin or vinblastine may cause local tissue injury, inflammation, and necrosis. Phlebitis at the IV site may occur. Skin changes with or without rash, hyperpigmentation, photosensitivity, radiation recall, and nail changes or loss have been seen. Alopecia is common.
- Neurotoxicity: Peripheral neuropathies occur as a result of toxicity to nerve fibers. Symptoms include absent deep tendon reflexes, numbness, weakness, myalgias, cramping, and late severe motor difficulties. Impotence may result in secondary to nerve damage.
- Reproduction: Drugs are teratogenic and mutagenic.

Initiate antiemetic protocol:	Moderately to highly emetogenic protocol.
Supportive drugs:	☐ pegfilgrastim (Neulasta) ☐ filgrastim (Neupogen)
	☐ epoetin alfa (Procrit) ☐ darbepoetin alfa (Aranesp)
Treatment schedule:	Chair time 1 hour on days 1 and 15. Repeat the cycle every 28 days.
Estimated number of visits:	Two visits per cycle. Request three cycles worth of visits.

Dose Calculation by: 1. _____ 2. _____

Physician _____ Date _____

Patient Name _____ ID Number _____

Diagnosis _____ Ht _____ / Wt _____ / M² _____

Single-Agent Regimens

Liposomal Daunorubicin (DaunoXome)

Baseline laboratory tests:	CBC: Chemistry
Baseline procedures or tests:	MUGA scan at baseline, at 320 mg/m^2 cumulative dose and every 160 mg/m^2 dose thereafter. Central line placement
Initiate IV:	0.9% sodium chloride
Premedicate:	5-HT$_3$ and dexamethasone 10–20 mg in 100 cc of NS
Administer:	**Liposomal Daunorubicin** _____ mg (40 mg/m^2) IV over 1 hour on day 1

- Available as a 2-mg/mL solution in 50-mg vials.
- Further dilute drug in D5W to a final concentration of 1 mg/mL. Solution is stable for 6 hours.
- Drug is a vesicant; administer with care as IV bolus over 60 minutes.

Major Side Effects

- Infusion Reaction: Occurs within the first 5 minutes of infusion and manifested by back pain, flushing, and tightness in the chest and throat. Observed in about 15% of patients and usually with the first infusion. Improves on termination of infusion and typically does not recur on reinstitution at a slower infusion rate.
- Bone Marrow Depression: Myelosuppression can be severe and affects the granulocytes primarily. Neutropenia (36%), concurrent antiretroviral, and antiviral agents may enhance this effect. Hold for granulocyte count < 750 cells/mm^3.
- Gastrointestinal Toxicities: Nausea and vomiting are usually mild to moderate and occur in 50% of patients. Mucositis and diarrhea are common but not dose limiting. Dose reduction required for abnormal liver function.
- Cardiac: Acutely, pericarditis and/or myocarditis, EKG changes, or arrhythmias. Chronic form is associated with a dose-dependent cardiomyopathy at cumulative doses of > 320 mg/m^2. Risk of cardiac toxicity increased with prior anthracycline use, pre-existing cardiac disease, or radiotherapy encompassing heart.
- Skin: Mild alopecia occurs in 6% of patients and moderate alopecia in 2% of patients. Folliculitis, seborrhea, and dry skin occur in > 5% of patients.
- Reproduction: Liposomal daunorubicin is embryotoxic.

Initiate antiemetic protocol:	Mildly to moderately emetogenic protocol.
Supportive drugs:	☐ pegfilgrastim (Neulasta) ☐ filgrastim (Neupogen)
	☐ epoetin alfa (Procrit) ☐ darbepoetin alfa (Aranesp)
Treatment schedule:	Chair time 2 hours on day 1. Repeat cycle every 14 days.
Estimated number of visits:	One visit per cycle. Request four cycles worth of visits.

Dose Calculation by: 1. _____   2. _____

_____
Physician

_____
Date

_____
Patient Name

_____
ID Number

_____
Diagnosis

_____ / _____ / _____
Ht   Wt   M^2

Liposomal Doxorubicin (DOXIL)

Baseline laboratory and tests:	CBC: Chemistry
Baseline procedures or tests:	MUGA scan
Initiate IV:	0.9% sodium chloride
Premedicate:	5-HT$_3$ and dexamethasone 10–20 mg in 100 cc of NS
Administer:	**Liposomal Doxorubicin** _____ mg (20 mg/m^2) IV on day 1

- Irritant
- Available as a 2-mg/mL solution in 20- or 50-mg vials.
- Further dilute drug doses up to 90 mg in 250 cc of D5W, use 500-mL D5W for doses > 90 mg.
- Administer at initial rate of 1 mg/mL to minimize risk of infusion reaction; if no reaction increase rate to complete administration in 1 hour.
- Diluted solution stable for 24 hours refrigerated.

Major Side Effects

- Infusion Reaction: Flushing, dyspnea, facial swelling, headache, back pain, tightness in the chest and throat, and/or hypotension. Usually occurs during first treatment and is seen in 5%–10% of patients. Resolves quickly after infusion stopped. Monitor vital signs for first 15–30 minutes. May administer coticosteroids or diphenhydramine before rechallenging, or have patient take steroids for 24 hours prior to the next administration.
- Bone Marrow Depression: Dose-limiting toxicity in the treatment of HIV-infected patients. Leukopenia occurs in 91% of patients, with anemia and thrombocytopenia less common.
- Gastrointestinal Toxicities: Nausea and vomiting are usually mild to moderate. Stomatitis is seen in 7% of patients and diarrhea in 8%; both are usually mild.
- GU: Red-orange discoloration of urine for up to 48 hours.
- Cardiac: Acutely, pericarditis and/or myocarditis, EKG changes, or arrhythmias. Not dose related. With high cumulative doses > 550 mg/m^2, cardiomyopathy may occur. Increased risk of cardiotoxicity when liposomal doxorubicin is given with Herceptin or mitomycin C. Risk of cardiac toxicity increased with prior anthracycline use, pre-existing cardiac disease, or radiotherapy encompassing heart and in patients > 70 years of age.
- Skin: Skin toxicity manifested as hand-foot syndrome with skin rash, swelling, erythema, pain, and/or desquamation. Seen in 3.4% of patients and is dose related. Hyperpigmentation of nails, skin rash, urticaria, and radiation recall occur. Alopecia seen in 9% of Kaposi's patients.
- Reproduction: Pregnancy category D. Breast feeding should be avoided.

Initiate antiemetic protocol:	Moderately to highly emetogenic protocol.	
Supportive drugs:	☐ pegfilgrastim (Neulasta)	☐ filgrastim (Neupogen)
	☐ epoetin alfa (Procrit)	☐ darbepoetin alfa (Aranesp)
Treatment schedule:	Chair time 2 hours on day 1. Repeat cycle every 21 days.	
Estimated number of visits:	One visit per cycle. Request four cycles worth of visits.	

Dose Calculation by: 1. _____   2. _____

_____   _____
Physician   Date

_____   _____
Patient Name   ID Number

_____   _____/_____/_____
Diagnosis   Ht   Wt   M^2

Paclitaxel (Taxol)

Baseline laboratory and tests:	CBC: Chemistry
Baseline procedures or tests:	N/A
Initiate IV:	0.9% sodium chloride
Premedicate:	Oral phenothiazines or 5-HT$_3$ in 100 cc of NS
	Diphenhydramine 25–50 mg and cimetidine 300 mg in 100 cc of NS
Administer:	**Paclitaxel** _____ mg (135 mg/m^2) IV over 3 hours on day 1. Repeat 3 times
	OR
Administer:	**Paclitaxel** _____ mg (100 mg/m^2) IV over 3 hours on day 1. Repeat every 2 weeks

- Available in 30-mg (6 mg/mL), 100-mg (16.7 mg/mL), and 300-mg (6-mg/mL) vials.
- Further dilute in NS or D5W to a final concentration of ≤ 1.2 mg/mL.
- Diluted solution stable for 27 hours at room temperature.
- **Use non-PVC containers and tubing with a 0.22-micron inline filter for administration.**

Major Side Effects

- Hypersensitivity Reaction: With anaphylaxis and severe hypersensitivity reactions in 2%–4%. Characterized by dyspnea, hypotension, andioedema, and generalized urticaria. May also see tachycardia, wheezing, and facial edema. Usually happens within first 2–3 minutes of infusion. Patients with mild reactions can be rechallenged after 24 hour corticosteroid prophylaxis. Patients with severe reactions should not be rechallenged. Premedicate as described. Monitor vital signs every 15 minutes for first hour of infusion.
- Bone Marrow Depression: Dose-limiting neutropenia with nadir at days 8–10 and recovery by days 15–21. Decreased the incidence of neutropenia with a 3-hour schedule when compared with a 24-hour schedule. G-CSF support is recommended.
- Gastrointestinal Toxicity: Mild to moderate nausea and vomiting, usually brief in duration. Mucositis and/or diarrhea seen in 30%–40% of patients. Mucositis is more common with the 24-hour schedule.
- Neurotoxicity: Dose limiting peripheral sensory neuropathy. Paresthesias and numbness in classic "stocking glove" pattern. Risk increases with cumulative doses. Loss of motor function, facial encephalopathy and seizures observed. Neurologic effects may be irreversible.
- Alopecia: A total loss of body hair occurs in nearly all patients.
- Reproduction: Pregnancy category D. Breast feeding should be avoided.

Initiate antiemetic protocol:	Mildly emetogenic protocol
Supportive drugs:	☐ pegfilgrastim (Neulasta) ☐ filgrastim (Neupogen)
	☐ epoetin alfa (Procrit) ☐ darbepoetin alfa (Aranesp)
Treatment schedule:	Chair time 4 hours. Repeat every 21 days as tolerated or until progression.
Estimated number of visits:	Two visits per cycle. Request three cycles worth of visits.

Dose Calculation by: 1. _____ 2. _____

_____

Physician

_____

Date

_____

Patient Name

_____

ID Number

_____

Diagnosis

_____ / _____ / _____

Ht   Wt   M^2

Interferon α-2a

Baseline laboratory and tests:	CBC: Chemistry (including LFTs)
Baseline procedures or tests:	N/A
Initiate IV:	N/A
Premedicate:	Oral phenothiazine or 5-HT$_3$ Acetaminophen
Administer:	**Interferon α-2a (Intron A)**_____ mg (36-million IU/m^2) SC or IM, daily for 8–12 weeks

• Available in 30 miu pen (30 miu in 1.5 ml).

OR

Interferon α-2b _____ mg (30-million IU/m^2) SC or IM three times weekly

Major Side Effects

• Flulike Symptoms: Fever, chills, headache, myalgias, and arthralgias. Occurs in 80%–90% of patients. Onset 3–4 hours after injection and lasting for up to 8–9 hours. Incidence decreases with subsequent injections. Symptoms can be managed with acetaminophen and increased oral fluid intake.

• Bone Marrow Depression: Myelosuppression with mild leukopenia and thrombocytopenia.

• Gastrointestinal Toxicities: Nausea and diarrhea are mild; vomiting is rare. Anorexia is seen in 46%–65% of patients and is cumulative and dose limiting. Taste alteration and xerostomia may occur.

• Renal/hepatic: Renal toxicity is uncommon and is manifested by mild proteinuria and hypocalcemia. Acute renal failure and nephrotic syndrome have been reported in rare instances. Mild transient elevations in serum transaminases. Dose-dependent toxicity is observed more frequently in the presence of pre-existing liver abnormalities.

• Cardiotoxicity: Chest pain, arrhythmias, and congestive heart failure are rare.

• Skin: Alopecia is partial. Dry skin, pruritus, and irritation at injection site seen.

• Ocular: Retinopathy with cotton-wool spots and small hemorrhages. Usually asymptomatic and resolves upon termination of therapy.

• Reproduction: Increased incidence of spontaneous abortions.

Initiate antiemetic protocol:	Mildly emetogenic protocol
Supportive drugs:	☐ pegfilgrastim (Neulasta) ☐ filgrastim (Neupogen) ☐ epoetin alfa (Procrit) ☐ darbepoetin alfa (Aranesp)
Treatment schedule:	Chair time 1 hour on day 1 for self-injection teaching
Estimated number of visits:	One visit per week for laboratories. Request 12 weeks worth of visits. May require extra visits for hydration.

Dose Calculation by: 1. _____   2. _____

_____   _____

Physician   Date

_____   _____

Patient Name   ID Number

_____   _____/ _____/ _____

Diagnosis   Ht   Wt   M^2

LEUKEMIA

Acute Lymphocytic Leukemia

Induction Therapy

Linker Regimen[1,203,204] 301

Daunorubicin: 50 mg/m^2 IV every 24 hours on days 1–3

Vincristine: 2 mg IV on days 1, 8, 15, and 22

Prednisone: 60 mg/m^2 PO divided into three doses on days 1–28

L-Asparaginase: 6000 U/m^2 IM on days 17–28

If bone marrow on day 14 is positive for residual leukemia,

Daunorubicin: 50 mg/m^2 IV on day 15

If bone marrow on day 28 is positive for residual leukemia,

Daunorubicin: 50 mg/m^2 IV on days 29 and 30

Vincristine: 2 mg IV on days 29 and 36

Prednisone: 60 mg/m^2 PO on days 29–42

L-Asparaginase: 6000 U/m^2 IM on days 29–35

Consolidation Therapy

Linker Regimen[1,203,204] 303

Treatment A (Cycles 1, 3, 5, and 7)

Daunorubicin: 50 mg/m^2 IV on days 1 and 2

Vincristine: 2 mg IV on days 1 and 8

Prednisone: 60 mg/m^2 PO on days 1–14

L-Asparaginase: 12,000 U/m^2 on days 2, 4, 7, 9, 11, and 14

Treatment B (Cycles 2, 4, 6, and 8)

Teniposide: 165 mg/m^2 IV on days 1, 4, 8, and 11

Cytarabine: 300 mg/m^2 IV on days 1, 4, 8, and 11

Treatment C (Cycle 9)

Methotrexate: 690 mg/m^2 IV over 42 hours

Leucovorin: 15 mg/m^2 IV every 6 hours for 12 doses beginning at 42 hours

Maintenance Therapy

Linker Regimen[1,203,204] 305

Methotrexate: 20 mg/m^2 PO weekly

6-Mercaptopurine: 75 mg/m^2 PO daily

Continue for a total of 30 months of complete response.

CNS Prophylaxis

Cranial irradiation: 1800 rad in 10 fractions over 12–14 days

Methotrexate: 12 mg IT weekly for 6 weeks

Begin within 1 week of complete response.

In patients with documented CNS involvement at time of diagnosis, intrathecal chemotherapy should begin during induction chemotherapy.

Methotrexate: 12 mg IT weekly for 10 doses

Cranial irradiation: 2800 rad

Induction (Weeks 1–4)

Cyclophosphamide: 1200 mg/m^2 IV on day 1

Daunorubicin: 45 mg/m^2 IV on days 1–3

Vincristine: 2 mg IV on days 1, 8, 15, and 22

Prednisone: 60 mg/m^2/day PO on days 1–21

L-Asparaginase: 6000 IU/m^2 SC on days 15, 18, 22, and 25

Early Intensification (Weeks 5–12)

Methotrexate: 15 mg IT on day 1

Cyclophosphamide: 1000 mg/m^2 IV on day 1

6-Mercaptopurine: 60 mg/m^2/day PO on days 1–4 and 8–11

Cytarabine: 75 mg/m^2 IV on days 1–14

Vincristine: 2 mg IV on days 15 and 22

L-Asparaginase: 6000 IU/m^2 SC on days 15, 18, 22, and 25

Repeat the early intensification cycle once.

CNS Prophylaxis and Interim Maintenance (Weeks 13–25)

Cranial irradiation: 2400 cGy on days 1–12

Methotrexate: 15 mg IT on days 1, 8, 15, 22, and 29

6-Mercaptopurine: 60 mg/m^2/day PO on days 1–70

Methotrexate: 20 mg/m^2 PO on days 36, 43, 50, 57, and 64

Late Intensification (Weeks 26–33)

Doxorubicin: 30 mg/m^2 IV on days 1, 8, and 15

Vincristine: 2 mg IV on days 1, 8, and 15

Dexamethasone: 10 mg/m^2/day PO on days 1–14

Cyclophosphamide: 1000 mg/m^2 IV on day 29

6-Thioguanine: 60 mg/m^2/day PO on days 29–42

Cytarabine: 75 mg/m^2 on days 29, 32, 36–39

Prolonged Maintenance (Continue Until 24 Months after Diagnosis)

Vincristine: 2 mg IV on day 1

Prednisone: 60 mg/m^2/day PO on days 1–5

Methotrexate: 20 mg/m^2 PO on days 1, 8, 15, and 22

6-Mercaptopurine: 80 mg/m^2/day PO on days 1–28

Repeat maintenance cycle every 28 days.

Hyper-CVAD Regimen[1,206] 311

Cyclophosphamide: 300 mg/m^2 IV over 3 hours every 12 hours for 6 doses on days 1–3

Mesna: 600 mg/m^2 IV over 24 hours on days 1–3 ending 6 hours after the last dose of cyclophosphamide

Vincristine: 2 mg IV on days 4 and 11

Doxorubicin: 50 mg/m^2 IV on day 4

Dexamethasone: 40 mg PO or IV on days 1–4 and 11–14

Alternate cycles every 21 days with the following:

(High dose-MTX-Ara-C)

Methotrexate: 200 mg/m^2 IV over 2 hours, followed by

800 mg/m^2 IV over 24 hours on day 1

Leucovorin: 15 mg IV every 6 hours for 8 doses, starting 24 hours after the completion of methotrexate infusion

Cytarabine: 3000 mg/m^2 IV over 2 hours every 12 hours for 4 doses on days 2–3

Methylprednisolone: 50 mg IV bid on days 1–3

Alternate four cycles of hyper-CVAD with four cycles of high-dose methotrexate and cytarabine therapy (HD-MTX-Ara-C) every three to four weeks.[1,206]

CNS Prophylaxis

Methotrexate: 12 mg IT on day 2

Cytarabine: 100 mg IT on day 8

Repeat with each cycle of chemotherapy, depending on the risk of CNS disease.

Supportive Care

Throughout treatment

Ciprofloxacin: 500 mg PO bid

Fluconazole: 200 mg/day PO

Acyclovir: 200 mg PO bid

G-CSF: 10 µg/kg/day starting 24 hours after the end of chemotherapy (i.e., on day 5 of hyper-CVAD therapy and on day 4 of high-dose methotrexate and cytarabine therapy)

Single-Agent Regimens

Clofarabine: 52 mg/m^2 IV for 5 days

Repeat cycle every 2–6 weeks.[1,207]

Induction Therapy

Linker Regimen: ALL

Baseline laboratory tests:	CBC: Chemistry, renal and liver functions
Baseline procedures or tests:	Bone marrow biopsy, central line placement, EKG, and MUGA if cardiac changes with induction therapy. Doses reduce with impaired functions.
Initiate IV:	NS. Consider central line.
Premedicate:	5-HT$_3$ and dexamethasone 20 mg IV
Administer:	**Daunorubicin** _____ 50 mg/m^2 IV on day 1, 2, and 3

- **Vesicant**
- Given through the side port of a free-flowing IV. Infuse over 1 hour only if patient has a central line. Maximum lifetime dose 550 mg/m^2.
- Available in 20 mg/5 mL or 50 mg/10 mL preservative-free vial. Further dilute with 10–15 mL of 0.9% sodium chloride before administration.
- Diluted solution stable for 24 hours protected from light.
- Incompatible with heparin and dexamethasone.

Vincristine _____ 2 mg IV on days 1, 8, 15, and 22

- Vesicant
- Given through the side port of a free-flowing IV.
- Available in 1 mg or 2 mg/mL vials. Keep refrigerated until ready to use.

Prednisone _____ 60 mg/m^2 PO divided into three doses on days 1–28

- Available in 1-, 5-, 20-, and 50-mg tablets.
- Take in the morning with food.

L-Asparaginase _____ 6000 U/m^2 IM on days 17–28

- Available in 10,000 IU/10 mL.
- Reconstituted solution is stable for 8 hours at room temperature. Do NOT administer more than 2 mL per IM injection.

If bone marrow on day 14 is positive for residual leukemia:

Administer:	**Daunorubicin** _____ 50 mg/m^2 IV on day 15

If bone marrow on day 28 is positive for residual leukemia:

Daunorubicin _____ 50 mg/m^2 IV on days 29 and 30

Administer:	**Vincristine** _____ 2 mg IV on days 29 and 36
	Prednisone _____ 60 mg/m^2 PO on days 29–42
	L-Asparaginase _____ 6000 U/m^2 m^2 IM on days 29–35

Major Side Effects	- Anaphylactic Reaction: Occurs in 20–30 of patients receiving L-asparaginase, incidence increases with subsequent doses. Occurs less often with IM doses.

- Bone Marrow Depression: Nadir at 10–14 days; leukopenia more common than thrombocytopenia. Teach self-care measures to minimize risk of infection and bleeding.
- Gastrointestinal (GI) Toxicities: Nausea and vomiting, anorexia, and mucositis. Autonomic neuropathy resulting in constipation and can lead to paralytic ileus.
- Cardiotoxicity: Irreversible congestive heart failure (CHF). Acute toxicity can occur within hours after administration. Have patients report dyspnea, shortness of breath, edema, or orthopnea. Daily weights.
- Mental Status: Lethargy, drowsiness, and somnolence with the L-asparaginase.
- Peripheral Neuropathy: Absent deep tendon reflexes, numbness, weakness, myalgias, jaw pain, diplopia, vocal cord paralysis, and metallic taste.
- GU Toxicity: Causes discoloration of urine (pink to red, red orange for up to 48 hours after administration).
- Tumor lysis syndrome occurring 1–5 days after initiation of treatment.
- Skin Alterations: Total alopecia, radiation recall, and sun sensitivity.

- Sexual dysfunction: mutagenic and potentially teratogenic, discuss contraception and sperm banking.

Initiate antiemetic protocol: Highly to moderately emetogenic protocol

Supportive drugs:

☐ G-CSF _____   ☐ Peg-G-CSF _____

☐ Epoetin Alfa/   ☐ Allopurinol _____
   Darbepoetin Alfa _____

☐ Antibiotic _____   ☐ Antifungal _____

Treatment schedule: Repeat cycle until remission (usually two to three cycles).

Chair time two hours on days 1, 2, 3, 8, 15, 22 and 17–28, 29, 30, 31, 32, 33, 34, 35, and 36.

Estimated number of visits: Five to seven days first week, daily, or every other day for CBC, may require hospitalization.

Dose Calculation by: 1. _____   2. _____

_____   _____
Physician   Date

_____   _____
Patient Name   ID Number

_____   _____/_____/_____
Diagnosis   Ht   Wt   M²

Consolidation Therapy

Linker Regimen: ALL

Treatment A (Cycles 1, 3, 5, and 7) Alternating with Treatment B (Cycles 2, 4, 6, and 8) Followed by Treatment C (Cycle 9)

Baseline laboratory tests: CBC: Chemistry, renal and liver functions

Baseline procedures or tests: Bone marrow biopsy, central line placement, EKG, and MUGA if cardiac changes with induction therapy. Doses reduce with impaired liver or renal functions.

Treatment Cycle A (Cycles 1, 3, 5, and 7)

Initiate IV: NS

Premedicate: 5-HT$_3$ and dexamethasone 20 mg IV

Administer: **Daunorubicin** _____ 50 mg/m^2 IV on days 1 and 2

- Given through the side port of a free-flowing IV.
- Infuse over 1 hour only if patient has a central line.
- Vesicant
- A maximum lifetime dose of 550 mg/m^2.
- Add 4-mL sterile water to vial for concentration of 5 mg/mL.
- Further dilute with 10–15 mL of 0.9% sodium chloride.
- Incompatible with heparin and dexamethasone.

Vincristine _____ 2 mg IV on days 1 and 8

- Given through the side port of a free-flowing IV.
- Vesicant

Prednisone _____ 60 mg/m^2 divided into three doses on days 1–14

L-Asparaginase: _____ 12,000 U/m^2 IM on days 2, 4, 7, 9, 11, and 14

- Available in 10,000 IU/10 mL.
- Reconstituted solution is stable for 8 hours at room temperature. Do NOT administer more than 2 mL per IM injection.

Treatment B (Cycles 2, 4, 6, and 8)

Administer: **Teniposide (Vumon)** _____ 165 mg/m^2 IV over at least 30–60 minutes on days 1, 4, 8, and 11

- 50-mg ampule, further dilute with NS or D5W for final concentration of 0.1–0.4 mg/mL. Concentrations of 1 mg/mL may precipitate faster and must be infused within 4 hours. Infuse over 30-60 minutes to avoid hypotension.
- Stable for 24 hours. Requires non-DEHP containers and tubing. Do not give if precipitate is seen. **Not compatible with heparin, flush line well with NS or D5W.**

Cytarabine (Ara-C) _____ 300 mg/m^2 IV on days 1, 4, 8, and 11

- Dilute in sterile water with benzyl alcohol and then further dilute in 50–100 mL of NS or D5W infused over 1 hour.
- Available in 100-mg, 500-mg, 1- and 2-gram vials. Solutions are 5 mg/mL.
- Stable for up to 192 days at room temperature.

Treatment C (Cycle 9)

Administer: **Methotrexate** _____ 690 mg/m^2 IV over 42 hours

- 250-mg vial, 25 mg/mL further diluted in NS.
- Reconstituted solution stable for 24 hours at room temperature.
- High-dose methotrexate requires leucovorin rescue.
- Drug interactions include aspirin, penicillins, NSAIDs, cephalosporins, and phenytoin; warfarin, 5-fluorouracil, thymidine, folic acid, and omeprazole.

Leucovorin _____ 15 mg/m^2 IV over 15 minutes every 6 hours for 12 doses beginning at 42 hours.

- Reconstitute vials with sterile water and further with NS or D5W beginning at 42 hours.
- Continue until MTX levels fall below 5×10^{-8}.

Major Side Effects

- Hypersensitivity/anaphylactic Reactions: Occurs in 20–30 of patients receiving L-asparaginase; incidence increases with subsequent doses and may result in death. Occurs less often with IM doses. Can also occur with teniposide infusion. Symptoms include chills, fever, flushing, and urticaria. Severe include tachycardia, bronchospasm, facial and tongue swelling, and hypotension.
- Myelosuppression dose limiting, onset 3–7 days. Teach self-care measures to minimize risk of infection and bleeding.
- GI Toxicities: Nausea and vomiting, anorexia; mucositis and stomatitis. Autonomic neuropathy resulting in constipation and can lead to paralytic ileus secondary to vincristine.
- Cardiotoxicity: Irreversible CHF. Acute toxicity can occur within hours after administration. Have patients report dyspnea, shortness of breath, edema, or orthopnea. Daily weights.
- CNS Changes: Lethargy, drowsiness, and somnolence with the L-asparaginase. Acute cerebral dysfunction with paresis, aphasia, behavioral abnormalities, and seizures in 5%–15% receiving high-dose therapy.
- Peripheral Neuropathy: Absent deep tendon reflexes, numbness, weakness, myalgias, jaw pain, diplopia, vocal cord paralysis, and metallic taste.
- GU Toxicity: Causes discoloration of urine (pink to red, red orange for up to 48 hours after administration). Acute renal failure, azotemia, urinary retention, and uric acid nephropathy can be seen with high-dose methotrexate.
- Tumor lysis syndrome occurring 1–5 days after initiation of treatment.
- Skin Alterations: Total alopecia, radiation recall, and sun sensitivity.
- Reproduction: mutagenic and potentially teratogenic, discuss contraception, and sperm banking.

Initiate antiemetic protocol: Highly to moderately emetogenic protocol

Supportive drugs:
- ☐ G-CSF _____
- ☐ Peg-G-CSF _____
- ☐ Epoetin Alfa/ Darbepoetin Alfa _____
- ☐ Allopurinol _____
- ☐ Antibiotic _____
- ☐ Antifungal _____

Treatment schedule: Visits for Treatment A, cycles 1, 3, 5, and 7

2 hours on days 1, 2, 4, 6, 8, 11, and 14

Visits for Treatment B, cycles 2, 4, 6, and 8

3 hours on days 1, 4, 8, and 11 followed by maintenance and CNS prophylaxis protocols

Estimated number of visits: Five to seven days first week, daily, or every other day for CBC, may require hospitalization.

Dose Calculation by: 1. _____ 2. _____

_____
Physician

_____
Date

_____
Patient Name

_____
ID Number

_____
Diagnosis

_____ / _____ / _____
Ht   Wt   M^2

Maintenance Therapy

Linker Regimen: ALL

Baseline laboratory and tests: CBC: Chemistry, renal and liver functions

Baseline procedures or tests: Bone marrow

Administer:

Methotrexate _____ 20 mg/m^2 PO weekly

- Available in 5-mg, 7.5-mg, 10-mg, 12.5-mg, and 15-mg tablets.
- Take at the same time each week.

6-Mercaptopurine: _____ 75 mg/m^2 PO daily (50-mg tablets)

- Take on an empty stomach; continue for a total of 30 months for complete response.
- Drug interactions—Anticoagulant effects of coumadin are inhibited. Monitor PT/INR. Allopurinol inhibits xantinine oxidase resulting in increased toxicities.

Major Side Effects

- Myelosuppression. Dose limiting.
- GI Toxicities: Nausea and vomiting, anorexia, mucositis, and stomatitis. Autonomic neuropathy resulting in constipation and can lead to paralytic ileus secondary to vincristine.
- CNS changes due to IT MTX: Dizziness, malaise, and blurred vision. May increase CSF pressure. Keep patient supine for at least 1 hour after IT injection to prevent headache. Brain XRT after MTX can result in neurologic changes. Liver function tests should be monitored while on oral methotrexate.
- Sensory Neuropathy: Loss of vibratory sensation, unsteady gate may occur.
- Reproduction: mutagenic and potentially teratogenic, discuss contraception, and sperm banking.

Dose Calculation by: 1: _____   2. _____

_____

Physician

_____

Patient Name

_____

Diagnosis

_____

Date

_____

ID Number

_____ / _____ / _____

Ht   Wt   M^2

CNS Prophylaxis

Linker Regimen

Administer:

Cranial irradiation _____ 1800 rad in 10 fractions over 12–14 days

Methotrexate _____ 12 mg IT weekly for 6 weeks

- Begin within 1 week of complete response.
- In patients with documented CNS involvement at time of diagnosis, intrathecal chemotherapy should begin during induction chemotherapy.

Cranial irradiation _____ 2800 rad

Methotrexate _____ 12 mg IT weekly for 10 doses

Major Side Effects

- Myelosuppression. Dose limiting.
- GI Toxicities: Nausea and vomiting, anorexia, mucositis, and stomatitis. Autonomic neuropathy resulting in constipation and can lead to paralytic ileus secondary to vincristine.
- CNS changes due to IT MTX: Dizziness, malaise, and blurred vision. May increase CSF pressure. Keep patient supine for at least 1 hour after IT injection to prevent headache. Brain XRT after MTX can result in neurologic changes. Liver function tests should be monitored while on oral methotrexate.
- Sensory Neuropathy: Loss of vibratory sensation, unsteady gate may occur.
- Reproduction: mutagenic and potentially teratogenic, discuss contraception, and sperm banking.

Initiate antiemetic protocol: Mildly emetogenic protocol.

Supportive drugs:

☐ G-CSF _____   ☐ Peg-G-CSF _____

☐ Epoetin Alfa/   ☐ Allopurinol _____
Darbepoetin Alfa _____

☐ Antibiotic _____   ☐ Antifungal _____

Treatment schedule: Weekly to monthly.

Estimated number of visits: One to four visits per month for CBC, weekly × 10 for IT methotrexate

Dose Calculation by: 1. _____ 2. _____

_____   _____
Physician   Date

_____   _____
Patient Name   ID Number

_____   _____ / _____ / _____
Diagnosis   Ht   Wt M^2

Larson Regimen: ALL

Baseline laboratory tests:	CBC: Chemistry, renal and liver functions
Baseline procedures or tests:	Bone marrow biopsy, central line placement, EKG, and MUGA if cardiac changes with induction therapy. Doses reduce with impaired liver or renal functions.

Induction: (Weeks 1–4)

Initiate IV:	NS
Premedicate:	5-HT$_3$ and dexamethasone 20 mg IV
Administer:	**Cyclophosphamide** _____ 1200 mg/m^2 IV over 2 hours on day 1

- Available in 500-mg, 1-, and 2-gram vials. Dilute with sterile water or bacteriostatic water for injection (sterile water or paraben preserved); shake well until solution is clear.
- Final concentration of 20 mg/mL.
- Further dilute into 250–500 mL of NS or D5W.
- Reconstituted solution is stable for 24 hours at room temperature and 6 days upon refrigeration.

Daunorubicin _____ 45 mg/m^2 IV on days 1–3

- Given through the side port of a free-flowing IV.
- Infuse over 1 hour only if patient has a central line.
- Vesicant
- Maximum lifetime dose of 550 mg/m^2.
- Add 4-mL sterile water to vial for concentration of 5 mg/mL.
- Further dilute with 10–15 mL of 0.9% sodium chloride. Incompatible with heparin and dexamethasone.
- Reconstituted solution is stable for 24 hours at room temperature and 48 hours upon refrigeration.

Vincristine _____ 2 mg IV on days 1, 8, 15, and 22

- Vesicant
- Given through the side port of a free-flowing IV.
- Available in 1-mg or 2-mg/mL vials. Keep refrigerated until ready to use.
- Vesicant

Prednisone _____ 60 mg/m^2 PO on days 1–21

- Available in 5-, 10-, 20-, and 50-mg tablets. Take in the morning with food.

L-Asparaginase _____ 6000 U/m^2 SC on days 15, 18, 22, and 25

- Available in 10,000 IU/10 mL.
- Reconstituted solution is stable for 8 hours at room temperature. Do NOT administer more than 2 mL per IM injection.

Larson Early Intensification (Weeks 5–12)

Administer:	**Methotrexate preservative-free solution** _____ 15 mg IT on day 1

- Preservative-free solution or preservative-free power reconstituted with sterile NS ONLY. Available in preservative-free solutions in 50-mg/2-mL, 100-mg/4-mL, 200-mg/8-mL, and 250-mg/10-mL vials.

Cyclophosphamide _____ 1000 mg/m^2/day over 2 hours on day 1

- Available in 500-mg, 1-, and 2-gram vials. Dilute with sterile water or bacteriostatic water for injection (sterile water or paraben preserved); shake well until solution is clear.
- Final concentration of 20 mg/mL.
- Further dilute into 250–500 mL of NS or D5W.

6-Mercaptopurine _____ 60 mg/m^2/day PO on days 1–4 and 8–11

- Available in 50-mg tablets. Take on an empty stomach; continue for a total of 30 months for complete response.

Cytarabine (Ara-C) _____ 75 mg/m^2 IV on days 1–14

- Dilute in sterile water with benzyl alcohol and then further dilute in 50–100 mL of NS or D5W infused over 1 hour.
- Available in 100-mg, 500-mg, 1-, and 2-gram vials. Solutions are 5 mg/mL.
- Stable for up to 192 days at room temperature.

Vincristine _____ 2 mg IV on days 15 and 22

- **Vesicant**
- Given through the side port of a free-flowing IV.
- Available in 1-mg or 2-mg/mL vials. Keep refrigerated until ready to use.

L-Asparaginase: _____ 6000 U/m^2 SC on days 15, 18, 22, and 25

- Available in 10,000 IU/10 mL.
- Reconstituted solution is stable for 8 hours at room temperature. Do NOT administer more than 2 mL per IM injection.

Repeat the early intensification cycle once.

Larson CNS Prophylaxis and Interim Maintenance (Weeks 13–25)

Administer:

Cranial irradiation _____ 2400 cGy on days 1–12

Methotrexate _____ 15 mg IT on days 1, 8, 15, 22, and 29

- Preservative-free solution or preservative-free power reconstituted with sterile NS ONLY. Available in preservative free solutions in 50-mg/2-mL, 100-mg/4-mL, 200-mg/8-mL, and 250-mg/10-mL vials.

6-Mercaptopurine _____ 60 mg/m^2/day PO on days 1–70

- Available in 50-mg tablets. Take on an empty stomach; continue for a total of 30 months for complete response.

Methotrexate _____ 20 mg/m^2 PO on days 36, 43, 50, 57, and 64

- Available in 5-mg, 7.5-mg, 10-mg, 12.5-mg, and 15-mg tablets.
- Take at the same time each week.

Larson Late Intensification (Weeks 26–33)

Administer:

Doxorubicin _____ 30 mg/m^2 IV on days 1, 8, and 15

- **Potent vesicant**
- Available as a 2-mg/mL solution. Given IV push through side port of free-flowing IV of NS or D5W.
- Doxorubicin will form a precipitate if mixed with heparin or 5-FU.
- Given IV push through the side port of a free-flowing IV.

Vincristine _____ 2 mg IV on days 1, 8, and 15

- **Vesicant**
- Given through the side port of a free-flowing IV.
- Available in 1-mg or 2-mg/mL vials. Keep refrigerated until ready to use.

Dexamethasone _____ 10 mg/m^2 PO on days 1–14.

- Available in 4-mg tablets. Take in the morning with food.

Cyclophosphamide _____1000 mg/m^2/day over 2 hours on day 29

- Available in 500-mg, 1-, and 2-gram vials. Dilute with sterile water or bacteriostatic water for injection (sterile water or paraben preserved); shake well until solution is clear.
- Final concentration of 20 mg/mL.
- Further dilute into 250–500 mL of NS or D5W.

6-Thioguanine _____ 60 mg/m^2/day PO on days 29–42.

- Available in 40-mg tablets. Take on an empty stomach.

Cytarabine (Ara-C) _____ 75 mg/m^2 IV on days 29, 32, and 36–39

- Dilute in sterile water with benzyl alcohol and then further dilute in 50–100 mL of NS or D5W infused over 1 hour.
- Available in 100-mg, 500-mg, 1-, and 2-gram vials. Solutions are 5 mg/mL.
- Stable for up to 192 days at room temperature.

Larson Prolonged Maintenance (Continue Until 24 Months after Diagnosis)

Administer:

Vincristine _____ 2 mg IV on day 1

- Vesicant
- Given through the side port of a free-flowing IV.
- Available in 1-mg or 2-mg/mL vials. Keep refrigerated until ready to use.

Prednisone _____ 60 mg/m^2 PO on days 1–5

- Available in 5-, 10-, 20-, and 50-mg tablets. Take in the morning with food.

Methotrexate _____ 20 mg/m^2 PO on days 1, 8, 15, and 22

- Available in 5-mg, 7.5-mg, 10-mg, 12.5-mg, and 15-mg tablets.
- Take at the same time each week.

6-Mercaptopurine _____ 80 mg/m^2/day PO on days 1–28

- Take on an empty stomach; continue for a total of 30 months for complete response (50-mg tablets).

Repeat maintenance cycle every 28 days.

Major Side Effects

- Hypersensitivity/anaphylactic Reactions: Occurs in 20–30 of patients receiving L-asparaginase; the incidence increases with subsequent doses. Occurs less often with IM doses. Symptoms include chills, fever, flushing, and urticaria. Severe include tachycardia, bronchospasm, facial and tongue swelling, and hypotension and death.
- Myelosuppression: Dose limiting, onset 3–7 days. Teach self-care measures to minimize risk of infection and bleeding.
- GI Toxicities: Nausea and vomiting, anorexia, mucositis, and stomatitis. Autonomic neuropathy resulting in constipation and can lead to paralytic ileus secondary to vincristine. Reversible cholestatic jaundice may develop after 2–5 months of treatment with 6-MP.
- Cardiotoxicity: Irreversible CHF. Acute toxicity can occur within hours after administration. Have patients report dyspnea, shortness of breath, edema, or orthopnea with daunorubicin. Evaluate cardiac function at baseline, before each course, at 550-mg/m^2 cumulative dose and every 160 mg/m^2 dose thereafter. Risk of cardiac toxicity increased with prior anthracycline use, pre-existing cardiac disease, or radiotherapy encompassing heart. Cardiac toxicity with doxorubicin as well, cumulative dose 550 mg/m^2. Daily weights.
- CNS Changes: Lethargy, drowsiness, and somnolence with the L-asparaginase. Acute cerebral dysfunction with paresis, aphasia, behavioral abnormalities, confusion, and seizures in 5%–15% receiving cytarabine high-dose therapy.
- CNS Changes Due to IT MTX: Dizziness, malaise, and blurred vision. May increase CSF pressure. Keep patient supine for at least 1 hour after IT injection to prevent headache. Brain XRT after MTX can result in neurologic changes.
- Peripheral Neuropathy: Absent deep tendon reflexes, numbness, weakness, myalgias, jaw pain, diplopia, vocal cord paralysis, and metallic taste.
- GU Toxicity: Doxorubicin and daunorubicin cause discoloration of urine (pink to red, red orange for up to 48 hours after administration). Hemorrhagic cystitis, dysuria, and frequency can be seen with cyclophosphamide. Tumor lysis syndrome can occur 1–5 days after initiation of treatment.
- Skin Alterations: Total alopecia, radiation recall, and sun sensitivity.
- Reproduction: Mutagenic and potentially teratogenic, discuss contraception, and sperm banking.

Initiate antiemetic protocol: Moderately to highly emetogenic protocol.

Supportive drugs:

☐ G-CSF _____   ☐ Peg-G-CSF _____

☐ Epoetin Alfa/   ☐ Allopurinol _____
   Darbepoetin Alfa _____

☐ Antibiotic _____   ☐ Antifungal _____

Treatment schedule:

Induction therapy: Visits days 1, 2, 3, 8, 15, 18, 22, and 25

Early intensification: Visits days 1–14, 15, 18, 22, and 25

CNS prophylaxis: Visits days 1, 8, 15, 22, and 29

Late intensification: Visits days 1, 8, 15, 29, 32, 36–39

Prolonged maintenance for 24 months: Visits day 1 every 28 days

Estimated number of visits: Five to seven days first week, daily, or every other day for CBC, may require hospitalization.

Dose Calculation by: 1. _____   2. _____

_____

Physician   Date

_____

Patient Name   ID Number

_____   _____/_____/_____

Diagnosis   Ht   Wt   M^2

Hyper-CVAD Regimen: ALL

Baseline laboratory tests: CBC: Chemistry, renal and liver functions

Baseline procedures or tests: Bone marrow biopsy with cytogenetics, immunophenotyping, or cytochemistry; HLA typing (in patients considering BMT) and donor search if indicated; FLT3 mutation evaluation; lumbar puncture, if symptomatic; central line placement

Posttreatment: Bone marrow biopsy 7–14 days after chemotherapy (7 days after last dose of G-CSF 7 to document remission).

Induction Therapy

Initiate IV: NS

Premedicate: 5-HT$_3$ and dexamethasone 20-mg IVPB over 10 minutes

Administer: **Cyclophosphamide** _____ 300 mg/m^2 IV over 3 hours every 12 hours for 6 doses on days 1–3

- Available in 500-mg, 1-, and 2-gram vials. Dilute with sterile water or bacteriostatic water for injection (sterile water or paraben preserved); shake well until solution is clear.
- Final concentration of 20 mg/mL.
- Further dilute into 250–500 mL of NS or D5W.
- Reconstituted solution is stable for 24 hours at room temperature and 6 days upon refrigeration.

Mesna _____ 600 mg/m^2 IV over 24 hours on days 1–3 ending 6 hours after the last dose of cyclophosphamide

- Available in 100-mg/mL 1000-mg vials.
- May further dilute in 250–1000 cc NS or D5W.
- Diluted solution is stable for 24 hours at room temperature.
- Refrigerate and use reconstituted solution within 6 hours.

Vincristine _____ 2 mg on days 4 and 11; IV push through side arm of free-flowing IV

- **Vesicant**
- Given through the side port of a free-flowing IV.
- Available in 1-mg or 2-mg/mL vials. Keep refrigerated until ready to use.

Doxorubicin _____ 50 mg/m^2 IV on day 4

- **Potent vesicant**
- Available as a 2-mg/mL solution. Given IV push through side port of free-flowing IV of NS or D5W.
- Doxorubicin will form a precipitate if mixed with heparin or 5-FU.
- Given IV push through the side port of a free-flowing IV.

Dexamethasone _____ 40 mg PO or IV on days 1–4 and 11–14

- Available in 5-, 10-, 20-, and 50-mg tablets. Take in the morning with food.
- Available IV as 4-mg or 10-mg/mL vials. Further dilute in 50–100 cc NS, as IV push dexamethasone causes peritoneal burning while drug is injected.

Alternate cycles every 21 days with the following:

Methotrexate _____ 200 mg/m^2 IV over 2 hours, followed by

Methotrexate _____ 800 mg/m^2 IV over 24 hours on day 1

- May further dilute in D5W or NS for infusion.
- Preservative-free solution or preservative-free power reconstituted with sterile NS ONLY. Available in preservative-free solutions in 50-mg/2-mL, 100-mg/4-mL, 200-mg/8-mL, and 250-mg/10-mL vials.

Leucovorin 15 mg _____ IV every 6 hours for 8 doses, starting 24 hours after the completion of methotrexate infusion

- Available in 10-mg/ml, 50-ml, 100-mg/20-mL, and 350-mg/30-mL vials.

- Maybe given IV push or IV infusion and can be further diluted in 100 to 250 cc NS.

Cytarabine _____ 3000 mg/m^2 IV over 2 hours every 12 hours for 4 doses on days 2–3

- Reconstitute with water with benzyl alcohol and then dilute with 0.9% sodium chloride or D5W.
- Reconstituted drug is stable for 48 hours at room temperature, 7 days refrigerated (fill pump for no more than 48-hour infusion and refill)

Methylprednisolone _____ 50-mg IV bid on days 1–3

- Available in 20-mg/mL, 40-mg/mL, and 80-mg/mL vials.

Alternate four cycles of hyper-CVAD with four cycles of high-dose methotrexate and cytarabine therapy.

CNS Prophylaxis

Hyper-CVAD Regimen: ALL

Administer:

Methotrexate _____ 12 mg IT on day 2

- Preservative-free solution or preservative-free power reconstituted with sterile NS ONLY. Available in preservative-free solutions in 50-mg/2-mL, 100-mg/4-mL, 200-mg/8-mL, and 250-mg/10-mL vials.

Cytarabine _____ IT on day 8

- Dilute in sterile water without preservative for intrathecal treatment.
- Available in 100-mg vial, dilute with sterile saline.

Repeat with each cycle of chemotherapy, depending on the risk of CNS disease.

Major Side Effects

- Bone Marrow Depression: Dose-limiting toxicity.
- GI Toxicities: Nausea and vomiting, anorexia; impaired skin/mucosal changes including maculopapular rash, 6–12 hours after infusion, stomatitis at days 7–10. Total alopecia at days 10–14.
- Cardiotoxicity: Dose limit 450–550 mg/m^2; arrhythmias and/or EKG changes, pericarditis or myocarditis. Usually transient and asymptomatic.
- GU Toxicities: Discoloration of urine from pink to red up to 48 hours.
- Neurotoxicity: At high doses includes cerebellar toxicity, including nystagmus, dysarthria, ataxia, slurred speech, or difficulty with fine-motor coordination, lethargy, or somnolence. Patients with rapidly rising creatinine caused by tumor lysis syndrome or neurotoxicity should discontinue the high-dose cytarabine.
- Saline or steroid drops to both eyes may be indicated for 24 hours after completion of high cytarabine.
- Tumor lysis syndrome occurring 1–5 days after initiation of treatment; treat with hydration and allopurinol.
- Reproduction: mutagenic and potentially teratogenic.

Supportive Care

Recommended as part of treatment plan

☐ Ciprofloxacin: 500 mg PO bid ☐ Fluconazole: 200 mg/day PO

☐ Acyclovir: 200 mg PO bid ☐ G-CSF: 10 μg/kg/day starting 24 hours after the end of chemotherapy (i.e., on day 5 of hyper-CVAD therapy and on day 4 of high-dose methotrexate and cytarabine therapy)

Initiate antiemetic protocol: Moderately to highly emetogenic protocol.

Treatment schedule: 4–5 hours on days 1–3 and 2 hours on day 4

Estimated number of visits: May require hospitalization; daily CBC.

Dose Calculation by: 1. _____   2. _____

_____   _____

Physician   Date

_____   _____

Patient Name   ID Number

_____   _____ / _____ / _____

Diagnosis   Ht   Wt   M^2

Single-Agent Regimens

Clofarabine: 52 mg/m2 IV for 5 days

Baseline laboratory test:	CBC: Chemistry, renal and liver functions
Monitor:	CBC, renal and liver functions throughout 5-day therapy
Baseline procedures or tests:	Bone marrow biopsy
Posttreatment:	Bone marrow biopsy
Initiate IV:	NS
Premedicate:	5-HT$_3$ and dexamethasone 20-mg IV
Administer:	**Clofarabine** _____ 52 mg/m^2 IV over 2 hours daily for 5 days with continuous IV fluids throughout the dosing course

- Available in 20-mL vial, 1 mg/mL.
- Withdraw drug using sterile 0.2 μm syringe filter.
- Dilute with NS or D5W or NS prior to infusion.
- Stable for 24 hours.

Major Side Effects

- Bone Marrow Depression: Dose-limiting toxicity. Febrile neutropenia occurs in 57% of patients, pyrexia in 41%. Infections include bacteremia, cellulites, herpes simplex, oral candidiasis, pneumonia, sepsis, and staphylococcal infections.
- Potential for dehydration, hypotension, and capillary leak syndrome
- GU Toxicities: Rapid lysis of tumor cells. Use allopurinol and adequate hydration to prevent renal toxicities.
- GI Toxicities: Nausea and vomiting occur in 75% and 83% of patients respectively, can be controlled with combination antiemetics. Anorexia occurs in 1/3 of patients and diarrhea is frequent, affecting 50% of patients. Constipation affects 21%. Hepatotoxicity and jaundice occur in 15% of patients.
- Skin Integrity: maculopapular rash, with or without fever, myalgias, bone pain, occasional chest pain, conjunctivitis, and malaise (cytarabine syndrome) may occur 6–12 hours after administration; corticosteroids used to treat/prevent syndrome. Mucosal inflammation and ulceration of anus/rectum may occur. Alopecia occurs.
- Edema, Fatigue, Lethargy and Pain: Edema 20%, fatigue 36%, injection site pain 14%, pain 19%, arthralgias 11%, pruritis 47%, pain in limbs and plantar erythrodysesthesia syndrome 13%.
- Reproduction: Drug is fetotoxic. All patients should be instructed on proper birth control and female patients should not breast feed.

Initiate antiemetic protocol:	Moderately to highly emetogenic protocol.

Supportive drugs:

☐ neupogen _____	☐ filgrastim _____
☐ aranesp _____	☐ procrit _____
☐ Allopurinol _____	☐ Antibiotic _____
☐ Antifungal _____	

Treatment schedule:	Chair time 3 hour on days 1–5 and continuous hydration over 24 hours, may require hospitalization
Estimated number of visits:	5 days in the first week; daily for blood counts.
	Repeat cycle every 2–6 weeks after recovery of all baseline organ functions.

Dose Calculation by: 1. _____   2. _____

_____   _____
Physician   Date

_____   _____
Patient Name   ID Number

_____   _____/_____/_____
Diagnosis   Ht   Wt M^2

LEUKEMIA

Acute Myelogenous Leukemia

Induction Regimens

Ara-C + Daunorubicin (7 + 3)[1,208] **318**

Cytarabine: 100 mg/m^2/day IV continuous infusion on days 1–7
Daunorubicin: 45 mg/m^2 IV on days 1–3

Ara-C + Idarubicin[1,209] **320**

Cytarabine: 100 mg/m^2/day IV continuous infusion on days 1–7
Idarubicin: 12 mg/m^2 IV on days 1–3

Ara-C + Doxorubicin[1,210] **322**

Cytarabine: 100 mg/m^2/day IV continuous infusion on days 1–7
Doxorubicin: 30 mg/m^2 IV on days 1–3

Consolidation Regimens

Ara-C + Daunorubicin (5 + 2)[1,215] **324**

Cytarabine: 100 mg/m^2/day IV continuous infusion on days 1–5
Daunorubicin: 45 mg/m^2 IV on days 1 and 2

Ara-C + Idarubicin[1,215] **326**

Cytarabine: 100-mg/m^2 IV continuous infusion on days 1–5
Idarubicin: 13-mg/m^2 IV on days 1 and 2
Repeat cycle every 21–28 days.

Single-Agent Regimens

Cladribine[1,216] **327**

Cladribine: 0.1-mg/kg/day IV continuous infusion on days 1–7

High-Dose Cytarabine **328**

Cytarabine: 3,000-mg/m^2 IV over 3 hours, every 12 hours on days 1, 3, and 5
Repeat cycle every 28 days.[1,217]

Gemtuzumab (Mylotarg) **330**

Gemtuzumab: 9-mg/m^2 IV as a 2-hour infusion

Repeat with a second dose 14 days after administration of the first dose.[1,219]

Premedicate with diphenhydramine 50-mg PO and acetaminophen 650–1000 mg PO at 1 hour before drug infusion. After the infusion is completed, give two additional doses of acetaminophen 650–1000 mg PO every 4 hours.

Relapsed AML

MV (Mitoxantrone + Etoposide)[1,213] **331**

Mitoxantrone: 10 mg/m^2/day IV push over 3 minutes on days 1–5

Etoposide: 100 mg/m^2/day IV over 1–2 hours on days 1–5

FLAG[1,214] **333**

Fludarabine: 30 mg/m^2/day IV over 30 minutes on days 1–5

Cytarabine: 2000 mg/m^2/day over 4 hours after completion of fludarabine on days 1–5

Neupogen: 5 mcg/kg/d day 0 (24 hours prior to starting chemotherapy until ANC recovery).

Induction Regimens

Ara-C + Daunorubicin (7 + 3)

Baseline laboratory tests:	CBC: Chemistry, renal and liver functions
Baseline procedures or tests:	Bone marrow biopsy, central line placement, MUGA if indicated
Initiate IV:	NS
Premedicate:	5-HT$_3$ and dexamethasone 20-mg IVPB over 10 minutes
Administer:	**Cytarabine** _____ 100-mg/m^2/day IV continuous infusion on days 1–7

- Available in 100-, 500-, 1000-, and 5000-mg multidose vials.
- Dilute in sterile water with benzyl alcohol and then further dilute with 50–100 mL of NS or D5W.
- For IT use or high dose, use preservative-free NS and use immediately.
- Stable 48 hours at room temperature and 7 days refrigerated.
- IV hydration at 150 per mL per hour with or without alkalinization, oral allopurinol, strict I & O, and daily weights.

Daunorubicin _____ 45-mg/m^2 IV on days 1–3.

- Given through the side port of a free-flowing IV. Infuse over 1 hour only if the patient has a central line.
- **Vesicant**
- Available in 20-mg vials with 100-mg mannitol for IV use. Add 4-mL sterile water to vial for concentration of 5 mg/mL. Reconstituted solution is stable for 24 hours at room temperature and 48 hours with refrigeration. Should protect from sunlight.
- Further dilute with 10–15 mL of NS.
- Incompatible with heparin and dexamethasone.

Major Side Effects

- Bone Marrow Depression: Dose-limiting toxicity.
- GI Toxicities: Nausea and vomiting in moderately emetogenic, anorexia; mucositis and diarrhea common within the first week, but not dose limiting.
- Skin Alteration: Hyperpigmentation of nails, rarely skin rash and urticaria. Radiation recall. Photosensitivity. Alopecia.
- Cardiotoxicity: Similar to but less severe than doxorubicin. EKG changes, pericarditis, and/or myocarditis. Usually transient and asymptomatic. Risk increases with dose of more than 550 mg/m^2.
- GU Toxicity: Red-orange discoloration of urine for 1–2 days after administration of daunorubicin.
- Neurotoxicity: At high doses includes cerebellar toxicity, including seizures, nystagmus, dysarthria, ataxia, slurred speech, or difficulty with fine-motor coordination, lethargy, or somnolence. Observe neurologic status, handwriting, or gait before and during cytarabine therapy.
- Ocular: Conjunctivitis can occur. Treat with corticosteroid eye drops.
- Tumor lysis syndrome occurring 1–5 days after initiation of treatment. Allopurinol and vigorous hydration recommended.
- Reproduction: Pregnancy category D. Breast feeding should be avoided.

Initiate antiemetic protocol:	Moderately to highly emetogenic protocol.
Supportive drugs:	☐ G-CSF_____ ☐ Peg-G-CSF_____ ☐ Epoetin Alfa/ Darbepoetin Alfa_____ ☐ Allopurinol_____ ☐ Antibiotic_____ ☐ Antifungal_____
Treatment schedule:	Chair time 1 hour on days 1–3, 30 minutes for pump refill days. Cycle does not repeat.
Estimated number of visits:	5–7 days first week, daily or every other day for blood counts. Request 21 days per treatment; may require hospitalization.

Dose Calculation by: 1. _____   2. _____

_____   _____
Physician   Date

_____   _____
Patient Name   ID Number

_____   _____ / _____ / _____
Diagnosis   Ht   Wt   M²

Ara-C + Idarubicin

Baseline laboratory tests:	CBC: Chemistry, renal and liver functions
Baseline procedures or tests:	Bone marrow biopsy, central line placement, MUGA if indiated
Initiate IV:	NS
Premedicate:	5-HT$_3$ and dexamethasone 20-mg IVPB over 10 minutes
Administer:	**Idarubicin** _____ 12-mg/m^2 slow IV push on days 1–3

- **Vesicant**
- Reconstitute with sodium chloride; final concentration 1 mg/1 mL.
- Further dilute in 100–250 cc of NS. Reconstituted solution stable for 3 days at room temperature.
- If patient has central line, infusion over 1 hour may cause less nausea and vomiting.

Cytarabine _____ 100-mg/m^2/day IV continuous infusion on days 1–7

OR

Cytarabine _____ 25-mg/m^2 IV push, followed by

Cytarabine _____ 200- mg/m^2/day IV continuous infusion on days 1–5. Irritant.

- Reconstitute with water with benzyl alcohol and then dilute with 0.9% sodium chloride or 5% dextrose.
- Reconstituted drug is stable for 48 hours at room temperature, 7 days refrigerated (fill pump for no more than 48-hour infusion and refill).
- Incompatible with heparin.

Major Side Effects	- Bone Marrow Depression: Dose-limiting toxicity.

- GI Toxicities: Nausea and vomiting moderately emetogenic. Anorexia, stomatitis, mucositis, and diarrhea common.
- Skin Alterations: Alopecia 77%; maculopapular rash 6–12 hours after infusion.
- Cardiotoxicity similar to but less severe than doxorubicin and daunorubicin. Idarubicin cummulative doses of > 150 mg/m^2 associated with decreased LVEF.
- GU Toxicity: Red-orange discoloration of urine for 1–2 days after administration of daunorubicin.
- Neurotoxicity: At high doses includes cerebellar toxicity, including seizures, nystagmus, dysarthria, ataxia, slurred speech, or difficulty with fine-motor coordination, lethargy, or somnolence.
- Tumor lysis syndrome occurring 1–5 days after the initiation of treatment. Allopurinol and vigorous hydration recommended.
- Reproduction: Mutagenic and potentially teratogenic.

Initiate antiemetic protocol:	Moderately to highly emetogenic protocol.
Supportive drugs:	☐ Neulasta _____ ☐ Neupogen _____
	☐ Procrit/Aranesp _____ ☐ Allopurinol _____
	☐ Antibiotic _____ ☐ Antifungal _____
Treatment schedule:	Chair time 1–2 hours on days 1–3, 30 minutes for pump refill days. Repeat cycle until remission (usually two to three cycles).
Estimated number of visits:	Five to seven days first week, daily or every other day for blood counts. Request 21 days per treatment; may require hospitalization.

Dose Calculation by: 1. _____   2. _____

_____   _____
Physician   Date

_____   _____
Patient Name   ID Number

_____   _____ / _____ / _____
Diagnosis   Ht   Wt   M²

Ara-C + Doxorubicin

Baseline laboratory and tests:	CBC: Chemistry, renal and liver functions
Baseline procedures or tests:	Bone marrow biopsy with cytogenetics, immunophenotyping, or cytochemistry; HLA typing (in patients considering BMT) and donor search if indicated; FLT3 mutation evaluation; lumbar puncture, if symptomatic; central line placement, MUGA
Posttreatment:	Bone marrow biopsy 7–14 days after chemotherapy (patient should be off G-CSF 7 days before bone marrow biopsy to document remission).
Initiate IV:	NS
Premedicate:	5-HT$_3$ and dexamethasone 20-mg IVPB over 10 minutes
Administer:	**Cytarabine** _____ 100-mg/m^2/day IV continuous infusion on days 1–7

- Dilute in sterile water with benzyl alcohol and then further dilute with 50–100 mL of 0.9% sodium. Stable 48 hours at room temperature and 7 days refrigerated chloride or D5W.
- IV hydration at 150 per mL per hour with or without alkalinization, oral allopurinol, strict I & O, and daily weights.

Doxorubicin _____ 30-mg/m^2 IV on days 1–3.

- Given through side port of free-flowing IV.
- **Vesicant**
- Available in 10-, 20-, 50-, 100-, and 150-mg vials and 200-mg multidose solution. Final concentration 2 mg/mL. May be further diluted in NS for prolonged infusions.

Major Side Effects

- Bone Marrow Depression: Dose-limiting toxicity. Daily CBC during chemotherapy and then every other day until WBCs are more than 500 per mcl, platelet transfusions as indicated.
- Chemistry Profile: Electrolytes, Cr, BUN, uric acid, and PO$_4$ daily to evaluate tumor lysis.
- GI Toxicities: Nausea and vomiting, anorexia; stomatitis, mucositis, and diarrhea.
- Skin Alterations: Total alopecia. Hyperpigmentation of nails, rarely skin rash and urticaria. Radiation recall.
- Cardiotoxicity: Dose limit 550 mg/m^2; EKG changes, pericarditis, and or myocarditis. Usually transient and mostly asymptomatic.
- GU Toxicities: Discoloration of urine from pink to red up to 48 hours. Hemorrhagic cystitis: Irritation of bladder wall capillaries occurs; preventable with appropriate hydration.
- Neurotoxicity: At high doses includes cerebellar toxicity, including nystagmus, dysarthria, ataxia, slurred speech, or difficulty with fine-motor coordination, lethargy, or somnolence. Patients with rapidly rising creatinine caused by tumor lysis syndrome or neurotoxicity should discontinue the high-dose cytarabine. Assess handwriting or gait before and during treatment.
- Ocular: Saline or steroid drops to both eyes may be indicated for 24 hours after completion of high cytarabine.
- Tumor lysis syndrome occurring 1–5 days after initiation of treatment; treat with hydration and allopurinol.
- Reproduction: mutagenic and potentially teratogenic.

Initiate antiemetic protocol:	Moderately to highly emetogenic protocol.
Supportive drugs:	☐ pegfilgrastim (Neulasta) ☐ filgrastim (Neupogen)
	☐ epoetin alfa (Procrit)/ darbepoetin alfa (Aranesp) ☐ Allopurinol _____
	☐ Antibiotic _____ ☐ Antifungal _____
Treatment schedule:	Chair time 1 hour on days 1–3 and 30 minutes for pump refill days
Estimated number of visits:	3–5 days on the first week, daily or every other day for blood counts

Dose Calculation by: 1. _____   2. _____

_____

Physician   Date

_____

Patient Name   ID Number

_____   _____ / _____ / _____

Diagnosis   Ht   Wt   M²

Consolidation Regimens

Ara-C + Daunorubicin (5 + 2)

Baseline laboratory tests:	CBC: Chemistry, renal and liver functions
Baseline procedures or tests:	Bone marrow biopsy, central line placement, MUGA if cardiac changes with induction therapy. Dose reductions with impaired hepatic functions.
Initiate IV:	NS
Premedicate:	5-HT$_3$ and dexamethasone 20-mg IVPB over 10 minutes
Administer:	**Cytarabine** _____ 100-mg/m^2/day IV continuous infusion on days 1–5

- Available in 100-, 500-, 1000-, and 5000-mg multidose vials. Dilute in sterile water with benzyl alcohol and then further dilute with 50–100 mL of NS or D5W. For IT use or high dose, immediately use preservative-free NS. Stable 48 hours at room temperature and 7 days refrigerated.
- IV hydration at 150/mL per hour with or without alkalinization. Oral allopurinol, strict I & O, and daily weights.

Daunorubicin _____ 45-mg/m^2 IV on days 1 and 2. Given through the side port of a free-flowing IV. Infuse over 1 hour only if the patient has a central line.

- **Vesicant**
- Available in 20-mg vials with 100-mg mannitol for IV use. Add 4 mL of sterile water to vial for concentration of 5 mg/mL. Reconstituted solution is stable for 24 hours at room temperature and 48 hours with refrigeration. Should protect from sunlight.
- Further dilute with 10–15 mL of NS.
- Incompatible with heparin and dexamethasone.

Major Side Effects	

- Bone Marrow Depression: Dose-limiting toxicity
- GI Toxicities: Nausea and vomiting in moderately emetogenic, anorexia; mucositis and diarrhea common within the first week, but not dose limiting.
- Skin Alteration: Hyperpigmentation of nails, rarely skin rash and urticaria. Radiation recall. Photosensitivity. Alopecia.
- Cardiotoxicity: Similar to but less severe than doxorubicin. EKG changes, pericarditis, and/or myocarditis. Usually transient and asymptomatic. Risk increases with dose > 550 mg/m^2.
- GU Toxicity: Red-orange discoloration of urine for 1–2 days after administration of daunorubicin.
- Neurotoxicity: At high doses includes cerebellar toxicity, including nystagmus, dysarthria, ataxia, slurred speech, or difficulty with fine-motor coordination, lethargy, or somnolence. Observe neurologic status, handwriting, or gait before and during cytarabine therapy.
- Ocular: Conjunctivitis can occur. Treat with corticosteroid eye drops.
- Tumor lysis syndrome occurring 1–5 days after initiation of treatment. Allopurinol and vigorous hydration recommended.
- Reproduction: Mutagenic and potentially teratogenic.

Initiate antiemetic protocol:	Moderately to highly emetogenic protocol.
Supportive drugs:	☐ Neulasta _____ ☐ Neupogen _____
	☐ Procrit/Aranesp _____ ☐ Allopurinol_____
	☐ Antibiotic _____ ☐ Antifungal _____
Treatment schedule:	Chair time 2 hours on days 1–2 and 30 minutes for pump refill days; given once after an induction regimen has been used.

Dose Calculation by: 1. _____   2. _____

_____

Physician _____   Date _____

Patient Name _____   ID Number _____

_____/_____/_____

Diagnosis _____   Ht _____ Wt _____ M^2 _____

Ara-C + Idarubicin

Baseline laboratories:	CBC: Chemistry, renal and liver functions
Baseline procedures or tests:	Bone marrow biopsy, central line placement
Initiate IV:	NS
Premedicate:	5-HT$_3$ and dexamethasone 20-mg IVPB over 10 minutes.
Administer:	**Idarubicin** _____ 13 mg/m^2 slow IV push on days 1 and 2.

- **Vesicant**

- Reconstitute with sodium chloride, final concentration 1 mg/1 mL.

- If patient has central line, infusion over 1 hour may cause less nausea and vomiting. Further dilute in 100–250 cc of NS.

Cytarabine _____ 100-mg/m^2/day IV continuous infusion on days 1–5

- IV continuous infusion days 1–5 (irritant).

- Reconstitute with water with benzyl alcohol and then dilute with NS or D5W.

- Reconstituted drug is stable for 48 hours at room temperature or 7 days refrigerated (fill pump for no more than 48 hour infusion and refill).

Major Side Effects

- Bone Marrow Depression: Dose limiting.

- GI Toxicities: Nausea and vomiting moderate to highly emetogenic, anorexia.

- Cardiotoxicity similar to but less severe than doxorubicin and daunorubicin. Idarubicin cumulative dose > 150 mg/m^2.

- GU Toxicities: Red-orange discoloration of urine for 1–2 days after administration of daunorubicin.

- Neurotoxicity: At high doses includes cerebellar toxicity, including seizures, nystagmus, dysarthria, ataxia, slurred speech, or difficulty with fine-motor coordination, lethargy, or somnolence.

- Tumor lysis syndrome occurring 1–5 days after initiation of treatment.

- Reproduction: Mutagenic and potentially teratogenic; discuss contraception and sperm banking.

Initiate antiemetic protocol:	Moderately to highly emetogenic protocol

Supportive drugs:

☐ G-CSF _____   ☐ Peg G-CSF _____
☐ Procrit/Aranesp _____   ☐ Allopurinol _____
☐ Antibiotic _____   ☐ Antifungal _____

Treatment schedule: Chair time 1–2 hours on days 1–3, 30 minutes for pump refill days. Repeat cycle until remission (usually two to three cycles).

Estimated number of visits: Five days in the first week and then daily or every other day for blood counts. Request 21–28 days per treatment, may require hospitalization.

Dose Calculation by: 1. _____ 2. _____

_____
Physician

_____
Date

_____
Patient Name

_____
ID Number

_____
Diagnosis

_____/_____/_____
Ht   Wt   M^2

Single-Agent Regimens

Cladribine (Leustatin)

Baseline laboratory tests:	CBC: Chemistry, renal and liver functions
Baseline procedures or tests:	Bone marrow biopsy, central line placement
Administer:	**Cladribine** _____ 0.1 mg/kg/day continuous infusion on days 1–7, one course

- Dilute 1:1 concentrated liquid in 500 mL of 0.9% NS per day. Unstable in D5W.
- Use a 22-μm filter when preparing the solution. Stable when diluted for 24 hours or refrigerated for 8 hours.

Major Side Effects

- Bone Marrow Depression: Nadir at 7–14 days, neutropenia is more common than anemia or thrombocytopenia. Increased risk for opportunistic infections, including fungal, herpes, and *Pneumocystis carinii*. Teach self-care measures to minimize risk of infection and bleeding.
- Tumor fever associated with fatigue, malaise, maligns, and arthralgias and chills.
- GI Toxicities: Nausea and vomiting mildly emetogenic, anorexia. Constipation and abdominal pain.
- Neurotoxicity: Headache, insomnia, and dizziness.
- Tumor lysis syndrome rare even with high tumor burden.
- Reproduction: Potentially mutagenic and teratogenic, discuss contraception and sperm banking.

Initiate antiemetic protocol:	Mildly emetogenic protocol.
Supportive drugs:	☐ G-CSF _____ ☐ Peg G-CSF _____
	☐ Procrit/Aranesp _____ ☐ Allopurinol _____
	☐ Antibiotic _____ ☐ Antifungal _____
Treatment schedule:	Chair time 1 hour on days 1–3, 30 minutes for pump refill days. Repeat cycle until remission (usually two to three cycles).
Estimated number of visits:	Seven days in the first week and then daily or every other day for blood counts.

Dose Calculation by: 1. _____ 2. _____

_____

Physician

_____

Patient Name

_____

Diagnosis

Date _____

ID Number _____

_____/_____/_____
Ht   Wt   M^2

High-Dose Cytarabine (HiDAC)

Baseline laboratory tests:	CBC: Chemistry, renal and liver functions
Baseline procedures or tests:	Bone marrow biopsy, central line placement
Posttreatment:	Bone marrow biopsy 7–14 days after chemotherapy (patient should be off G-CSF 7 days before bone marrow biopsy to document remission).
Initiate IV:	NS
Premedicate:	5-HT$_3$ and dexamethasone 20-mg IV
	Saline, methylcellulose, or steroid eye drops, OU q6h, with cytarabine and continuing 48–72 hours after the last cytarabine dose is completed.

Administer:

Cytarabine _____ 3000-mg/m^2/day IV over 1–2 hours every 12 hours on days 1, 2, and 3
OR

Cytarabine _____ 3000-mg/m^2/day IV over 1–2 hours every 12 hours on days 1, 3, and 5
OR

Cytarabine _____ 3000-mg/m^2/day IV over 1–2 hours every 12 hours on days 1–6.
OR

Cytarabine _____ 2000-mg/m^2/day IV over 1–2 hours every 12 hours on days 1–6.

- Dilute in sterile water with benzyl alcohol and then further dilute with 50–100 mL of NS or D5W.
- IV hydration at 150/mL per hour with/without alkalinization, oral allopurinol; strict I & O, daily weights. Stable 48 hours at room temperature and 7 days refrigerated.

Drug interactions: Decreases efficacy of gentamicin and digoxin.

Major Side Effects

- Bone Marrow Depression: Nadir biphasic, WBCs fall within 24 hours, nadir on day 7–10, platelets drop by day 5, nadir on day 15–24, with recovery in 10 days.
- Daily CBC during chemotherapy and then every other day until WBCs > 500 per mcl, platelet transfusions as indicated.
- Chemistry Profile: electrolytes, creatinine, BUN, uric acid, and PO$_4$ daily during treatment to evaluate tumor lysis.
- GI Toxicities: Nausea and vomiting, anorexia; impaired skin/mucosal changes including maculopapular rash, 6–12 hours after infusion, stomatitis at days 7–10, total alopecia on days 10–14.
- Neurotoxicity: At high doses includes cerebellar toxicity, including seizures, nystagmus, dysarthria, ataxia, slurred speech, or difficulty with fine-motor coordination, lethargy, or somnolence. Assess baseline neurologic status and cerebellar function (coordinated movements such as handwriting and gait) before and during therapy. If cerebellar toxicity develops, treatment must be discontinued.
- Patients with rapidly rising creatinine due to tumor lysis syndrome or neurotoxicity should discontinue the high-dose cytarabine.
- Tumor Lysis Syndrome: Occurs 1–5 days after initiation of treatment. Pretreat with hydration and allopurinol.
- Reproduction: Mutagenic and potentially teratogenic. Discuss contraception and sperm banking.

Initiate antiemetic protocol:	Moderately to highly emetogenic protocol.
Supportive drugs:	☐ G-CSF _____ ☐ Peg-G-CSF _____
	☐ Epoetin Alfa/ Darbepoetin Alfa _____ ☐ Allopurinol _____
	☐ Antibiotic _____ ☐ Antifungal _____
Treatment schedule:	Repeat cycle every 28 days or 1 week after marrow recovery.
Estimated number of visits:	Patients usually require hospitalization. Daily or every other day for blood counts.

Dose Calculation by: 1. _____   2. _____

_____

Physician

_____

Patient Name

_____

Diagnosis

_____

Date

_____

ID Number

_____ / _____ / _____

Ht   Wt   M²

Gemtuzumab (Mylotarg)

Baseline laboratory tests:	CBC: Chemistry
Posttreatment:	CBC at least weekly or BID
Initiate IV:	9NS
Premedicate:	5-HT$_3$ and dexamethasone 20-mg IV
	1 hour before treatment: Diphenhydramine 50-mg PO and acetaminophen 650–1000 mg PO
	Acetaminophen 650–1000 mg at completions of infusion and then Q 4 hours

Administer: **Gemtuzumab** _____ 9-mg/m^2 IV as a 2-hour infusion

- Available in 5-mg vials. Dilute in 5-mL sterile water to a final concentration of 1 mg/mL, and mix gently DO NOT SHAKE.
- Diluted solution is stable for 8 hours with refrigeration and when protected from light. Further dilute into a 100-mL bag of NS, and place the bag in an ultraviolet-protected bag. Use the medication immediately.
- Use a 1.2-micron filter. Do not administer by IVP or bolus.

Major Side Effects

- Myelosuppression; dose-limiting toxicity. With neutropenia and thrombocytopenia.
- Infusion-related Symptoms: Fever, chills, nausea, and vomiting. Urticaria, skin rash, fatigue, headache, diarrhea, dyspnea, and/or hypotension. Usually observed in the first 2 hours after infusion. Transient hypotension can be observed up to 6 hours after the infusion.
- Gastrointestinal Toxicities: Nausea and vomiting is mild to moderate. Mucositis and stomatitis mild. Transient increases in LFTs. Diarrhea seen in 38% of patients.
- Infusion Reaction: Flushing, facial swelling, headache, dyspnea, and/or hypotension can be related to rate of infusion.
- Reproduction: Pregnancy category D: Breastfeeding should be avoided.

Initiate antiemetic protocol: Moderately emetogenic.

Supportive drugs:

☐ G-CSF_____   ☐ Peg-G-CSF _____
☐ Procrit/Aranesp _____   ☐ Allopurinol_____
☐ Antibiotic _____   ☐ Antifungal _____

Treatment schedule: Repeat with a second dose 14 days after administration of the first dose.

Estimated number of visits: Two visits per week for 12 weeks.

Dose Calculation by: 1. _____   2. _____

_____
Physician

_____
Patient Name

_____
Diagnosis

_____
Date

_____
ID Number

_____/ _____/ _____
Ht   Wt   M^2

Relapse AML

MV (Mitoxantrone [M], Etoposide [V])

Baseline laboratory and test:	CBC: Chemistry, renal and liver functions
Baseline procedures or tests:	Bone marrow biopsy, central line placement, MUGA
Initiate IV:	NS
Premedicate:	5-HT$_3$ and dexamethasone 20-mg IV
Administer:	**Mitoxantrone** _____ 10-mg/m^2/day IV days 1–5, IV push over 3 minutes

OR

IV infusion over 30 minutes.

- **Vesicant**
- Supplied as 2-mg/mL solution. Should be diluted in at least 50 mL with either NS or D5W. Multimode vial stable for 7 days at room temperature or 14 days refrigerated. Mitoxantrone is not a vesicant, but rare cases of extravasation have been reported.

Etoposide _____ 100-mg/m^2/day IV over 1 hour on days 1–5

- (VePesid) 5 cc/100 mg; Etopophos reconstitute with 5–10 mL on NS, D5W, sterile water or bacteriostatic sterile water, or bacteriostatic NS with benzyl alcohol to 20 or 10 mg/mL, respectively. Further dilute to a final concentration NS or D5W to 0.1 mg/mL. Reconstituted solution is stable for 24 hours at room temperature or refrigerated.

Major Side Effects

- Myelosuppression: Dose-limiting toxicity.
- Hypersensitivity Reaction: Etoposide can result in chills, fever bronchospasm, tachycardia, facial and tongue swelling, and hypotension
- GI Toxicities: Nausea and vomiting, anorexia; mucositis, diarrhea
- Cardiotoxicity: CHF with decreased LVEF (less than 3%), increased cardiotoxicity with cumulative dose > 180 mg/m^2.
- GU Toxicity: Urine will be green blue for 24 hours; sclera may become discolored blue.
- Skin Alterations: Radiation recall. Blue discoloration of fingernails and sclera for 1–2 days after treatment.
- Alopecia: Total hair loss.
- Tumor lysis syndrome, consider treating with hydration and allopurinol.
- Reproduction: mutagenic and potentially teratogenic, discuss contraception and sperm banking.

Initiate antiemetic protocol:	Moderately to highly emetogenic protocol.
Supportive drugs:	☐ G-CSF _____ ☐ Peg-G-CSF _____
	☐ Epoetin Alfa/ Darbepoetin Alfa _____ ☐ Allopurinol _____
	☐ Antibiotic _____ ☐ Antifungal _____
Treatment schedule:	Chair time 2 hours on days 1–5; second cycle may be given if remission is not achieved
Estimated number of visits:	Days 1–4 in the first week, daily or every other day for blood counts; request 21 days per treatment, may require hospitalization.

Dose Calculation by: 1. _____   2. _____

_____   _____
Physician   Date

_____   _____
Patient Name   ID Number

_____   _____ / _____ / _____
Diagnosis   Ht   Wt M^2

FLAG: Fludarabine, Cytarabine(Ara-C), G-CSF

Baseline laboratory tests:	CBC: Chemistry, renal and liver functions
Baseline procedures or tests:	Bone marrow biopsy, central line placement
Initiate IV:	NS
Premedicate:	5-HT$_3$ and dexamethasone 20-mg IV
Administer:	**Fludarabine** _____ 30-mg/m^2/day IV on days 1–5 over 30 minutes

* Dilute with 2 mL of sterile water for a final concentration of 25 mg/mL.

* Further dilute in 100 mL of NS or D5W. Drug should be used within 8 hours.

Cytarabine _____ 2000-mg/m^2/day IV on days 1–5 over 4 hours, given 3.5 hours after the end of the fludarabine infusion.

* Dilute in sterile water with benzyl alcohol and then further dilute with 50–100 mL of 0.9% sodium chloride or D5W. IV hydration at 150 mL per hour with or without alkalinization, oral allopurinol, strict I & O, daily weights. Stable 48 hours at room temperature and 7 days refrigerated.

G-CSF _____ 5-mcg/kg SQ on day 0 and then 300-mcg SQ until ANC recovery

Major Side Effects

* Myelosuppression: Dose-limiting toxicity

* Neurotoxicity: Observed with high doses. Presents as weakness, agitation, confusion, progressive encephalopathy cortecal blindness, seizures and/or coma.

* Pulmonary Toxicities: Pneumonia occurs in 16%–22% of patients. Pulmonary hypersensitivity reaction characterized by dyspnea, cough, and interstitial pulmonary infiltrates.

* Immunosuppression: Decrease in CD4+ and CD8+, increasing risk for opportunistic infections (fungus, herpes, and *Pneumocystis carinii*).

* Patients with rapidly rising creatinine caused by tumor lysis syndrome or neurotoxicity should discontinue the high-dose cytarabine, tumor lysis syndrome consider treating with hydration and allopurinol.

* GI Toxicities: Nausea and vomiting, anorexia; mucositis, diarrhea.

* Alopecia: Total hair loss. Maculopapular rash, erythema, and pruritus.

* Reproduction: mutagenic and potentially teratogenic, discuss contraception and sperm banking.

Initiate antiemetic protocol:	Highly emetogenic protocol.
Supportive drugs:	☐ G-CSF _____ ☐ Peg-G-CSF _____
	☐ Epoetin Alfa/ ☐ Allopurinol _____
	Darbepoetin Alfa _____
	☐ Antibiotic _____ ☐ Antifungal _____
Treatment schedule:	Chair time 1–2 hours on days 1–3; the second cycle may be given if remission is not achieved.
Estimated number of visits:	Days 1–4 in the first week and daily or every other day for blood counts. Request 21 days per treatment, may require hospitalization.

Dose Calculation by: 1. _____ 2. _____

_____

Physician   Date

_____

Patient Name   ID Number

_____

Diagnosis   Ht _____ / Wt _____ / M^2 _____

LEUKEMIA

Acute Promyelocytic Leukemia (APL)

Single Agents

Induction: 0.15-mg/kg/d IV until bone marrow remission, not to exceed 60 doses

Consolidation: 0.15 mg/kg/d for 25 doses over a period of up to 5 weeks

ATRA: 45-mg/m^2 PO daily in one to two divided doses

ATRA: 45 mg/m^2 PO daily

Idarubicin: 12 mg/m^2 IV on days 2, 4, 6, and 8

Single Agents

Arsenic Trioxide (Trisenox)

Baseline laboratory tests:	CBC: Chemistry panel (including Mg^{2+}) and LFTs,
Baseline procedures or tests:	12-lead EKG
Initiate IV:	Normal saline
Premedicate:	Oral $5HT_3$ or phenothiazine if nausea occurs.
Administer:	Induction:

Arsenic Trioxide _____(0.15 mg/kg/d) IV daily until bone marrow remission, not to exceed 60 doses

Consolidation:

Arsenic Trioxide _____(0.15 mg/kg/d) IV daily for 25 doses over a period of up to 5 weeks

- Available in 10-mL, single-use ampules containing 10 mg of arsenic trioxide, at a concentration of 1 mg/mL.
- Further dilute in 100–250 cc D5W or 0.9% sodium chloride injection, USP.
- Give IV over 1–2 hours (or up to 4 hours if acute vasomotor reactions occur).
- Drug is chemically and physically stable for 24 hours at room temperature and 48 hours when refrigerated. However, does not contain any preservatives, so unused portions should be discarded.

Major Side Effects:

- Vasomotor Reactions: Symptoms include flushing, tachycardia, dizziness, and lightheadedness. Increasing the infusion time to 4 hours usually resolves these symptoms. Stop infusion for tachycardia and/or hypotension. Resume at decreased rate after resolution. Headaches can also occur, treat with acetaminophen as needed.
- APL Differentiation Syndrome: Characterized by fever, dyspnea, weight gain, pulmonary infiltrates, and pleural or pericardial effusions, with or without leukocytosis. Can be fatal. At the first suggestion, high-dose steroids should be instituted (dexamethasone 10-mg IV bid) for at least 3 days or longer until signs and symptoms abate. Most patients do not require termination of arsenic trioxide therapy during treatment of the syndrome.
- Cardiotoxicities: Drug can cause QT interval prolongation and complete atrioventricular block. Prolonged QT interval can progress to a torsade de pointes-type fatal ventricular arrhythmia. Patients with history of QT prolongation, concomitant administration of drugs that prolong the QT interval, CHF, administration of potassium-wasting diuretics, and conditions resulting in hypokalemia or hypomagnesemia such as concurrent administration of amphotericin B. EKGs should be done weekly, more often if abnormal.
- Fluid/electrolyte Imbalance: Hypokalemia occurs in about 50% of patients, hypomagnesemia and hyperglycemia also commonly occur. Edema seen in 40% of patients. Less commonly, hyperkalemia, hypocalcemia, hypoglycemia, and acidosis occur. Potassium levels should be kept > 4.0 mEq/dL and magnesium > 1.8 mg/dL during arsenic trioxide therapy.
- Hematologic Effects: Leukocytosis seen in 50%–60% of patients with a gradual increase in WBC that peaks between 2 and 3 weeks after starting therapy. Usually resolves spontaneously without treatment and/or complications. Anemia (14%), thrombocytopenia (19%), and neutropenia (10%). Disseminated intravascular coagulation (DIC) occurred in 8% of patients.
- GI Toxicities: Nausea is most common (75%) and is usually mild, followed by vomiting (58%), abdominal pain (58%), diarrhea (53%), constipation (28%), anorexia (23%), dyspepsia (10%), abdominal tenderness or distention (8%), and dry mouth (8%).
- Hepatic Toxicities: Increased hepatic transaminases ALT and AST seen.
- Renal Toxicities: Use with caution in patients with renal impairment. Kidney is the main route of elimination of arsenic.
- Respiratory Toxicities: Cough is common. Other symptoms include dyspnea, epistaxis, hypoxia, pleural effusion, postnasal drip, wheezing, decreased breath sounds, crepitations, rales/crackles, hemoptysis, tachypnea, and rhonchi.

- Musculoskeletal: Arthralgias (33%), myalgias (25%), bone pain (23%), back pain (18%), neck pain, and pain in limbs (13%).
- Sensory/perception: Fatigue was reported by 63% of patients. Headache, insomnia, and pareshtesias common. Dizziness, tremors, seizures, somnolence, and (rarely) coma can occur.
- Skin: Dermatitis common. Pruritis, ecchymosis, dry skin, erythema, hyperpigmentation, and urticaria also reported. Injection site reactions (pain, erythema, and edema) can occur.
- Reproduction: Pregnancy category D.

Initiate antiemetic protocol: Mildly emetogenic protocol.

Supportive drugs:

☐ Neulasta   ☐ Neupogen
☐ Imodium   ☐ Procrit
☐ Aranesp   ☐ Lomotil

Treatment schedule: Chair time 2 hours daily until bone marrow remission, then 2 hours daily for 25 doses.

Estimated number of visits: Maximum of 85 visits per complete treatment course.

Dose Calculation by: 1. _____   2. _____

_____

Physician _____   Date _____

Patient Name _____   ID Number _____

Diagnosis _____   Ht _____ / Wt _____ / M^2 _____

ATRA (All-Trans-Retinoic Acid, Vesanoid, Tretinoin)

Baseline laboratory tests:	CBC: Chemistry, renal and liver functions
Monitor:	CBC, coagulation studies, liver functions, triglyceride, and cholesterol levels frequently throughout therapy
Baseline procedures or tests:	Bone marrow biopsy
Posttreatment:	Bone marrow biopsy at 5–6 weeks from the start of induction therapy
Administer:	**ATRA (Tretinoin)** _____ 45 mg/m² PO daily in one to two divided doses.

- (10-mg tablets) Protect from light.
- Absorption enhanced when taken with food.
- Use with caution in patients with caution in patients with pre-existing hypertriglyceridemia, diabetes mellitus, obesity, or predisposition to excessive alcohol intake.

Drug interactions: Drugs that induce cytochrome P450 hepatic enzyme system: rifampin glucocorticoids, phenobarbital, and pentobarbital.

Drugs that inhibit the enzyme system: ketoconazole, cimetidine, erythromycin, verapamil, diltiazem, and cyclosporin

Major Side Effects

- Alteration in oxygenation occurs in approximately 25% of patients, varies in severity, but has resulted in death. More commonly seen with WBC > 10,000 per mm³. Usually seen with the first treatment. Signs and symptoms include fever, dyspnea, weight gain, pulmonary infiltrates, pleural, and/or pericardial effusions. Access VS, weight and pulmonary exam at each visit. Give high-dose steroids (e.g., dexamethasone 10-mg IV every 12 hours × 3 days).
- Bone Marrow Depression: Dose-limiting toxicity.
- Vitamin A Toxicity: Headache, benign intracranial hypertension with papilledema can occur, earache or ear "fullness," fever, skin/mucous membrane dryness, pruritus, increased sweating, and visual disturbances.
- CNS Toxicity: Dizziness, anxiety, paresthesias, depression, confusion, and agitation.
- GI Toxicities: Nausea and vomiting, anorexia; stomatitis is usually mild; diarrhea infrequent and mild. Gastrointestinal bleeding/hemorrhage in up to 34% of patients, abdominal pain, diarrhea, and constipation may also occur.
- Skin Integrity: Alopecia about 30% in about 3 weeks, darkening of nail beds, skin ulcer/necrosis, sensitivity to light, and radiation recall.
- Circulatory disturbances include arrhythmia, flushing, hypotension, and phlebitis. Cardiotoxicity is similar characteristically but less severe than with daunorubicin and doxorubicin. Access cardiac status before treatment.
- Reproduction: Teratogenic. Discuss contraception and sperm banking.

Initiate antiemetic protocol:	Mild to moderately emetogenic protocol
Supportive drugs:	

☐ G-CSF _____   ☐ Peg-G-CSF _____

☐ Epoetin Alfa/   ☐ Allopurinol _____
 Darbepoetin Alfa _____

☐ Antibiotic _____   ☐ Antifungal _____

Estimated number of visits:	Three to five days first week, daily or every other day for blood counts

Dose Calculation by: 1. _____   2. _____

_____
Physician

_____
Patient Name

_____
Diagnosis

_____
Date

_____
ID Number

_____ / _____ / _____
Ht   Wt   M²

AIDA (All-Trans-Retinoic Acid, Idarubicin): Acute Promyelocytic Leukemia Only

Baseline laboratory test:	CBC: Chemistry, renal and liver functions
Monitor:	CBC: Coagulation studies, LFTs, triglyceride, and cholesterol levels frequently throughout therapy
Baseline procedures or tests:	Bone marrow biopsy
Posttreatment:	Bone marrow biopsy 5–6 weeks from the start of induction therapy
Initiate IV:	NS
Premedicate:	5-HT$_3$ and dexamethasone 20-mg IV
Administer:	**ATRA** _____ 45-mg/m^2 PO daily (10-mg tablets); protect from light.

* Absorption enhanced when taken with food.

Idarubicin _____ 12-mg/m^2 slow IV push through side port of free-flowing IV on days 2, 4, 6, and 8

* Vesicant. If patient has a central line, a slower infusion over 1 hour may cause less N and V.

* Available in 20-mg lyophilized vials for IV use only. Reconstitute with 20 mL of water for injection, final concentration 1 mg/1 mL, for central line infusion; further dilute in 100–250 cc of NS. Reconstituted solution is stable for 3 days at room temperature.

* Dose reduced for renal dysfunction. For hepatic dysfunction, give 50% of dose, if serum bili is 2.5 mg/dL; do not give if serum bili is > 5 mg/dL.

Drug interactions: Drugs that induce cytochrome P450 hepatic enzyme system include rifampin, glucocorticoids, phenobarbital, and pentobarbital. Drugs that inhibit the enzyme system include ketoconazole, cimetidine, erythromycin, verapamil, diltiazem, and cyclosporin.

Major Side Effects:

* Bone Marrow Depression: Dose-limiting toxicity.

* Alteration in oxygenation occurs in approximately 25% of patients; varies in severity but has resulted in death. Signs and symptoms include fever, dyspnea, weight gain, pulmonary infiltrates, and pleural and/or pericardial effusions. Access VS, weight, and pulmonary exam at each visit. Give high-dose steroids (e.g., dexamethasone 10-mg IV every 12 hours × 3 days).

* Vitamin A Toxicity: Headache, benign intracranial hypertension with papilledema can occur, earache or ear "fullness," fever, skin/mucous membrane dryness, pruritus, increased sweating, and visual disturbances.

* CNS Toxicity: Dizziness, anxiety, paresthesias, depression, confusion, and agitation.

* GI Toxicities: Nausea and vomiting mild to moderate. Anorexia; stomatitis and diarrhea are common but not severe. Gastrointestinal bleeding/hemorrhage in up to 34% of patients, abdominal pain, diarrhea, or constipation.

* Skin Integrity: Alopecia about 30% in about 3 weeks, darkening of nail beds, skin ulcer/necrosis, sensitivity to light, and radiation recall.

* Circulatory disturbances include arrhythmia, flushing, hypotension, and phlebitis. Cardiotoxicity is similar characteristically but less severe than with daunorubicin and doxorubicin. Assess cardiac status before treatment.

* GU Toxicities: Discoloration of urine from pink to red up to 48 hours.

* Reproduction: Gonadal and fertility may be permanent or transient. Discuss contraception and sperm banking.

Initiate antiemetic protocol:	Mild to moderately emetogenic protocol.
Supportive drugs:	☐ G-CSF _____ ☐ Peg-G-CSF _____
	☐ Epoetin Alfa/ Darbepoetin Alfa _____ ☐ Allopurinol _____
	☐ Antibiotic _____ ☐ Antifungal _____
Treatment schedule:	Chair time 1 hour on days 1–3 and 30 minutes for pump refill days.
Estimated number of visits:	Three to five days in the first week; daily or every other day for blood counts.

Dose Calculation by: 1. _____   2. _____

_____   _____
Physician   Date

_____   _____
Patient Name   ID Number

_____   _____/_____/_____
Diagnosis   Ht   Wt   M²

LEUKEMIA

Chronic Lymphocytic Leukemia

Combination Regimens

Cyclophosphamide: 400-mg/m^2 PO on days 1–5 (or 800-mg/m^2 IV on day 1)

Vincristine: 1.4-mg/m^2 IV on day 1 (maximum dose, 2 mg)

Prednisone: 100-mg/m^2 PO on days 1–5

Repeat cycle every 21 days.[1,221]

Cyclophosphamide: 1000-mg/m^2 IV on day 1

Fludarabine: 20-mg/m^2 IV on days 1–5

Bactrim DS: One tablet PO bid

Repeat cycle every 21–28 days.[1,222]

Fludarabine: 30-mg/m^2 IV on days 1–5

Prednisone: 30-mg/m^2 PO on days 1–5

Repeat cycle every 28 days.[1,223]

Chlorambucil: 30-mg/m^2 PO on day 1

Prednisone: 80-mg PO on days 1–5

Repeat cycle every 2 weeks.[1,221]

Fludarabine: 25-mg/m^2 IV on days 1–5

Rituxan: 375-mg/m^2 IV on day 5.

Repeat cycle every 28 days.[1,224]

Fludarabine: 25-mg/m^2 IV on days 1–3

Rituxan: 375-mg/m^2 IV on day 1 first cycle only

Rituxan: 500-mg/m^2 IV on day 5 all subsequent cycles

Cyclophosphamide: 250-mg/m^2 IV on days 1–3

Repeat cycle every 28 days.[1,225]

Single-Agent Regimens

Alemtuzumab: 30-mg/day IV, three times per week
Repeat weekly for up to a maximum of 23 weeks.[1,226]
Premedicate with diphenhydramine 50-mg PO and
Acetaminophen 625-mg PO 30 minutes before drug infusion.
Patients should be placed on Bactrim DS PO bid and
Famciclovir 250-mg PO bid from day 8 through 2 months after
  completion of therapy.

Chlorambucil: 6–14 mg/day PO as induction therapy and then 0.7-mg/kg
  PO for 2–4 days
Repeat cycle every 21 days.[1,227]

Cladribine: 0.09-mg/kg/day IV continuous infusion on days 1–7
Repeat cycle every 28–35 days.[1,228]

Fludarabine: 20–30 mg/m^2 IV on days 1–5
Repeat cycle every 28 days.[1,229]

Prednisone: 20–30 mg/m^2/day PO for 1–3 weeks.[1,230]

Combination Regimens

CVP (Cyclophosphamide, Vincristine, Prednisone)

Baseline laboratory tests:	CBC: Chemistry, renal and liver functions
Baseline procedures or tests:	Bone marrow biopsy, central line placement
Posttreatment:	Bone marrow biopsy (stop G-CSF 7 days before bone marrow biopsy)
Initiate IV:	NS
Premedicate:	5-HT$_3$ and dexamethasone 20-mg IVPB over 10 minutes
Administer:	**Cyclophosphamide** _____ 400-mg/m^2 PO on days 1–5

OR

Cyclophosphamide _____ 800-mg/m^2 IV over 1 hour on day 1

- Available in 500-mg, 1-, and 2-gram vials. Dilute with sterile water or bacteriostatic water for injection (sterile water or paraben preserved); shake well until solution is clear.
- Final concentration of 20 mg/mL.
- Further dilute into 250–500 mL of NS or D5W.
- Reconstituted solution is stable for 24 hours at room temperature and 6 days upon refrigeration.

Vincristine _____ 2 mg on days 4 and 11; IV push through side arm of free-flowing IV

Prednisone _____ 100-mg PO or IV on days 1–5 (taper prednisone dose)

Major Side Effects

- Bone Marrow Depression: Dose-limiting toxicity.
- GI Toxicities: Nausea and vomiting, anorexia, stomatitis, and gastric irritation.
- Hemorrhagic Cystitis: Irritation of bladder wall capillaries; preventable with hydration.
- GU Toxicities: Discoloration of urine from pink to red up to 48 hours.
- Neurotoxicites: Peripheral neuropathy including numbness, weakness, myalgias, and cramping. Jaw pain and paralytic ileus may also occur. May require discontinuation of vincristine. Impotency may also occur.
- Alopecia: Complete hair loss is possible.
- Tumor lysis syndrome can occur if WBC is elevated. Prevent with allopurinol and hydration.
- Steroid Toxicities: Sodium and water retention, Cushingoid changes, behavioral changes, including emotional lability, insomnia, mood swings, and euphoria. Muscle weakness and loss with prolonged use. May increase glucose and sodium and decrease potassium and affect warfarin dose.
- Reproduction: Mutagenic and potentially teratogenic.

Initiate antiemetic protocol:	Moderately emetogenic protocol.
Supportive drugs:	☐ G-CSF _____ ☐ Peg-G-CSF _____
	☐ Epoetin Alfa/ ☐ Allopurinol _____
	Darbepoetin Alfa _____
	☐ Antibiotic _____ ☐ Antifungal _____
Treatment schedule:	Chair time 2 hours on day 1. Repeat cycle every 21 days.
Estimated number of visits:	Weekly until remission.

Dose Calculation by: 1. _____   2. _____

_____   _____
Physician   Date

_____   _____
Patient Name   ID Number

                                              _____/ _____/ _____
Diagnosis   Ht   Wt   M^2

CF-Cyclophosphamide, Fludarabine, Bactrim DS

Baseline laboratory tests:	CBC: Chemistry, renal and liver functions
Baseline procedures or tests:	Bone marrow biopsy, central line placement
Initiate IV:	NS
Premedicate:	5-HT$_3$ and dexamethasone 20-mg IV
Administer:	**Cyclophosphamide** _____ 1000-mg/m^2 IV over 1 hour on day 1

- Available in 500-mg, 1-, and 2-gram vials. Dilute with sterile water or bacteriostatic water for injection (sterile water or paraben preserved); shake well until solution is clear.
- Final concentration of 20 mg/mL.
- Further dilute into 250–500 mL of NS or D5W.
- Reconstituted solution is stable for 24 hours at room temperature and 6 days upon refrigeration.

Fludarabine _____ 20-mg/m^2/day IV on days 1–5 over 30 minutes

- Dilute with 2 mL of sterile water for final concentration of 25 mg/mL.
- Further dilute in 100 mL NS or D5W. The drug should be used within 8 hours.

Bactrim DS: One tablet PO BID

Major Side Effects

- Myelosuppression: Nadir occurs in 7–14 days and includes red blood cells.
- Neurotoxicity: Agitation, confusion, and visual disturbances have occurred.
- Immunosuppression: Decrease in CD4+ and CD8+, increasing risk for opportunistic infections (fungus, herpes, and *Pneumocystis carinii*).
- GI Toxicities: Nausea and vomiting, anorexia; mucositis, diarrhea
- Hemorrhagic Cystitis: Irritation of bladder wall capillaries; preventable with hydration.
- Skin Alterations: Alopecia. Total hair loss. Maculopapular skin rash, erythema and pruritis.
- Tumor lysis syndrome can occur if WBC is elevated. Prevent with allopurinol and hydration.
- Reproduction: Mutagenic and potentially teratogenic, discuss contraception and sperm banking.

Initiate antiemetic protocol:	Moderately emetogenic protocol.
Supportive drugs:	☐ G-CSF _____ ☐ Peg-G-CSF _____
	☐ Epoetin Alfa/ Darbepoetin Alfa _____ ☐ Allopurinol _____
	☐ Antibiotic _____ ☐ Antifungal _____
Treatment schedule:	Chair time 2 hours on day 1 and 1 hour on days 2–5.
Estimated number of visits:	Daily for five days and then weekly. Repeat the schedule every 21–28 days.

Dose Calculation by: 1. _____   2. _____

_____
Physician

_____
Date

_____
Patient Name

_____
ID Number

_____
Diagnosis

_____ / _____ / _____
Ht   Wt   M^2

FP-Fludarabine, Prednisone

Baseline laboratory tests:	CBC: Chemistry, renal and liver functions
Baseline procedures or tests:	Bone marrow biopsy, central line placement
Initiate IV:	NS
Premedicate:	5-HT$_3$ IV
Administer:	**Fludarabine** _____ 30-mg/m^2/day IV on days 1–5 over 30 minutes

- Dilute with 2-mL sterile water for final concentration of 25 mg/mL.
- Further dilute in 100-mL NS or D5W. The drug should be used within 8 hours.

Prednisone: _____ 30-mg PO on days 1–5

Major Side Effects

- Myelosuppression: Nadir occurs in 7–14 days and includes red blood cells.
- Neurotoxicity: Agitation, confusion, and visual disturbances have occurred.
- Immunosuppression: Decrease in CD4+ and CD8+, increasing risk for opportunistic infections (fungus, herpes, and *Pneumocystis carinii*).
- Pulmonary Toxicities: Pneumonia occurs in 16%–22% of patients. Pulmonary hypersensitivity reaction characterized by dyspnea, cough, and interstitial pulmonary infiltrates.
- Steroid Toxicities: Sodium and water retention, Cushingoid changes, and behavioral changes, including emotional lability, insomnia, mood swings, and euphoria. Muscle weakness and loss with prolonged use. May increase glucose and sodium and decrease potassium and affect warfarin dose.
- GI Toxicities: Nausea and vomiting, anorexia; mucositis, diarrhea.
- Skin Alterations, Alopecia. Total hair loss. Maculapapular skin rash, erythema, and pruritis.
- Reproduction: Mutagenic and potentially teratogenic, discuss contraception and sperm banking.

Initiate antiemetic protocol:	Mildly emetogenic protocol.
Supportive drugs:	☐ G-CSF _____ ☐ Peg-G-CSF _____
	☐ Epoetin Alfa/ Darbepoetin Alfa _____ ☐ Allopurinol _____
	☐ Antibiotic _____ ☐ Antifungal _____
Treatment schedule:	Chair time 1–2 hours on days 1–5
Estimated number of visits:	Daily for five days and then weekly. Repeat the schedule every 28 days.

Dose Calculation by: 1. _____   2. _____

_____
Physician

_____
Date

_____
Patient Name

_____
ID Number

_____
Diagnosis

_____/ _____/ _____
Ht   Wt   M^2

CP Pulse—Chlorambucil, Prednisone

Baseline laboratory tests:	CBC: Chemistry, renal and liver functions
Baseline procedures or tests:	Bone marrow biopsy
Administer:	**Chlorambucil:** _____ 30-mg/m^2 PO on day 1 every 2 weeks
	• Available 2 mg brown film-coated tablets.
	Prednisone: _____ 80-mg PO on days 1–5 every 2 weeks

Major Side Effects

- Bone Marrow Depression: Neutropenia after the third week, teach self-care measures to minimize risk of infection and bleeding.
- GI Toxicities: Nausea and vomiting are rare. Anorexia and weight loss may occur.
- Pulmonary Toxicities: Pulmonary fibrosis and pneumonitus dose related and potentially life threatening.
- Skin Alteration: Skin rash on face, scalp, and trunk seen in early stage of therapy.
- Tumor lysis syndrome can occur if WBCs are elevated.
- Steroid Toxicities: Sodium and water retention, Cushingoid changes, and behavioral changes, including emotional lability, insomnia, mood swings, and euphoria. Muscle weakness and loss with prolonged use. May increase glucose and sodium and decrease potassium and affect warfarin dose.
- Reproduction: Mutagenic and potentially teratogenic.

Initiate antiemetic protocol:	Mildly emetogenic protocol.
Treatment schedule:	Repeat the cycle every 2 weeks.
Chair time:	None
Estimated number of visits:	Weekly or every other week for CBC.

Dose Calculation by: 1. _____   2. _____

_____

Physician   Date

_____

Patient Name   ID Number

_____   _____/_____/_____

Diagnosis   Ht   Wt   M^2

Fludarabine + Rituxan

Baseline laboratory tests:	CBC: Chemistry, renal and liver functions
Baseline procedures or tests:	Bone marrow biopsy, central line placement
Initiate IV:	NS
Premedicate:	5-HT$_3$ and dexamethasone 10–20 mg IV in 100 cc of NS over 20 minutes.
	Diphenhydramine 25–50 mg and cimetidine 300-mg IV in 100 cc of NS over 20 minutes

Administer:

Fludarabine _____ 25-mg/m^2/day IV on days 1–5

- Dilute with 2-mL sterile water for a final concentration of 25 mg/mL.
- Further dilute in 100 mL of NS or D5W. The drug should be used within 8 hours.

Rituximab _____ 50-mg/m^2/day IV over 4 hours without rate escalation, day 1 (first cycle only)

Rituximab _____ 325-mg/m^2/day IV on day 3 (first cycle only)

- Use rate escalation: start at 50-mg/hr, increasing to maximum of 400 mg/hr.

Rituximab _____ 375-mg/m^2/day IV, day 5 and day 1 on cycles 2–6

- Start rate escalation with 100 mg/hr up to 400 mg/hr.
- Dilute with NS or D5W to a final concentration of 1–4 mg/mL (infusion rates are easier to calculate if solution is 1:1 concentration). Antibodies are fragile; do not shake vial or bag. Do not use a filter. Stable at room temperature for 24 hours.

Major Side Effects

- Myelosuppression: Severe and cumulative, nadir day 13
- Hypersensitivity Reactions: Occur within 30 minutes to 2 hours; most commonly seen with first infusion of Rituxan and patients with high tumor burden characterized by fever, chills, rigors, back pain, flushing, bronchospasms, angioedema, and hypotension. Usually resolves when infused stopped. Premedicate with acetaminophen, diphenhydramine, and corticosteroids. Ensure emergency medications are available (antihistamines, corticosteroids, epinephrine, and bronchodilators). When symptoms resolve, resume infusion at 50% of the previous infusion rate. Monitor vital signs frequently.
- Immunosuppression: Decrease in CD4+ and CD8+, increasing risk for opportunistic infections (fungus, herpes, and *Pneumocystis carinii*).
- Tumor lysis syndrome can occur if WBC is elevated or large tumor burden. Prevent with allopurinol and hydration 150 mL/hr with or without alkalinization.
- Fatigue: Secondary to anemia.
- Neurotoxicity: Agitation, confusion, and visual disturbances have occurred.
- Pulmonary Toxicities: Pneumonia occurs in 16%–22% of patients. Pulmonary hypersensitivity reaction characterized by dyspnea, cough, and interstitial pulmonary infiltrates.
- GI Toxicities: Nausea and vomiting, anorexia; mucositis, diarrhea.
- Reproduction: Mutagenic and potentially teratogenic, discuss contraception and sperm banking.

Initiate antiemetic protocol:	Mildly emetogenic protocol.
Supportive drugs:	☐ G-CSF _____ ☐ Peg-G-CSF _____
	☐ Epoetin Alfa/ ☐ Allopurinol _____
	Darbepoetin Alfa _____
	☐ Antibiotic _____ ☐ Antifungal _____
Treatment schedule:	Chair time 1 hour on day on fludarabine only days and 5–8 hours for rituxan days
Estimated number of visits:	Daily for five days. Repeat schedule every 28 days for six cycles.
Restage:	If a CR, PR, or Sable disease is obtained, give the following:

Rituximab _____ 375-mg/m^2/day IV every week × 4 weeks

- Start rate escalation with 100 mg/hr up to 400 mg/hr.

Dose Calculation by: 1. _____   2. _____

_____   _____
Physician   Date

_____   _____
Patient Name   ID Number

_____   _____ / _____ / _____
Diagnosis   Ht   Wt   M²

Fludarabine + Cyclophosphamide + Rituxan

Baseline laboratory tests:	CBC: Chemistry, renal and liver functions
Baseline procedures or tests:	Bone marrow biopsy, central line placement
Initiate IV:	NS
Premedicate:	5-HT$_3$ IV with dexamethasone 10–20 mg in 100 cc of NS over 20 minutes
	Diphenhydramine 25–50 mg and cimetidine 300 mg in 100 cc NS over 20 minutes

Administer:

Fludarabine _____ 25-mg/m^2/day IV on days 2–4 of cycle 1

Fludarabine _____ 25-mg/m^2/day IV on days 1–3 of cycles 2–6

- Dilute with 2 mL of sterile water for a final concentration of 25 mg/mL.
- Further dilute in 100 mL of NS or D5W. The drug should be used within 8 hours.

Cyclophosphamide _____ 250 mg/m^2 on days 2–4 of cycle 1

Cyclophosphamide _____ 250 mg/m^2 on days 1–3 of cycles 2–6

Rituximab _____ 375-mg/m^2/day IV, day 1 of cycle 1

- Start at 50 mg/hr with rate escalation 50 mg/hr up to 400 mg/hr.

Rituximab _____ 500-mg/m^2/day IV on day 1 on cycles 2–6

- Start rate escalation with 100 mg/hr up to 400 mg/hr.
- Dilute with NS or D$_5$W to a final concentration of 1–4 mg/mL (infusion rates easier to calculate if solution is 1:1 concentration).
- Antibodies are fragile; do not shake vial or bag. Do not use a filter. Stable at room temperature for 24 hours.

Major Side Effects

- Myelosuppression: Severe and cumulative, nadir day 13.
- Hypersensitivity Reactions: Occur within 30 minutes to 2 hours, most commonly seen with the first infusion of Rituxan, and patients with high tumor burden characterized by fever, chills, rigors, back pain, flushing, bronchospasms, angioedema, and hypotension. Usually resolves when infused stopped. Premedicate with acetaminophen, diphenhydramine, and corticosteroids. Ensure that emergency medications are available (antihistamines, corticosteroids, epinephrine, and bronchodilators). When symptoms resolve, resume infusion at 50% of the previous infusion rate. Monitor vital signs frequently.
- Immunosuppression: Decrease in CD4+ and CD8+, increasing risk for opportunistic infections (fungus, herpes, and *Pneumocystis carinii*).
- Tumor lysis syndrome can occur if WBC is elevated or large tumor burden. Prevent with allopurinol and hydration 150 mL/hr with or without alkalinization.
- Fatigue: Secondary to anemia.
- Hemorrhagic cystitis: Irritation of bladder wall capillaries; preventable with hydration.
- Neurotoxicity: Agitation, confusion, and visual disturbances have occurred.
- Pulmonary Toxicities: Pneumonia occurs in 16%–22% of patients. Pulmonary hypersensitivity reaction characterized by dyspnea, cough, and interstitial pulmonary infiltrates.
- GI Toxicities: Nausea and vomiting, anorexia; mucositis, diarrhea.
- Reproduction: Mutagenic and potentially teratogenic, discuss contraception and sperm banking.

Initiate antiemetic protocol:	Mildly emetogenic protocol.
Supportive drugs:	Allopurinol 300 mg daily × 7 days for cycle 1
	Septa DS twice weekly for patients at high risk of myelosuppression
	Famciclovir 500 mg daily
	☐ G-CSF _____ ☐ Peg-G-CSF _____
	☐ Epoetin Alfa/Darbepoetin Alfa _____
Treatment schedule:	Chair time 1 hour for fludarabine; 5–8 hours on rituxan days.
Estimated number of visits:	Daily for three to four days. Repeat schedule every 28 days for six cycles.

Dose Calculation by: 1. _____ 2. _____

_____

Physician

_____

Patient Name

_____

Diagnosis

Date

ID Number

_____/_____/_____

Ht   Wt   M²

Single-Agent Regimens

Alemtuzumab (Campath)

Baseline laboratory tests: CBC: Chemistry, renal and liver functions

Baseline procedures or tests: Bone marrow biopsy, central line placement

Initiate IV: NS

Premedicate: 5-HT$_3$ and dexamethasone 10-mg IV

Acetaminophen 650 mg and diphenhydramine 50 mg

Administer: **Alemtuzumab** _____ 30-mg IV over 2 hours three times a week

- Initiate dosing at 3-mg IV daily.
- When tolerated (infusion-related toxicities are less than grade 2).
- Increase to 10-mg IV three times per week.
- When tolerated (infusion-related toxicities are less than grade 2), increase to the maintenance dose of 30-mg IV three times per week.
- Available in 30-mg ampule, draw up with filtered needle and dilute in 100 mL of NS or D5W.
- Use within 8 hours.

Contraindications: Patients with active systemic infections, HIV-positive, AIDS, or known type 1 hypersensitivity or anaphylactic reactions

Supportive drugs recommended starting on day 8:

Anti-infective prophylaxis: Bactrim DS and trimethoprim

☐ G-CSF _____   ☐ Peg-G-CSF _____

☐ Epoetin Alfa/   ☐ Allourinol _____
  Darbepoetin Alfa _____   ☐ Antifungal _____

☐ Antibiotic Bactrim and Trimethoprim recommended

Major Side Effects

- Hypersensitivity Reactions: Most often seen in the first week of therapy. Fever, chills, rigors, nausea and vomiting, urticaria, skin rash, fatigue, headache, diarrhea, dyspnea, and/or hypotension. Stop the drug if reaction occurs; may treat with steroids; meperidine for rigors. Usually resolves in 20 minutes.
- Myelosuppression: Dose-limiting toxicity. Dramatic drop in WBCs during the first week. Opportunistic infections common, including *Pneumocystis carinii* pneumonia, pulmonary aspergillus, and herpes simplex infections.
- Tumor Lysis Syndrome: May occur with high WBCs or high tumor burden. Prevent with allopurinol and hydration.
- Alteration in Comfort: Pain, headache, asthenia, dysphasias, and dizziness.
- Reproduction: Not studied in pregnant women, but IgG can cross the placental barrier and may cause B- and T-cell depletion in the fetus. Breastfeeding should be avoided.

Initiate antiemetic protocol: Mildly emetogenic protocol.

Treatment schedule: Chair time 2–3 hours on days 1–3–5.

Estimated number of visits: Daily for 3 days per week for 8–12 weeks, weekly CBC and CD4+. CBC more frequent if counts are low.

Dose Calculation by: 1. _____ 2. _____

_____
Physician

_____
Date

_____
Patient Name

_____
ID Number

_____
Diagnosis

_____/ _____/ _____
Ht   Wt   M^2

Chlorambucil

Baseline laboratory tests: CBC: Chemistry, renal and liver functions

Baseline procedures or tests: Bone marrow biopsy

Administer: **Chlorambucil** _____ 0.1–0.2 mg/kg/day (equals 4–8 mg/m^2/day) for 3–6 weeks as required

Then intermittent therapy:

Chlorambucil _____ 0.4 mg/kg/day for 5 days PO; repeat every 14–28 days, increasing dose by 0.1 mg/kg until control of lymphocytosis or toxicity is observed.

- Available in 2-mg tablets.

OR

Chlorambucil _____ 6–14 mg/day PO as induction therapy and then 0.7-mg/kg PO for 2–4 days (repeat every 28–35 days).

Major Side Effects
- Bone Marrow Depression: Neutropenia after third week, teach self-care measures to minimize risk of infection and bleeding. Myelosuppression dose limiting.
- Pulmonary Toxicities: Pulmonary fibrosis and pneumonitis dose related–rare.
- GI Toxicities: Nausea and vomiting are rare. Anorexia and weight loss may occur.
- Reproduction: Mutagenic and potentially teratogenic.

Initiate antiemetic protocol: Mildly emetogenic protocol if necessary.

Treatment schedule: Repeat cycle every 28 days.

Chair time: None

Estimated number of visits: Weekly or every other week for CBC.

Dose Calculation by: 1. _____   2. _____

_____

Physician

_____

Date

_____

Patient Name

_____

ID Number

_____

Diagnosis

_____ / _____ / _____

Ht   Wt   M^2

Cladribine (Leustatin, 2-CdA): CLL

Baseline laboratory tests:	CBC: Chemistry, renal and liver functions
Baseline procedures or tests:	Bone marrow biopsy, central line placement
Initiate IV:	NS
Administer:	**Cladribine** _____ 0.09-mg/kg/day IV continuous infusion on days 1–7

- Use 22-dilute with NS, dilute in minimum of 100 mL, stable for 24 hours.
- DO NOT use D5W.

Major Side Effects

- Myelosuppression: Nadir occurs in 7–14 days, recovery by weeks 3–5. Increased risk of opportunistic infections.
- Immunosuppression: Decrease in CD4+ and CD8+, increasing risk for opportunistic infections (fungus, herpes, and *Pneumocystis carinii*).
- Tumor lysis syndrome can occur if WBC is elevated or large tumor burden. Prevent with allopurinol and hydration 150 mL/hr with or without alkalinization.
- Fatigue: Secondary to anemia.
- GI Toxicities: Mild nausea and vomiting, anorexia; constipation, diarrhea.
- Neurotoxicites: Headache, insomnia, and dizziness.
- Skin Integrity: Rash, pruritus, or injection site reactions.
- Reproduction: Mutagenic and potentially teratogenic, discuss contraception and sperm banking.

Initiate antiemetic protocol:	Mildly emetogenic protocol.
Supportive drugs:	☐ G-CSF _____ ☐ Peg-G-CSF _____
	☐ Epoetin Alfa/ ☐ Allopurinol _____
	Darbepoetin Alfa _____
	☐ Antibiotic _____ ☐ Antifungal _____
Treatment schedule:	Chair time 1 hour on day 1, pump dc day 8. Repeat cycle every 28–35 days.
Estimated number of visits:	Daily for seven days and then weekly CBC.

Dose Calculation by: 1. _____ 2. _____

_____
Physician

_____
Date

_____
Patient Name

_____
ID Number

_____
Diagnosis

_____ / _____ / _____
Ht   Wt   M²

Fludarabine

Baseline laboratory tests:	CBC: Chemistry, renal and liver functions
Baseline procedures or tests:	Bone marrow biopsy, central line placement
Initiate IV:	NS
Premedicate:	5-HT$_3$ IV
Administer:	**Fludarabine** _____ 20–30 mg/m^2/day IV on days 1–5

- Available 50 mg vial.
- Dilute with 2 mL of sterile water for final concentration of 25 mg/mL.
- Further dilute in 100 mL of NS or D5W. The drug should be used within 8 hours.

Major Side Effects

- Myelosuppression: Severe and cumulative, nadir day 13.
- Immunosuppression: Decrease in CD4+ and CD8+, increasing risk for opportunistic infections (fungus, herpes, and *Pneumocystis carinii*).
- Fatigue: Secondary to anemia.
- Neurotoxicity: Agitation, confusion, and visual disturbances have occurred.
- Pulmonary Toxicities: Pneumonia occurs in 16%–22% of patients. Pulmonary hypersensitivity reaction characterized by dyspnea, cough, and interstitial pulmonary infiltrates.
- GI Toxicities: Nausea and vomiting, anorexia; mucositis, diarrhea.
- Reproduction: Mutagenic and potentially teratogenic, discuss contraception and sperm banking.

Initiate antiemetic protocol:	Mildly emetogenic protocol.
Supportive drugs:	☐ G-CSF _____ ☐ Peg-G-CSF _____
	☐ Epoetin Alfa/ ☐ Allopurinol _____
	Darbepoetin Alfa _____
	☐ Antibiotic _____ ☐ Antifungal _____
Treatment schedule:	Chair time 1 hour on days 1–5.
Estimated number of visits:	Daily for 5 days and then weekly. Repeat schedule every 28 days.

Dose Calculation by: 1. _____   2. _____

_____

Physician

_____

Patient Name

_____

Diagnosis

_____

Date

_____

ID Number

_____/ _____/ _____
Ht   Wt   M^2

Prednisone

Baseline laboratory tests: CBC: Chemistry, renal and liver functions

Baseline procedures or tests: Bone marrow biopsy

Administer:

Prednisone _____ 20–30 mg/m^2/day PO for 1–3 weeks

OR

Prednisone _____ 60–100 mg/m^2/day PO for 3–6 weeks

- Take with food.

Major Side Effects

- GI Toxicities: Gastric irritation, increased appetite.
- Steroid Toxicities: Sodium and water retention, Cushingoid changes, behavioral changes, including emotional lability, insomnia, mood swings, and euphoria. May increase glucose and sodium and decrease potassium and affect warfarin dose.
- Musculoskeletal Changes: Muscle weakness, loss of muscle mass, osteoporosis, and pathologic fractures with prolonged use.
- Perceptual Alterations: Cataracts or glaucoma may develop.

Chair time: None

Estimated number of visits: Weekly or every other week for CBC.

Dose Calculation by: 1. _____ 2. _____

_____   _____
Physician   Date

_____   _____
Patient Name   ID Number

_____   _____/_____   _____/_____
Diagnosis   Ht   Wt   M^2

LEUKEMIA

Chronic Myelogenous Leukemia

Combination Regimens

Interferon α-2b: 5×10^6 IU/m^2 SC daily

Cytabarabine: 20-mg/m^2 SC daily for 10 days

Repeat cytarabine on a monthly basis.[1,231]

The dose of interferon should be reduced by 50% when the neutrophil count drops below 1500/mm^3, the platelet count drops below 100,000/mm^3, or both.

Interferon and cytarabine should both be discontinued when the neutrophil count drops below 1000/mm^3, the platelet count drops below 50,000/mm^3, or both.

Single-Agent Regimens

Imatinib: 400-mg/day PO (chronic phase) 600-mg/day PO (accelerated phase blast crisis)

Continue treatment until disease progression.[1,232]

Busulfan: 1.8-mg/m^2/day PO.[1,233]

Hydroxyurea: 1–5 g/day PO.[1,234]

Interferon 9 million units SQ per day, three times per week for up to 1–1.5 years.[1,235]

Sprycel: 70 mg PO twice daily.[236a,236b]

Combination Regimens

Interferon + Cytarabine (Ara-C)

Baseline laboratory tests:	CBC: Chemistry, renal and liver functions
Baseline procedures or tests:	Bone marrow biopsy
Administer:	

Interferon α-2b _____ 5×10^6 IU/m^2 SQ daily

- Available in single dose prefilled syringes 3, 6, and 9 million units.
- Do not freeze or shake.
- Stable for 1 month refrigerated.

Cytarabine _____ 20-mg/m^2 SQ daily for 10

- Dilute in sterile water with benzyl alcohol and then further dilute with 50–100 mL of 0.9% sodium. Stable 48 hours at room temperature and 7 days refrigerated chloride or D5W.
- IV hydration at 150 per mL per hour with or without alkalinization, oral allopurinol, strict I & O, and daily weights.
- Reconstitute with water with benzyl alcohol; stable for 48 hours at room temperature.

Major Side Effects
- Bone Marrow Depression: Interferon should be reduced by 50% when neutrophil count drops below 1500 per mm^3, the platelet count drops below 100,000 per m^3, or both. Both drugs should be discontinued with neutrophils less than 1000 mm^3, platelets less than 50,000 mm^3, or both. Teach self-care measures to minimize risk of infection and bleeding.
- Flulike Syndrome: Chills 3–6 hours after interferon. Fatigue, malaise, headache, and myalgias are cumulative and dose limiting.
- Thrombophlebitis, pain at the injection site, should be treated with warm compresses.
- GI Toxicities: Nausea and vomiting, anorexia, xerostomia, and mild diarrhea.
- Partial alopecia.
- Tumor lysis syndrome occurring 1–5 days after the initiation of treatment.
- Reproduction: Mutagenic and potentially teratogenic.

Initiate antiemetic protocol:	Mildly to moderately emetogenic protocol.
Supportive drugs:	☐ pegfilgrastim (Neulasta) ☐ filgrastim (Neupogen)
	☐ Procrit/Aranesp _____ ☐ Allopurinol_____
	☐ Antibiotic _____ ☐ Antifungal _____
Treatment schedule:	Repeat cycle every 28 days.
Chair time:	May be administered in the office or self-administered.
Estimated number of visits:	Weekly or every other week for CBC.

Dose Calculation by: 1. _____ 2. _____

_____

Physician   Date

_____

Patient Name   ID Number

_____

Diagnosis   Ht _____/ Wt _____/ M^2

Single-Agent Regimens

Imatinib (Gleevec): CML

Baseline laboratory tests:	CBC: Chemistry, renal and liver functions
Baseline procedures or tests:	Bone marrow biopsy
Administer:	**Imatinib** _____ 400–800 mg per day

- 400-mg/day single dose for patients in chronic phase CML.
- 600-mg/day single dose for patients in accelerated phase or blast crisis.
- Treatment continues as long as patient derives benefit from drug.
- If disease progression, failure of hematologic response after 3 months, or loss of hematologic remission, increase dose to 600-mg/day (chronic CML) or to 800-mg/day given as 400-mg BID (accelerated or blast crisis).
- Available in 100- and 400-mg tablets.

Drug interactions: Ketoconazole, itraconazole, erythromycin, and clarithromycin may increase imatinib plasma concentrations, dexamethasone, phenytoin, carbamazepine, rifampicin, phenobarbital, and St. John's Wort. Do not coadminister ketoconazole.

Cyclosporine, pimozide plasma levels may increase; triazolo-benzadiazepines, dihydropyridine calcium channel blockers, HMG-CoA reductase inhibitors may also have increased serum levels.

Warfarin metabolism is inhibited with imitinab. Use low molecular weight heparin.

Major Side Effects

- Bone Marrow Depression: Median duration 2–3 weeks and thrombocytopenia 3–4 weeks. Teach self-care measures to minimize risk of infection and bleeding.
- GI Toxicities: Nausea and vomiting are mild to moderate. Diarrhea and dyspepsia may also occur.
- Fluid Retention: Common, especially in the older and primarily periorbital and lower extremity edema. May require diuretics. Pleural effusions, ascites, pulmonary edema and weight gain. More common in accelerated phase.
- Alteration in Comfort: Muscle cramps, musculoskeletal pain, headaches, fatigue, arthralgias, and abdominal pain.
- Rash may occur with pruritus.
- Reproduction: Mutagenic and potentially teratogenic.

Initiate antiemetic protocol:	Mildly to moderately emetogenic protocol.
Treatment schedule:	Daily
Chair time:	None
Estimated number of visits:	Weekly or every other week for CBC and then monthly.

Dose Calculation by: 1. _____   2. _____

_____
Physician

_____
Patient Name

_____
Diagnosis

_____
Date

_____
ID Number

_____ / _____ / _____
Ht   Wt M^2

Busulfan (Myleran)

Baseline laboratory tests:	CBC: Chemistry, renal and liver functions
Baseline procedures or tests:	Bone marrow biopsy
Administer:	**Busulfan** _____ 4–8 mg or 1.8 mg/m^2 per day for 2–3 weeks remission induction
Maintenance:	**Busulfan** _____ 1–3 mg/m^2 PO daily or 0.05-mg/kg PO daily for maintenance

- Hold when leukocyte count reaches 15,000 per μL; resume when total leukocyte count is 50,000 per μL; maintenance dose of 1–3 mg qd used if remission lasts less than 3 months.
- Available in 2-mg scored tablets.

Major Side Effects

- Bone Marrow Depression: Dose-limiting toxicity.
- Tumor lysis syndrome can occur if WBC is elevated. Prevent with allopurinol and hydration.
- GI Toxicities: Nausea and vomiting are common but mild. Mucositis dose related and may require interruption of therapy.
- Skin Alterations: Hyperpigmentation of skin, especially increases on the hands and nail beds. Skin rash and pruritis also observed.
- Pulmonary Toxicities: Cough, dyspnea and fever can be seen after long-term therapy.
- Neurotoxicities: Insomnia, anxiety, dizziness, and depression are most common.
- Reproduction: Mutagenic and potentially teratogenic.

Initiate antiemetic protocol:	Mildly emetogenic protocol.
Treatment schedule:	Daily
Chair time:	None
Estimated number of visits:	Weekly for CBC and then monthly.

Dose Calculation by: 1. _____ 2. _____

_____
Physician

_____
Patient Name

_____
Diagnosis

_____
Date

_____
ID Number

_____/ _____/ _____
Ht   Wt   M^2

Hydroxyurea

Baseline laboratory tests:	CBC: Chemistry, renal and liver functions
Baseline procedures or tests:	Bone marrow biopsy
Administer:	**Hydroxyurea** _____ 1–5 g/day PO, adjusted to keep WBC about 20–30 $\times$ 10^9/L
Major Side Effects	• Available in 500-mg caplets

- Bone Marrow Depression: Median duration 2–3 weeks and thrombocytopenia 3–4 weeks. Teach self-care measures to minimize risk of infection and bleeding.
- GI Toxicities: Nausea and vomiting are mild to moderate. Diarrhea and dyspepsia may also occur. Dose limiting toxicity.
- Fluid Retention: Common, especially in the older population and primarily periorbital and lower extremity edema. May require diuretics.
- Alteration in Comfort: Muscle cramps, musculoskeletal pain, headaches, fatigue, arthralgias, and abdominal pain. Drowsiness and confusion.
- Skin Alterations: Maculopopular rash, facial, and acral erythemia, hyperpigmentation, dry skin with atrophy and pruritis. Radiation recall.
- Reproduction: Mutagenic and potentially teratogenic.

Initiate antiemetic protocol:	Mildly to moderately emetogenic protocol.
Treatment schedule:	Daily
Chair time:	None
Estimated number of visits:	Weekly or every other week for CBC and then monthly.

Dose Calculation by: 1. _____ 2. _____

_____
Physician

_____
Date

_____
Patient Name

_____
ID Number

_____
Diagnosis

_____/ _____/ _____
Ht   Wt M^2

Interferon α-2b

Baseline laboratory tests:	CBC: Chemistry, renal and liver functions
Baseline procedures or tests:	Bone marrow biopsy
Administer:	**Interferon α-2b** _____ 9-million units SQ per day

Major Side Effects

- Available in single dose prefilled syringes 3, 6, and 9 million units.
- Bone Marrow Depression: Teach self-care measures to minimize the risk of infection and bleeding.
- Flulike Syndrome: Chills 3–6 hours after interferon. Fatigue, malaise, headache, and myalgias are cumulative and dose limiting.
- CNS Effects: Dizziness, confusion, and decreased mental status and depression.
- Thrombophlebitis, pain at the injection site, should be treated with warm compresses.
- GI Toxicities: Nausea and vomiting, anorexia, xerostomia, and mild diarrhea.
- Partial alopecia.
- Reproduction: Mutagenic and potentially teratogenic.

Initiate antiemetic protocol: Mildly to moderately emetogenic protocol.

Supportive drugs:

☐ G-CSF _____   ☐ Peg-G-CSF _____

☐ Epoetin Alfa/   ☐ Allopurinol _____
  Darbepoetin Alfa _____

☐ Antibiotic _____   ☐ Antifungal _____

Treatment schedule: Continue SQ injections 3 days per week for up to 1–1.5 years.

Estimated number of visits: Weekly or every other week for CBC.

Dose Calculation by: 1. _____   2. _____

_____   _____
Physician   Date

_____   _____
Patient Name   ID Number

_____   _____/ _____/ _____
Diagnosis   Ht   Wt   M²

Dasatinib (Sprycel): CML

Baseline laboratory tests:	CBC: Chemistry, renal and liver functions
Baseline procedures or tests:	Bone marrow biopsy
Administer:	**Sprycel** _____ 70 mg PO twice per day with or without food

- Treatment continues as long as patient derives benefit from drug.
- Available in 20-, 50-, and 70-mg tablets.
- Do not take within 2 hours of antacids, do not crush or cut tablets.

Drug interactions:

Ketoconazole, itraconazole, erythromycin, and clarithromycin, ritonavir, atazanavir, indinavir, nefazondone, nelfinavir, saquinavir and telithromycin may increase plasma concentrations.

Dexamethasone, phenytoin, carbamazepine, rifampicin, and phenobarbital may decrease plasma levels. Antacids should be avoided or taken 2 hours after administration of Sprycel. Proton pump inhibitors should be avoided. Drugs that may have their plasma concentration include: alfentanil, astemizole, terfenadine, cisapride, cyclosporine, fentanyl, pimoside, quinidine, sirolims, tacrolimus or ergot alkaloids and should be administered with caution.

Major Side Effects

- Bone Marrow Depression: Severe (grade 3 & 4) thrombocytopenia, neutropenia and anemia. Monitor CBC weekly $\times$ 2 months, then monthly.
- Bleeding Related Events: CNS bleed seen in 1%, GI bleed seen in 7% of patients.
- GI Toxicities: Nausea and vomiting are mild to moderate. Diarrhea and dyspepsia may also occur.
- Fluid Retention: Severe in 9% of patients including pleural effusion and pericardial effusion. May require diuretics.
- Cardiac: Prolongation of QT interval. Monitor potassium and magnesemium levels.
- Rash may occur with pruritus.
- Reproductive: Pregnancy Category D. Breast feeding should be avoided.

Initiate antiemetic protocol:	Mildly to moderately emetogenic protocol.
Treatment schedule:	Daily
Chair time:	None
Estimated number of visits:	Weekly for CBC for 2 months then monthly.

Dose Calculation by: 1. _____   2. _____

_____

Physician

_____

Patient Name

_____

Diagnosis

_____

Date

_____

ID Number

_____ / _____ / _____

Ht   Wt   M^2

LEUKEMIA

Hairy Cell Leukemia

_____   _____

Physician   Date

_____   _____

Patient Name   ID Number

_____   _____/ _____/ _____

Diagnosis   Ht   Wt   M^2

LEUKEMIA

Hairy Cell Leukemia

Cladribine: 0.09-mg/kg/day IV continuous infusion on days 1–7
Administer one cycle.[1,236]

Pentostatin: 4-mg/m^2 IV on day 1
Repeat cycle every 14 days for 6 cycles.[1,237]

Interferon α-2a: 3-million units SC or IM, three times per week
Continue treatment for up to 1 to 1.5 years.[1,238]

Cladribine (Leustatin, 2-CdA)

Baseline laboratory tests:	CBC: Chemistry, renal and liver functions
Baseline procedures or tests:	Bone marrow biopsy, central line placement
Initiate IV:	NS
Administer:	**Cladribine** _____ 0.09-mg/kg/day IV continuous infusion on days 1–7

- Use 22-dilute with NS, dilute in minimum of 100 mL, stable for 24 hours.
- DO NOT USE D5W.

Major Side Effects

- Myelosuppression: Nadir occurs in 7–14 days, recovery by weeks 3–5. Increased risk of opportunistic infections.
- Immunosuppression: Decrease in CD4+ and CD8+, increasing risk for opportunistic infections (fungus, herpes, and *Pneumocystis carinii*).
- Fatigue: Secondary to anemia.
- GI Toxicities: Mild nausea and vomiting, anorexia; constipation, diarrhea.
- Neurotoxicites: Headache, insomnia, and dizziness.
- Flulike Symptoms: Fever, fatigue, malaise, myalgias, arthralgias, and chills. Incidence decreases with continued therapy.
- Skin Integrity: Rash, pruritus, or injection site reactions.
- Reproduction: Mutagenic and potentially teratogenic, discuss contraception and sperm banking.

Initiate antiemetic protocol:	Mildly emetogenic protocol.
Supportive drugs:	☐ G-CSF _____ ☐ Peg-G-CSF _____
	☐ Epoetin Alfa/ ☐ Allopurinol _____
	Darbepoetin Alfa _____
	☐ Antibiotic _____ ☐ Antifungal _____
Treatment schedule:	Chair time 1 hour on day 1, pump dc day 8 one cycle.
Estimated number of visits:	Daily for seven days, then weekly CBC.

Dose Calculation by: 1. _____   2. _____

_____   _____
Physician   Date

_____   _____
Patient Name   ID Number

_____   _____/ _____/ _____
Diagnosis   Ht   Wt   M^2

Pentostatin

Baseline laboratory tests:	CBC: Chemistry, renal and liver functions
Baseline procedures or tests:	Bone marrow biopsy
Initiate IV:	NS
Administer:	**Pentostatin** _____ 4-mg/m^2 IV on day 1

- Available in single dose vials of 10 mg.
- Dilute with 5 mL of sterile water for a concentration of 2 mg/mL. May be given IV push or as bolus diluted in 25–50 mL of NS or D5W over 30 minutes. Solution is stable at room temperature for 8 hours.

Major Side Effects

- Myelosuppression: Increased risk of opportunistic infections. Dose limiting toxicity.
- Fatigue: Secondary to anemia.
- GI Toxicities: Moderate nausea and vomiting, anorexia.
- Allergic Hypersensitivity Reaction: Fever, chills, myalgias, and arthralgias.
- Neurologic Toxicities: Headache, lethargy, and fatigue.
- Immunosuppression: Decrease in CD4+ and CD8+, increasing risk for opportunistic infections (fungus, herpes, and *Pneumocystis carinii*).
- Reproduction: Mutagenic and potentially teratogenic, discuss contraception and sperm banking.

Initiate antiemetic protocol: Moderately emetogenic protocol.

Supportive drugs:

☐ G-CSF _____   ☐ Peg-G-CSF _____
☐ Epoetin Alfa/   ☐ Allopurinol _____
   Darbepoetin Alfa _____
☐ Antibiotic _____ ☐ Antifungal _____

Treatment schedule: Chair time 1 hour on day 1; treat every other week for six cycles or two cycles beyond complete remission. Do not treat for more than 1 year.

Estimated number of visits: Every other week until remission.

Dose Calculation by: 1. _____   2. _____

_____   _____
Physician   Date

_____   _____
Patient Name   ID Number

_____   _____/ _____/ _____
Diagnosis   Ht   Wt   M^2

Interferon

Baseline laboratory tests:	CBC: Chemistry, renal and liver functions
Baseline procedures or tests:	Bone marrow biopsy
Administer:	**Interferon α-2a** _____ 3-million units SQ per day 3 days per week
Major Side Effects	

- Available in single dose prefilled syringes 3, 6, and 9 million units.
- Do not freeze or shake.
- Stable for 1 month refrigerated.
- Bone Marrow Depression: Teach self-care measures to minimize risk of infection and bleeding.
- Flulike Syndrome: Chills 3–6 hours after interferon. Fatigue, malaise, headache, and myalgias are cumulative and dose limiting.
- CNS Effects: Dizziness, confusion, and decreased mental status and depression.
- Thrombophlebitis, pain at the injection site, should be treated with warm compresses.
- GI Toxicities: Nausea and vomiting, anorexia, xerostomia, and mild diarrhea.
- Partial alopecia.
- Reproduction: Mutagenic and potentially teratogenic.

Initiate antiemetic protocol:	Mildly to moderately emetogenic protocol.
Supportive drugs:	☐ G-CSF _____ ☐ Peg-G-CSF _____
	☐ Epoetin Alfa/ ☐ Allopurinol _____
	Darbepoetin Alfa _____
	☐ Antibiotic _____ ☐ Antifungal _____
Treatment schedule:	Continue SQ injections 3 days per week for up to 1–1.5 years.
Estimated number of visits:	Weekly or every other week for CBC.

Dose Calculation by: 1. _____   2. _____

_____   _____
Physician   Date

_____   _____
Patient Name   ID Number

_____   _____ / _____ / _____
Diagnosis   Ht   Wt   M^2

LUNG CANCER

Non–Small Cell Lung Cancer

ADJUVANT THERAPY
Combination Therapy

Paclitaxel + Carboplatin..372

Paclitaxel: 175-mg/m^2 IV over 3 hours on day 1
Carboplatin: Area under the curve (AUC) of 6, IV on day 1
Repeat cycle every 21 days for 4 cycles.[1,239]

Vinorelbine + Cisplatin...373

Vinorelbine: 25-mg/m^2 IV weekly for 16 weeks
Cisplatin: 50-mg/m^2 IV on days 1 and 8.
Repeat cisplatin every 28 days for 4 cycles.[1,240]

METASTATIC DISEASE
Combination Regimens

Carboplatin + Paclitaxel..374

Carboplatin: AUC of 6, IV on day 1
Paclitaxel: 175-mg/m^2 IV over 3 hours on day 1
Repeat cycle every 21 days.[1,241]
It is important to administer paclitaxel first, followed by carboplatin.

Cisplatin + Paclitaxel...375

Cisplatin: 80-mg/m^2 IV on day 1
Paclitaxel: 175-mg/m^2 IV over 3 hours on day 1
Repeat cycle every 21 days.[1,242]
Important to administer paclitaxel first, followed by cisplatin

Docetaxel + Carboplatin..377

Docetaxel: 75-mg/m^2 IV on day 1
Carboplatin: AUC of 6, IV on day 1
Repeat cycle every 21 days.[1,243]

Docetaxel + Cisplatin **379**

Docetaxel: 75-mg/m^2 IV on day 1
Cisplatin: 75-mg/m^2 IV on day 1
Repeat cycle every 21 days.[1,244]

Docetaxel + Gemcitabine **381**

Docetaxel: 100-mg/m^2 IV on day 8
Gemcitabine: 1100-mg/m^2 IV on days 1 and 8
Repeat cycle every 21 days.[1,245]
Granulocyte colony stimulating factor (G-CSF) support is required from
days 9 to 15.

Gemcitabine + Cisplatin **383**

Gemcitabine: 1250-mg/m^2 IV on days 1 and 8
Cisplatin: 100-mg/m^2 IV on day 1
Repeat cycle every 21 days.[1,246]

Gemcitabine + Carboplatin **384**

Gemcitabine: 1000-mg/m^2 IV on days 1 and 8
Carboplatin: AUC of 5, IV on day 1
Repeat cycle every 21 days.[1,247]

Gemcitabine + Vinorelbine **386**

Gemcitabine: 1200-mg/m^2 IV on days 1 and 8
Vinorelbine: 30-mg/m^2 IV on days 1 and 8
Repeat cycle every 21 days.[1,248]

Vinorelbine + Cisplatin **387**

Vinorelbine: 30-mg/m^2 IV on days 1, 8, and 15
Cisplatin: 120-mg/m^2 IV on day 1
Repeat cycle every 28 days.[1,249]

Vinorelbine + Carboplatin **388**

Vinorelbine: 25-mg/m^2 IV on days 1 and 8
Carboplatin: AUC of 6, IV on day 1
Repeat cycle every 28 days.[1,250]

Etoposide (VP-16): 120-mg/m^2 IV on days 1–3
Cisplatin: 60-mg/m^2 IV on day 1
Repeat cycle every 21–28 days.[1,251]

Cisplatin: 50-mg/m^2 IV on days 1, 8, 29, and 36
Etoposide: 50-mg/m^2 IV on days 1–5 and 29–33
Administer concurrent thoracic radiation therapy, followed 4–6 weeks
  after the completion of combined modality therapy by
Docetaxel: 75-mg/m^2 IV on day 1
Repeat cycle every 21 days for three cycles.[1,252] The dose of docetaxel can be
  escalated to 100-mg/m^2 IV on subsequent cycles in the absence of toxicity.

Single-Agent Regimens

Paclitaxel: 225-mg/m^2 IV over 3 hours on day 1
Repeat cycle every 21 days.[1,253]
OR
Paclitaxel: 80–100-mg/m^2 IV weekly for 3 weeks
Repeat cycle every 28 days after a 1-week rest.[1,254]

Docetaxel: 75-mg/m^2 IV on day 1
Repeat cycle every 21 days.[1,255]
OR
Docetaxel: 36-mg/m^2 IV weekly for 6 weeks
Repeat cycle every 8 weeks after 2-week rest.[1,256]
Premedicate with dexamethasone 8 mg PO at 12 hours and immediately
  before docetaxel infusion and 12 hours after each dose.

Pemetrexed: 500-mg/m^2 IV over 10–30 minutes every 21 days.[1,257]

Gemcitabine: 1000-mg/m^2 IV on days 1, 8, and 15
Repeat cycle every 28 days.[1,258]

Topotecan **398**

Topotecan: 1.5-mg/m^2 IV on days 1–5
Repeat cycle every 21 days.[1,259]

Vinorelbine **399**

Vinorelbine: 25-mg/m^2 IV every 7 days
Repeat every 7 days.[1,260]

Gefitinib (Iressa) **400**

Gefitinib: 250 mg/day PO
Continue treatment until disease progression.[1,261]

Erlotinib (Tarceva) **401**

Erotinib: 150-mg PO
Continue until disease progression.[1,262]

ADJUVANT THERAPY
Combination Therapy

Paclitaxel + Carboplatin

Baseline laboratory tests: CBC: Chemistry

Baseline procedures or tests: N/A

Initiate IV: 0.9% sodium chloride

Premedicate: 5-HT$_3$ and dexamethasone 10–20 mg in 100 cc of normal saline (NS)
Diphenhydramine 25–50 mg and cimetidine 300 mg in 100 cc of NS

Administer: **Paclitaxel** _____mg (175 mg/m^2) IV over 3 hours on day 1

- Available in 30 mL, 6 mg/mL; 100 mL, 16.7 mg/mL and 300.
- Final concentration is ± 1.2 mg/mL.
- Stable for up to 27 hours at room temperature in 0.3–1.2 mg/mL solutions.
- **Use non-PVC containers and tubing with a 0.22-micron inline filter to administer.**

Carboplatin _____mg (AUC 6) IV on day 1

- Available in 50, 150, and 450 lyophilized powder or 450 and 600 premixed vial.
- Do not use aluminum needles, because precipitate will form.
- Give carboplatin **after** paclitaxel to decrease toxicities.
- Reconstitute with D5W or 0.9% sodium chloride to final concentration of 1–4 mg/mL.
- Reconstituted solution stable for 8 hours at room temperature.

Major Side Effects

- Hypersensitivity Reaction: Paclitaxel (30%–40%). Premedicate as described. Increased risk of hypersensitivity reactions in patients receiving more than seven courses of carboplatin therapy. Characterized by dyspnea, hypotension, angiodema, usticoria, skin rash, pruritis, tachycardim, wheezing, and facial edema. Patients with mild reactions can be rechallenged.
- Bone Marrow Depression: Neutropenia, thrombocytopenia, and anemia are cumulative and dose related. Can be dose limiting. G-CSF support recommended.
- Gastrointestinal (GI) Toxicities: Moderate to severe nausea and vomiting may be acute or delayed. Mucositis and/or diarrhea occur in 30%–40% of patients.
- Renal: Nephrotoxicity less common than with cisplatin and rarely symptomatic.
- Neurotoxicity: Sensory neuropathy with numbness and paresthesias; dose related. More frequent with longer infusions and at doses of > 175 mg/m^2.
- Alopecia: Total loss of body hair occurs in nearly all patients.
- Reproduction: Pregnancy category D. Breast feeding should be avoided.

Initiate antiemetic protocol: Moderately to highly emetogenic protocol.

Supportive drugs:
☐ pegfilgrastim (Neulasta) ☐ filgrastim (Neupogen)
☐ epoetin alfa (Procrit) ☐ darbepoetin alfa (Aranesp)

Treatment schedule: Chair time 5 hours on day 1. Repeat cycle every 21 days for 4 cycles.

Estimated number of visits: Two visits per cycle. Request three cycles worth of visits.

Dose Calculation by: 1. _____   2. _____

_____
Physician

_____
Patient Name

_____
Diagnosis

_____
Date

_____
ID Number

_____/_____/_____
Ht   Wt   M^2

Vinorelbine + Cisplatin

Baseline laboratory tests:	CBC: Chemistry (including Mg^{2+})
Baseline procedures or tests:	N/A
Initiate IV:	0.9% sodium chloride
Premedicate:	5-HT_3 and dexamethasone 10–20 mg in 100 cc of NS
Administer:	**Vinorelbine** _____mg (25 mg/m^2) IV on weekly for 16 weeks

- **Vesicant**.
- Available in 10 mg/mL in 1- or 5-mL single use vials.
- Further dilute to a final concentration in syringe 1.5–3.0 or IV bag of 0.5–3.0 mg/mL.
- Infuse diluted drug IV over 6–10 minutes into sidearm port of a freely flowing IV, either peripherally or via central line (preferred). Use port closest to the IV bag. Not the patient.
- Flush vein with at least 75–125 mL of IV solution after infusion.
- Reconstituted solution is stable for 24 hours refrigerated.

Cisplatin _____mg (50 mg/m^2) IV on days 1 and 8.

- Available in 100-mL vials. 1-mg/1-mL concentrations.
- Do not use aluminum needles, as precipitate will form.
- Further dilute solution with 250 cc or more NS.
- 100-mL vial stable for 28 days protected from light, 7 days under florescent light.

Major Side Effects

- Bone Marrow Depression: Neutropenia, thrombocytopenia, and anemia are dose related and can be dose limiting.
- GI Toxicities: Moderate to severe nausea and vomiting may be acute or delayed. Constipation, diarrhea, stomatitis, and anorexia may be seen. Metallic taste to foods.
- Neurotoxicity: Severe neuropathy with numbness, tingling, and sensory loss in arms and legs. Proprioception and vibratory sense and loss of motor function can occur. Paresthesias are dose related and can be severe, requiring pain medication or neurontin. Ototoxicity occurs in > 30% beginning with high-frequency hearing.
- Renal: Dose-limiting toxicity and may be cumulative and presents at 10–20 days. May result in necrosis of proximal and distal renal tubules preventing reabsorption of Mg^{2+}, Ca^{2+}, and K^+. Can be avoided with adequate hydration, diuresis as well as slower infusion time.
- Skin: Extravasation of vinorelbine may cause local tissue injury and inflammation. Alopecia likely.
- Reproduction: Pregnancy category D. Breast feeding should be avoided.

Initiate antiemetic protocol:	Moderately to highly emetogenic protocol.
Supportive drugs:	☐ pegfilgrastim (Neulasta) ☐ filgrastim (Neupogen)
	☐ epoetin alfa (Procrit) ☐ darbepoetin alfa (Aranesp)
Treatment schedule:	Chair time 3 hours on day 1 and 1 hour on days 8 and 15. Repeat cisplatin every 28 days for 4 cycles (1 hour for vinorelbine weekly for 16 weeks).
Estimated number of visits:	Weekly. Request three cycles worth of visits.

Dose Calculation by: 1. _____   2. _____

_____   _____
Physician   Date

_____   _____
Patient Name   ID Number

_____   _____/_____/_____
Diagnosis   Ht   Wt   M^2

METASTATIC DISEASE
Combination Regimens

Carboplatin + Paclitaxel

Baseline laboratory tests:	CBC: Chemistry
Baseline procedures or tests:	N/A
Initiate IV:	0.9% sodium chloride
Premedicate:	5-HT$_3$ and dexamethasone 10–20 mg in 100 cc of normal saline (NS)
	Diphenhydramine 25–50 mg and cimetidine 300 mg in 100 cc of NS
Administer:	**Paclitaxel** _____ mg (175 mg/m^2) IV over 3 hours on day 1

- Available in 30 mL, 6 mg/mL; 100 mL, 16.7 mg/mL and 300.
- Final concentration is ± 1.2 mg/mL.
- Stable for up to 27 hours at room temperature in 0.3–1.2 mg/mL solutions.
- **Use non-PVC containers and tubing with a 0.22-micron inline filter to administer.**

Carboplatin _____ mg (AUC 6) IV on day 1

- Available in 50, 150, and 450 lyophilized powder or 450 and 600 premixed vial.
- Do not use aluminum needles, because precipitate will form.
- Give carboplatin **after** paclitaxel to decrease toxicities.
- Reconstitute with D5W or 0.9% sodium chloride to final concentration of 1–4 mg/mL.
- Reconstituted solution stable for 8 hours at room temperature.

Major Side Effects

- Hypersensitivity Reaction: Paclitaxel (30%–40%). Premedicate as described. Increased risk of hypersensitivity reactions in patients receiving more than seven courses of carboplatin therapy. Characterized by dyspnea, hypotension, angiodema, usticoria, skin rash, pruritis, tachycardim, wheezing, and facial edema. Patients with mild reactions can be rechallenged.
- Bone Marrow Depression: Neutropenia, thrombocytopenia, and anemia are cumulative and dose related. Can be dose limiting. G-CSF support recommended.
- Gastrointestinal (GI) Toxicities: Moderate to severe nausea and vomiting may be acute or delayed. Mucositis and/or diarrhea occur in 30%–40% of patients.
- Renal: Nephrotoxicity less common than with cisplatin and rarely symptomatic.
- Neurotoxicity: Sensory neuropathy with numbness and paresthesias; dose related.
- Alopecia: Total loss of body hair occurs in nearly all patients.
- Reproduction: Pregnancy category D. Breast feeding should be avoided.

Initiate antiemetic protocol:	Moderately to highly emetogenic protocol.
Supportive drugs:	☐ pegfilgrastim (Neulasta) ☐ filgrastim (Neupogen)
	☐ epoetin alfa (Procrit) ☐ darbepoetin alfa (Aranesp)
Treatment schedule:	Chair time 5 hours on day 1. Repeat cycle every 21 days until disease progression.
Estimated number of visits:	Two visits per cycle. Request three cycles worth of visits.

Dose Calculation by: 1. _____ 2. _____

_____
Physician

_____
Date

_____
Patient Name

_____
ID Number

_____
Diagnosis

_____ / _____ / _____
Ht   Wt   M^2

Cisplatin + Paclitaxel

Baseline laboratory tests:	CBC: Chemistry (including Mg^{2+}) and CEA
Baseline procedures or tests:	Central line placement
Initiate IV:	0.9% sodium chloride
Premedicate:	5-HT_3 and dexamethasone in 100 cc of NS (days 1 and 2)
	Diphenhydramine 25–50 mg and cimetidine 300 mg in 100 cc of NS (day 1 only)
Administer:	Paclitaxel _____mg (175 mg/m^2) IV over 3 hours on day 1

- Available in 30 mg (6 mg/mL), 100 mg (16.7 mg/mL) and 300 mg (6 mg/ mL) vials.
- Stable for up to 27 hours at room temperature in 0.3–1.2 mg/mL solutions.
- Further dilute in 250–500 cc NS or D5W. Final concentration is $\pm$ 1.2 mg/mL.
- **Use non-PVC tubing and containers and a 0.22-micron inline filter to administer.**

Cisplatin _____mg (80 mg/m^2) IV on day 1

- Available in 100-mL vials. 1-mg/1-mL concentrations.
- Do not use aluminum needles, as precipitate will form.
- Further dilute solution with 250 cc or more NS.
- 100-mL vial stable for 28 days protected from light, 7 days under florescent light.

Paclitaxel must be administered first, followed by cisplatin.

Repeat the cycle every 21 days.

Major Side Effects	

- Hypersensitivity Reaction: Paclitaxel and cisplatin, with anaphylaxis and severe hypersensitivity reactions in 2%–4%. Characterized by dyspnea, hypotension, andioedema, and generalized urticaria. May also see tachycardia, wheezing, and facial edema. Patients with mild reactions can be rechallenged after 24 hour corticosteroid prophylaxis. Patients with severe reactions should not be rechallenged. Monitor vitals signs every 15 minutes for the first hour. Premedicate as described.
- Bone Marrow Depression: Neutropenia, thrombocytopenia, and anemia are cumulative and dose related. Can be dose limiting. G-CSF support recommended.
- GI Toxicities: Nausea and vomiting may be severe and will occur in 100% of patients if antiemetics are not given. May be acute (within 1 or more hours, lasting for 8–24 hours or delayed occurring 24–72 hours after cisplatin). Taste alterations and anorexia occur with long-term use. Metallic taste to food.
- Renal: Dose-limiting toxicity and may be cumulative and presents at 10–20 days. May result in necrosis of proximal and distal renal tubules preventing reabsorption of Mg^{2+}, Ca^{2+}, and K^V. Can be avoided with adequate hydration, diuresis as well as slower infusion time.
- Neurotoxicity: Severe neuropathy with numbness, tingling, and sensory loss in arms and legs. Proprioception and vibratory sense and loss of motor function can occur. Paresthesias are dose related and can be severe, requiring pain medication or neurontin. Ototoxicity occurs in >30% beginning with high-frequency hearing.
- Alopecia: Total loss of body hair occurs in nearly all patients.
- Reproduction: Pregnancy category D. Breast feeding should be avoided.

Initiate antiemetic protocol:	Moderately to highly emetogenic protocol.
Supportive drugs:	☐ pegfilgrastim (Neulasta) ☐ filgrastim (Neupogen)
	☐ epoetin alfa (Procrit) ☐ darbepoetin alfa (Aranesp)
Treatment schedule:	Chair time 5 hours on day 1. Repeat every 21 days.
Estimated number of visits:	Two visits per cycle.

Dose Calculation by: 1. _____ 2. _____

_____   _____
Physician   Date

_____   _____
Patient Name   ID Number

_____   _____ / _____ / _____
Diagnosis   Ht   Wt   M^2

Docetaxel + Carboplatin

Baseline laboratory tests:	CBC: Chemistry (including Mg^{2+}) and CEA
Baseline procedures or tests:	N/A
Initiate IV:	0.9% sodium chloride
Premedicate:	Dexamethasone 8-mg PO bid for 3 days, starting the day before treatment; 5-HT_3 and dexamethasone 10–20 mg in 100 cc of NS on day of treatment

Administer:

Docetaxel _____mg (75 mg/m^2) IV on day 1

- Available in 20- or 80-mg doses; comes with own diluent. Do not shake.
- Reconstituted vials stable at room temperature or refrigerated for 8 hours.
- Further dilute in 250 cc of D5W or 0.9% sodium chloride.
- **Use non-PVC containers and tubings to administer. No filter needed.**

Carboplatin _____mg (AUC 6) IV on day 1

- Available in 50-mg, 150-mg, and 450-mg lyophilized powder; dilute with sterile water. Also available in 50-mg and 150-mg 10-mg/mLg/mL solution; 450-mg and 600-mg 10-mg/mL multidose vials stable for 15 days after first use.
- Do not use aluminum needles, as precipitate will form.
- Further dilute in 250–1000 cc 0.9% sodium chloride.
- Chemically stable for 24 hours, discard after 8 hours because of lack of bacteriostatic perservative.
- Give carboplatin **after** paclitaxel to decrease toxicities.

Major Side Effects

- Hypersensitivity Reaction: Docetaxel and carboplatin, with anaphylaxis and severe hypersensitivity reactions in 2%–4%. Characterized by dyspnea, hypotension, andioedema, and generalized urticaria. May also see tachycardia, wheezing, and facial edema. Patients with mild reactions can be rechallenged after 24-hour corticosteroid prophylaxis. Patients with severe reactions should not be rechallenged. Monitor vitals signs every 15 minutes for the first hour. Carboplatin can cause rash, flushing, urticaria, erythema, and pruritus. Bronchospasm and hypotension are uncommon, but risk increases from 1% to 27% in patients receiving more than seven courses of carboplatin-based therapy. Premedicate as indicated.
- Bone Marrow Depression: Neutropenia, thrombocytopenia, and anemia are dose related and can be dose limiting. Risk of thrombocytopenia is severe.
- GI Toxicities: Moderate to severe nausea and vomiting within first 6–24 hours. Reversible hepatic dysfunction mild to moderate. Monitor SGOT, SGPT, and bili.
- Renal: Nephrotoxicity less common than with cisplatin and rarely symptomatic, especially when well hydrated. Decreases Mg^{2+}, K^+, Ca^{2+}, and Na^+.
- Fluid Balance: Fluid retention is a cumulative toxicity that may occur with docetaxel. Characterized by peripheral edema, pleural effusions, dyspnea at rest, cardiac tamponade, or ascites. Pre-treatment with dexamethasone as above may minimize the effect.
- Neuropathy: Peripheral neuropathy may affect up to 49% of patients (severe 5.5%). Sensory alterations are paresthesias in a glove-and-stocking distribution and numbness. There is an increased risk in patients > 65 years old or in those previously treated with cisplatin and receiving prolonged carboplatin treatment.
- Skin: Alopecia is common. Maculopapular, violaceous/erythematous and pruritic rash may occur with docetaxel. Changes in nails may occur in 11%–40% of patients and may include onycholysis (loss of nail). Keep nails clean, use nail hardeners or Tea Tree Oil. Lotrimin if indicated.
- Reproduction: Drugs are mutagenic and teratogenic.

Initiate antiemetic protocol:	Moderately to highly emetogenic protocol.
Supportive drugs:	☐ pegfilgrastim (Neulasta) ☐ filgrastim (Neupogen)
	☐ epoetin alfa (Procrit) ☐ darbepoetin alfa (Aranesp)
Treatment schedule:	Chair time 4 hours on day 1. Repeat cycle every 21 days.
Estimated number of visits:	Two visits per cycle. Request four cycles worth of visits.

Dose Calculation by: 1. _____   2. _____

_____

Physician

_____

Patient Name

_____

Diagnosis

_____

Date

_____

ID Number

_____ / _____ / _____

Ht   Wt   M^2

Docetaxel + Cisplatin

Baseline laboratory tests:	CBC: Chemistry (including Mg^{2+}) and CEA
Baseline procedures or tests:	Central line placement
Initiate IV:	0.9% sodium chloride
Premedicate:	Dexamethasone 8-mg PO bid for 3 days, starting the day before treatment; 5-HT$_3$ and dexamethasone 10–20 mg in 100 cc of NS day of treatment

Administer:

Docetaxel _____mg (75 mg/m^2) IV on day 1

- Comes in 20- or 80-mg blister packs with own diluent. Do not shake. Final concentration 10 mg/mL.
- Reconstituted vials stable at room temperature or refrigerate for 8 hours.
- Further dilute in 250 cc of D5W or 0.9% sodium chloride. Thoroughly mix by manual rotation.
- Use non-PVC containers and tubing to administer. Filter NOT necessary.

Cisplatin _____mg (75 mg/m^2) IV on day 1

- Available in 100-mL vials. 1-mg/1-mL concentrations.
- Do not use aluminum needles, as precipitate will form.
- Further dilute solution with 250 cc or more NS.
- 100-mL vial stable for 28 days protected from light, 7 days under florescent light.

Major Side Effects

- Hypersensitivity Reaction: Docetaxel and cisplatin, with anaphylaxis and severe hypersensitivity reactions in 2%–4%.Characterized by dyspnea, hypotension, andioedema, and generalized urticaria. May also see tachycardia, wheezing, and facial edema. Patients with mild reactions can be rechallenged after 24-hour corticosteroid prophylaxis. Patients with severe reactions should not be rechallenged. Monitor vitals signs every 15 minutes for the first hour. Premedicate as described.
- Bone Marrow Depression: Neutropenia, thrombocytopenia, and anemia are dose related and can be dose limiting. Nadir at day 7.
- GI Toxicities: Moderate-to-severe nausea and vomiting may be acute or delayed. Metallic taste to food.
- Neurotoxicity: Severe neuropathy with numbness, tingling, and sensory loss in arms and legs. Proprioception and vibratory sense and loss of motor function can occur. Paresthesias are dose related and can be severe, requiring pain medication or neurontin. Ototoxicity occurs in > 30% beginning with high-frequency hearing.
- Renal: Dose-limiting toxicity and may be cumulative and presents at 10–20 days. May result in necrosis of proximal and distal renal tubules preventing reabsorption of Mg^{2+}, Ca^{2+}, and K^+. Can be avoided with adequate hydration, diuresis as well as slower infusion time.
- Fluid Balance: Fluid retention is a cumulative toxicity that may occur with docetaxel. Characterized by peripheral edema, pleural effusions, dyspnea at rest, cardiac tamponade, or ascites. Pre-treatment with dexamethasone as above may minimize the effect.
- Skin: Alopecia is common. Maculopapular, violaceous/erythematous and pruritic rash may occur with docetaxel. Changes in nails may occur in 11%–40% of patients and may include onycholysis (loss of nail). Keep nails clean, use nail hardeners or Tea Tree Oil. Lotrimin if indicated.
- Reproduction: Pregnancy category D. Breast feeding should be avoided.

Initiate antiemetic protocol:	Moderately to highly emetogenic protocol.
Supportive drugs:	☐ pegfilgrastim (Neulasta) ☐ filgrastim (Neupogen)
	☐ epoetin alfa (Procrit) ☐ darbepoetin alfa (Aranesp)
Treatment schedule:	Chair time 4 hours on day 1. Repeat cycle every 21 days.
Estimated number of visits:	Two visits per cycle. Request four cycles worth of visits. May require extra visits for hydration.

Dose Calculation by: 1. _____   2. _____

_____

Physician   Date

_____

Patient Name   ID Number

_____   _____ / _____ / _____

Diagnosis   Ht   Wt   M²

Docetaxel + Gemcitabine

Baseline laboratory tests:	CBC: Chemistry panel, and liver function tests (LFTs)
Baseline procedures or tests:	N/A
Initiate IV:	0.9% sodium chloride
Premedicate:	Oral phenothiazine

OR

5-HT$_3$ and dexamethasone 10 mg in 100 cc of NS and dexamethasone 8-mg PO bid for 3 days, starting the day before treatment

Administer:

Docetaxel _____ mg (100 mg/m^2) IV on day 8

- Comes in 20- or 80-mg blister packs with own diluent. Do not shake. Thoroughly mix by manual rotation. Final concentration 10 mg/mL.
- Reconstituted vials stable at room temperature or refrigerate for 8 hours.
- Further dilute in 250 cc of D5W or 0.9% sodium chloride.
- Use non-PVC containers and tubing to administer. No filter needed.

Gemcitabine _____ mg (1100 mg/m^2) IV on days 1 and 8 over 30 minutes

- Available in 200-mg/10-mL or 1-g/50-mL vials (20-mg/mL).
- Further dilute in 0.9% sodium chloride.
- Reconstituted solution is stable 24 hours at room temperature. Do NOT refrigerate, because precipitate will form.

Major Side Effects

- Hypersensitivity Reaction: Docetaxel with anaphylaxis and severe hypersensitivity reactions in 2%–4%. Characterized by dyspnea, hypotension, andioedema, and generalized urticaria. May also see tachycardia, wheezing, and facial edema. Patients with mild reactions can be rechallenged after 24-hour corticosteroid prophylaxis. Patients with severe reactions should not be rechallenged. Monitor vitals signs every 15 minutes for the first hour. Premedicate as described.
- Hematologic: Myelosuppression is dose limiting. G-CSF support required from days 9–15. Thrombocytopenia grades 3–4 are more common in the elderly.
- GI Symptoms: Mild to moderate nausea and vomiting, diarrhea, and mucositis.
- Neurotoxicity: Severe neuropathy with numbness, tingling, and sensory loss in arms and legs. Proprioception and vibratory sense and loss of motor function can occur. Paresthesias are dose related and can be severe, requiring pain medication or neurontin. Ototoxicity occurs in > 30% beginning with high-frequency hearing.
- Flulike Syndrome (20%) with fever 6–12 hours after treatment.
- Hepatic: Elevation of serum transaminase and bilirubin levels.
- Fluid Balance: Fluid retention is a cumulative toxicity that may occur with docetaxel. Characterized by peripheral edema, pleural effusions, dyspnea at rest, cardiac tamponade, or ascites. Pre-treatment with dexamethasone as above may minimize the effect.
- Skin: Alopecia is common. Maculopapular, violaceous/erythematous and pruritic rash may occur with docetaxel. Changes in nails may occur in 11%–40% of patients and may include onycholysis (loss of nail). Keep nails clean, use nail hardeners or Tea Tree Oil. Lotrimin if indicated.
- Reproduction: Pregnancy category D. Breast feeding should be avoided.

Initiate antiemetic protocol:	Mildly to moderately emetogenic protocol
Supportive drugs:	☐ pegfilgrastim (Neulasta) ☐ filgrastim (Neupogen)
	☐ epoetin alfa (Procrit) ☐ darbepoetin alfa (Aranesp)
Treatment schedule:	Chair time 1 hour on day 1 and 2 hours on day 8. Repeat cycle every 21 days.
Estimated number of visits:	Three visits per cycle. Request four cycles worth of visits.

Dose Calculation by: 1. _____   2. _____

_____   _____
Physician   Date

_____   _____
Patient Name   ID Number

_____   _____ / _____ / _____
Diagnosis   Ht   Wt   M^2

Gemcitabine + Cisplatin

Baseline laboratory tests:	CBC: Chemistry panel (including Mg^{2+}) and LFTs
Baseline procedures or tests:	N/A
Initiate IV:	0.9% sodium chloride
Premedicate:	5-HT$_3$ and dexamethasone 10–20 mg in 100 cc of NS
Administer:	**Gemcitabine** _____ mg (1250 mg/m^2) IV over 30 minutes on days 1 and 8

- Available in 200-mg/10-mL or 1-g/50-mL vials (20-mg/mL).
- Further dilute in 0.9% sodium chloride.
- Reconstituted solution is stable 24 hours at room temperature. Do NOT refrigerate, because precipitate will form.

Cisplatin _____ mg (100 mg/m^2) IV on day 1

- Available in 100-mL vials. 1-mg/1-mL concentrations.
- Do not use aluminum needles, as precipitate will form.
- Further dilute solution with 250 cc or more NS.
- 100-mL vial stable for 28 days protected from light, 7 days under florescent light.

Major Side Effects

- Hematologic: Leukopenia (63%), thrombocytopenia (36%), and anemia (73%), with grade 3 and 4 thrombocytopenia more common in older patients. Myelosuppression is dose limiting. Nadir occurs in 10–14 days with recovery at 21 days. Prolonged infusion time (> 60 minutes) is associated with higher toxicities.
- GI Symptoms: Moderate-to-severe nausea and vomiting that may be acute or delayed. Diarrhea and/or mucositis (15%–20%). Metallic taste to food.
- Flulike Syndrome (20%) with fever in absence of infection 6–12 hours after treatment (40%).
- Neurotoxicity: Severe neuropathy with numbness, tingling, and sensory loss in arms and legs. Proprioception and vibratory sense and loss of motor function can occur. Paresthesias are dose related and can be severe, requiring pain medication or neurontin. Ototoxicity occurs in > 30% beginning with high-frequency hearing.
- Renal: Dose-limiting toxicity and may be cumulative and presents at 10–20 days. May result in necrosis of proximal and distal renal tubules, preventing reabsorption of Mg^{2+}, Ca^{2+}, and K^+. Can be avoided with adequate hydration, diuresis as well as slower infusion time.
- Hepatic: Elevation of serum transaminase and bilirubin levels.
- Skin: Pruritic, maculopapular skin rash, usually involving trunk and extremities, occurs in 30% of patients. Alopecia.
- Use in pregnancy: Embryotoxic; women of childbearing potential should avoid becoming pregnant during treatment.

Initiate antiemetic protocol:	Moderately to highly emetogenic protocol.
Supportive drugs:	☐ pegfilgrastim (Neulasta) ☐ filgrastim (Neupogen)
	☐ epoetin alfa (Procrit) ☐ darbepoetin alfa (Aranesp)
Treatment schedule:	Chair time 3 hours on day 1, and 1 hour on day 8. Repeat cycle every 21 days.
Estimated number of visits:	Two visits per cycle. Request three cycles worth of visits.

Dose Calculation by: 1. _____   2. _____

_____
Physician

_____
Date

_____
Patient Name

_____
ID Number

_____
Diagnosis

_____ / _____ / _____
Ht   Wt   M^2

Gemcitabine + Carboplatin

Baseline laboratory tests:	CBC: Chemistry panel (with LFTs)
Baseline procedures or tests:	N/A
Initiate IV:	0.9% sodium chloride
Premedicate:	5-HT$_3$ and dexamethasone 10–20 mg in 100 cc of NS
	Diphenhydramine 25–50 mg and cimetidine 300 mg in 100 cc of NS

Administer:

Gemcitabine _____mg (1000 mg/m^2) IV on days 1 and 8 over 30 minutes

- Available in 200-mg/10-mL or 1-g/50-mL vials (20-mg/mL).
- Further dilute in 0.9% sodium chloride.
- Reconstituted solution is stable 24 hours at room temperature. Do NOT refrigerate, because precipitate will form.

Carboplatin _____ mg (AUC 5) IV on day 1

- Available in 50-mg, 150-mg, and 450-mg lyophilized powder; dilute with sterile water. Also available in 50-mg and 150-mg 10-mg/mLg/mL solution; 450-mg and 600-mg 10-mg/mL multidose vials stable for 15 days after first use.
- Do not use aluminum needles, as precipitate will form.
- Further dilute in 250–1000 cc 0.9% sodium chloride.
- Chemically stable for 24 hours, discard after 8 hours because of lack of bacteriostatic perservative.
- Give carboplatin **after** paclitaxel to decrease toxicities.

Major Side Effects

- Hypersensitivity Reaction: Anaphylaxis and severe hypersensitivity reactions in 2%–4%. Characterized by dyspnea, hypotension, andioedema, and generalized urticaria. May also see tachycardia, wheezing, and facial edema. Patients with mild reactions can be rechallenged after 24-hour corticosteroid prophylaxis. Patients with severe reactions should not be rechallenged. Monitor vitals signs every 15 minutes for the first hour. Premedicate as described. The risk increases in patients receiving more than seven courses of carboplatin therapy.
- Bone Marrow Depression: Neutropenia, thrombocytopenia, and anemia are cumulative and dose related. Can be dose limiting. G-CSF recommended. Thrombocytopenia grades 3–4 are more common in the elderly.
- GI Toxicities: Moderate to severe nausea and vomiting, acute or delayed. Mucositis and diarrhea seen. Elevation of serum transaminase and bilirubin levels.
- Flulike Syndrome: Flulike symptoms with fever in absence of infection 6–12 hours after treatment.
- Fluid Balance: Fluid retention is a cumulative toxicity that may occur with docetaxel. Characterized by peripheral edema, pleural effusions, dyspnea at rest, cardiac tamponade, or ascites. Pre-treatment with dexamethasone as above may minimize the effect.
- Neurotoxicity: Severe neuropathy with numbness, tingling, and sensory loss in arms and legs. Proprioception and vibratory sense and loss of motor function can occur. Paresthesias are dose related and can be severe, requiring pain medication or neurontin. Ototoxicity occurs in > 30% beginning with high-frequency hearing.
- Renal: Not as severe as with cisplatin. Altered renal function preventing reabsorption of Mg^{2+}, Ca^{2+}, and K$^+$. Can be avoided with adequate hydration, diuresis as well as slower infusion time.
- Skin: Pruritic, maculopapular skin rash, usually involving trunk and extremities. Alopecia.
- Reproduction: Pregnancy category D. Breast feeding should be avoided.

Initiate antiemetic protocol:	Moderately to highly emetogenic protocol.

Supportive drugs:

☐ pegfilgrastim (Neulasta)	☐ filgrastim (Neupogen)
☐ epoetin alfa (Procrit)	☐ darbepoetin alfa (Aranesp)

Treatment schedule: Chair time 3 three hours on day 1 and 1 hour on day 8. Repeat cycle every 21 days.

Estimated number of visits: Three visits per cycle. Request four cycles worth of visits.

Dose Calculation by: 1. _____   2. _____

_____   _____
Physician   Date

_____   _____
Patient Name   ID Number

_____   _____/_____/_____   _____
Diagnosis   Ht   Wt   M²

Gemcitabine + Vinorelbine

Baseline laboratory tests:	CBC: Chemistry panel, and LFTs
Baseline procedures or tests:	N/A
Initiate IV:	0.9% sodium chloride
Premedicate:	5-HT$_3$ and dexamethasone 10 mg in 100 cc of NS
Administer:	**Gemcitabine** _____ mg (1200 mg/m^2) IV on days 1 and 8 over 30 minutes

- Available in 200-mg/10-mL or 1-g/50-mL vials (20-mg/mL).
- Further dilute in 0.9% sodium chloride.
- Reconstituted solution is stable 24 hours at room temperature. Do NOT refrigerate, because precipitate will form.

Vinorelbine _____ mg (30 mg/m^2) IV on days 1 and 8

- **Vesicant**
- Available in 10 mg/mL in 1- or 5-mL single-use vials.
- Further dilute to a final concentration in syringe 1.5–3.0 or IV bag of 0.5–3.0 mg/mL
- Infuse diluted drug IV over 6–10 minutes into sidearm port of a freely flowing IV, either peripherally or via central line (preferred). Use port closest to the IV bag, not the patient.
- Flush vein with at least 75–125 mL of IV solution after infusion.
- Reconstituted solution is stable for 24 hours refrigerated.

Major Side Effects

- Hematologic: Myelosuppression is dose limiting. Prolonged infusion time (> 60 minutes) with gemcitabine is associated with higher toxicities.
- GI Symptoms: Mild-to-moderate nausea and vomiting. Constipation, diarrhea, and mucositis seen.
- Flulike Syndrome (20%) with fever in absence of infection 6–12 hours after treatment (40%).
- Neurotoxicity: Usually mild to moderate neuropathy is 25% but incidence increased if patient had prior vinca alkaloids. Constipation may occur in 29% of patients.
- Hepatic: Elevation of serum transaminase and bilirubin levels.
- Skin: Extravasation of vinorelbine may cause local tissue injury and inflammation. Pruritic, maculopapular skin rash, usually involving trunk and extremities. Edema is seen in 30% of patients. Alopecia is rare.
- Reproduction: Pregnancy category D. Breast feeding should be avoided.

Initiate antiemetic protocol:	Mildly to moderately emetogenic protocol.
Supportive drugs:	☐ pegfilgrastim (Neulasta) ☐ filgrastim (Neupogen)
	☐ epoetin alfa (Procrit) ☐ darbepoetin alfa (Aranesp)
Treatment schedule:	Chair time 2 hours on days 1 and 8. Repeat cycle every 21 days.
Estimated number of visits:	Three visits per cycle. Request four cycles worth of visits.

Dose Calculation by: 1. _____   2. _____

_____
Physician

_____
Patient Name

_____
Diagnosis

_____
Date

_____
ID Number

_____/_____/_____
Ht   Wt   M^2

Vinorelbine + Cisplatin

Baseline laboratory tests:	CBC: Chemistry (including Mg^{2+})
Baseline procedures or tests:	N/A
Initiate IV:	0.9% sodium chloride
Premedicate:	5-HT$_3$ and dexamethasone 10–20 mg in 100 cc of NS
Administer:	Vinorelbine _____ mg (30 mg/m^2) IV on days 1, 8, and 15

- **Vesicant**
- Available in 10 mg/mL in 1- or 5-mL single-use vials.
- Further dilute to a final concentration in syringe 1.5–3.0 or IV bag of 0.5–3.0 mg/mL.
- Infuse diluted drug IV over 6–10 minutes into sidearm port of a freely flowing IV, either peripherally or via central line (preferred). Use port closest to the IV bag, not the patient.
- Flush vein with at least 75–125 mL of IV solution after infusion.
- Reconstituted solution is stable for 24 hours refrigerated.

Cisplatin _____ mg (120 mg/m^2) IV on day 1

Available in 100-mL vials. 1-mg/1-mL concentrations.

- Do not use aluminum needles, as precipitate will form.
- Further dilute solution with 250 cc or more NS.
- 100-mL vial stable for 28 days protected from light, 7 days under florescent light.

Major Side Effects

- Bone Marrow Depression: Neutropenia, thrombocytopenia, and anemia are dose related and can be dose limiting.
- GI Toxicities: Moderate to severe nausea and vomiting may be acute or delayed. Constipation, diarrhea, stomatitis, and anorexia may be seen.
- Neurotoxicity: Severe neuropathy with numbness, tingling, and sensory loss in arms and legs. Proprioception and vibratory sense and loss of motor function can occur. Paresthesias are dose related and can be severe, requiring pain medication or neurontin. Ototoxicity occurs in > 30% beginning with high-frequency hearing.
- Renal: Dose-limiting toxicity and may be cumulative and presents at 10–20 days. May result in necrosis of proximal and distal renal tubules preventing reabsorption of Mg^{2+}, Ca^{2+}, and K^+. Can be avoided with adequate hydration, diuresis as well as slower infusion time.
- Skin: Extravasation of vinorelbine may cause local tissue injury and inflammation. Alopecia likely.
- Reproduction: Pregnancy category D. Breast feeding should be avoided.

Initiate antiemetic protocol:	Moderately to highly emetogenic protocol.
Supportive drugs:	☐ pegfilgrastim (Neulasta) ☐ filgrastim (Neupogen)
	☐ epoetin alfa (Procrit) ☐ darbepoetin alfa (Aranesp)
Treatment schedule:	Chair time 3 hours on day 1 and 1 hour on days 8 and 15. Repeat cycle every 28 days.
Estimated number of visits:	Three visits per cycle. Request three cycles worth of visits.

Dose Calculation by: 1. _____   2. _____

_____
Physician

_____
Patient Name

_____
Diagnosis

_____
Date

_____
ID Number

_____ / _____ / _____
Ht   Wt   M^2

Vinorelbine + Carboplatin

Baseline laboratory tests:	CBC: Chemistry (including Mg^{2+})
Baseline procedures or tests:	N/A
Initiate IV:	0.9% sodium chloride
Premedicate:	5-HT$_3$ and dexamethasone 10–20 mg in 100 cc of NS

Administer: **Vinorelbine** _____mg (25 mg/m^2) IV on days 1 and 8.

- Vesicant
- Available in 10 mg/mL in 1- or 5-mL single-use vials.
- Further dilute to a final concentration in syringe 1.5–3.0 or IV bag of 0.5–3.0 mg/mL.
- Infuse diluted drug IV over 6–10 minutes into sidearm port of a freely flowing IV, either peripherally or via central line (preferred). Use port closest to the IV bag, not the patient.
- Flush vein with at least 75–125 mL of IV solution after infusion.
- Reconstituted solution is stable for 24 hours refrigerated.

Carboplatin _____ (AUC 6) IV on day 1

- Available in 50-mg, 150-mg, and 450-mg lyophilized powder; dilute with sterile water. Also available in 50-mg and 150-mg 10-mg/mLg/mL solution; 450-mg and 600-mg 10-mg/mL multidose vials stable for 15 days after first use.
- Do not use aluminum needles, as precipitate will form.
- Further dilute in 250–1000 cc 0.9% sodium chloride.
- Chemically stable for 24 hours, discard after 8 hours because of lack of bacteriostatic perservative.
- Give carboplatin **after** paclitaxel to decrease toxicities.

Major Side Effects

- Hypersensitivity Reaction: Carboplatin with anaphylaxis and severe hypersensitivity reactions in 2%–4%. Characterized by dyspnea, hypotension, andioedema, and generalized urticaria. May also see tachycardia, wheezing, and facial edema. Patients with mild reactions can be rechallenged after 24-hour corticosteroid prophylaxis. Patients with severe reactions should not be rechallenged. Monitor vitals signs every 15 minutes for the first hour. Premedicate as described. Risk increases from 1% to 27% in patients receiving more than seven courses of carboplatin-based therapy.
- Bone Marrow Depression: Neutropenia, thrombocytopenia, and anemia are dose related and can be dose limiting.
- GI Toxicities: Moderate-to-severe nausea and vomiting within first 24 hours. Constipation, diarrhea, stomatitis, and anorexia may be seen.
- Renal: Nephrotoxicity less common than with cisplatin and rarely symptomatic.
- Electrolyte Imbalance: Decreases Mg^{2+}, K^+, Ca^{2+}, and Na^+.
- Skin: Extravasation of vinorelbine may cause local tissue injury and inflammation. Alopecia likely.
- Neurotoxicity: Usually mild to moderate neuropathy is 25% but incidence increased if patient had prior vinca alkaloids. Constipation may occur in 29% of patients.
- Reproduction: Pregnancy category D. Breast feeding should be avoided.

Initiate antiemetic protocol:	Moderately to highly emetogenic protocol.
Supportive drugs:	☐ pegfilgrastim (Neulasta) ☐ filgrastim (Neupogen) ☐ epoetin alfa (Procrit) ☐ darbepoetin alfa (Aranesp)
Treatment schedule:	Chair time 3 hours on day 1 and 1 hour on day 8. Repeat cycle every 28 days.
Estimated number of visits:	Three visits per cycle. Request three cycles worth of visits.

Dose Calculation by: 1. _____ 2. _____

_____

Physician

Date

_____

Patient Name

ID Number

_____

Diagnosis

Ht _____/_____ Wt _____/_____ M^2

Etoposide + Cisplatin

Baseline laboratory tests:	CBC: Chemistry (including Mg^{2+}) and CEA
Baseline procedures or tests:	N/A
Initiate IV:	0.9% sodium chloride
Premedicate:	5-HT_3 and dexamethasone 10–20 mg in 100 cc of NS
Administer:	**Etoposide** _____ mg (120 mg/m^2) IV on days 1–3

- Available in 100-mg vials; when reconstituted with 5 or 10 mL of NS, D5W, or sterile water with benzyl alcohol makes a 20- or 10-mg/mL solution. Also available in solution as a 20-mg/mL concentration.
- May be further diluted in NS or D5W to final concentration of 0.1 mg/mL.
- Diluted drug is stable 96 hours in glass and 48 hours in plastic containers at room temperature.

Cisplatin _____ mg (60 mg/m^2) IV on day 1

- Available in 100-mL vials. 1-mg/1-mL concentrations.
- Do not use aluminum needles, as precipitate will form.
- Further dilute solution with 250 cc or more NS.
- 100-mL vial stable for 28 days protected from light, 7 days under florescent light.

Major Side Effects

- Allergic reaction: Bronchospasm, with or without fever, chills. Hypotension may occur during rapid infusion of etoposide. Anaphylaxis may occur but is rare.
- Bone Marrow Depression: Myelosuppression can be a dose-limiting toxicity.
- GI Toxicities: Moderate to severe nausea and vomiting. May be acute (first 24 hours) or delayed (> 24 hours). Mucositis and diarrhea are rare. Metallic taste to food.
- Neurotoxicity: Severe neuropathy with numbness, tingling, and sensory loss in arms and legs. Proprioception and vibratory sense and loss of motor function can occur. Paresthesias are dose related and can be severe, requiring pain medication or neurontin. Ototoxicity occurs in > 30% beginning with high-frequency hearing.
- Renal: Dose-limiting toxicity and may be cumulative and presents at 10–20 days. May result in necrosis of proximal and distal renal tubules, preventing reabsorption of Mg^{2+}, Ca^{2+}, and K^+. Can be avaoided with adequate hydration, diuresis as well as slower infusion time.
- Skin: Alopecia. Etoposide is a radiosensitizer and an irritant. Patients receiving high-dose therapy may develop bullae on the skin (similar to Stevens-Johnson Syndrome).
- Reproduction: Pregnancy category D. Breast feeding should be avoided.

Initiate antiemetic protocol:	Moderately to highly emetogenic protocol.
Supportive drugs:	☐ pegfilgrastim (Neulasta) ☐ filgrastim (Neupogen)
	☐ epoetin alfa (Procrit) ☐ darbepoetin alfa (Aranesp)
Treatment schedule:	Chair time 3 hours on day 1 and 1 hour on days 2–3. Repeat cycle every 21–28 days.
Estimated number of visits:	Four visits per cycle. Request three cycles worth of visits.

Dose Calculation by: 1. _____   2. _____

Physician _____   Date _____

Patient Name _____   ID Number _____

Diagnosis _____   _____/_____/_____
Ht   Wt   M^2

Etoposide + Cisplatin + Docetaxel

Baseline laboratory tests:	CBC: Chemistry (including Mg^{2+})
Baseline procedures or tests:	N/A
Initiate IV:	0.9% sodium chloride
Premedicate:	5-HT_3 and dexamethasone 10–20 mg in 100 cc of NS
	Docetaxel: Dexamethasone 8-mg bid for 3 days starting the day before treatment

Administer:

Etoposide _____ mg (50 mg/m^2) IV on days 1–5 and 29–33

- Available in 100-mg vials; when reconstituted with 5 or 10 mL of NS, D5W, or sterile water with benzyl alcohol makes a 20- or 10-mg/mL solution. Also available in solution as a 20-mg/mL concentration.
- May be further diluted in NS or D5W to final concentration of 0.1 mg/mL.
- Diluted drug is stable 96 hours in glass and 48 hours in plastic containers at room temperature.

Cisplatin _____ mg (50 mg/m^2) IV on days 1, 8, 29, and 36

- Available in 100-mL vials. 1-mg/1-mL concentrations.
- Do not use aluminum needles, as precipitate will form.
- Further dilute solution with 250 cc or more NS.
- 100-mL vial stable for 28 days protected from light, 7 days under florescent light.

Administer concurrent thoracic radiotherapy, 4–6 weeks after the completion of combined modality therapy follow with:

Docetaxel _____ mg (75 mg/m^2) IV on day 1

- Available in 20- or 80-mg blister pack with own diluent. Do not shake.
- Reconstituted vials stable at room temperature or refrigerated for 8 hours.
- Use non-PVC containers and tubing to administer. No filter needed.

Major Side Effects

- Allergic Reaction: Bronchospasm, with or without fever, chills. Hypotension may occur during rapid infusion of etoposide. Anaphylaxis may occur but is rare. Severe hypersensitivity reactions with docetaxel in 2%–3% of patients. Premedication with dexamethasone recommended.
- Bone Marrow Depression: Myelosuppression can be a dose-limiting toxicity.
- GI Toxicities: Moderate-to-severe nausea and vomiting with etoposide and cisplatin. May be acute (first 24 hours) or delayed (> 24 hours). Mild-to-moderate nausea and vomiting with docetaxel. Mucositis and diarrhea are rare. Metallic taste to food.
- Neurotoxicity: Severe neuropathy with numbness, tingling, and sensory loss in arms and legs. Proprioception and vibratory sense and loss of motor function can occur. Paresthesias are dose related and can be severe, requiring pain medication or neurontin. Ototoxicity occurs in > 30% beginning with high-frequency hearing.
- Renal: Dose-limiting toxicity and may be cumulative and presents at 10–20 days. May result in necrosis of proximal and distal renal tubules, preventing reabsorption of Mg^{2+}, Ca^{2+}, and K^+. Can be avoided with adequate hydration, diuresis as well as slower infusion time.
- Fluid Balance: Fluid retention is a cumulative toxicity that may occur with docetaxel. Characterized by peripheral edema, pleural effusions, dyspnea at rest, cardiac tamponade, or ascites. Pre-treatment with dexamethasone as above may minimize the effect.
- Skin: Alopecia.
- Reproduction: Pregnancy category D. Breast feeding should be avoided.

Initiate antiemetic protocol:	Moderately to highly emetogenic protocol.
Supportive drugs:	☐ pegfilgrastim (Neulasta) ☐ filgrastim (Neupogen)
	☐ epoetin alfa (Procrit) ☐ darbepoetin alfa (Aranesp)
Treatment schedule:	Chair time 3 hours on days 1, 8, 29, and 36; 1 hour on days 4–5 and 30–33. Etoposide cycle 36 days, rest 4–6 weeks; then repeat docetaxel every 21 days for three cycles.
Estimated number of visits:	Twelve visits first cycle, three visits second cycle.

Dose Calculation by: 1. _____ 2. _____

_____

Physician   Date

_____

Patient Name   ID Number

_____

Diagnosis   Ht ___/___ Wt ___/___ M²

Single-Agent Regimens

Paclitaxel

Baseline laboratory tests:	CBC: Chemistry (including Mg^{2+}) and CEA
Baseline procedures or tests:	N/A
Initiate IV:	0.9% sodium chloride
Premedicate:	5-HT_3 and dexamethasone 10–20 mg in 100 cc of NS
	Diphenhydramine 25–50 mg and cimetidine 300 mg in 100 cc of NS
Administer:	**Paclitaxel** _____mg (225 mg/m^2) IV over 3 hours on day 1 every 3 weeks.
	OR
	Paclitaxel _____mg (80–100 mg/m^2) IV over 3 hours on day 1 weekly for 3 weeks. Repeat cycle every 28 days after 1 week rest.

- Available in 30-mg (6 mg/mL), 100-mg (16.7 mg/mL) and 300-mg (6 mg/mL) vials.
- Further dilute in 250–500 cc NS or D5W. Final concentration is 1.2 mg/mL.
- **Use non-PVC tubing and containers and a 0.22-micron inline filter to administer.**

Major Side Effects

- Hypersensitivity Reaction: Occurs in 20%–40% of patients. Characterized by generalized skin rash, flushing, erythema, hypotension, dyspnea, and/or bronchospasm. Usually occurs within the first 2–3 minutes of infusion and almost always within the first 10 minutes. Premedicate as described.
- Bone Marrow Depression: Dose-limiting neutropenia with nadir at days 8–10 and recovery by days 15–21. Decreased incidence of neutropenia with 3-hour schedule when compared with 24-hour schedule. G-CSF support recommended.
- GI Toxicity: Nausea and vomiting occur in 52% of patients, mild and preventable with anitemetics. Diarrhea in 38% of patients and stomatitis in 31%.
- Neurotoxicity: Severe neuropathy with numbness, tingling, and sensory loss in arms and legs. Proprioception and vibratory sense and loss of motor function can occur. Paresthesias are dose related and can be severe, requiring pain medication or neurontin. More frequent with longer infusions and at doses > 175 mg/m^2.
- Ototoxicity occurs in > 30% beginning with high-frequency hearing.
- Alopecia: Total loss of body hair occurs in nearly all patients.
- Reproduction: Pregnancy category D. Breast feeding should be avoided.

Initiate antiemetic protocol:	Mildly emetogenic protocol.
Supportive drugs:	☐ pegfilgrastim (Neulasta) ☐ filgrastim (Neupogen)
	☐ epoetin alfa (Procrit) ☐ darbepoetin alfa (Aranesp)
Treatment schedule:	Chair time 4 hours every 3 weeks for 3 hour infusion and high dose. Repeat every 21 days. 2 hour chair time for weekly dosing for 3 weeks with 1 week rest. Repeat every 28 days.
Estimated number of visits:	Two visits per cycle. Request three cycles worth of visits.

Dose Calculation by: 1. _____   2. _____

_____
Physician

_____
Date

_____
Patient Name

_____
ID Number

_____
Diagnosis

_____/ _____/ _____
Ht   Wt   M^2

Docetaxel

Baseline laboratory tests:	CBC: Chemistry (including Mg^{2+})
Baseline procedures or tests:	Central line placement
Initiate IV:	0.9% sodium chloride
Premedicate:	Dexamethasone 8-mg PO 12 hours and immediately before docetaxel infusion and 12 hours after each dose.
	Oral phenothiazine or 5-HT$_3$

Administer:

Docetaxel _____mg (75 mg/m^2) IV on day 1 every 3 weeks

OR

Docetaxel _____mg (36 mg/m^2) IV weekly for 6 weeks

- Comes in 20- or 80-mg blister packs with own diluent. Do not shake. Reconstituted vials stable at room temperature or refrigerated for 8 hours.
- Further dilute in 250 cc of D5W or 0.9% sodium chloride.
- Use non-PVC containers and tubing to administer. No filter needed

Major Side Effects

- Hypersensitivity Reaction: Docetaxel with anaphylaxis and severe hypersensitivity reactions in 2%–4%. Characterized by dyspnea, hypotension, andioedema, and generalized urticaria. May also see tachycardia, wheezing, and facial edema. Patients with mild reactions can be rechallenged after 24-hour corticosteroid prophylaxis. Patients with severe reactions should not be rechallenged. Monitor vitals signs every 15 minutes for the first hour. Premedicate as described.
- Bone Marrow Depression: Neutropenia is dose limiting with nadir at days 7–10 and recovery by day 14. Thrombocytopenia and anemia are also seen.
- GI Toxicities: Nausea and vomiting is mild to moderate. Mucositis and diarrhea seen in 40% of patients.
- Neurotoxicity: Sensory neuropathy with numbness and paresthesias; dose related. More frequent with longer infusions and peripheral neuropathy may affect up to 49% of patients. Sensory alterations are paresthesias in a glove-and-stocking distribution and numbness.
- Fluid Balance: Fluid retention syndrome. Symptoms include weight gain, peripheral and/or generalized edema, pleural effusion, and ascites. Seen in about 50% of patients. Premedication with dexamethasone effective in preventing or minimizing occurrences.
- Skin: Alopecia. Etoposide is a radiosensitizer and an irritant. Patients receiving high-dose therapy may develop bullae on the skin (similar to Stevens-Johnson Syndrome).
- Hyperlacrimation: Epiphor or hyperlacrimation of tear ducts. Use aritificial tears and/or steroid ophthalmic solution. Severe cases may require the placement of lacrimal duct stents.
- Reproduction: Pregnancy category D. Breast feeding should be avoided.

Initiate antiemetic protocol:	Mildly to moderately emetogenic protocol.
Supportive drugs:	☐ pegfilgrastim (Neulasta) ☐ filgrastim (Neupogen)
	☐ epoetin alfa (Procrit) ☐ darbepoetin alfa (Aranesp)

Treatment schedule:

Chair time 2 hours on day 1. Repeat cycle every 21 days.

OR

Chair time 2 hours on day 1. Repeat cycle every 8 weeks after 2-week rest.

Estimated number of visits: Two visits per cycle for three week protocol. Six visits per cycle for weekly protocol. Request three cycles worth of visits.

Dose Calculation by: 1. _____   2. _____

_____   _____
Physician   Date

_____   _____
Patient Name   ID Number

_____   _____/_____/_____
Diagnosis   Ht   Wt   M²

Pemetrexed (Alimta)

Baseline laboratory tests:	CBC: Chemistry panel, creatinine clearance
Baseline procedures or tests:	N/A
Initiate IV:	NS
Premedicate:	Dexamethasone 4-mg PO bid for 3 days, starting the day before treatment

Folic acid 1-mg (350–1,000 mg) PO qd, starting 5 days before the first treatment and ending 21 days after the last dose of pemetrexed.

Vitamin B$_{12}$ 1000-mcg IM during the week preceding the first dose and every three cycles thereafter (may be given the same day as pemetrexed second dose only).

Oral phenothiazine or 5-HT$_3$

Administer: **Pemetrexed** _____mg (500 mg/m^2) IV over 10 minutes on day 1

- Available in 500-mg single-use vials for reconstitution.
- Reconstitute with 20 mL of 0.9% sodium chloride (preservative free) for a final concentration of 25 mg/mL.
- Further dilute in 100 cc of NS.
- Discard any unused portion.

Major Side Effects

- Bone Marrow Toxicities: Myelosuppression is dose-limiting toxicity. Dose reductions or treatment delay may be necessary for subsequent doses. Instruct patient to take vitamin B$_{12}$ and folic acid supplements to minimize hematologic toxicities.
- GI Toxicities: Nausea, vomiting, and diarrhea, usually mild to moderate. Mild anorexia, stomatitis, and pharyngitis seen. Instruct patient to take vitamin B$_{12}$ and folic acid supplements to minimize GI toxicities.
- Renal/hepatic: Patients with renal or hepatic impairment may require dose adjustment.
- Skin: Pruritus and rash in 22% of patients. Premedication with dexamethasone if effective in preventing or minimizing symptoms.
- Reproduction: Pregnancy category D. Breast feeding should be avoided.

Initiate antiemetic protocol:	Mildly to moderately emetogenic protocol.
Supportive drugs:	☐ pegfilgrastim (Neulasta) ☐ filgrastim (Neupogen)
	☐ epoetin alfa (Procrit) ☐ darbepoetin alfa (Aranesp)
Treatment schedule:	Chair time 1 hour on day 1. Repeat cycle every 21 days until disease progression.
Estimated number of visits:	Two visits per cycle. Request six cycles worth of treatments.

Dose Calculation by: 1. _____ 2. _____

_____
Physician

Date

_____
Patient Name

ID Number

_____
Diagnosis

_____/ _____/ _____
Ht   Wt   M^2

Gemcitabine

Baseline laboratory tests:	CBC: Chemistry panel and LFTs
Baseline procedures or tests:	N/A
Initiate IV:	0.9% sodium chloride
Premedicate:	Oral phenothiazine
	OR
	5-HT$_3$ and dexamethasone 10 mg in 100 cc of NS

Administer: **Gemcitabine** _____ mg (1000 mg/m^2) IV on days 1, 8, and 15 over 30 minutes

- Available in 200-mg/10-mL or 1-g/50-mL vials, (20-mg/mL).
- Further dilute in 0.9% sodium chloride.
- Reconstituted solution is stable 24 hours at room temperature. Do NOT refrigerate, because precipitate will form.

Major Side Effects

- Myelosuppression: Leukopenia (63%), thrombocytopenia (36%), and anemia (73%), with grade 3 and 4 thrombocytopenia more common in older patients. Myelosuppression is dose limiting. Nadir occurs in 10–14 days with recovery at 21 days. Prolonged infusion time (> 60 minutes) is associated with higher toxicities.
- GI Symptoms: Mild-to-moderate nausea and vomiting (70%), diarrhea, and/or mucositis (15%–20%).
- Flulike Syndrome (20%) with fever in absence of infection 6–12 hours after treatment (40%).
- Hepatic: (Transient) Elevation of serum transaminase and bilirubin levels.
- Skin: Pruritic, maculopapular skin rash, usually involving trunk and extremities. Edema is seen in 30% of patients. Alopecia is rare.
- Reproduction: Pregnancy category D. Breast feeding should be avoided.

Initiate antiemetic protocol:	Mildly to moderately emetogenic protocol.
Supportive drugs:	☐ pegfilgrastim (Neulasta) ☐ filgrastim (Neupogen)
	☐ epoetin alfa (Procrit) ☐ darbepoetin alfa (Aranesp)
Treatment schedule:	Chair time 1 hour on days 1, 8, and 15. Repeat cycle every 28 days.
Estimated number of visits:	Three visits per cycle. Request three cycles worth of visits.

Dose Calculation by: 1. _____   2. _____

_____
Physician

_____
Date

_____
Patient Name

_____
ID Number

_____
Diagnosis

_____ / _____ / _____
Ht   Wt   M^2

Topotecan

Baseline laboratory tests:	CBC: Chemistry panel, LFTs, and CA 19-9
Baseline procedures or tests:	N/A
Initiate IV:	0.9% sodium chloride
Premedicate:	5-HT$_3$ and dexamethasone 10 mg in 100 cc of NS
Administer:	**Topotecan** _____ mg (1.5 mg/m^2) IV on days 1–5

- Available as a 4-mg single-dose vial.
- Reconstitute vial with 4 mL of sterile water for injection.
- Further dilute in 0.9% sodium chloride or D5W.
- Use immediately.

Major Side Effects

- Myelosuppression: Severe grade 4 myelosuppression seen during the first course of therapy in 60% of patients. Dose-limiting toxicity. Typical nadir occurs at days 7–10, with full recovery by days 21–28. If severe neutropenia occurs, reduce dose by 0.25 mg/m^2 for subsequent doses or may use G-CSF to prevent neutropenia 24 hours after last day of topotecan therapy.

- GI Toxicities: Mild to moderate nausea and vomiting, dose related. Occurs in 60%–80% of patients. Diarrhea occurs in 42% of patients, and constipation occurs in 39%. Abdominal pain may occur in 33% of patients.

- Flulike Symptoms: Headache, fever, malaise, arthralgias, and myalgias.

- Hepatic Toxicity: Evidence of increased drug toxicity in patients with low protein level and hepatic dysfunction. Dose reductions may be necessary.

- Renal: Use with caution in patients with abnormal renal function. Dose reduction is necessary in this setting. Microscopic hematuria seen in 10% of patients.

- Skin: Alopecia.

- Reproduction: Pregnancy category D. Breast feeding should be avoided.

Initiate antiemetic protocol:	Mildly to moderately emetogenic protocol.
Supportive drugs:	☐ pegfilgrastim (Neulasta) ☐ filgrastim (Neupogen)
	☐ epoetin alfa (Procrit) ☐ darbepoetin alfa (Aranesp)
Treatment schedule:	Chair time 1 hour on days 1–5. Repeat every 21 days until disease progression.
Estimated number of visits:	Six visits per course. Request three courses.

Dose Calculation by: 1. _____   2. _____

Physician _____   Date _____

Patient Name _____   ID Number _____

Diagnosis _____   Ht _____ / Wt _____ / M^2 _____

Vinorelbine

Baseline laboratory tests:	CBC: Chemistry
Baseline procedures or tests:	N/A
Initiate IV:	0.9% sodium chloride
Premedicate:	Oral phenothiazine or 5-HT$_3$
Administer:	**Vinorelbine** _____ mg (25 mg/m^2) IV weekly

- **Vesicant**
- Available in 10 mg/mL in 1- or 5-mL single-use vials.
- Further dilute to a final concentration in syringe 1.5–3.0 or IV bag of 0.5–3.0 mg/mL.
- Infuse diluted drug IV over 6–10 minutes into sidearm port of a freely flowing IV, either peripherally or via central line (preferred). Use port closest to the IV bag, not the patient.
- Flush vein with at least 75–125 mL of IV solution after infusion.
- Reconstituted solution is stable for 24 hours refrigerated.

Major Side Effects

- Bone Marrow Depression: Leukopenia is dose-limiting toxicity. Nadir at 7–10 days. Severe thrombocytopenia and anemia are uncommon.
- GI Toxicities: Nausea and vomiting are mild in IV dosing with an incidence of 44%. Stomatitis is mild to moderate with < 20% incidence. Constipation (35%), diarrhea (17%), and anorexia (< 20%) also seen.
- Skin: Extravasation of vinorelbine may cause local tissue injury and inflammation. Alopecia observed in 10%–15% of patients.
- Neurotoxicity: Usually mild to moderate neuropathy is 25% but incidence increased if patient had prior vinca alkaloids. Constipation may occur in 29% of patients.
- Reproduction: Pregnancy category D. Breast feeding should be avoided.

Initiate antiemetic protocol:	Mildly emetogenic protocol.
Supportive drugs:	☐ pegfilgrastim (Neulasta) ☐ filgrastim (Neupogen) ☐ epoetin alfa (Procrit) ☐ darbepoetin alfa (Aranesp)
Treatment schedule:	Chair time 1 hour weekly. Repeat cycle every week until disease progression.
Estimated number of visits:	Weekly. Request 12 cycles worth of visits.

Dose Calculation by: 1. _____   2. _____

_____
Physician

_____
Patient Name

_____
Diagnosis

_____
Date

_____
ID Number

_____ / _____ / _____
Ht   Wt   M^2

Gefitinib (Iressa)

Baseline laboratory tests:	CBC: Chemistry
Baseline procedures or tests:	N/A
Premedicate:	Oral phenothiazine or 5-HT$_3$
Administer:	**Gefitinib** 250-mg/day PO

- Available in 250-mg tablets, 30 per bottle.
- Taken with or without food.
- Available to patients:
  1. who are currently or have previously taken the drug and are benefiting
  2. previously enrolled patients or new patients in non-investigational (IND) clinical trials
  3. through the Iressa access program.

Major Side Effects

- Interstitial Lung Disease: Seen in 1% of patients with a 33% mortality. Symptoms include dyspnea, sometimes with cough or low-grade fever, rapidly becoming more severe.
- GI Toxicities: Mild to moderate diarrhea occurred in 48% of patients. Drug may be interrupted for up to 14 days with severe diarrhea. Nausea and vomiting only 13%.
- Skin Alterations: Rash occurred in 43% of patients, acne in 25%, dry skin and pruritis also seen. May interrupt drug for 14 days until rash resolves before resuming drug.
- Cardiovascular: Elevations in blood pressure, especially in those with underlying hypertension.
- Visual Alterations: Amblyopia occurred in 2% of patients and conjunctivitis in 1%.
- Reproduction: Pregnancy category D. Breast feeding should be avoided.

Initiate antiemetic protocol:	Mildly emetogenic protocol.
Treatment schedule:	Continue treatment until disease progression.[1,262]
Estimated number of visits:	One visit per cycle. Request 12 cycles worth of visits.

Dose Calculation by: 1. _____   2. _____

Physician _____   Date _____

Patient Name _____   ID Number _____

Diagnosis _____   _____/_____/_____
                                      Ht   Wt   M^2

Erlotinib (Tarceva)

Baseline laboratory tests:	CBC: Chemistry
Baseline procedures or tests:	N/A
Premedicate:	Oral phenothiazine or 5-HT$_3$
Administer:	**Tarceva** (erlotinib) 150-mg/day PO

- Available in 150-, 100-, and 25-mg tablets.
- Take on an empty stomach.

Major Side Effects

- Skin Alterations: Rash, from Maculopapular to pustular on the face, neck, chest, back, and arms, affecting up to 75% of patients. Most rashes are mild to moderate, beginning on day 8–10, maximizing in intensity by week 2, and gradually resolving by week 2. Use of skin treatments such as corticorsteriods, topical clindamycin, or minocycline have been used with varying results.
- GI Toxicities: Diarrhea is seen in 54% of patients, and is mild to moderate, only 6% grade 3.
- Visual Alterations: Conjuctivitis and dry eyes may occur and are mild to moderate (grade 1–2).
- Interstitial Lung Disease: Seen in 1% of patients with a 33% mortality. Symptoms include dyspnea, sometimes with cough or low-grade fever, rapidly becoming more severe. This is a class effect. Drug should be stopped immediately in patients with worsening or unexplained pulmonary symptoms.
- Drug Interactions: Inducers of the CYP3A4 pathway may increase metabolism of erlotinib and decrease plasma concentrations; and inhibitors of the CYP3A4 pathway may increase the metabolism of erlotinib and increase plasma concentrations. Patients taking coumadin should have PT/INR monitored closely.
- Reproduction: Pregnancy category D. Breast feeding should be avoided.

Initiate antiemetic protocol:	Mildly emetogenic protocol.
Treatment schedule:	Erlotinib: 150-mg PO
	Continue until disease progression
Estimated number of visits:	One visit per cycle. Request 12 cycles worth of visits.

Dose Calculation by: 1. _____ 2. _____

_____   _____
Physician   Date

_____   _____
Patient Name   ID Number

_____   _____ / _____ / _____
Diagnosis   Ht   Wt   M^2

LUNG CANCER

Small-Cell Lung Cancer

Combination Regimens

Etoposide: 80-mg/m^2 IV on days 1–3
Cisplatin: 80-mg/m^2 IV on day 1
Repeat cycle every 21 days.[1,263]

Etoposide: 100-mg/m^2 IV on days 1–3
Carboplatin: AUC of 6, IV on day 1
Repeat cycle every 28 days.[1,264]

Irinotecan: 60-mg/m^2 IV on days 1, 8, and 15
Cisplatin: 60-mg/m^2 IV on day 1
Repeat cycle every 28 days.[1,265]

Carboplatin: AUC of 6, IV on day 1
Paclitaxel: 200-mg/m^2 IV over 3 hours on day 1
Etoposide: 50 mg alternating with 100 mg PO on days 1–10
Repeat cycle every 21 days.[1,266]

Cyclophosphamide: 1000-mg/m^2 IV on day 1
Doxorubicin: 40-mg/m^2 IV on day 1
Vincristine: 1-mg/m^2 IV on day 1 (maximum, 2 mg)
Repeat cycle every 21 days.[1,267]

Cyclophosphamide: 1000-mg/m^2 IV on day 1
Doxorubicin: 45-mg/m^2 IV on day 1
Etoposide: 50-mg/m^2 IV on days 1–5
Repeat cycle every 21 days.[1,268]

Single-Agent Regimens

Etoposide: 160-mg/m^2 PO on days 1–5
Repeat cycle every 28 days.[1,269]

OR

Etoposide: 50-mg/m^2 PO bid on days 1–21
Repeat cycle as tolerated.[1,270]

Paclitaxel: 80–100-mg/m^2 IV weekly for 3 weeks
Repeat cycle every 28 days.[1,2721]

Topotecan: 1.5-mg/m^2 IV on days 1–5
Repeat cycle every 21 days.[1,272]

Combination Regimens

Etoposide + Cisplatin

Baseline laboratory tests:	CBC: Chemistry (including Mg^{2+}) and CEA
Baseline procedures or tests:	N/A
Initiate IV:	0.9% sodium chloride
Premedicate:	5-HT$_3$ and dexamethasone 10–20 mg in 100 cc of NS
Administer:	**Etoposide** _____ mg (80 mg/m^2) IV on days 1–3

- Available in 100-mg vials; when reconstituted with 5 or 10 mL of NS, D5W, or sterile water with benzyl alcohol makes a 20- or 10-mg/mL solution. It is also available in solution as a 20-mg/mL concentration.
- May be further diluted in NS or D5W to final concentration of 0.1 mg/mL.

Cisplatin _____ mg (80 mg/m^2) IV on day 1

- Available in 100-mL vials. 1-mg/1-mL concentrations
- Do not use aluminum needles, as precipitate will form.
- Further dilute solution with 250 cc or more NS.
- 100-mL vial stable for 28 days protected from light, 7 days under florescent light.

Major Side Effects

- Allergic Reaction: Bronchospasm, with or without fever, chills. Hypotension may occur during rapid infusion of etoposide. Anaphylaxis may occur but is rare.
- Bone Marrow Depression: Myelosuppression can be a dose-limiting toxicity.
- GI Toxicities: Moderate to severe nausea and vomiting. May be acute (first 24 hours) or delayed (> 24 hours). Mucositis and diarrhea are rare. Metallic taste to food
- Neurotoxicity: Severe neuropathy with numbness, tingling, and sensory loss in arms and legs. Proprioception and vibratory sense and loss of motor function can occur. Paresthesias are dose related and can be severe, requiring pain medication or neurontin. Ototoxicity occurs in > 30% beginning with high-frequency hearing.
- Renal: Dose-limiting toxicity and may be cumulative and presents at 10–20 days. May result in necrosis of proximal and distal renal tubules, preventing reabsorption of Mg^{2+}, Ca^{2+}, and K^+. Can be avoided with adequate hydration, diuresis as well as slower infusion time.
- Skin: Alopecia.
- Reproduction: Pregnancy category D. Breast feeding should be avoided.

Initiate antiemetic protocol:	Moderately to highly emetogenic protocol.
Supportive drugs:	☐ pegfilgrastim (Neulasta) ☐ filgrastim (Neupogen) ☐ epoetin alfa (Procrit) ☐ darbepoetin alfa (Aranesp)
Treatment schedule:	Chair time 4 hours on day 1 and 2 hours on days 2–3. Repeat cycle every 21 days.
Estimated number of visits:	Four visits per cycle. Request three cycles worth of visits.

Dose Calculation by: 1. _____   2. _____

_____

Physician

_____

Patient Name

_____

Diagnosis

_____

Date

_____

ID Number

_____ / _____ / _____

Ht   Wt   M^2

Etoposide + Carboplatin

Baseline laboratory tests:	CBC: Chemistry (including Mg^{2+}) and CEA
Baseline procedures or tests:	N/A
Initiate IV:	0.9% sodium chloride
Premedicate:	5-HT_3 and dexamethasone 10–20 mg in 100 cc of NS
Administer:	**Etoposide** _____ mg (100 mg/m^2) IV on days 1–3

- Available in 100-mg vials; when reconstituted with 5 or 10 mL of NS, D5W, or sterile water with benzyl alcohol makes a 20- or 10-mg/mL solution. Also available in solution as a 20-mg/mL concentration.
- May be further diluted in NS or D5W to final concentration of 0.1 mg/mL.

Carboplatin _____ mg (AUC 6) IV on day 1

- Available in 50-mg, 150-mg, and 450-mg lyophilized powder; dilute with sterile water. Also available in 50-mg and 150-mg 10-mg/mLg/mL solution; 450-mg and 600-mg 10-mg/mL multidose vials stable for 15 days after first use.
- Do not use aluminum needles, as precipitate will form.
- Further dilute in 250–1000 cc 0.9% sodium chloride.
- Chemically stable for 24 hours, discard after 8 hours because of lack of bacteriostatic perservative.
- Give carboplatin **after** paclitaxel to decrease toxicities.

Major Side Effects

- Allergic Reaction: Bronchospasm, with or without fever, chills. Hypotension may occur during rapid infusion of etoposide. Anaphylaxis may occur but is rare. Rash, urticaria, erythema, and pruritus with carboplatin. Bronchospasm and hypotension are uncommon, but risk increases in patients receiving more than seven courses of carboplatin-based therapy.
- Bone Marrow Depression: Myelosuppression can be a dose-limiting toxicity.
- GI Toxicities: Moderate to severe nausea and vomiting occurs within the first 24 hours. Mucositis and diarrhea are rare.
- Renal: Nephrotoxicity less common than with cisplatin and rarely symptomatic.
- Electrolyte Imbalance: Decreases Mg^{2+}, K^+, Ca^{2+}, and Na^+.
- Neurotoxicity: Dose-limiting toxicity, usually in the form of peripheral sensory neuropathy. Paresthesias and numbness in a classic "stocking glove" pattern.
- Skin: Alopecia.
- Reproduction: Pregnancy category D. Breast feeding should be avoided.

Initiate antiemetic protocol:	Moderately to highly emetogenic protocol.
Supportive drugs:	☐ pegfilgrastim (Neulasta) ☐ filgrastim (Neupogen)
	☐ epoetin alfa (Procrit) ☐ darbepoetin alfa (Aranesp)
Treatment schedule:	Chair time 3 hours on day 1 and 2 hours on days 2–3. Repeat cycle every 28 days.
Estimated number of visits:	Four visits per cycle. Request three cycles worth of visits.

Dose Calculation by: 1. _____   2. _____

_____   _____
Physician   Date

_____   _____
Patient Name   ID Number

_____   _____ / _____ / _____
Diagnosis   Ht   Wt   M^2

Irinotecan + Cisplatin

Baseline laboratory tests:	CBC: Chemistry panel
Baseline procedures or tests:	N/A
Initiate IV:	D5W and water
Premedicate:	$5HT_3$ and dexamethasone 20 mg in 100 cc of D5W
	Atropine 0.25–1.0 mg IV unless contraindicated

Administer:

Irinotecan _____ mg (60 mg/m^2) IV in 500 cc of D5W over 90 minutes on days 1, 8, and 15

- Available in 100-mg vials.
- Store unopened vials at room temperature and protect from light.
- Dilute and mix drug in D5W (preferred) or NS.
- Diluted drug is stable for 24 hours at room temperature. If diluted in D5W, stable for 48 hours if refrigerated and protected from light.

Cisplatin _____ mg (60 mg/m^2) IV in 1000 cc of NS on day 1

- Available in 100-mL vials. 1-mg/1-mL concentrations
- Do not use aluminum needles, as precipitate will form.
- Further dilute solution with 250 cc or more NS.
- 100-mL vial stable for 28 days protected from light, 7 days under florescent light.

Major Side Effects

- GI Toxicities: Irinotecan can cause early diarrhea, most likely a cholinergic effect, can be managed with atropine before therapy. Late diarrhea observed in 22% of patients; it can be severe and should be treated aggressively. Nausea and vomiting in 35%–60% of patients, with 17% experiencing grade 3–4 nausea and 13% experiencing grade 3–4 vomiting.
- Bone Marrow Depression: Neutropenia can be dose limiting. GCSF recommended.
- Renal: Dose-limiting toxicity and may be cumulative and presents at 10–20 days. May result in necrosis of proximal and distal renal tubules, preventing reabsorption of Mg^{2+}, Ca^{2+}, and K^+. Can be avoided with adequate hydration, diuresis as well as slower infusion time.
- Alopecia: Mild.
- Reproduction: Pregnancy category D. Breast feeding should be avoided.

Initiate antiemetic protocol:	Moderately to highly emetogenic protocol.

Supportive drugs:

☐ pegfilgrastim (Neulasta) ☐ filgrastim (Neupogen)
☐ loperamide (Imodium) ☐ epoetin alfa (Procrit)
☐ darbepoetin alfa (Aranesp) ☐ diphenoxylate/atropine sulfate (Lomotil)

Treatment schedule: Chair time 4 hours weekly for 4 weeks. Repeat cycle every 28 days for 6 cycles as tolerated or until disease progression.

Estimated number of visits: Four visits per cycle. Request three to six cycles worth of visits.

Dose Calculation by: 1. _____ 2. _____

_____
Physician

_____
Date

_____
Patient Name

_____
ID Number

_____
Diagnosis

_____ / _____ / _____
Ht   Wt   M^2

Carboplatin + Paclitaxel + Etoposide

Baseline laboratory tests:	CBC: Chemistry
Baseline procedures or tests:	N/A
Initiate IV:	0.9% sodium chloride
Premedicate:	5-HT$_3$ and dexamethasone 10–20 mg in 100 cc of NS
	Diphenhydramine 25–50 mg and cimetidine 300 mg in 100 cc of NS
	Oral phenothiazine or 5-HT$_3$ before etoposide days 4–10

Administer:

Paclitaxel _____ mg (200 mg/m^2) IV over 3 hours on day 1

- Available in 30-mg (6 mg/mL), 100-mg (16.7 mg/mL), and 300-mg (6 mg/mL) vials.
- Further dilute in 250–500 cc NS or D5W. Final concentration is ± 1.2 mg/mL.
- **Use non-PVC tubing and containers and a 0.22-micron inline filter to administer.**

Carboplatin _____ mg (AUC 6) IV on day 1

- Available in 50-mg, 150-mg, and 450-mg lyophilized powder; dilute with sterile water. Also available in 50-mg and 150-mg 10-mg/mLg/mL solution; 450-mg and 600-mg 10-mg/mL multidose vials stable for 15 days after first use.
- Do not use aluminum needles, as precipitate will form.
- Further dilute in 250–1000 cc 0.9% sodium chloride.
- Chemically stable for 24 hours, discard after 8 hours because of lack of bacteriostatic perservative
- Give carboplatin **after** paclitaxel to decrease toxicities

Etoposide 50 mg alternating with 100 mg PO on days 1–10

- Available in 50- and 100-mg capsules.
- Store in refrigerator.
- Monitor patients taking warfarin; it can elevate prothrombin time (PT)/international normalized ratio.

Major Side Effects

- Hypersensitivity Reaction: Paclitaxel and carboplatin, with anaphylaxis and severe hypersensitivity reactions in 30%–40%. Characterized by dyspnea, hypotension, andioedema, and generalized urticaria. May also see tachycardia, wheezing, and facial edema. Patients with mild reactions can be rechallenged after 24-hour corticosteroid prophylaxis. Patients with severe reactions should not be rechallenged. Monitor vitals signs every 15 minutes for the first hour. Premedicate as described. Increased risk of hypersensitivity reactions in patients receiving more than seven courses of carboplatin therapy.
- Bone Marrow Depression: Neutropenia, thrombocytopenia, and anemia are cumulative and dose related. Can be dose limiting. G-CSF support recommended.
- GI Toxicities: Moderate to severe nausea and vomiting may be acute or delayed. Mucositis and/or diarrhea seen in 30%–40% of patients.
- Neurotoxicity: Severe neuropathy with numbness, tingling, and sensory loss in arms and legs. Proprioception and vibratory sense and loss of motor function can occur. Paresthesias are dose related and can be severe, requiring pain medication or neurontin. Ototoxicity occurs in > 30% beginning with high-frequency hearing.
- Renal: Dose-limiting toxicity and may be cumulative and presents at 10–20 days. May result in necrosis of proximal and distal renal tubules, preventing reabsorption of Mg^{2+}, Ca^{2+}, and K$^+$. Can be avoided with adequate hydration, diuresis as well as slower infusion time.
- Alopecia: Total loss of body hair occurs in nearly all patients.
- Reproduction: Pregnancy category D. Breast feeding should be avoided.

Initiate antiemetic protocol:	Moderately to highly emetogenic protocol.
Supportive drugs:	☐ pegfilgrastim (Neulasta) ☐ filgrastim (Neupogen)
	☐ epoetin alfa (Procrit) ☐ darbepoetin alfa (Aranesp)
Treatment schedule:	Chair time 5 hours on day 1. Repeat cycle every 21 days until disease progression.
Estimated number of visits:	Two visits per cycle. Request three cycles worth of visits.

Dose Calculation by: 1. _____ 2. _____

_____

Physician   Date

_____   _____

Patient Name   ID Number

_____   _____/_____/_____

Diagnosis   Ht   Wt   M^2

Cyclophosphamide + Doxorubicin + Vincristine (CAV)

Baseline laboratory tests:	CBC: Chemistry and LFTs
Baseline procedures or tests:	Multigated angiogram (MUGA) scan
Initiate IV:	0.9% sodium chloride
Premedicate:	5-HT$_3$ and dexamethasone 20 mg in 100 cc of NS.
Administer:	**Cyclophosphamide** _____ mg (1000 mg/m^2) IV on day 1

* Available in 100-, 200-, 500-, 1000-, and 2000-mg vials.
* Dilute with sterile water to a concentration of 20 mg/mL and shake well to ensure that solution is completely dissolved.
* Reconstituted solution stable for 24 hours at room temperature and 6 days if refrigerated.

Doxorubicin _____ mg (40 mg/m^2) IV on day 1

* **Potent vesicant**
* Available as a 2-mg/mL solution.
* Doxorubicin will form a precipitate if it is mixed with heparin or 5-fluorouracil.

Vincristine _____ mg (1 mg/m^2) IV on day 1 (maximum dose 2 mg)

* **Vesicant**
* Available in 1-, 2-, and 5-mg vials, 1 mg/mL.
* Refrigerate vials until use.
* Given as an IV push through side port of a freely flowing IV.

Major Side Effects	

* Bone Marrow Depression: Leukopenia, thrombocytopenia, and anemia seen; may be severe.
* GI Toxicities: Nausea and vomiting are moderate to severe and can be acute or delayed. Stomatitis and diarrhea incidence 10%, but is not dose limiting. Constipation, abdominal pain, or paralytic ileus as a result of nerve toxicity.
* Cardiac: Acutely, pericarditis-myocarditis syndrome may occur. With high cumulative doses > 550 mg/m^2, cardiomyopathy may occur. Cyclophosphamide may increase the risk of doxorubicin-induced cardiotoxicity.
* Neurotoxicities: Peripheral neuropathies as a result of toxicity to nerve fibers. Cranial nerve dysfunction may occur (rare), as well as jaw pain, diplopia, vocal cord paresis, mental depression, and metallic taste.
* Hepatic: Use with caution in patients with abnormal liver function. Dose reduction is required in the presence of liver dysfunction.
* Bladder Toxicities: Hemorrhagic cystitis, dysuria, and urinary frequency. Red-orange discoloration of urine; resolves by 24–48 hours. Provide adequate hydration.
* Skin: Extravasation of vesicants causes severe tissue destruction. Hyperpigmentation, photosensitivity, and radiation recall occur. Complete alopecia.
* Reproduction: Pregnancy category D. Breast feeding should be avoided. Impotence may occur.

Initiate antiemetic protocol:	Moderately to highly emetogenic protocol.
Supportive drugs:	☐ pegfilgrastim (Neulasta) ☐ filgrastim (Neupogen)
	☐ epoetin alfa (Procrit) ☐ darbepoetin alfa (Aranesp)
Treatment schedule:	Chair time 2 hours on day 1. Repeat cycle every 21 days.
Estimated number of visits:	Two visits per cycle. Request four cycles worth of visits.

Dose Calculation by: 1. _____   2. _____

_____   _____

Physician   Date

_____   _____

Patient Name   ID Number

_____   _____/_____/_____

Diagnosis   Ht   Wt M^2

Cyclophosphamide + Doxorubicin + Etoposide (CAE)

Baseline laboratory tests:	CBC: Chemistry panel (including Mg^{2+}), and LFTs
Baseline procedures or tests:	MUGA scan
Initiate IV:	0.9% sodium chloride
Premedicate:	5-HT$_3$ and dexamethasone 10–20 mg in 100 cc of NS
Administer:	

Cyclophosphamide _____ mg (1000 mg/m^2) IV on day 1

- Available in 100-, 200-, 500-, 1000-, and 2000-mg vials.
- Dilute with sterile water, and shake well to ensure that solution is completely dissolved.
- Reconstituted solution stable for 24 hours at room temperature and 6 days if refrigerated.

Doxorubicin _____ (45 mg/m^2) IV on day 1

- **Potent vesicant**
- Available in 2-mg/mL solution; no need to further dilute.
- Given IV push through the sidearm port of a freely flowing IV.

Etoposide _____ (50 mg/m^2) IV over 30–60 minutes on days 1–5

- Available in 20-mg/mL solution.
- May be further diluted with NS or D5W.
- Stability is dependent on final concentration. A concentration of 0.2 mg/mL is stable for 48 hours in a plastic container at room temperature or 96 hours in a glass container at room temperature (under normal fluorescent light).

Major Side Effects

- Bone Marrow Depression: Neutropenia, thrombocytopenia, and anemia. Effects are dose related. GCSF support recommended.
- GI Toxicities: Moderate to severe nausea and vomiting may be acute or delayed. Mucositis can occur.
- Bladder Toxicities: Hemorrhagic cystitis, dysuria, and urinary frequency. Red-orange discoloration of urine; resolves by 24–48 hours. Provide adequate hydration
- Skin: Tissue necrosis with extravasation. Hyperpigmentation, radiation recall, and nail changes are seen. Alopecia will occur.
- Cardiovascular: Hypotension may occur with rapid infusion of etoposide. Cardiomyopathy may occur with high cumulative doses of doxorubicin.
- Reproduction: Pregnancy category D. Breast feeding should be avoided.

Initiate antiemetic protocol:	Moderately to highly emetogenic protocol.
Supportive drugs:	☐ pegfilgrastim (Neulasta) ☐ filgrastim (Neupogen)
	☐ epoetin alfa (Procrit) ☐ darbepoetin alfa (Aranesp)
Treatment schedule:	Chair time 4 hours on day 1 and 2 hours on days 2–5. Repeat cycle every 21 days.
Estimated number of visits:	Six visits per cycle; request three cycles worth. May require extra visits for hydration.

Dose Calculation by: 1. _____   2. _____

_____   _____
Physician   Date

_____   _____
Patient Name   ID Number

_____   _____/_____/_____
Diagnosis   Ht   Wt   M^2

Single-Agent Regimens

Etoposide

Baseline laboratory tests:	CBC: Chemistry, LFTs, and CA 19-9
Baseline procedures or tests:	N/A
Initiate IV:	N/A
Premedicate:	Oral phenothiazine or 5-HT$_3$
Administer:	**Etoposide** _____mg (160 mg/m^2/day) PO on days 1–5
	OR
	Etoposide _____mg (50 mg/m^2) PO bid on days 1–21

- Available in 50- or 100-mg capsules for oral use.
- May give as a single dose up to 400 mg; > 400 mg, divide dose into two to four doses.
- Store in refrigerator.

Major Side Effects

- Bone Marrow Depression: Nadir 10–14 days after drug dose. Neutropenia may be severe.
- GI Toxicities: Nausea and vomiting occur in 30%–40% of patients and are generally mild to moderate. More commonly observed with oral administration. Metallic taste to food.
- Skin: Alopecia observed in nearly two thirds of patients.
- Neurotoxicities: Peripheral neuropathies may occur but are uncommon and mild.
- Reproduction: Pregnancy category D. Breast feeding should be avoided.

Initiate antiemetic protocol:	Mildly emetogenic protocol.
Supportive drugs:	☐ pegfilgrastim (Neulasta) ☐ filgrastim (Neupogen)
	☐ epoetin alfa (Procrit) ☐ darbepoetin alfa (Aranesp)
Treatment schedule:	No chair time. Repeat cycle every 28 days as tolerated or until disease progression.
Estimated number of visits:	One visit per cycle. Request three cycles worth of visits.

Dose Calculation by: 1. _____   2. _____

_____

Physician

Date _____

_____

Patient Name

ID Number _____

_____

Diagnosis

Ht _____ / Wt _____ / M^2 _____

Paclitaxel

Baseline laboratory tests:	CBC: Chemistry (including Mg^{2+}) and CEA
Baseline procedures or tests:	N/A
Initiate IV:	0.9% sodium chloride
Premedicate:	5-HT$_3$ and dexamethasone 10–20 mg in 100 cc of NS
	Diphenhydramine 25–50 mg and cimetidine 300 mg in 100 cc of NS

Administer: **Paclitaxel** _____ mg (80–100 mg/m²) IV weekly for 3 weeks

- Available in 30-mg (6 mg/mL), 100-mg (16.7 mg/mL), and 300-mg (6 mg/ mL) vials.
- Further dilute in 250–500 cc NS or D5W. Final concentration is $\pm$ 1.2 mg/mL.
- **Use non-PVC tubing and containers and a 0.22-micron inline filter to administer.**

Major Side Effects

- Hypersensitivity Reaction: Occurs in 20%–40% of patients. Characterized by generalized skin rash, flushing, erythema, hypotension, dyspnea, and/or bronchospasm. Usually occurs within the first 2–3 minutes of infusion and almost always within the first 10 minutes. Premedicate as described.
- Bone Marrow Depression: Dose-limiting neutropenia with nadir at days 8–10 and recovery by days 15–21. Decreased incidence of neutropenia with 3-hour schedule when compared with 24-hour schedule. G-CSF support recommended.
- GI Toxicity: Nausea and vomiting occur in 52% of patients, mild and preventable with anitemetics. Diarrhea in 38% of patients and stomatitis in 31%.
- Neurotoxicity: Severe neuropathy with numbness, tingling, and sensory loss in arms and legs. Proprioception and vibratory sense and loss of motor function can occur. Paresthesias are dose related and can be severe, requiring pain medication or neurontin. More frequent with longer infusions and at doses > 175 mg/m².
- Ototoxicity occurs in > 30% beginning with high-frequency hearing.
- Alopecia: Total loss of body hair occurs in nearly all patients.
- Reproduction: Pregnancy category D. Breast feeding should be avoided.

Initiate antiemetic protocol:	Mildly emetogenic protocol.
Supportive drugs:	☐ pegfilgrastim (Neulasta) ☐ filgrastim (Neupogen)
	☐ epoetin alfa (Procrit) ☐ darbepoetin alfa (Aranesp)
Treatment schedule:	Chair time 4 hours per week every 3 weeks. Repeat cycle every 28 days.
Estimated number of visits:	Two visits per cycle. Request three cycles worth of visits.

Dose Calculation by: 1. _____   2. _____

_____
Physician

_____
Date

_____
Patient Name

_____
ID Number

_____
Diagnosis

_____/_____/_____
Ht   Wt   M²

Topotecan

Baseline laboratory tests:	CBC: Chemistry panel, LFTs, and CA 19-9
Baseline procedures or tests:	N/A
Initiate IV:	0.9% sodium chloride
Premedicate:	5-HT$_3$ and dexamethasone 10 mg in 100 cc of NS
Administer:	**Topotecan** _____ mg (1.5 mg/m^2) IV over at least 30 minutes on days 1–5

Available as a 4-mg single-dose vial.

- Reconstitute vial with 4 mL of sterile water for injection.
- Further dilute in 0.9% sodium chloride or D5W.
- Use immediately.

Major Side Effects

- Myelosuppression: Severe grade 4 myelosuppression seen during the first course of therapy in 60% of patients. Dose-limiting toxicity. Typical nadir occurs at days 7–10 with full recovery by days 21–28. If severe neutropenia occurs, reduce dose by 0.25 mg/m^2 for subsequent doses or may use G-CSF to prevent neutropenia 24 hours after last day of topotecan therapy.
- GI Toxicities: Mild to moderate nausea and vomiting, dose related. Occurs in 60%–80% of patients. Diarrhea occurs in 42% of patients, and constipation occurs in 39%. Abdominal pain may occur in 33% of patients.
- Flulike Symptoms: Headache, fever, malaise, arthralgias, and myalgias.
- Hepatic Toxicity: Evidence of increased drug toxicity in patients with low protein level and hepatic dysfunction. Dose reductions may be necessary.
- Renal: Use with caution in patients with abnormal renal function. Dose reduction is necessary in this setting. Microscopic hematuria seen in 10% of patients.
- Skin: Alopecia.
- Reproduction: Pregnancy category D. Breast feeding should be avoided.

Initiate antiemetic protocol:	Mildly to moderately emetogenic protocol.
Supportive drugs:	☐ pegfilgrastim (Neulasta) ☐ filgrastim (Neupogen)
	☐ epoetin alfa (Procrit) ☐ darbepoetin alfa (Aranesp)
Treatment schedule:	Chair time 1 hour on days 1–5. Repeat every 21 days until disease progression.
Estimated number of visits:	Six visits per course. Request three courses.

Dose Calculation by: 1. _____   2. _____

_____
Physician

_____
Patient Name

_____
Diagnosis

_____
Date

_____
ID Number

_____/_____/_____
Ht   Wt   M^2

LYMPHOMA

Hodgkin's Disease

L

Combination Regimens

Doxorubicin: 25-mg/m^2 IV on days 1 and 15
Bleomycin: 10-U/m^2 IV on days 1 and 15
Vinblastine: 6-mg/m^2 IV on days 1 and 15
Dacarbazine: 375-mg/m^2 IV on days 1 and 15
Repeat cycle every 28 days.[1,273]

Nitrogen mustard: 6-mg/m^2 IV on days 1 and 8
Vincristine: 1.4-mg/m^2 IV on days 1 and 8
Procarbazine: 100-mg/m^2 PO on days 1–14
Prednisone: 40-mg/m^2 PO on days 1–14
Repeat cycle every 28 days.[1, 274]

Nitrogen mustard: 6-mg/m^2 IV on days 1 and 8
Vincristine: 1.4-mg/m^2 IV on day 1 (maximum dose 2 mg)
Procarbazine: 100-mg/m^2 PO on days 1–14
Prednisone: 40-mg/m^2 PO on days 1–14
Doxorubicin: 35-mg/m^2 IV on day 8
Bleomycin: 10-U/m^2 IV on day 8
Hydrocortisone: 100-mg IV given before bleomycin
Vinblastine: 6-mg/m^2 IV on day 8
Repeat cycle every 28 days.[1,275]

See MOPP and ABVD regimens outlined earlier.

Nitrogen mustard: 6-mg/m^2 IV on day 1

Doxorubicin: 25-mg/m^2 IV on days 1 and 15

Vinblastine: 6-mg/m^2 IV on days 1 and 15

Vincristine: 1.4-mg/m^2 IV on days 8 and 22 (maximum 2 mg)

Bleomycin: 5-U/m^2 IV on days 8 and 22

Etoposide: 60-mg/m^2 IV on days 15 and 16

Prednisone: 40-mg/m^2 PO every other day, taper starting day 10

Repeat cycle every 28 days.[1,276]

Bleomycin: 10-U/m^2 IV on day 8

Etoposide: 100-mg/m^2 IV on days 1–3

Doxorubicin: 25-mg/m^2 IV on day 1

Cyclophosphamide: 650-mg/m^2 IV on day 1

Vincristine: 1.4-mg/m^2 IV on day 8 (maximum dose 2 mg)

Procarbazine: 100-mg/m^2 PO on days 1–7

Prednisone: 40-mg/m^2 PO on days 1–14

Repeat cycle every 21 days.[1,277]

Bleomycin: 10-U/m^2 IV on day 8

Etoposide: 200-mg/m^2 IV on days 1–3

Doxorubicin: 35-mg/m^2 IV on day 1

Cyclophosphamide: 1200-mg/m^2 IV on day 1

Vincristine: 1.4-mg/m^2 IV on day 8 (maximum dose 2 mg)

Procarbazine: 100-mg/m^2 PO on days 1–7

Prednisone: 40-mg/m^2 PO on days 1–14

Repeat cycle every 21 days.[1,278]

G-CSF 5 µg/kg/day SC starting on day 8 and continuing until neutrophil recovery.

Etoposide: 200-mg/m^2 IV on days 1–5

Vincristine: 2-mg/m^2 IV on day 1 (maximum dose 2 mg)

Doxorubicin: 50-mg/m^2 IV on day 2

Repeat cycle every 28 days.[1,279]

Etoposide: 120-mg/m^2 IV on days 1, 8, and 15
Vinblastine: 4-mg/m^2 IV on days 1, 8, and 15
Cytarabine: 30-mg/m^2 IV on days 1, 8, and 15
Cisplatin: 40-mg/m^2 IV on days 1, 8, and 15
Repeat cycle every 28 days.[1,280]

BCNU: 60-mg/m^2 IV on day 1
Etoposide: 75-mg/m^2 IV on days 2–5
Cytarabine: 100-mg/m^2 IV every 12 hours on days 2–5
Melphalan: 30-mg/m^2 IV on day 6
Repeat cycle every 4–6 weeks.[1,281]

Single-Agent Regimen

Gemcitabine: 1250-mg/m^2 IV on days 1, 8, and 15
Repeat cycle every 28 days.[1,282]

Combination Regimens

Doxorubicin, Bleomycin, Vinblastine, Dacarbazine (ABVD)

Baseline laboratory tests: CBC: Chemistry, sedimentation rate, and MUGA

Laboratory tests: CBC before each treatment, central line placement

Premedicate: 5-HT$_3$, dexamethasone, and acetaminophen

Administer: **Doxorubicin:** _____ 25-mg/m^2 IV push on days 1 and 15

- Available as 2 mg/mL. Refrigerated. Given IV push through a free-flowing IV.

Bleomycin: _____ 10-U/m^2 IV push on days 1 and 15

- A test dose of 2 U is recommended before the first dose to detect hypersensitivity.

- Available as a powder in 15- or 30-unit sizes. Dilute powder in NS or sterile water 1–5 cc for the 15-unit vial and 2–10 cc for the 30-unit vial. Should NOT be diluted in D5W.

- Stable for 24 hours when diluted with NS.

- Given IV push or further diluted in NS and infused or pushed over at least 10 minutes.

- Reduce dose with impaired renal function.

Vinblastine _____ 6-mg/m^2 IV push days 1 and 15.

- Vesicant

- Available in 1-mg/mL, 10-mg vials, refrigerated.

- Dilute with 10 mL of bacteriostatic water NS with benzyl alcohol.

- Should be clear and free of particulate matter.

- Given slow IV push over 1–2 minutes through side port of freely flowing IV.

Dacarbazine _____ 375-mg/m^2 IVPB over at least 1 hour on days 1 and 15.

- Vesicant

- Available in 100- and 200-mg vials, refrigerated.

- Add sterile water or NS to vial.

- Avoid exposure to light.

- Reconstituted solution should be yellow. Discard if solution turns pink or red.

Major Side Effects

- Myelosuppression: May be severe. Teach self-care measures to minimize risk of infection and bleeding. GCSF support may be needed.

- GI Toxicities: Nausea, vomiting, and anorexia, moderately to highly emetogenic. Mucositis and stomatitis. Constipation and paralytic ileus secondary to autonomic neuropathy.

- Flulike Symptoms: Fever, chills, malaise, myalgias, and arthralgias. May last for several days after treatment.

- Cardiotoxicity: Doxorubicin dose limit 450–550 mg/m^2. Arrhythmias and/or EKG changes, pericarditis, or myocarditis. Usually transient and asymptomatic.

- Genitourinary (GU) toxicities: Discoloration of urine from pink to red up to 48 hours.

- Neurotoxicity: Peripheral neuropathy, including numbness, weakness, myalgias, and late severe motor difficulties. Jaw pain.

- Pulmonary Toxicity: Pneumonitis occurs with Bleomycin in 10% of patients. Risk factors include age > 70 years, dose > 400 U.

- Skin Alterations: Alopecia total, hyperpigmentation of nail beds and dermal crease of hands, greatest in dark-skinned individuals. Radiation recall.

- Reproduction: Pregnancy category D. Breast feeding should be avoided. Discuss sperm banking.

Initiate antiemetic protocol: Mildly to moderately emetogenic protocol.

Supportive drugs:

☐ G-CSF _____ neupogen   ☐ pegfilgrastim (Neulasta)

☐ epoetin alfa (Procrit)/   ☐ Allopurinol_____
darbepoetin alfa (Aranesp)_____

☐ Antibiotic _____   ☐ Antifungal _____

Treatment schedule: Repeat cycle every 28 days for four to six cycles.

Estimated number of visits: Every other week.

Chair time: Chair time 2–3 hours on days 1 and 15.

Dose Calculation by: 1. _____   2. _____

_____   _____

Physician   Date

_____   _____

Patient Name   ID Number

_____   _____ / _____ / _____

Diagnosis   Ht   Wt   M^2

Nitrogen Mustard, Vincristine, Procarbazine, Prednisone (MOPP)

Baseline laboratory tests:	CBC: Chemistry, sedimentation rate
	Draw blood before each chemotherapy administration
Premedicate:	5-HT$_3$ and dexamethasone
Administer:	**Nitrogen mustard** _____ 6-mg/m^2 IV push on days 1 and 8

- Add 10 mL of sterile water or NS for final concentration of 1 mg/1 mL.
- Prepare immediately before administrations (within 15 minutes).
- Powerful vesicant; avoid contact with skin or eyes or inhaling powder.
- Given IV push through the side port of a freely flowing IV.

Vincristine _____ 1.4-mg/m^2 IV push on days 1 and 8. Maximum dose 2 mg.

- Available in 1-, 2-, and 5-mg vial. 1 mg/mL. Keep refrigerated.
- Vesicant
- Given IV push through a free-flowing IV.

Procarbazine _____ 100-mg/m^2 PO on days 1–14

- Available in 50-mg tablets.

Prednisone _____ 40-mg/m^2 PO on days 1–14 taper: _____

Major Side Effects

- Myelosuppression: May be severe and dose-limiting toxicity.
- GI Toxicities: Nausea, vomiting, anorexia, and taste alterations; highly emetogenic. Mucositis and stomatitis. Constipation and paralytic ileus secondary to autonomic neuropathy. Antabuse-like reaction with alcohol and procarbazine. Monoamine oxidase (MAO) inhibitor activity. Avoid the following foods: beer, wine, cheese, brewer's yeast, chicken liver, and bananas.
- Cardiotoxicity: Decreased bioavailability of digoxin with procarbazine.
- Flulike Syndrome: Fever, chills, sweating, lethargy, myalgias, and arthralgias common.
- Neurotoxicity: Peripheral neuropathy, including numbness, weakness, myalgias, and late severe motor difficulties. Jaw pain. Tinnitus, deafness, and other signs of eighth cranial nerve damage. Central nervous system (CNS) toxicity with paresthesias, neuropathies, ataxia, lethargy, headache, confusion, and/or seizures.
- Steroid Toxicities: Sodium and water retention, cushingoid changes, hyperglycemia, hypokalemia, and increased sodium level. Warfarin and insulin doses may need to be increased. Muscle weakness, loss of muscle mass, osteoporosis, and pathologic fractures with prolonged use. Mood changes, euphoria, headache, insomnia, depression, and psychosis. Cataracts or glaucoma may develop.
- Pulmonary Toxicity: Pneumonitis in 10% of patients. Risk factors include age > 70, dose > 400 U.
- Skin Alterations: Alopecia total, hyperpigmentation of nail beds and dermal crease of hands, greatest in dark-skinned individuals. Radiation recall. Sun sensitivity.
- Reproduction: Pregnancy category D. Breast feeding should be avoided. Discuss sperm banking.

Initiate antiemetic protocol:	Moderately to highly emetogenic protocol.
Supportive drugs:	☐ G-CSF (neupogen) _____ ☐ pegfilgrastim (Neulasta)
	☐ epoetin alfa (Procrit)/ ☐ Allopurinol
	darbepoetin alfa (Aranesp)
	☐ Antibiotic _____ ☐ Antifungal
Treatment schedule:	Repeat cycle every 28 days for four to six cycles.
Estimated number of visits:	16
Chair time:	Chair time 1 hour on days 1 and 15.

Dose Calculation by: 1. _____   2. _____

_____   _____
Physician   Date

_____   _____
Patient Name   ID Number

_____   _____/_____/_____
Diagnosis   Ht   Wt   M²

MOPP/ABVD Hybrid

Baseline laboratory tests:	CBC: Chemistry, sedimentation rate, MUGA
Laboratory tests:	CBC before each treatment
Premedicate:	5-HT$_3$, dexamethasone, and acetaminophen
Administer:	

Nitrogen mustard: _____ 6-mg/m^2 IV push on days 1 and 8.

- Powerful vesicant; avoid contact with skin and eyes or inhaling powder.
- Add 10 mL of sterile water or NS for final concentration 1 mg/1 mL.
- Prepare immediately before administration (within 15 minutes). Given IV push through the side port of a freely flowing IV.

Vincristine: _____ 1.4-mg/m^2 IV on day 1. Maximum dose 2 mg.

- Vesicant.
- Available in 1 mg/mL 1-, 2-, and 5-mg vial, refrigerated. Given IV push through a free-flowing IV.

Procarbazine: _____ 100-mg/m^2 PO on days 1–14

- Available in 50-mg capsules.

Prednisone: _____ 40-mg/m^2 PO on days 1–14; take with breakfast.

Doxorubicin: 35-mg/m^2 IV on day 8

- Potent Vesicant
- Available as 2 mg/mL.
- Refrigerated. Given IV push through a free-flowing IV.

Bleomycin: _____ 10-units/m^2 IV push day 8

- A test dose of 2 U is recommended before the first dose to detect hypersensitivity.
- Available as a powder in 15- or 30-unit sizes. Dilute powder in NS or sterile water 1–5 cc for the 15-unit vial and 2–10 cc for the 30-unit vial. Should NOT be diluted in D5W.
- Stable for 24 hours when diluted with NS.
- Given IV push or further diluted in NS and infused or pushed over at least 10 minutes.
- Reduce dose with impaired renal function

Hydrocortisone: _____ 100-mg IV given before bleomycin (not needed if dexamethasone given as an antiemetic)

Vinblastine: _____ 6-mg/m^2 IV on day 8

- Vesicant
- 10-mg vial, 1 mg/mL. Refrigerated.
- Rapid push through a free-flowing IV.

Major Side Effects

- Myelosuppression: May be severe and dose limiting.
- GI Toxicities: Nausea, vomiting, and anorexia; moderate to highly emetogenic. Mucositis and stomatitis. Constipation and paralytic ileus secondary to autonomic neuropathy. Antabuse-like reaction with alcohol and procarbazine. MAO inhibitor activity. Avoid the following foods: beer, wine, cheese, brewer's yeast, chicken liver, and bananas.
- Cardiotoxicity: Dose limit 450–550 mg/m^2; decreased bioavailability of digoxin with procarbazine.
- Flulike Syndrome: Fever, chills, sweating, lethargy, myalgias, and arthralgias common.
- GU Toxicities: Discoloration of urine from pink to red up to 48 hours.
- Neurotoxicity: Peripheral neuropathy, including numbness, weakness, myalgias, and late severe motor difficulties. Jaw pain. CNS toxicity with paresthesias, neuropathies, ataxia, lethargy, headache, confusion, and/or seizures.
- Steroid Toxicities: Sodium and water retention, cushingoid changes, hyperglycemia, hypokalemia, and increased sodium levels. Warfarin and insulin doses may need to be increased. Muscle weakness, loss of muscle mass, osteoporosis, and pathologic fractures with prolonged use. Mood changes, euphoria, headache, insomnia, depression, and psychosis. Cataracts or glaucoma may develop.

- Pulmonary Toxicity: Pneumonitis in 10% of patients. Risk factors include age > 70, dose > 400 U.
- Skin Alterations: Alopecia total, hyperpigmentation of nail beds and dermal crease of hands, greatest in dark-skinned individuals. Radiation recall. Sun sensitivity.
- Reproduction: Pregnancy category D. Breast feeding should be avoided. Discuss sperm banking.

Initiate antiemetic protocol: Mildly to moderately emetogenic protocol.

Supportive drugs:

☐ G-CSF _____ neupogen   ☐ pegfilgrastim (Neulasta)

☐ epoetin alfa (Procrit)/   ☐ Allopurinol_____
darbepoetin alfa (Aranesp)_____

☐ Antibiotic _____   ☐ Antifungal _____

Treatment schedule: Repeat cycle every 28 days for four to six cycles.

Estimated number of visits: Every other week for six weeks.

Chair time: Chair time 2 hours on days 1 and 15.

Dose Calculation by: 1. _____   2. _____

_____   _____

Physician   Date

_____   _____

Patient Name   ID Number

_____ /_____ /_____

Diagnosis   Ht   Wt   M^2

MOPP Alternating with ABVD (see MOPP and ABVD regimens outlined previously)

Stanford V

Baseline laboratory tests:	CBC: Chemistry, sedimentation rate, and MUGA
Laboratory tests:	CBC before each treatment
Premedicate:	5-HT$_3$, dexamethasone, and acetaminophen
Administer:	**Nitrogen mustard:** _____ 6-mg/m^2 IV on day 1

  - Add 10 mL of sterile water or NS for final concentration of 1 mg/1 mL.
  - Prepare immediately before administrations (within 15 minutes). Given as an IV push through side port of freely flowing IV.
  - Powerful vesicant; avoid contact with skin and eyes or inhaling powder.

Doxorubicin: _____ 25-mg/m^2 IV on days 1 and 15
  - Potent vesicant
  - Available as 2 mg/mL. Refrigerated. Given IV push through a free-flowing IV.

Vinblastine: _____ 6-mg/m^2 IV on days 1 and 15. Reduce to 4–6 mg/m^2 on weeks 9 and 12 if age > 50 years.
  - Vesicant
  - 10-mg vial, 1 mg/mL. Refrigerated.
  - Rapid push through a free-flowing IV.

Vincristine: _____1.4-mg/m^2 IV on days 8 and 22 (maximum dose 2 mg). Reduce to 1 mg/m^2 on weeks 9 and 12 if age > 50 years.
  - Available in 1 mg/mL 1-, 2-, and 5-mg vial.
  - Given IV push through sidearm of freely flowing IV.
  - Keep refrigerated.
  - Vesicant
  - Given IV push through a free-flowing IV.

Bleomycin: _____ 5 units/m^2 IV push on days 8 and 22
  - A test dose of 2 U is recommended before the first dose to detect hypersensitivity.
  - Available as a powder in 15- or 30-unit sizes. Dilute powder in NS or sterile water 1–5 cc for the 15-unit vial and 2–10 cc for the 30-unit vial. Should NOT be diluted in D5W.
  - Stable for 24 hours when diluted with NS.
  - Given IV push or further diluted in NS and infused or pushed over at least 10 minutes.
  - Reduce dose with impaired renal function.

Etoposide: _____ 60-mg/m^2 IV infusion on days 15 and 16
  - Available in 500- and 1000-mg vials, 20 mg/mL.
  - Further dilute with NS or D5W to 0.1-mg/mL final concentration.
  - Give over 30–60 minutes to minimize risk of hypotension.
  - Stable 48 hours at room temperature.
  - Enhances warfarin action by increasing PT.
  - Dose modification for increased bilirubin level or creatinine clearance.

Prednisone: _____ 40-mg/m^2 PO every other day. Taper starting on week 10.
  - Take with breakfast.

Prophylactic: Bactrim DS PO bid, **acyclovir** 200-mg PO tid

Major Side Effects
  - Myelosuppression: May be severe. Teach self-care measures to minimize risk of infection and bleeding.
  - Hypersensitivity Reactions: Characterized by hypotension, bronchospasms, or wheezing may occur with bleomycin and etoposide.
  - GI Toxicities: Nausea, vomiting, and anorexia; moderate to highly emetogenic. Mucositis and stomatitis. Constipation and paralytic ileus secondary to autonomic neuropathy.

- Cardiotoxicity: Dose limit 450–550 mg/m². Arrhythmias and/or EKG changes, pericarditis, or myocarditis. Usually transient and asymptomatic.
- Flulike Syndrome: Fever, chills, sweating, lethargy, myalgias, and arthralgias common.
- GU Toxicities: Discoloration of urine from pink to red up to 48 hours.
- Neurotoxicity: Peripheral neuropathy, including numbness, weakness, myalgias, and late severe motor difficulties. Jaw pain.
- Pulmonary Toxicity: Pneumonitis occurs in 10% of patients. Risk factors include age > 70, dose > 400 U.
- Skin Alterations: Total alopecia, hyperpigmentation of nail beds and dermal crease of hands, greatest in dark-skinned individuals. Radiation recall. Sun sensitivity.
- Reproduction: Pregnancy category D. Breast feeding should be avoided. Discuss sperm banking.

Initiate antiemetic protocol: Moderately to highly emetogenic protocol.

Supportive drugs:

☐ G-CSF _____ neupogen   ☐ pegfilgrastim (Neulasta) + G-CSF _____

☐ epoetin alfa (Procrit)/ darbepoetin alfa (Aranesp) ___   ☐ Bactrim DS PO BID, ☐ Acyclovir 200-mg PO TID

☐ Allopurinol _____   ☐ Antibiotic _____

☐ Antifungal _____

Treatment schedule: Repeat cycle every 28 days for three cycles.

Estimated number of visits: Weekly chemotherapy for 16 visits.

Chair time: Chair time 1–2 hours weekly.

Dose Calculation by: 1. _____ 2. _____

_____   _____
Physician   Date

_____   _____
Patient Name   ID Number

_____ / _____ / _____
Diagnosis   Ht   Wt   M²

Bleomycin, Etoposide, Doxorubicin, Cyclophosphamide, Vincristine, Procarbazine, Prednisone (BEACOPP)

Baseline laboratory tests:	CBC: Chemistry, sedimentation rate, and MUGA
Laboratory tests:	CBC before each treatment
Premedicate:	5-HT$_3$, dexamethasone, and acetaminophen
Administer:	**Bleomycin:** _____ 10-units/m^2 IV push on day 8

- A test dose of 2 U is recommended before the first dose to detect hypersensitivity.
- Available as a powder in 15- or 30-unit sizes. Dilute powder in NS or sterile water 1–5 cc for the 15-unit vial and 2–10 cc for the 30-unit vial. Should NOT be diluted in D5W.
- Stable for 24 hours when diluted with NS.
- Given IV push or further diluted in NS and infused or pushed over at least 10 minutes.
- Reduce dose with impaired renal function.

Etoposide: _____ 100-mg/m^2 IV infusion on days 1–3

- Available in 100-mg/5-mL vials, 20 mg/mL.
- Further dilute with NS or D5W to 0.1-mg/mL final concentration.
- Give over 30–60 minutes to minimize the risk of hypotension.
- Stable at 48 hours at room temperature.
- Enhances warfarin action by increasing PT.
- Dose modification for increased bilirubin level or creatinine clearance.

Doxorubicin: _____ 25-mg/m^2 IV on day 1

- Vesicant
- Available as 2 mg/mL.
- Refrigerated.
- Given IV push through a free-flowing IV.

Cyclophosphamide: _____ 650-mg/m^2 IV on day 1

- Dilute with sterile water or bacteriostatic water for injection or paraben preserved; shake well until solution is clear.
- Final concentration equals 20 mg/mL.
- Further dilute into NS or D5W 250–500 mL.

Vincristine: _____ 1.4-mg/m^2 IV on day 8 (maximum dose 2 mg)

- Vesicant
- Available in 1 mg/mL 1-, 2-, and 5-mg vials.
- Keep refrigerated.
- Given IV push through a free-flowing IV.

Procarbazine _____ 100-mg/m^2 PO on days 1–7

- Available in 50-mg tablets.

Prednisone: _____ 40-mg/m^2 PO on days 1–14.

- Take with breakfast.

Major Side Effects

- Myelosuppression: Dose-limiting toxicity. Teach self-care measures to minimize risk of infection and bleeding.
- Hypersensitivity Reactions: Characterized by hypotension, bronchospasms, or wheezing may occur with bleomycin and etoposide.
- GI Toxicities: Nausea, vomiting, and anorexia; moderately to highly emetogenic. Mucositis and stomatitis. Constipation and paralytic ileus secondary to autonomic neuropath. Antabuse-like reaction with alcohol and procarbazine. MAO inhibitor activity. Avoid the following foods: beer, wine, cheese, brewer's yeast, chicken liver, and bananas.
- Cardiotoxicity: Doxorubicin dose limit 450–550 mg/m^2. Arrhythmias and/or EKG changes, pericarditis, or myocarditis. Usually transient and asymptomatic.
- Flulike Syndrome: Fever, chills, sweating, lethargy, myalgias, and arthralgias common.

- GU Toxicities: Discoloration of urine from pink to red up to 48 hours. Hemorrhagic cystitis or irritation of bladder wall capillaries; it is preventable with appropriate hydration.
- Neurotoxicity: Peripheral neuropathy, including numbness, weakness, myalgias, and late severe motor difficulties. Jaw pain. CNS toxicity with paresthesias, neuropathies, ataxia, lethargy, headache, confusion, and/or seizures.
- Steroid Toxicities: Sodium and water retention, cushingoid changes, hyperglycemia, hypokalemia, and increased sodium level. Warfarin and insulin doses may need to be increased. Muscle weakness, loss of muscle mass, osteoporosis, and pathologic fractures with prolonged use. Mood changes, euphoria, headache, insomnia, depression, and psychosis. Cataracts or glaucoma may develop.
- Pulmonary Toxicity: Pneumonitis occurs in 10% of patients. Risk factors include age > 70, dose > 400 U.
- Skin Alterations: Alopecia total, hyperpigmentation of nail beds and dermal crease of hands, greatest in dark-skinned individuals. Radiation recall. Sun sensitivity.
- Reproduction: Pregnancy category D. Breast feeding should be avoided. Discuss sperm banking.

Initiate antiemetic protocol: Moderately to highly emetogenic protocol

Supportive drugs:
☐ G-CSF _____   ☐ pegfilgrastim (Neulasta)
☐ epoetin alfa (Procrit)/   ☐ Allopurinol _____
darbepoetin alfa (Aranesp) _____
☐ Antibiotic _____   ☐ Antifungal _____

Treatment schedule: Repeat cycle every 21 days.

Estimated number of visits: Five visits every 3 weeks.

Chair time: Chair time 1–3 hours day 1; 2 hours days 2 and 3; 1 hour day 8.

Dose Calculation by: 1. _____ 2. _____

_____

Physician _____   Date _____

_____

Patient Name _____   ID Number _____

_____

Diagnosis _____   Ht _____/ Wt _____/ M² _____

Bleomycin, Etoposide, Doxorubicin, Cyclophosphamide, Vincristine, Procarbazine, Prednisone (BEACOPP Escalated)

Baseline laboratory tests: CBC: Chemistry, sedimentation rate, and MUGA.

Laboratory tests: CBC before each treatment

Premedicate: 5-HT$_3$, dexamethasone, and acetaminophen

Administer: **Bleomycin:** _____ 10-units/m^2 IV push day 8

- A test dose of 2 U is recommended before the first dose to detect hypersensitivity.
- Available as a powder in 15- or 30-unit sizes. Dilute powder in NS or sterile water 1–5 cc for the 15-unit vial and 2–10 cc for the 30-unit vial. Should NOT be diluted in D5W.
- Stable for 24 hours when diluted with NS.
- Given IV push or further diluted in NS and infused or pushed over at least 10 minutes.
- Reduce dose with impaired renal function.

Etoposide: _____ 200-mg/m^2 IV infusion on days 1–3

- Available in 500- and 1000-mg vials, 20 mg/mL.
- Further dilute with NS or D5W to 0.1-mg/mL final concentration.
- Give over 30–60 minutes to minimize risk of hypotension.
- Stable 48 hours at room temperature.
- Enhances warfarin action by increasing PT.
- Dose modification for increased bilirubin level or creatinine clearance.

Doxorubicin: _____ 35-mg/m^2 IV on day 1

- Vesicant
- Available as 2 mg/mL.
- Refrigerated.
- Given IV push through a free-flowing IV.

Cyclophosphamide: _____ 1200-mg/m^2 IV on day 1

- Dilute with sterile water or bacteriostatic water for injection (paraben preserved only).
- Shake well until solution is clear.
- Final concentration equals 20 mg/mL.
- Further dilute into NS or D5W 250–500 mL.

Vincristine: _____ 1.4-mg/m^2 IV on day 8 (maximum dose 2 mg)

- Vesicant
- Available in 1 mg/mL 1-, 2-, and 5-mg vial.
- Keep refrigerated.
- Given IV push through a free-flowing IV.

Procarbazine _____ 100-mg /m^2 PO on days 1–7

- Available in 50-mg tablets.

Prednisone: _____ 40-mg/m^2 PO on days 1–14.

- Take with breakfast.
- Repeat cycle every 21 days. G-CSF, at 5-μg/kg/day SQ, starting at day 8 and continuing until neutrophil recovery.

Major Side Effects

- Myelosuppression: Dose-limiting toxicity. Teach self-care measures to minimize risk of infection and bleeding. GCSF recommended.
- Hypersensitivity Reactions: Characterized by hypotension, bronchospasms, or wheezing may occur with bleomycin and etoposide.
- GI Toxicities: Nausea, vomiting, and anorexia; moderately to highly emetogenic. Mucositis and stomatitis. Constipation and paralytic ileus secondary to autonomic neuropathy Antabuse-like reaction with alcohol and procarbazine. MAO inhibitor activity. Avoid the following foods: beer, wine, cheese, brewer's yeast, chicken liver, and bananas.

- Cardiotoxicity: Dose limit 450–550 mg/m^2. Arrhythmias and/or EKG changes, pericarditis, or myocarditis. Usually transient and asymptomatic.
- Flu-like Syndrome: Fever, chills, sweating, lethargy, myalgias, and arthralgias common.
- GU Toxicities: Discoloration of urine from pink to red up to 48 hours. Hemorrhagic cystitis or irritation of bladder wall capillaries; preventable with appropriate hydration.
- Neurotoxicity: Peripheral neuropathy, including numbness, weakness, myalgias, and late severe motor difficulties. Jaw pain. CNS toxicity with paresthesias, neuropathies, ataxia, lethargy, headache, confusion, and/or seizures.
- Steroid Toxicities: Sodium and water retention, cushingoid changes, hyperglycemia, hypokalemia, and increased sodium level. Warfarin and insulin doses may need to be increased. Muscle weakness, loss of muscle mass, osteoporosis, and pathological fractures with prolonged use. Mood changes, euphoria, headache, insomnia, depression, and psychosis. Cataracts or glaucoma may develop.
- Pulmonary Toxicity: Pneumonitis occurs in 10% of patients. Risk factors include age > 70, dose > 400 U.
- Skin Alterations: Alopecia total, hyperpigmentation of nail beds and dermal crease of hands, greatest in dark-skinned individuals. Radiation recall. Sun sensitivity.
- Reproduction: Pregnancy category D. Breast feeding should be avoided. Discuss sperm banking.

Initiate antiemetic protocol: Moderately to highly emetogenic protocol.

Supportive drugs:

☐ G-CSF _____   ☐ pegfilgrastim (Neulasta)

☐ epoetin alfa (Procrit)/   ☐ Allopurinol_____
   darbepoetin alfa (Aranesp)_____

☐ Antibiotic _____   ☐ Antifungal _____

Treatment schedule: Repeat cycle every 21 days.

Estimated number of visits: Five visits every 3 weeks.

Chair time: Chair time 1–3 hours day 1; 2 hours days 2 and 3; 1 hour day 8.

Dose Calculation by: 1. _____ 2. _____

Physician _____ Date _____

Patient Name _____ ID Number _____

Diagnosis _____ Ht _____ / Wt _____ / M^2 _____

Etoposide, Vincristine, Doxorubicin (EVA)

Baseline laboratory tests:	CBC: Chemistry, sedimentation rate, and MUGA
Laboratory tests:	CBC before each treatment
Premedicate:	5-HT$_3$ and dexamethasone
Administer:	

Etoposide: _____ 200-mg/m^2 IV infusion on days 1–5

- Available in 500- and 1000-mg vials, 20 mg/mL.
- Further dilute with NS or D5W to 0.1-mg/mL final concentration.
- Give over 30–60 minutes to minimize risk of hypotension.
- Stable 48 hours at room temperature.
- Enhances warfarin action by increasing PT.
- Dose modification for increased bilirubin level or creatinine clearance.

Vincristine: _____ 2-mg IV on day 1 (maximum dose, 2 mg)

- Available in 1-, 2-, and 5-mg vial.
- Keep refrigerated.
- **Vesicant**
- Given IV push through a free-flowing IV.

Doxorubicin: _____ 50-mg/m^2 IV on day 2

- **Vesicant**
- Available as 2 mg/mL.
- Refrigerated.
- Given IV push through a free-flowing IV.
- Repeat cycle every 28 days.

Major Side Effects

- Myelosuppression: May be severe. Teach self-care measures to minimize risk of infection and bleeding.
- Hypersensitivity Reactions: Characterized by hypotension, bronchospasms, or wheezing may occur with etoposide.
- GI Toxicities: Nausea, vomiting, and anorexia; moderately to highly emetogenic. Mucositis and stomatitis. Constipation and paralytic ileus secondary to autonomic neuropathy.
- Cardiotoxicity: Doxorubicin dose limit 450–550 mg/m^2. Arrhythmias and/or EKG changes, pericarditis, or myocarditis. Usually transient and asymptomatic.
- GU Toxicities: Discoloration of urine from pink to red up to 48 hours.
- Neurotoxicity: Peripheral neuropathy, including numbness, weakness, myalgias, and late severe motor difficulties. Jaw pain.
- Skin Alterations: Total alopecia, hyperpigmentation of nail beds and dermal crease of hands, greatest in dark-skinned individuals. Radiation recall. Sun sensitivity.
- Reproduction: Pregnancy category D. Breast feeding should be avoided. Discuss sperm banking.

Initiate antiemetic protocol:	Moderately to highly emetogenic protocol.
Supportive drugs:	☐ G-CSF (Neupogen) _____ ☐ pegfilgrastim (Neulasta)
	☐ epoetin alfa (Procrit)/ ☐ Allopurinol_____
	darbepoetin alfa (Aranesp)_____
	☐ Antibiotic _____ ☐ Antifungal _____
Treatment schedule:	Repeat cycle every 28 days.
Estimated number of visits:	Six visits per cycle.
Chair time:	Chair time 2–3 hours day 1; 2 hours day 2–5.

Dose Calculation by: 1. _____   2. _____

_____

Physician   Date

_____

Patient Name   ID Number

_____

Diagnosis   Ht _____ / Wt _____ / M² _____

Etoposide, Vinblastine, Cytarabine, Cisplatin (EVAP)

Baseline laboratory tests:	CBC: Chemistry panel (especially blood urea nitrogen [BUN], Cr, Na^+, Mg^{2+}, Ca^{2+}, K), sedimentation rate, and MUGA.
Premedicate:	5-HT_3 and dexamethasone
Administer:	

Etoposide: _____ 120-mg/m^2 IV infusion on days 1, 8, and 15

- Available in 500- and 1000-mg vials, 20 mg/mL.
- Further dilute with NS or D5W to 0.1-mg/mL final concentration.
- Give over 30–60 minutes to minimize risk of hypotension.
- Stable 48 hours at room temperature.
- Enhances warfarin action by increasing PT.
- Dose modification for increased bilirubin level or creatinine clearance.

Vinblastine: _____ 4-mg/m^2 IV on days 1, 8, and 15.

- Vesicant
- 10-mg vial, 1 mg/mL.
- Refrigerated.
- Rapid push through a free-flowing IV.

Cytarabine _____ 30-mg/m^2 IV over 1–2 hours on days 1, 8, and 15.

- Irritant.
- Reconstitute with water with benzyl alcohol, then dilute with 0.9% sodium chloride or D5W.
- Reconstituted drug is stable for 48 hours at room temperature, 7 days refrigerated (fill pump for no more than 48-hour infusion and refill).

Cisplatin _____ 40-mg/m^2 IV on days 1, 8, and 15

- Available in 100-mg vials, 1-mg/mL concentration.
- Further dilute to 100–1000 mL with NS.
- Do NOT mix with D5W.
- Avoid aluminum needles.
- Stable for 24 hours at room temperature.
- Reduces renal clearance of etoposide and decreases effect of phenytoin.
- Cisplatin is inactivated in the presence of alkaline solutions containing sodium bicarbonate.

Major Side Effects

- Myelosuppression: May be severe. Teach self-care measures to minimize risk of infection and bleeding.
- Hypersensitivity Reactions: Characterized by hypotension, bronchospasms, or wheezing may occur with etoposide. Hypersensitivity reactions can occur with cisplatin.
- GI Toxicities: Nausea, vomiting and anorexia, metallic taste of foods; moderate to highly emetogenic. Mucositis and stomatitis. Constipation and paralytic ileus secondary to autonomic neuropathy can occur.
- Potential Renal Damage: Dose-limiting toxicity with cisplatin. Can be prevented by adequate hydration and diuresis.
- Neurotoxicity: Dose limiting. Effects on renal function dose related and seen in 10–20 days after therapy. Peripheral neuropathy, including numbness, weakness, myalgias, and late severe motor difficulties. Jaw pain. At high doses includes cerebellar toxicity, including nystagmus, dysarthria, ataxia, slurred speech, difficulty with fine motor coordination, lethargy, or somnolence. Ototoxicity: High-frequency hearing loss and tinnitus.
- Renal: Dose-limiting toxicity and may be cumulative and presents at 10–20 days. May result in necrosis of proximal and distal renal tubules preventing reabsorption of Mg^{2+}, Ca^{2+}, and K^+. Can be avoided with adequate hydration, diuresis as well as slower infusion time.
- Skin Alterations: Total alopecia, hyperpigmentation of nail beds and dermal crease of hands, greatest in dark-skinned individuals. Radiation recall. Sun sensitivity.

- Reproduction: Pregnancy category D. Breast feeding should be avoided. Discuss sperm banking.

Initiate antiemetic protocol: Moderately to highly emetogenic protocol.

Supportive drugs:
☐ G-CSF (Neupogen)_____   ☐ pegfilgrastim (Neulasta)
☐ epoetin alfa (Procrit)/   ☐ Allopurinol_____
darbepoetin alfa (Aranesp)_____
☐ Antibiotic _____   ☐ Antifungal _____

Treatment schedule: Repeat cycle every 28 days.

Estimated number of visits: Weekly chemotherapy, for 16 visits.

Chair time: Chair time 2–3 hours.

Dose Calculation by: 1. _____   2. _____

_____

Physician   Date

_____

Patient Name   ID Number

_____ / _____ / _____

Diagnosis   Ht   Wt   M^2

Carmustine (BCNU), Etoposide, Cytarabine, Melphalan (Mini-BEAM)

Baseline laboratory tests:	CBC: Chemistry panel (especially BUN, Cr, Na$^+$, Mg^{2+}, Ca^{2+}, K), sedimentation rate, and pulmonary function tests
Premedicate:	5-HT$_3$ and dexamethasone
Administer:	**Carmustine:** _____ 60-mg/m^2 IV over 1–2 hours on day 1

- Add sterile alcohol to vial, and dilute with sterile water.
- Further dilute with 100–250 mL of D5W or NS.
- Reconstituted solution stable for 8 hours at room temperature and 24 hours refrigerated.
- Cimetidine and amphotericin B increase toxicity, and carmustine decreases plasma levels of digoxin and phenytoin.

Etoposide: _____ 75-mg/m^2 IV infusion on days 2–5

- Available in 500- and 1000-mg vials, 20 mg/mL.
- Further dilute with NS or D5W to 0.1-mg/mL final concentration.
- Give over 30–60 minutes to minimize risk of hypotension.
- Stable for 48 hours at room temperature.
- Enhances warfarin action by increasing PT.
- Dose modification for increased bilirubin level or creatinine clearance.

Cytarabine _____ 100-mg/m^2 IV every 12 hours over 1–2 hours on days 2–5.

- Irritant.
- Reconstitute with water with benzyl alcohol, and then dilute with NS or D5W.
- Reconstituted drug is stable for 48 hours at room temperature.

Melphalan: _____ 30-mg/m^2 IV over 30–45 minutes on day 6.

- Irritant.
- 50-mg vial diluted with provided diluent, to a final concentration of 5 mg/mL.
- Further dilute in 100–150 mL of NS.
- Use 0.45-µ filter.
- Stable for 1 hour at room temperature.
- Dose reductions for abnormal renal function.

Major Side Effects

- Myelosuppression: May be severe, delayed, and prolonged. Teach self-care measures to minimize risk of infection and bleeding.
- Hypersensitivity Reactions: Characterized by hypotension, bronchospasms, or wheezing may occur with etoposide and melphalan. Hypersensitivity reactions can occur with cisplatin.
- GI Toxicities: Nausea, vomiting, and anorexia, metallic taste of foods; moderate to highly emetogenic. Mucositis and stomatitis. Constipation and paralytic ileus secondary to autonomic neuropathy can occur. Watch LFT changes.
- Neurotoxicity: Dose limiting. Effects on renal function dose related and seen 10–20 days after therapy. Peripheral neuropathy, including numbness, weakness, myalgias, and late severe motor difficulties. Jaw pain. At high doses includes cerebellar toxicity, including nystagmus, dysarthria, ataxia, slurred speech, difficulty with fine motor coordination, lethargy, or somnolence.
- Electrolyte Imbalance: Hypomagnesemia, hypocalcemia, and hypokalemia.
- Pulmonary Toxicity: Dose related > 1400 mg carmustine. Presents with cough and dyspnea. Obtain baseline pulmonary function tests. Chest x-ray study shows pulmonary infiltrates.
- Ototoxicity: High-frequency hearing loss and tinnitus.
- Skin Alterations: Total alopecia, hyperpigmentation of nail beds and dermal crease of hands, greatest in dark-skinned individuals. Radiation recall. Sun sensitivity.
- Reproduction: Pregnancy category D. Breast feeding should be avoided. Discuss sperm banking.

Initiate antiemetic protocol:	Moderately to highly emetogenic protocol.

Supportive drugs:

☐ G-CSF (Neupogen)_____

☐ pegfilgrastim (Neulasta)

☐ epoetin alfa (Procrit)/
   darbepoetin alfa (Aranesp)_____

☐ Allopurinol_____

☐ Antibiotic _____

☐ Antifungal _____

Treatment schedule: Repeat cycle every 28 days.

Estimated number of visits: Seven visits per cycle. Request 3–6 cycles of visits.

Chair time: Chair time 3 hours day 1–5; 1–2 hours day 6.

Dose Calculation by: 1. _____ 2. _____

_____   _____
Physician   Date

_____   _____
Patient Name   ID Number

_____   ____/____/____
Diagnosis   Ht   Wt   M²

Single-Agent Regimen

Gemcitabine (Gemzar)

Baseline laboratory tests:	CBC: Chemistry, LFTs, and RFTs
Initiate IV:	NS
Premedicate:	5-HT$_3$ and dexamethasone
Administer:	**Gemcitabine** _____ 1250-mg/m^2 IV infusion on days 1, 8, and 15

- Available in 200- and 1000-mg vial. 40 mg/mL.
- Reconstitute with 5 mL of preservative-free NS for 200-mg vial and 25 mL of NS for 1-g vial.
- Shake vial until mixture is dissolved.
- Concentration is 38 mg/mL.
- Further dilute in 250–500 cc NS and infuse over 30 minutes. May cause some irritation with infusion.

Major Side Effects

- Myelosuppression: Dose-limiting toxicity, with grade 3 and 4 neutropenia, thrombocytopenia.
- GI Toxicities: Nausea and vomiting, anorexia, stomatitis, and diarrhea.
- Flulike Syndrome: Transient febrile episodes. Treat with acetaminophen.
- Skin Alterations: Erythematous, pruritic, and/or maculopapular, appearing on neck and extremities. Edema mild to moderate and not related to renal, hepatic, or cardiac impairment. Alopecia occurs in about 15% of patients and is reversible.
- Reproduction: Pregnancy category D. Breast feeding should be avoided.

Initiate antiemetic protocol: Mildly to moderately emetogenic protocol.

Supportive drugs:

☐ G-CSF (Neupogen) _____	☐ pegfilgrastim (Neulasta)
☐ epoetin alfa (Procrit)/ darbepoetin alfa (Aranesp)_____	☐ Allopurinol_____
☐ Antibiotic _____	☐ Antifungal _____

Treatment schedule:	Repeat every 28 days.
Estimated number of visits:	Weekly
Chair time:	1 hour

Dose Calculation by: 1. _____ 2. _____

_____

Physician

Date _____

_____

Patient Name

ID Number _____

_____

Diagnosis

Ht _____/ Wt _____/ M^2 _____

LYMPHOMA

Non-Hodgkin's Lymphoma

LOW-GRADE
Combination Regimens

Cyclophosphamide: 400-mg/m^2 PO on days 1–5 (or 800-mg/m^2 IV on day 1)

Vincristine: 1.4-mg/m^2 IV on day 1 (maximum 2 mg)

Prednisone: 100-mg/m^2 PO on days 1–5

Repeat cycle every 21 days.[1,283]

Cyclophosphamide: 750-mg/m^2 IV on day 1

Mitoxantrone: 10-mg/m^2 IV on day 1

Vincristine: 1.4-mg/m^2 IV on day 1 (maximum 2 mg)

Prednisone: 50-mg/m^2 PO on days 1–5

Repeat cycle every 21 days.[1,284]

Fludarabine: 25-mg/m^2 IV on days 1–3

Mitoxantrone: 10-mg/m^2 IV on day 1

Dexamethasone: 20-mg PO on days 1–5

Bactrim DS: 1 tablet PO bid, three times per week

Repeat cycle every 21 days.[1,285]

Fludarabine: 20-mg/m^2 IV on days 1–5

Cyclophosphamide: 1000-mg/m^2 IV on day 1

Bactrim DS: 1 tablet PO bid

Repeat cycle every 21–28 days.[1,286]

Cyclophosphamide: 750-mg/m^2 IV on day 1

Doxorubicin: 50-mg/m^2 IV on day 1

Vincristine: 1.4-mg/m^2 IV on day 1 (maximum 2 mg)

Prednisone: 100-mg/m^2 PO on days 1–5

Repeat cycle every 21 days.[1,287]

INTERMEDIATE-GRADE

Cyclophosphamide: 750-mg/m^2 IV on day 1
Doxorubicin: 50-mg/m^2 IV on day 1
Vincristine: 1.4-mg/m^2 IV on day 1 (maximum 2 mg)
Prednisone: 100-mg PO on days 1–5
Repeat cycle every 21 days.[1,287]

Cyclophosphamide: 750-mg/m^2 IV on day 1
Mitoxantrone: 10-mg/m^2 IV on day 1
Vincristine: 1.4-mg/m^2 IV on day 1 (maximum 2 mg)
Prednisone: 100-mg PO on days 1–5
Repeat cycle every 21 days.[1,288]

Etoposide: 50-mg/m^2/day IV continuous infusion on days 1–4
Prednisone: 60-mg/m^2 PO on days 1–5
Vincristine: 0.4-mg/m^2/day IV continuous infusion on days 1–4
Cyclophosphamide: 750-mg/m^2 IV on day 5; begin after infusion
Doxorubicin: 10-mg/m^2/day IV continuous infusion on days 1–4
Bactrim DS: One tablet PO bid three times per week
Repeat cycle every 21 days.[1,289]

Etoposide: 50-mg/m^2/day IV continuous infusion on days 1–4
Prednisone: 60-mg/m^2 PO bid on days 1–5
Vincristine: 0.4-mg/m^2/day IV continuous infusion on days 1–4
Cyclophosphamide: 750-mg/m^2 IV on day 5; begin after infusion
Doxorubicin: 10-mg/m^2/day IV continuous infusion on days 1–4
Rituximab: 375-mg/m^2 IV on day 0 prior to continuous infusion
Bactrin DS: 1 tablet PO bid 3 times per week
Repeat cycle every 21 days.[1,290]

Methotrexate: 400-mg/m^2 IV on weeks 2, 6, and 10

Leucovorin: 15-mg/m^2 PO every 6 hours for 6 doses, beginning 24 hours after methotrexate

Doxorubicin: 50-mg/m^2 IV on weeks 1, 3, 5, 7, 9, and 11

Cyclophosphamide: 350-mg/m^2 IV on weeks 1, 3, 5, 7, 9, and 11

Vincristine: 1.4-mg/m^2 IV on weeks 2, 4, 6, 8, 10, and 12

Prednisone: 75-mg/day PO for 12 weeks with taper over the last 2 weeks

Bleomycin: 10-U/m^2 IV on weeks 4, 8, and 12

Bactrim DS: One tablet PO bid

Ketoconazole: 200-mg/day PO

Administer one cycle.[1,291]

Methotrexate: 200-mg/m^2 IV on days 8 and 15

Leucovorin: 10-mg/m^2 PO every 6 hours for 8 doses beginning 24 hours after methotrexate

Bleomycin: 4-U/m^2 IV on day 1

Doxorubicin: 45-mg/m^2 IV on day 1

Cyclophosphamide: 600-mg/m^2 IV on day 1

Vincristine: 1-mg/m^2 IV on day 1 (maximum 2 mg)

Dexamethasone: 6-mg/m^2 PO on days 1–5

Repeat cycle every 21 days.[1,292]

Prednisone: 60-mg/m^2 PO on days 1–14

Doxorubicin: 25-mg/m^2 IV on day 1

Cyclophosphamide: 650-mg/m^2 IV on day 1

Etoposide: 120-mg/m^2 IV on day 1

Cytarabine: 300-mg/m^2 IV on day 8

Bleomycin: 5-U/m^2 IV on day 8

Vincristine: 1.4-mg/m^2 IV on day 8

Methotrexate: 120-mg/m^2 IV on day 8

Leucovorin rescue: 25-mg/m^2 PO every 6 hours for 6 doses beginning 24 hours after methotrexate

Bactrim DS: One tablet PO bid on days 1–21

Repeat cycle every 21 days.[1,293]

HIGH-GRADE

Cyclophosphamide: 1200-mg/m^2 IV on day 1

Doxorubicin: 40-mg/m^2 IV on day 1

Vincristine: 1.4-mg/m^2 IV on day 1 (maximum 2 mg)

Prednisone: 40-mg/m^2 PO on days 1–5

Methotrexate: 300-mg/m^2 IV on day 10 for 1 hour and then 60-mg/m^2 IV on days 10 and 11 for 41 hours

Leucovorin rescue: 15-mg/m^2 IV every 6 hours for 8 doses, starting 24 hours after methotrexate on day 12

Intrathecal cytarabine: 30-mg/m^2 IT on day 7, cycle 1 only; 45-mg/m^2 IT on day 7 all subsequent cycles

Intrathecal methotrexate: 12.5-mg IT on day 10, all cycles

Repeat cycle every 28 days.[1,294]

OR

Cyclophosphamide: 800-mg/m^2 IV on day 1 and 200-mg/m^2 IV on days 2–5

Doxorubicin: 40-mg/m^2 IV on day 1

Vincristine: 1.5-mg/m^2 IV on days 1 and 8 in cycle 1 and on days 1, 8, and 15 in cycle 3

Methotrexate: 1200-mg/m^2 IV over 1 hour, followed by 240 mg/m^2/hour for the next 23 hours on day 10

Leucovorin: 192-mg/m^2 IV starting at hour 36 after the start of the methotrexate infusion and 12-mg/m^2 IV every 6 hours thereafter until serum methotrexate (MTX) levels < 50 nM

CNS Prophylaxis

Cytarabine: 70-mg IT on days 1 and 3

Methotrexate: 12-mg IT on day 15

Alternate Regimen A with Regimen B for 4 cycles.

Ifosfamide: 1500-mg/m^2 IV on days 1–5

Etoposide: 60-mg/m^2 IV on days 1–5

Cytarabine: 2-g/m^2 IV every 12 hours on days 1 and 2 for a total of four doses

Methotrexate: 12-mg IT on day 5

Cyclophosphamide: 1200-mg/m^2 IV on day 1

Doxorubicin: 40-mg/m^2 IV on day 1

Vincristine: 1.4-mg/m^2 IV on day 1 (maximum 2 mg)

Prednisone: 40-mg/m^2 PO on days 1–5

Methotrexate: 3-g/m^2 IV over 6 hours on day 10

Leucovorin rescue: 25-mg/m^2 IV or PO every 6 hours for 12 doses
  beginning 24 hours after methotrexate

Intrathecal methotrexate: 12-mg IT on days 1 and 10

Repeat cycle every 21 days.[1,296]

MANTLE CELL LYMPHOMA

Bortezomib: 1.5-mg/m^2 IV on days 1, 4, 8, and 11

Repeat cycle every 21 days.[1,297]

CD20$^+$, B-CELL LYMPHOMAS

Cyclophosphamide: 750-mg/m^2 IV on day 1

Doxorubicin: 50-mg/m^2 IV on day 1

Vincristine: 1.4-mg/m^2 IV on day 1 (maximum 2 mg)

Prednisone: 40-mg/m^2 PO on days 1–5

Rituximab: 375-mg/m^2 IV on day 1

Repeat cycle every 21 days.[1,298]

Rituximab is to be administered first, followed by cyclophosphamide,
  doxorubicin, and vincristine.

OR

Cyclophosphamide: 750-mg/m^2 IV on day 3

Doxorubicin: 50-mg/m^2 IV on day 3

Vincristine: 1.4-mg/m^2 IV on day 3 (maximum 2 mg)

Prednisone: 100-mg PO on days 3–7

Rituximab: 375-mg/m^2 IV on day 1

Repeat cycle every 21 days.[1,299]

Salvage Regimens

Etoposide: 40-mg/m^2 IV on days 1–4

Methylprednisolone: 500-mg IV on days 1–4

Cisplatin: 25-mg/m^2/day IV continuous infusion on days 1–4

Cytarabine: 2000-mg/m^2 IV on day 5 after completion of cisplatin and etoposide

Repeat cycle every 21 days.[1,300]

Cisplatin: 100-mg/m^2 IV on day 1

Cytarabine: 2000-mg/m^2 IV over 2 hours every 12 hours for 2 doses on day 1

Dexamethasone: 40-mg PO on days 1–14

Repeat cycle every 3–4 weeks.[1,301]

Ifosfamide: 5000-mg/m^2 IV continuous infusion for 24 hours on day 2

Etoposide: 100-mg/m^2 IV on days 1–3

Carboplatin: AUC of 5.0, IV on day 2

Mesna: 5000-mg/m^2 IV in combination with ifosfamide dose

Repeat cycle every 14 days.[1,302]

G-CSF is administered at 5 µg/kg on days 5–12.

Mesna: 1330-mg/m^2 IV administered at same time as ifosfamide on days 1–3 and then 500-mg IV 4 hours after ifosfamide on days 1–3

Ifosfamide: 1330-mg/m^2 IV on days 1–3

Mitoxantrone: 8-mg/m^2 IV on day 1

Etoposide: 65-mg/m^2 IV on days 1–3

Repeat cycle every 21 days.[1,303]

LOW-GRADE
Combination Regimens

Cyclophosphamide, Vincristine, Prednisone (CVP)

Baseline laboratory tests:	SMAC, CBC: sedimentation rate
Initiate IV:	NS
Premedicate:	5-HT$_3$ and dexamethasone
Administer:	

Cyclophosphamide _____ 400-mg/m^2 PO on days 1–5 (or 800 mg/m^2 on day 1)

* Take with breakfast.
* Available in 25- and 50-mg tablets.
* OR IV at same doses.
* Dilute with sterile water or bacteriostatic water for injection (sterile water paraben preserved); shake well until solution is clear.
* Final concentration equals 20 mg/mL.
* Further dilute into NS or D5W 250–500 mL.
* Increases effect of anticoagulants and decreases digoxin levels.

Vincristine: _____ 1.4-mg/m^2 IV on day 1 (maximum dose 2 mg)

* Vesicant
* Available in 1 mg/mL 1-, 2-, and 5-mg vial.
* Keep refrigerated.
* Given IV push through a free-flowing IV.

Prednisone: _____ 100-mg/m^2 PO on days 1–5

* Take with breakfast.

Major Side Effects

* Myelosuppression: Dose-limiting toxicity. Nadir day 10–14.
* GI Toxicities: Nausea and vomiting, anorexia; mucositis, diarrhea
* GU Toxicities: Hemorrhagic cystitis or irritation of bladder wall capillaries; preventable with appropriate hydration.
* Neurotoxicity: Peripheral neuropathy, including numbness, weakness, myalgias, and late severe motor difficulties. Jaw pain.
* Steroid Toxicities: Sodium and water retention, cushingoid changes, hyperglycemia, hypokalemia, and increased sodium level. Warfarin and insulin doses may need to be increased. Muscle weakness, loss of muscle mass, osteoporosis, and pathologic fractures with prolonged use. Mood changes, euphoria, headache, insomnia, depression, and psychosis. Cataracts or glaucoma may develop.
* Skin Alterations: Alopecia, hyperpigmentation of nails and skin, and transverse ridging of nails may occur.
* Reproduction: Pregnancy category D. Breast feeding should be avoided.

Initiate antiemetic protocol after chemotherapy.

Supportive drugs:	☐ pegfilgrastim (Neulasta)_____ ☐ filgrastim (Neupogen) _____
	☐ epoetin alfa (Procrit)/ darbepoetin alfa (Aranesp) _____ ☐ Allopurinol_____
	☐ Antibiotic _____ ☐ Antifungal _____
Treatment schedule:	Repeat cycle every 21–28 days for four cycles.
Estimated number of visits:	8–12 over 4 months. Chair time 2 hours.

Dose Calculation by: 1. _____   2. _____

_____

Physician   Date

_____

Patient Name   ID Number

_____   _____/_____/_____

Diagnosis   Ht   Wt   M²

Cyclophosphamide, Mitoxantrone (Novantrone), Vincristine (Oncovin), Prednisone (CNOP)

Baseline laboratory tests:	SMAC, CBC: sedimentation rate MUGA
Initiate IV:	NS
Premedicate:	5-HT$_3$ and dexamethasone
Administer:	**Cyclophosphamide** _____ 750-mg/m^2 IV on day 1

- Dilute with sterile water or bacteriostatic water for injection (sterile water or paraben preserved); shake well until solution is clear.
- Final concentration equals 20 mg/mL.
- Further dilute into NS or D5W 250–500 mL.

Mitoxantrone _____ 10-mg/m^2 IV on day 1.

- Nonvesicant.
- IV push over 3 minutes through the side arm of a free-flowing IV or IV infusion over 5–30 minutes.
- Available in 20 mg in 10-mL dark blue solution. May be diluted in D5W or NS. Stable at room temperature for 48 hours. Incompatible with heparin.

Vincristine: _____ 1.4-mg/m^2 IV on day 1 (maximum dose 2 mg)

- Available in 1-, 2-, and 5-mg vial.
- Keep refrigerated.
- **Vesicant.**
- Given IV push through a free-flowing IV.

Prednisone: _____ 50-mg/m^2 PO on days 1–5

- Take with breakfast.

Major Side Effects

- Myelosuppression: Dose-limiting toxicity.
- Cardiotoxicity: Less than that of doxorubicin or daunorubicin. Patients with cumulative dose 140 mg/m^2 with no prior anthracycline exposure; 120 mg/m^2 with prior exposure, at greater risk.
- GI Toxicities: Nausea and vomiting, anorexia; mucositis, diarrhea.
- GU Toxicities: Hemorrhagic cystitis or irritation of bladder wall capillaries; preventable with appropriate hydration. Urine will be green-blue for 24 hours. Sclera may become discolored blue.
- Neurotoxicity: Peripheral neuropathy, including numbness, weakness, myalgias, and late severe motor difficulties. Jaw pain.
- Steroid Toxicities: Sodium and water retention, cushingoid changes, hyperglycemia, hypokalemia, and increased sodium level. Warfarin and insulin doses may need to be increased. Muscle weakness, loss of muscle mass, osteoporosis, and pathologic fractures with prolonged use. Mood changes, euphoria, headache, insomnia, depression, and psychosis. Cataracts or glaucoma may develop.
- Skin Alterations: Alopecia, hyperpigmentation of nails and skin, and transverse ridging of nails may occur.
- Reproduction: Pregnancy category D. Breast feeding should be avoided. Discuss contraception and sperm banking.

Supportive drugs:	☐ pegfilgrastim (Neulasta)_____ ☐ filgrastim (Neupogen) _____
	☐ epoetin alfa (Procrit)/ ☐ Allopurinol_____
	darbepoetin alfa (Aranesp) _____
	☐ Antibiotic _____ ☐ Antifungal _____
Initiate antiemetic protocol after chemotherapy:	Moderately emetogenic.
Treatment schedule:	Repeat cycle every 21 days.
Estimated number of visits:	Day 1 and at nadir for each cycle. Chair time 2 hours.

Dose Calculation by: 1. _____ 2. _____

_____

Physician _____ Date _____

_____

Patient Name _____ ID Number _____

_____ / _____ / _____

Diagnosis _____ Ht _____ Wt _____ M²

Fludarabine, Mitoxantrone (Novantrone), Dexamethasone (FND)

Baseline laboratory tests:	SMAC, CBC: sedimentation rate, baseline MUGA
Initiate IV:	NS
Premedicate:	5-HT$_3$ and dexamethasone
Administer:	

Fludarabine _____ 25-mg/m^2 IV infused over 30 minutes on days 1–3

- Mix 50-mg vial with 2 cc of sterile water for final concentration of 25 mg/mL.
- Further dilute in at least 100 mL of D5W or NS.
- Reconstituted solution stable for 8 hours.

Mitoxantrone _____ 10-mg/m^2 IV on day 1.

- Nonvesicant
- IV push over 3 minutes through the side arm of a free-flowing IV or IV infusion over 5–30 minutes.
- Available in 20 mg in 10-mL dark blue solution. May be diluted in D5W or NS. Stable at room temperature for 48 hours. Incompatible with heparin.

Dexamethasone: _____ 20-mg PO on days 1–5

- Take with breakfast.

Bactrim DS: 1 tablet PO bid, 3 time per week

Major Side Effects

- Myelosuppression: Dose-limiting toxicity. Severe and cumulative.
- Cardiotoxicity: Less than that of doxorubicin or daunorubicin. Patients with cumulative dose 140 mg/m^2 with no prior anthracycline exposure; 120 mg/m^2 with prior exposure, at greater risk.
- Fatigue: Secondary to anemia, appropriate iron diet, red blood cell growth factor, and/or transfusions may be necessary.
- GI Toxicities: Nausea and vomiting, anorexia; mucositis, diarrhea.
- Tumor lysis syndrome occurring 1–5 days after initiation of treatment; treat with hydration and allopurinol. Metallic taste during infusion of Fludarabine.
- GU Toxicities: Urine will be green-blue for 24 hours. Sclera may become discolored blue.
- Neurotoxicity: Peripheral neuropathy, including numbness, weakness, myalgias, and late severe motor difficulties. Jaw pain. Agitation, confusion, visual disturbances have also occurred.
- Pulmonary Toxicities: Pneumonia and pulmonary hypersensitivity reactions characterized by cough, dyspnea, and interstitial infiltrate.
- Steroid Toxicities: Sodium and water retention, cushingoid changes, hyperglycemia, hypokalemia, and increased sodium level. Warfarin and insulin doses may need to be increased. Muscle weakness, loss of muscle mass, osteoporosis, and pathologic fractures with prolonged use. Mood changes, euphoria, headache, insomnia, depression, and psychosis. Cataracts or glaucoma may develop.
- Skin Alterations: Alopecia, hyperpigmentation of nails and skin, and transverse ridging of nails may occur. Dry skin, photosensitivity, and hyperpigmentation of infused vein.
- Reproduction: Pregnancy category D. Breastfeeding should be avoided. Discuss contraception and sperm banking.

Supportive drugs:	☐ pegfilgrastim (Neulasta)_____ ☐ filgrastim (Neupogen) _____
	☐ epoetin alfa (Procrit)/darbepoetin alfa (Aranesp) _____
	☐ Allopurinol_____ ☐ Antibiotic _____
	☐ Antifungal _____
Initiate antiemetic protocol after chemotherapy:	Moderately emetogenic
Treatment schedule:	Repeat cycle every 21 days.
Estimated number of visits:	Four visits per cycle. Ask for 3–6 cycles worth of visits. Chair time 1–2 hours.

Dose Calculation by: 1. _____   2. _____

_____

Physician   Date

_____

Patient Name   ID Number

_____ / _____ / _____

Diagnosis   Ht   Wt M^2

Fludarabine, Cyclophosphamide (FC)

Baseline laboratory tests:	SMAC, CBC: sedimentation rate
Initiate IV:	NS
Premedicate:	5-HT$_3$ and dexamethasone
Administer:	**Fludarabine** _____ 20-mg/m^2 IV infused over 30 minutes on days 1–5

- Mix 50-mg vial with 2 cc of sterile water for final concentration of 25 mg/mL.
- Further dilute in at least 100 mL of D5W or NS.
- Reconstituted solution stable for 8 hours.

Cyclophosphamide _____ 1000-mg/m^2 IV on day 1

- Dilute with sterile water or bacteriostatic water for injection (sterile water orparaben preserved); shake well until solution is clear.
- Final concentration equals 20 mg/mL.
- Further dilute into NS or D5W 250–500 mL.

Bactrim DS: 1 tablet PO bid

Major Side Effects

- Myelosuppression: Dose-limiting toxicity. Severe and cumulative.
- Fatigue: Secondary to anemia; appropriate iron diet, red blood cell growth factor, and/or transfusions may be necessary.
- GI Toxicities: Nausea and vomiting, anorexia; mucositis, diarrhea.
- Tumor lysis syndrome occurring 1–5 days after initiation of treatment; treat with hydration and allopurinol.
- GU Toxicities: Discoloration of urine from pink to red up to 48 hours. Hemorrhagic cystitis or irritation of bladder wall capillaries; preventable with appropriate hydration.
- Neurotoxicity: Objective weakness and paresthesias as well as agitation, confusion, and visual disturbances have occurred.
- Pulmonary Toxicities: Pneumonia and pulmonary hypersensitivity reactions characterized by cough, dyspnea, and interstitial infiltrate.
- Steroid Toxicities: Sodium and water retention, cushingoid changes, hyperglycemia, hypokalemia, and increased sodium level. Warfarin and insulin doses may need to be increased. Muscle weakness, loss of muscle mass, osteoporosis, and pathologic fractures with prolonged use. Mood changes, euphoria, headache, insomnia, depression, and psychosis. Cataracts or glaucoma may develop.
- Skin Alterations: Alopecia, hyperpigmentation of nails and skin, and transverse ridging of nails may occur. Dry skin, photosensitivity, and hyperpigmentation of infused vein.
- Reproduction: Pregnancy category D. Breast feeding should be avoided. Discuss contraception and sperm banking.

Supportive drugs:

☐ pegfilgrastim (Neulasta)_____ ☐ filgrastim (Neupogen) _____

☐ epoetin alfa (Procrit)/ ☐ Allopurinol_____
darbepoetin alfa (Aranesp) _____

☐ Antibiotic _____ ☐ Antifungal _____

Initiate antiemetic protocol after chemotherapy:	Moderately emetogenic.
Treatment schedule:	Repeat cycle every 21–28 days.
Estimated number of visits:	Days 1–5 and weekly to monitor CBC each cycle. Request 3 cycles worth of visits. Chair time 2 hours.

Dose Calculation by: 1. _____   2. _____

_____
Physician

Date _____

_____
Patient Name

ID Number _____

_____
Diagnosis

Ht _____ / Wt _____ / M² _____

Cyclophosphamide, Doxorubicin, Vincristine, Prednisone (CHOP)

Baseline laboratory tests:	CBC: Chemistry, sedimentation rate, and MUGA
Premedicate:	5-HT$_3$ and dexamethasone
Initiate IV:	NS
Administer:	

Cyclophosphamide: _____ 750-mg/m^2 IV on day 1
- Dilute with sterile water or bacteriostatic water for injection (paraben preserved only); shake well until solution is clear.
- Final concentration equals 20 mg/mL.
- Further dilute into NS or D5W 250–500 mL.

Doxorubicin: _____ 50-mg/m^2 IV on day 1
- Vesicant
- Available as 2 mg/mL.
- Refrigerated.
- Given IV push through a free-flowing IV.

Vincristine: _____ 1.4-mg/m^2 IV push on day 1 (maximum dose 2 mg)
- Vesicant
- Available in 1 mg/mL 1-, 2-, and 5-mg vials.
- Refrigerated.
- Given IV push through a free-flowing IV.

Prednisone: _____ 100-mg PO on days 1 through 5; then taper to 0
- Take with breakfast.

Major Side Effects
- Myelosuppression: Moderate to severe. GCSF recommended.
- GI Toxicities: Nausea and vomiting, anorexia; mucositis, diarrhea.
- GU Toxicities: Discoloration of urine from pink to red up to 48 hours. Hemorrhagic cystitis or irritation of bladder wall capillaries; preventable with appropriate hydration.
- Cardiotoxicity: Doxorubicin dose limit 450–550 mg/m^2. Arrhythmias and/or EKG changes, pericarditis, or myocarditis. Usually transient and asymptomatic.
- Neurotoxicity: Peripheral neuropathy, including numbness, weakness, myalgias, and late severe motor difficulties. Jaw pain.
- Steroid Toxicities: Sodium and water retention, cushingoid changes, hyperglycemia, hypokalemia, and increased sodium level. Warfarin and insulin doses may need to be increased. Muscle weakness, loss of muscle mass, osteoporosis, and pathologic fractures with prolonged use. Mood changes, euphoria, headache, insomnia, depression, and psychosis. Cataracts or glaucoma may develop.
- Reproduction: Pregnancy category D. Breast feeding should be avoided. Discuss contraception and sperm banking.

Supportive Drugs:
- ☐ pegfilgrastim (Neulasta)_____
- ☐ filgrastim (Neupogen) _____
- ☐ epoetin alfa (Procrit)/ darbepoetin alfa (Aranesp) _____
- ☐ Allopurinol_____
- ☐ Antibiotic _____
- ☐ Antifungal _____

Initiate antiemetic protocol after chemotherapy:	Moderately to highly emetogenic protocol.
Treatment schedule:	Repeat every 21 days for six cycles.
Estimated number of visits:	Two visits per cycle. Request 4–6 months of visits. Chair time 2 hours.

Dose Calculation by: 1. _____   2. _____

_____

Physician

_____

Patient Name

_____

Diagnosis

_____

Date

_____

ID Number

_____ / _____ / _____

Ht   Wt   M^2

INTERMEDIATE-GRADE

Cyclophosphamide, Doxorubicin, Vincristine, Prednisone (CHOP)

Baseline laboratory tests:	CBC: Chemistry, sedimentation rate, and MUGA
Premedicate:	5-HT$_3$ and dexamethasone
Initiate IV:	NS
Administer:	**Cyclophosphamide:** _____ 750-mg/m^2 IV on day 1

- Dilute with sterile water or bacteriostatic water for injection (paraben preserved only); shake well until solution is clear.
- Final concentration equals 20 mg/mL.
- Further dilute into NS or D5W 250–500 mL.

Doxorubicin: _____ 50-mg/m^2 IV on day 1

- Vesicant
- Available as 2 mg/mL.
- Refrigerated.
- Given IV push through a free-flowing IV.

Vincristine: _____1.4-mg/m^2 IV push on day 1 (maximum dose 2 mg)

- Vesicant
- Available in 1 mg/mL 1-, 2-, and 5-mg vials.
- Refrigerated.
- Given IV push through a free-flowing IV.

Prednisone: _____100-mg PO on days 1 through 5; then taper to 0

- Take with breakfast.

Major Side Effects

- Myelosuppression: Moderate to severe. GCSF recommended.
- GI Toxicities: Nausea and vomiting, anorexia; mucositis, diarrhea.
- GU Toxicities: Discoloration of urine from pink to red up to 48 hours. Hemorrhagic cystitis or irritation of bladder wall capillaries; preventable with appropriate hydration.
- Cardiotoxicity: Doxorubicin dose limit 450–550 mg/m^2. Arrhythmias and/or EKG changes, pericarditis, or myocarditis. Usually transient and asymptomatic.
- Neurotoxicity: Peripheral neuropathy, including numbness, weakness, myalgias, and late severe motor difficulties. Jaw pain.
- Steroid Toxicities: Sodium and water retention, cushingoid changes, hyperglycemia, hypokalemia, and increased sodium level. Warfarin and insulin doses may need to be increased. Muscle weakness, loss of muscle mass, osteoporosis, and pathologic fractures with prolonged use. Mood changes, euphoria, headache, insomnia, depression, and psychosis. Cataracts or glaucoma may develop.
- Reproduction: Pregnancy category D. Breast feeding should be avoided. Discuss contraception and sperm banking.

Supportive Drugs:

☐ pegfilgrastim (Neulasta)_____   ☐ filgrastim (Neupogen) _____

☐ epoetin alfa (Procrit)/   ☐ Allopurinol_____
  darbepoetin alfa (Aranesp) _____

☐ Antibiotic _____   ☐ Antifungal _____

Initiate antiemetic protocol after chemotherapy:	Moderately to highly emetogenic protocol.
Treatment schedule:	Repeat every 21 days for six cycles.
Estimated number of visits:	Two visits per cycle. Request 4–6 months of visits. Chair time 2 hours.

Dose Calculation by: 1. _____ 2. _____

_____

Physician   Date

_____   _____

Patient Name   ID Number

_____   ___/___/___ _____

Diagnosis   Ht   Wt   M²

Cyclophosphamide, Mitoxantrone (Novantrone), Vincristine (Oncovin), Prednisone (CNOP)

Baseline laboratory tests:	SMAC, CBC: sedimentation rate
Initiate IV:	NS
Premedicate:	5-HT$_3$ and dexamethasone
Administer:	**Cyclophosphamide** _____ 750-mg/m^2 IV on day 1

- Dilute with sterile water or bacteriostatic water for injection (sterile water or paraben preserved); shake well until solution is clear.
- Final concentration equals 20 mg/mL.
- Further dilute into NS or D5W 250–500 mL.

Mitoxantrone _____ 10-mg/m^2 IV on day 1.

- Nonvesicant.
- IV push over 3 minutes through the side arm of a free-flowing IV or IV infusion over 5–30 minutes.
- Available in 20 mg in 10-mL dark blue solution. May be diluted in D5W or NS. Stable at room temperature for 48 hours. Incompatible with heparin.

Vincristine: _____ 1.4-mg/m^2 IV on day 1 (maximum dose 2 mg)

- Available in 1-, 2-, and 5-mg vial.
- Keep refrigerated.
- **Vesicant**
- Given IV push through a free-flowing IV.

Prednisone: _____ 100 mg PO on days 1–5

- Take with breakfast.

Major Side Effects

- Myelosuppression: Dose-limiting toxicity.
- Cardiotoxicity: Less than that of doxorubicin or daunorubicin. Patients with cumulative dose 140 mg/m^2 with no prior anthracycline exposure; 120 mg/m^2 with prior exposure, at greater risk.
- GI Toxicities: Nausea and vomiting, anorexia; mucositis, diarrhea.
- GU Toxicities: Hemorrhagic cystitis or irritation of bladder wall capillaries; preventable with appropriate hydration. Urine will be green-blue for 24 hours. Sclera may become discolored blue.
- Neurotoxicity: Peripheral neuropathy, including numbness, weakness, myalgias, and late severe motor difficulties. Jaw pain.
- Steroid Toxicities: Sodium and water retention, cushingoid changes, hyperglycemia, hypokalemia, and increased sodium level. Warfarin and insulin doses may need to be increased. Muscle weakness, loss of muscle mass, osteoporosis, and pathologic fractures with prolonged use. Mood changes, euphoria, headache, insomnia, depression, and psychosis. Cataracts or glaucoma may develop.
- Skin Alterations: Alopecia, hyperpigmentation of nails and skin, and transverse ridging of nails may occur.
- Reproduction: Pregnacy category D. Breast feeding should be avoided. Discuss contraception and sperm banking.

Supportive drugs:	☐ pegfilgrastim (Neulasta)_____ ☐ filgrastim (Neupogen) _____
	☐ epoetin alfa (Procrit)/ ☐ Allopurinol_____
	darbepoetin alfa (Aranesp) _____
	☐ Antibiotic _____ ☐ Antifungal _____
Initiate antiemetic protocol after chemotherapy:	Moderately emetogenic.
Treatment schedule:	Repeat cycle every 21 days.
Estimated number of visits:	Day 1 and at nadir for each cycle. Chair time 2 hours.

Dose Calculation by: 1. _____   2. _____

Physician _____   Date _____

Patient Name _____   ID Number _____

Diagnosis _____   Ht _____/ Wt _____/ M²

Etoposide, Prednisone, Vincristine, Cyclophosphamide, Doxorubicin (EPOCH)

Baseline laboratory tests:	CBC: Chemistry, sedimentation rate, and MUGA
Laboratory tests:	CBC: Chemistry, RFTs, and LFTs before each treatment
Premedicate:	5-HT$_3$, dexamethasone
Administer:	

Etoposide _____ 50-mg/m^2/d IV continuous infusion on days 1–4

- 100 mg/5mL.
- Reconstitute etopophos with 5–10 mL of NS, D5W, sterile water, bacteriostatic sterile water, or bacteriostatic NS with benzyl alcohol to 20 mg/mL or 10 mg/mL, respectively.
- Further dilute to final concentration NS or D5W to 0.1 mg/mL 250–500 cc

Prednisone: _____ 60-mg/m^2/day PO on days 1–5.

- Take with breakfast.

Vincristine: _____ 0.4-mg/m^2/day IV continuous infusion on days 1–4.

- Maximum dose, 2 mg.
- Available in 1 mg/mL 1-, 2-, and 5-mg vials.
- Keep refrigerated.
- **Vesicant.** Give through side port of freely flowing IV, as continuous infusion use patent central line.

Doxorubicin: _____ 10 mg/m^2/day continuous infusion on days 1–4

- **Vesicant.** Must give continuous infusion with patent central line.
- Available as 2 mg/mL.
- Refrigerated.
- Etoposide, Viscristine, and Doxorubicin compatible in same solution for continuous infusion.

Cyclophosphamide: _____ 750-mg/m^2 IV on day 5

- Dilute with sterile water or bacteriostatic water for injection (paraben preserved only); shake well until solution is clear.
- Final concentration equals 20 mg/mL.
- Further dilute into NS or D5W 250–500 mL.

Bactrim DS: _____1 tablet PO bid, 3 times per week.

Major Side Effects

- Myelosuppression: Dose-limiting toxicity.
- GI Toxicities: Nausea, vomiting, and anorexia; moderately to highly emetogenic. Mucositis, stomatitis, and diarrhea. Constipation and paralytic ileus secondary to autonomic neuropathy.
- Cardiotoxicity: Dose limit 450–550 mg/m^2. Arrhythmias and/or EKG changes, pericarditis, or myocarditis. Usually transient and asymptomatic.
- Steroid Toxicities: Sodium and water retention, cushingoid changes, hyperglycemia, hypokalemia, and increased sodium level. Warfarin and insulin doses may need to be increased. Muscle weakness, loss of muscle mass, osteoporosis, and pathologic fractures with prolonged use. Mood changes, euphoria, headache, insomnia, depression, and psychosis. Cataracts or glaucoma may develop.
- Hypersensitivity Reaction: Characterized by hypotension, bronchospasms, or wheezing may occur with etoposide. Occur more frequently with first dose of etoposide, may premedicate with dexamethasone, cinetidine, and/or diphenhydra mix.
- GU Toxicities: Discoloration of urine from pink to red up to 48 hours. Hemorrhagic cystitis or irritation of bladder wall capillaries; preventable with appropriate hydration.
- Neurotoxicity: Peripheral neuropathy, including numbness, weakness, myalgias, and late severe motor difficulties. Jaw pain.
- Skin Alterations: Total alopecia, hyperpigmentation of nail beds and dermal crease of hands, greatest in dark-skinned individuals. Radiation recall. Sun sensitivity.
- Reproduction: Pregnancy category D. Breast feeding should be avoided. Discuss contraception and sperm banking.

Initiate antiemetic protocol: Moderately to highly emetogenic protocol.
Supportive drugs: □ G-CSF (Neupogen) _____   □ pegfilgrastim (Neulasta)
 □ epoetin alfa (Procrit)/   □ Allopurinol_____
 darbepoetin alfa (Aranesp)_____
 □ Antibiotic _____   □ Antifungal _____
Treatment schedule: Repeat cycle every 21 days.
Estimated number of visits: Six visits per cycle. Request 3 cycles worth of visits.
Chair time: One hour day 1–4; 2–3 hours day 5.

Dose Calculation by: 1. _____   2. _____

_____
Physician   Date

_____
Patient Name   ID Number

_____/_____/_____
Diagnosis   Ht   Wt   M²

Etoposide, Prednisone, Vincristine, Cyclophosphamide, Doxorubicin + Rituximab (EPOCH + Rituximab)

Baseline laboratory tests:	CBC: Chemistry, sedimentation rate, MUGA
Laboratory tests:	CBC: Chemistry, RFT, and LFTs before each treatment
Premedicate:	5-HT$_3$, dexamethasone
Administer:	

Rituximab: _____ 375-mg/m^2 IV on day 0 (pull Rituximab protocol for administration)

- To be administered day 1 before continuous infusion.

Etoposide _____ 50-mg/m^2/d IV continuous infusion on days 1–4

- 100 mg/5mL.
- Reconstitute etopophos with 5–10 mL of NS, D5W, sterile water, bacteriostatic sterile water, or bacteriostatic NS with benzyl alcohol to 20 mg/mL or 10 mg/mL, respectively.
- Further dilute to final concentration NS or D5W to 0.1 mg/mL.

Prednisone: _____ 60-mg/m^2/day PO on days 1– 5.

- Take with breakfast.

Vincristine: _____ 0.4-mg/m^2/day IV continuous infusion on days 1–4

- Maximum dose 2 mg.
- Available in 1 mg/mL 1-, 2-, and 5-mg vials.
- Keep refrigerated.
- **Vesicant**

Doxorubicin: _____ 10 mg/m^2/day continuous infusion on days 1–4

- Available as 2 mg/mL.
- Refrigerated.
- Given as continuous infusion through patent central line. Avoid extravasation.
- Etoposide, vincristine, and doxorubicin can be mixed in same solution for continuous infusion.

Cyclophosphamide: _____ 750-mg/m^2 IV on day 5

- Dilute with sterile water or bacteriostatic water for injection (paraben preserved only); shake well until solution is clear.
- Final concentration 20 mg/mL.
- Further dilute into NS or D5W 250–500 mL.

Bactrim DS: _____1 tablet PO bid, 3 times per week.

Major Side Effects

- Myelosuppression: Dose-limiting toxicity.
- GI Toxicities: Nausea, vomiting, and anorexia; moderately to highly emetogenic. Mucositis, stomatitis, and diarrhea. Constipation and paralytic ileus secondary to autonomic neuropathy.
- Cardiotoxicity: Dose limit 450–550 mg/m^2. Arrhythmias and/or EKG changes, pericarditis, or myocarditis. Usually transient and asymptomatic.
- Steroid Toxicities: Sodium and water retention, cushingoid changes, hyperglycemia, hypokalemia, and increased sodium level. Warfarin and insulin doses may need to be increased. Muscle weakness, loss of muscle mass, osteoporosis, and pathologic fractures with prolonged use. Mood changes, euphoria, headache, insomnia, depression, and psychosis. Cataracts or glaucoma may develop.
- Hpersensitivity Reactions: Characterized by hypotension, bronchospasms, or wheezing may occur with etoposide. More frequent with first dose and faster infusions. May premedicate with dexamethasone, diphenhydramine, and/or cinetidine.
- GU Toxicities: Discoloration of urine from pink to red up to 48 hours. Hemorrhagic cystitis or irritation of bladder wall capillaries; preventable with appropriate hydration.
- Neurotoxicity: Peripheral neuropathy, including numbness, weakness, myalgias, and late severe motor difficulties. Jaw pain.

- Skin Alterations: Total alopecia, hyperpigmentation of nail beds and dermal crease of hands, greatest in dark-skinned individuals. Radiation recall. Sun sensitivity.
- Reproduction: Pregnancy category D. Breast feeding should be avoided. Discuss sperm banking.

Initiate antiemetic protocol: Highly to moderately emetogenic protocol.

Supportive drugs:
☐ G-CSF (Neupogen) _____   ☐ pegfilgrastim (Neulasta)
☐ epoetin alfa (Procrit)/   ☐ Allopurinol_____
darbepoetin alfa (Aranesp)_____
☐ Antibiotic _____   ☐ Antifungal _____

Treatment schedule: Repeat cycle every 21 days.

Estimated number of visits: Four visits in five weeks. Request visits for 3–6 cycles.

Chair time: 1 hour on Monday, Thursday, and Friday during week 1 and nadir. Chair time 4–6 hours day 0; 1–2 hours day 1–4.

Dose Calculation by: 1. _____ 2. _____

_____
Physician

_____
Patient Name

_____
Diagnosis

_____
Date

_____
ID Number

_____/_____/_____
Ht   Wt   M²

Methotrexate, Doxorubicin, Cyclophosphamide, Vincristine, Prednisone, Bleomycin (MACOP-B)

Baseline laboratory tests:	CBC: Chemistry, sedimentation rate, and MUGA
Laboratory tests:	CBC before each treatment
Premedicate:	5-HT$_3$, dexamethasone, and acetaminophen
Administer:	**MTX** _____ 400-mg/m^2 IV on weeks 2, 6, and 10

- 250-mg vial further diluted in NS. Reconstituted solution stable for 24 hours at room temperature. High-dose methotrexate requires leucovorin rescue. Drug interactions include aspirin, penicillins, nonsteroidal anti-inflammatory drugs (NSAIDs), cephalosporins, phenytoin warfarin, 5-fluorouracil, thymidine, folic acid, and omeprazole. Vigorously hydrate; moderate dose of MTX.

Leucovorin: _____ 15-mg/m^2 PO every 6 hours for 6 doses, beginning 24 hours after methotrexate

Doxorubicin: _____ 50-mg/m^2 IV on weeks 1, 3, 5, 7, 9, and 11

- Vesicant
- Available as 2 mg/mL.
- Refrigerated.
- Given IV push through a free-flowing IV or IV infusion through central line.

Cyclophosphamide: _____ 350-mg/m^2 IV on weeks 1, 3, 5, 7, 9, and 11

- Dilute with sterile water or bacteriostatic water for injection (paraben preserved only); shake until solution is clear.
- Final concentration equals 20 mg/mL.
- Further dilute into NS or D5W 250–500 mL.

Vincristine: _____1.4-mg/m^2 IV on weeks 2, 4, 6, 8, 10, and 12

- Maximum dose 2 mg.
- Vesicant
- Available in 1 mg/mL 1-, 2-, and 5-mg vials.
- Keep refrigerated.
- Given IV push through a free-flowing IV.

Prednisone: _____ 75-mg/day PO for 12 weeks; taper over the last 2 weeks

- Take with breakfast.

Bleomycin: _____ 10-units/m^2 IV on weeks 4, 8, and 12

- A test dose of 2 U is recommended before the first dose to detect hypersensitivity.
- Available as a powder in 15- or 30-unit sizes. Dilute powder in NS or sterile water 1–5 cc for the 15-unit vial and 2–10 cc for the 30-unit vial. Should NOT be diluted in D5W.
- Stable for 24 hours when diluted with NS.
- Given IV push or further diluted in NS and infused or pushed over at least 10 minutes. Dilute in NS or sterile water.
- Reduce dose with impaired renal function.

Bactrim DS: _____ 1 tablet PO bid **Ketoconazole:** _____ 200-mg/day PO

Major Side Effects

- Myelosuppression: Dose-limiting toxicity.
- GI Toxicities: Nausea, vomiting, and anorexia; moderately to highly emetogenic. Mucositis and stomatitis can be severe. Constipation and paralytic ileus secondary to autonomic neuropath.
- Cardiotoxicity: Dose limit 450–550 mg/m^2. Arrhythmias and/or EKG changes, pericarditis, or myocarditis. Usually transient and asymptomatic.
- Flulike Syndrome: Fever, chills, sweating, lethargy, myalgias, and arthralgias common.
- GU Toxicities: Discoloration of urine from pink to red up to 48 hours. Hemorrhagic cystitis or irritation of bladder wall capillaries; preventable with appropriate hydration. Acute renal failure, azotemia, urinary retention, and uric acid nephropathy.

- Neurotoxicity: Peripheral neuropathy, including numbness, weakness, myalgias, and late severe motor difficulties. Jaw pain. CNS toxicity with paresthesias, neuropathies, ataxia, lethargy, headache, confusion, and/or seizures.
- Steroid Toxicities: Sodium and water retention, cushingoid changes, hyperglycemia, hypokalemia, and increased sodium level. Warfarin and insulin doses may need to be increased. Muscle weakness, loss of muscle mass, osteoporosis, and pathologic fractures with prolonged use. Mood changes, euphoria, headache, insomnia, depression, and psychosis. Cataracts or glaucoma may develop.
- Pulmonary Toxicity: Pneumonitis in 10% of patients. Risk factors include age > 70, dose > 400 U.
- Skin Alterations: Total alopecia, hyperpigmentation of nail beds and dermal crease of hands, greatest in dark-skinned individuals. Radiation recall. Sun sensitivity.
- Reproduction: Pregnancy category D. Breast feeding should be avoided. Discuss sperm banking.

Initiate antiemetic protocol: Moderately to highly emetogenic protocol.

Supportive drugs:
- ☐ G-CSF _____
- ☐ epoetin alfa (Procrit)/ darbepoetin alfa (Aranesp)_____
- ☐ Antibiotic _____
- ☐ pegfilgrastim (Neulasta)
- ☐ Allopurinol_____
- ☐ Antifungal _____

Treatment schedule: Administer one cycle.

Estimated number of visits: Weekly for 12 weeks.

Chair time: Chair time 2–3 hours.

Dose Calculation by: 1. _____ 2. _____

_____ _____
Physician   Date

_____ _____
Patient Name   ID Number

_____ / _____ / _____
Diagnosis   Ht   Wt   M²

Methotrexate, Bleomycin, Doxorubicin, Cyclophosphamide, Vincristine, Dexamethasone (m-BACOD)

Baseline laboratory tests:	CBC: Chemistry, sedimentation rate, and MUGA
Laboratory tests:	CBC before each treatment
Premedicate:	$5-HT_3$, dexamethasone, and acetaminophen
Administer:	**Methotrexate** _____ 200-mg/m^2 IV on days 8 and 15

- 250-mg vial further diluted in NS.
- Reconstituted solution stable for 24 hours at room temperature.
- High-dose methotrexate requires leucovorin rescue.
- Drug interactions include aspirin, penicillins, NSAIDs, cephalosporins, phenytoin, warfarin, 5-fluorouracil, thymidine, folic acid, and omeprazole. Vigorously hydrate; moderate dose of MTX.

Leucovorin: _____ 10-mg/m^2 PO every 6 hours for 8 doses, beginning 24 hours after methotrexate.

Bleomycin: _____ 4-units/m^2 IV on day 1

- A test dose of 2 U is recommended before the first dose to detect hypersensitivity.
- Available as a powder in 15- or 30-unit sizes. Dilute powder in NS or sterile water 1–5 cc for the 15-unit vial and 2–10 cc for the 30-unit vial. Should NOT be diluted in D5W.
- Stable for 24 hours when diluted with NS.
- Given IV push or further diluted in NS and infused or pushed over at least 10 minutes
- Reduce dose with impaired renal function.

Doxorubicin: _____ 45-mg/m^2 IV on day 1

- **Vesicant**
- Available as 2 mg/mL.
- Refrigerated.
- Given IV push through a free-flowing IV or IV infusion through central line.

Cyclophosphamide: _____ 600-mg/m^2 IV on day 1

- Dilute with sterile water or bacteriostatic water for injection (paraben preserved only); shake until solution is clear.
- Final concentration equals 20 mg/mL.
- Further dilute into NS or D5W 250–500 mL.

Vincristine: _____1-mg/m^2 IV on day 1 (maximum 2 mg)

- Maximum dose 2 mg.
- Vesicant.
- Available in 1-, 2-, and 5-mg vials.
- Keep refrigerated.
- Given IV push through a free-flowing IV.

Dexamethasone: _____ 6-mg/m^2 PO on days 1–5

- Take with breakfast.

Major Side Effects

- Myelosuppression: Dose-limiting toxicity.
- GI Toxicities: Nausea, vomiting, and anorexia; moderately to highly emetogenic. Mucositis and stomatitis can be severe. Constipation and paralytic ileus secondary to autonomic neuropath.
- Cardiotoxicity: Dose limit 450–550 mg/m^2. Arrhythmias and/or EKG changes, pericarditis, or myocarditis. Usually transient and asymptomatic.
- Flulike Syndrome: Fever, chills, sweating, lethargy, myalgias, and arthralgias common.
- GU Toxicities: Discoloration of urine from pink to red up to 48 hours. Hemorrhagic cystitis or irritation of bladder wall capillaries; preventable with appropriate hydration. Acute renal failure, azotemia, urinary retention, and uric acid nephropathy.
- Neurotoxicity: Peripheral neuropathy, including numbness, weakness, myalgias, and late severe motor difficulties. Jaw pain. CNS toxicity with paresthesias, neuropathies, ataxia, lethargy, headache, confusion, and/or seizures.

- Steroid Toxicities: Sodium and water retention, cushingoid changes, hyperglycemia, hypokalemia, and increased sodium level. Warfarin and insulin doses may need to be increased. Muscle weakness, loss of muscle mass, osteoporosis, and pathologic fractures with prolonged use. Mood changes, euphoria, headache, insomnia, depression, and psychosis. Cataracts or glaucoma may develop.

- Pulmonary Toxicity: Pneumonitis in 10% of patients. Risk factors include age > 70, dose > 400 U.

- Skin Alterations: Total alopecia, hyperpigmentation of nail beds and dermal crease of hands, greatest in dark-skinned individuals. Radiation recall. Sun sensitivity.

- Reproduction: Pregnancy category D. Breast feeding should be avoided. Discuss sperm banking.

Initiate antiemetic protocol:	Highly to moderately emetogenic protocol.
Supportive drugs:	☐ G-CSF (Neupogen)_____ ☐ pegfilgrastim (Neulasta)
	☐ epoetin alfa (Procrit)/ ☐ Allopurinol_____
	darbepoetin alfa (Aranesp)_____
	☐ Antibiotic _____ ☐ Antifungal _____
Treatment schedule:	Repeat cycle every 21 days.
Estimated number of visits:	Three visits per cycle.
Chair time:	Chair time 2–3 hours on day 1, and 1 hour on days 8 and 15.

Dose Calculation by: 1. _____   2. _____

_____

Physician   Date

_____

Patient Name   ID Number

_____

Diagnosis   Ht _____/ Wt _____/ M²

ProMACE/CytaBOM

Baseline laboratory tests:	CBC: Chemistry, sedimentation rate, and MUGA
Laboratory tests:	CBC: Chemistry, RFTs, and LFTs before each treatment
Premedicate:	5-HT$_3$, dexamethasone
Administer:	

Prednisone: _____ 60-mg/m^2/day PO on days 1–14

- Take with breakfast.

Doxorubicin: _____ 25-mg/m^2 IV on day 1

- Available as 2 mg/mL.
- Refrigerated.
- Given IV push through a free-flowing IV.

Cyclophosphamide: _____ 650-mg/m^2 IV on day 1

- Dilute with sterile water or bacteriostatic water for injection (paraben preserved only); shake well until solution is clear.
- Final concentration equals 20 mg/mL.
- Further dilute into NS or D5W 250–500 mL.

Etoposide _____ 120-mg/m^2/d IV on day 1

- 5 cc/100 mg, 20 mg/mL.
- Etoposide reconstitute with 5–10 mL of NS, D5W, sterile water, bacteriostatic sterile water, or bacteriostatic NS with benzyl alcohol to 20 mg/mL or 10 mg/mL, respectively.
- Further dilute to final concentration NS or D5W to 0.1 mg/mL.

Cytarabine _____ 300-mg/m^2/day IV on day 8

- Dilute in sterile water with benzyl alcohol, then further dilute with 50–100 mL of 0.9% sodium chloride or D5W.
- IV hydration at 150 mL per hour with or without alkalinization, oral allopurinol, strict intake and output recording, and daily weights.
- Stable 48 hours at room temperature and 7 days refrigerated.

Bleomycin: _____ 5-units/m^2 IV push day 8.

- A test dose of 2 U is recommended before the first dose to detect hypersensitivity.
- Available as a powder in 15- or 30-unit sizes. Dilute powder in NS or sterile water 1–5 cc for the 15-unit vial and 2–10 cc for the 30-unit vial. Should NOT be diluted in D5W.
- Stable for 24 hours when diluted with NS.
- Given IV push or further diluted in NS and infused or pushed over at least 10 minutes.
- Reduce dose with impaired renal function.

Vincristine: _____ 1.4-mg/m^2/day IV continuous infusion on days 1–4

- Maximum dose, 2 mg.
- Available in 1-, 2-, and 5-mg vials.
- Keep refrigerated.
- **Vesicant**

Methotrexate _____ 120-mg/m^2 IV on day 8

- A 250-mg vial further diluted in NS.
- Reconstituted solution stable for 24 hours at room temperature.
- High-dose methotrexate requires leucovorin rescue. Drug interactions include aspirin, penicillins, NSAIDs, cephalosporins, phenytoin, warfarin, 5-fluorouracil, thymidine, folic acid, and omeprazole.

Leucovorin _____ 25-mg/m^2 PO every 6 hours for six doses, beginning 24 hours after methotrexate

Major Side Effects

- Myelosuppression: Dose-limiting toxicity.
- GI Toxicities: Nausea, vomiting, and anorexia; moderately to highly emetogenic. Mucositis, stomatitis, and diarrhea. Constipation and paralytic ileus secondary to autonomic neuropathy.

- Cardiotoxicity: Dose limit 450–550 mg/m^2. Arrhythmias and/or EKG changes, pericarditis, or myocarditis. Usually transient and asymptomatic.
- Steroid Toxicities: Sodium and water retention, cushingoid changes, hyperglycemia, hypokalemia, and increased sodium level. Warfarin and insulin doses may need to be increased. Muscle weakness, loss of muscle mass, osteoporosis, and pathologic fractures with prolonged use. Mood changes, euphoria, headache, insomnia, depression, and psychosis. Cataracts or glaucoma may develop.
- Hypersensitivity Reactions: Characterized by hypotension, bronchospasms, or wheezing may occur with etoposide.
- GU Toxicities: Discoloration of urine from pink to red up to 48 hours. Hemorrhagic cystitis or irritation of bladder wall capillaries; preventable with appropriate hydration.
- Neurotoxicity: Peripheral neuropathy, including numbness, weakness, myalgias, and late severe motor difficulties. Jaw pain. At high doses, cerebellar toxicity, including nystagmus, dysarthria, ataxia, slurred speech, difficulty with fine motor coordination, lethargy, or somnolence. Patients with rapidly rising creatinine level due to tumor lysis syndrome or neurotoxicity should discontinue the high-dose cytarabine.
- Tumor lysis syndrome occurring 1–5 days after initiation of treatment; treat with hydration and allopurinol.
- Skin Alterations: Total alopecia, hyperpigmentation of nail beds and dermal crease of hands, greatest in dark-skinned individuals. Radiation recall. Sun sensitivity.
- Reproduction: Pregnancy category D. Breast feeding should be avoided. Discuss sperm banking.

Initiate antiemetic protocol:	Moderately to highly emetogenic protocol.
Supportive drugs:	☐ G-CSF (Neupogen)_____ ☐ pegfilgrastim (Neulasta)
	☐ epoetin alfa (Procrit)/ ☐ Allopurinol_____
	darbepoetin alfa (Aranesp)_____
	☐ Antibiotic _____ ☐ Antifungal _____
Treatment schedule:	Repeat cycle every 21 days.
Estimated number of visits:	Four visits per cycle. Request 4–6 cycles worth of visits.
Chair time:	Three hours day 1 and 3 hours day 8.

Dose Calculation by: 1. _____   2. _____

_____   _____
Physician   Date

_____   _____
Patient Name   ID Number

_____   _____/_____/_____
Diagnosis   Ht   Wt   M^2

HIGH-GRADE

Magrath Protocol (Burkitt's Lymphoma)

Baseline laboratory tests:	CBC: Chemistry, sedimentation rate, MUGA, Ommaya reservoir placement vs lumbar puncture every cycle.
Laboratory tests:	CBC: Chemistry, RFTs, and LFTs before each treatment
Premedicate:	5-HT$_3$, dexamethasone, and acetaminophen
Administer:	**Cyclophosphamide:** _____ 1200-mg/m^2 IV on day 1

- Dilute with sterile water or bacteriostatic water for injection (paraben preserved only); shake well until solution is clear.
- Final concentration equals 20 mg/mL.
- Further dilute into NS or D5W 250–500 mL.

Doxorubicin: _____ 40-mg/m^2 IV on day 1

- Vesicant
- Available as 2 mg/mL.
- Refrigerated.
- Given IV push through a free-flowing IV.

Vincristine: _____1.4-mg/m^2 IV on day 1 (maximum dose 2 mg)

- **Vesicant**
- Available in 1-, 2-, and 5-mg vials.
- Keep refrigerated.
- IV push through a free-flowing IV.

Prednisone: _____ 40-mg/m^2 PO on days 1–5

- Take with breakfast.

Methotrexate _____ 300-mg/m^2 IV on day 10 for 1 hour and then

Methotrexate _____ 60-mg/m^2 on days 10 and 11 for 41 hours

- 250-mg vial further diluted in NS.
- Reconstituted solution stable for 24 hours at room temperature.
- High-dose methotrexate requires leucovorin rescue and adequate hydration.
- Drug interactions include aspirin, penicillins, NSAIDs, cephalosporins, phenytoin, warfarin, 5-fluorouracil, thymidine, folic acid, and omeprazole.

Leucovorin rescue _____ 15-mg/m^2 IV over 15 minutes every 6 hours for 8 doses starting 24 hours after methotrexate on day 12

- Reconstitute vials with sterile water and further with NS or D5W.

Intrathecal cytarabine_____ 30-mg/m^2 IT on day 7, cycle 1 only; _____ 45-mg/m^2 IT on day 7 all subsequent cycles

- Use **preservative-free NS** to dilute. **Must use immediately after reconstitution**. Discard unused drug.
- Available in 100-mg vials.

Intrathecal methotrexate _____ 12.5-mg IT on day 10, all cycles

- Use **preservative-free NS** to dilute. **Must use immediately after reconstitution**. Discard unused drug.
- Available in 50-mg and 250-preservative free vials.

Major Side Effects

- Myelosuppression: Dose-limiting toxicity.
- GI Toxicities: Nausea, vomiting, and anorexia; moderately to highly emetogenic. Mucositis and stomatitis. Constipation and paralytic ileus secondary to autonomic neuropathy. Diarrhea is common and an indication to interrupt therapy of methotrexate. Transient increases in LFTs can be seen with methotrexate.
- Cardiotoxicity: Dose limit 450–550 mg/m^2. Arrhythmias and/or EKG changes, pericarditis, or myocarditis. Usually transient and asymptomatic.

- GU Toxicities: Discoloration of urine from pink to red up to 48 hours. Hemorrhagic cystitis or irritation of bladder wall capillaries; preventable with appropriate hydration. Monitor BUN and creatinine levels because methotrexate can precipitate in renal tubules, resulting in acute tubular necrosis.

- Neurotoxicity: Peripheral neuropathy with vincristine, including numbness, weakness, myalgias, and late severe motor difficulties. Jaw pain. CNS toxicity with paresthesias, neuropathies, dizziness, blurred vision, ataxia, lethargy, headache, confusion, and/or seizures. Intrathecal chemotherapy can increase cerebrospinal fluid pressure.

- Steroid Toxicities: Sodium and water retention, cushingoid changes, hyperglycemia, hypokalemia, and increased sodium level. Warfarin and insulin doses may need to be increased; muscle weakness, loss of muscle mass, osteoporosis, and pathologic fractures with prolonged use. Mood changes, euphoria, headache, insomnia, depression, and psychosis. Cataracts or glaucoma may develop.

- Skin Alterations: Total alopecia, hyperpigmentation of nail beds and dermal crease of hands, greatest in dark-skinned individuals. Radiation recall. Photosensitivity.

- Tumor lysis syndrome occurring 1–5 days after initiation of treatment; treat with hydration and allopurinol.

- SIADH: May occur with high-dose cyclophosphamide. Monitor serum Na^+ level, intake and output, and daily weights.

- Reproduction: Pregnancy category D. Breast feeding should be avoided.

Initiate antiemetic protocol: Moderately to highly emetogenic protocol.

Supportive drugs:
☐ G-CSF (Neupogen)_____   ☐ pegfilgrastim (Neulasta)
☐ epoetin alfa (Procrit)/   ☐ Allopurinol_____
  darbepoetin alfa (Aranesp)_____
☐ Antibiotic _____   ☐ Antifungal _____

Treatment schedule: Repeat cycle every 28 days.
Estimated number of visits: Five visits every 3 weeks.
Chair time: Chair time 2–3 hours. 2 hours day 1; 2 hours day 10; 1 hour day 7.

Dose Calculation by: 1. _____ 2. _____

_____
Physician   Date

_____
Patient Name   ID Number

_____
Diagnosis   Ht _____/ Wt _____/ M^2 _____

Cyclophosphamide + Doxorubicin + Vincristine + Methotrexate + Leucovorin (Regimen A-CODOX-M) (Small Non-Cleaved and Burkitt's Lymphoma)

Baseline laboratory tests: CBC: Chemistry, sedimentation rate, MUGA, Ommaya reservoir placement vs lumbar puncture each cycle.

Laboratory tests: CBC: Chemistry, RFTs, and LFTs before each treatment

Premedicate: 5-HT$_3$ and dexamethasone IV

Administer:

Cyclophosphamide: _____ 800-mg/m^2 IV on day 1

Cyclophosphamide _____ 200-mg/m^2 IV on days 2–5

- Dilute with sterile water or bacteriostatic water for injection (paraben preserved only); shake well until solution is clear.
- Final concentration equals 20 mg/mL.
- Further dilute into NS or D5W 250–500 mL.

Doxorubicin: _____ 40-mg/m^2 IV on day 1

- **Vesicant**
- Available as 2 mg/mL.
- Refrigerated.
- Given IV push through a free-flowing IV.

Vincristine: _____ 1.5-mg/m^2 IV push through free-flowing IV on days 1 and 8 in cycle 1; days 1, 8, and 15 in cycle 3. Maximum dose 2 mg.

- **Vesicant**
- Available in 1 mg/mL 1-, 2-, and 5-mg vials.
- Keep refrigerated.

Methotrexate _____ 1200-mg/m^2 IV over 1 hour on day 10, followed by

Methotrexate _____ 240-mg/m^2/hour for the next 23 hours on day 10

- 250-mg vial further diluted in NS.
- Reconstituted solution stable for 24 hours at room temperature.
- High-dose methotrexate requires leucovorin rescue and adequate hydration.
- Drug interactions include aspirin, penicillins, NSAIDs, cephalosporins, phenytoin; warfarin, 5-fluorouracil, thymidine, folic acid, and omeprazole.

Leucovorin rescue _____ 192-mg/m^2 IV on day 11, starting 36 hours after the start of the methotrexate infusion

Leucovorin _____ 12-mg/m^2 IV every 6 hours until serum MTX levels < 50 nM

- Reconstitute vials with sterile water and further with NS or D$_5$W.

CNS Prophylaxis

Intrathecal cytarabine _____ 70-mg/m^2 IT on days 1 and 3

- Use **preservative-free NS** to dilute. **Must use immediately after reconstitution.**
- Discard unused drug.
- Available in 100-mg vials.

Intrathecal methotrexate _____ 12-mg IT on day 15

- Use **preservative-free NS** to dilute. **Must use immediately after reconstitution.**
- Discard unused drug.
- Available in 50- and 250-mg preservative-free vials.

Major Side Effects

- Myelosuppression: Dose-limiting toxicity.
- GI Toxicities: Nausea, vomiting, and anorexia; moderately to highly emetogenic. Mucositis and stomatitis. Constipation and paralytic ileus secondary to autonomic neuropathy. Diarrhea is common and an indication to interrupt therapy of methotrexate. Transient increases in LFTs can be seen with methotrexate.
- Cardiotoxicity: Dose limit 450–550 mg/m^2. Arrhythmias and/or EKG changes, pericarditis, or myocarditis. Usually transient and asymptomatic.

- GU Toxicities: Discoloration of urine from pink to red up to 48 hours. Hemorrhagic cystitis or irritation of bladder wall capillaries; preventable with appropriate hydration. Monitor BUN and creatinine levels because methotrexate can precipitate in renal tubules, resulting in acute tubular necrosis. Hemorrhagic cystitis, hematuria, frequency preventable with uroprotection and hydration of 2–3 L per day. Monitor BUN and serum creatinine levels.

- Neurotoxicity: Peripheral neuropathy with vincristine, including numbness, weakness, myalgias, and late severe motor difficulties. Jaw pain. CNS toxicity with paresthesias, neuropathies, dizziness, blurred vision, ataxia, lethargy, headache, confusion, and/or seizures. Intrathecal chemotherapy can increase cerebrospinal fluid pressure.

- Skin Alterations: Total alopecia, hyperpigmentation of nail beds and dermal crease of hands, greatest in dark-skinned individuals. Radiation recall. Photosensitivity.

- Tumor lysis syndrome occurring 1–5 days after initiation of treatment; treat with hydration and allopurinol.

- SIADH: May occur with high-dose cyclophosphamide. Monitor serum Na$^+$, intake and output, and daily weights.

- Reproduction: Pregnancy category D. Breast feeding should be avoided.

Alternate with
Ifosfamide, Etoposide, Cytarabine (Regimen B-IVAC)

Administer:

Ifosfamide _____1500-mg/m^2 IV on days 1–5

- Available in 1- and 3-g vials.
- Reconstitute with sterile water.
- Further dilute to concentrations of 6–20 mg/mL in D5W or NS.
- Stable for 24 hours refrigerated.
- Phenobarbital, phenytoin, cimetidine, and allopurinol increase toxicity.
- Ifosfamide may enhance anticoagulant effects of warfarin.

Etoposide _____ 60-mg/m^2/d IV over 1–2 hours on days 1–5

- VePesid 5 cc/100 mg; reconstitute etopophos with 5–10 mL of NS, D5W, sterile water, bacteriostatic sterile water, or bacteriostatic NS with benzyl alcohol to 20 mg/mL or 10 mg/mL, respectively. Further dilute to final concentration NS or D5W to 0.1 mg/mL. Stability is dose concentration dependent from 8–96 hours.

Cytarabine _____ 2-g/m^2/day IV over 2 hours q 12 hours on days 1 and 2 for a total of four doses

- Dilute in sterile water with benzyl alcohol, then further dilute with 50–100 mL of 0.9% sodium chloride or D5W.
- Stable 48 hours at room temperature and 7 days refrigerated.
- IV hydration at 150/mL per hour with or without alkalinization, oral allopurinol, strict intake and output, and daily weights.

Methotrexate _____ 12-mg IT on day 5

- 250-mg vial further diluted in NS.
- Reconstituted solution stable for 24 hours at room temperature.
- High-dose methotrexate requires leucovorin rescue and adequate hydration.
- Drug interactions include aspirin, penicillins, NSAIDs, cephalosporins, phenytoin; warfarin, 5-fluorouracil, thymidine, folic acid, and omeprazole.

Major Side Effects

- Myelosuppression: Dose-limiting toxicity.
- GI Toxicities: Nausea, vomiting, and anorexia; moderately to highly emetogenic. Mucositis and stomatitis. Constipation and paralytic ileus secondary to autonomic neuropathy. Diarrhea is common and an indication to interrupt therapy of methotrexate. Transient increases in LFTs can be seen with methotrexate.
- Nephrotoxicity: Patients with renal dysfunction are at risk. Monitor electrolyte, BUN, and creatinine values.

- Cerebellar Toxicity: High doses of cytarabine can result in cerebellar toxicity, including nystagmus, dysarthria, ataxia, slurred speech, difficulty with fine motor coordination, lethargy, or somnolence. Assess baseline neurologic status and cerebellar function (coordinated movements, such as handwriting and gait) before and during therapy. If cerebellar toxicity develops, treatment must be discontinued.

- Skin Alterations: Alopecia with total hair loss. Sterile phlebitis may occur at injection site. Hyperpigmentation, dermatitis, and nail ridging may occur. Total alopecia.

- Sensory/perceptual alterations: Lethargy and confusion at high doses of ifosfamide, usually lasting 1–8 hours; reversible.

- Reproduction: Pregnancy category D. Breast feeding should be avoided.

Initiate antiemetic protocol: Moderately to highly emetogenic protocol.

Supportive drugs:

☐ G-CSF (Neupogen)_____   ☐ pegfilgrastim (Neulasta)

☐ epoetin alfa (Procrit)/   ☐ Allopurinol_____
darbepoetin alfa (Aranesp)_____

☐ Antibiotic _____   ☐ Antifungal _____

Treatment schedule:

Regimen A–3 hours day 1 and 8; 1 hour day 2–5 and day 15.

Regimen B–3 hours day 1 and 2; 1 hour day 5.

Alternate Regimen A with Regimen B for 4 cycles.

Estimated number of visits: Requests 15–20 visits per cycle. May need hospitalization for every 12-hour treatment.

Dose Calculation by: 1. _____   2. _____

_____   _____
Physician   Date

_____   _____
Patient Name   ID Number

_____   _____/_____   _____/_____   _____
Diagnosis   Ht   Wt   M²

Stanford Regimen (Small Non-Cleaved Cell and Burkitt's Lymphoma)

Baseline laboratory tests:	CBC: Chemistry, sedimentation rate, MUGA
Laboratory tests:	CBC: Chemistry, RFTs, and LFTs before each treatment
Premedicate:	5-HT$_3$, dexamethasone
Administer:	**Cyclophosphamide:** _____ 1200-mg/m^2 IV on day 1

- Dilute with sterile water or bacteriostatic water for injection (paraben preserved only); shake well until solution is clear.
- Final concentration equals 20 mg/mL.
- Further dilute into NS or D5W 250–500 mL.

Doxorubicin: _____ 40-mg/m^2 IV on day 1

- Available as 2 mg/mL.
- Refrigerated.
- Given IV push through a free-flowing IV

Vincristine: _____1.4-mg/m^2 IV on day 1 (maximum dose 2 mg)

- Available in 1-, 2-, and 5-mg vials.
- Keep refrigerated.
- **Vesicant**.
- Given IV push through a free-flowing IV.

Prednisone: _____ 40-mg/m^2 PO on days 1–5

- Take with breakfast.

Methotrexate _____ 3000-mg/m^2 IV over 6-hour day on day 10

- 250-mg vial further diluted in NS.
- Reconstituted solution stable for 24 hours at room temperature.
- High-dose methotrexate requires leucovorin rescue and adequate hydration.
- Drug interactions include aspirin, penicillins, NSAIDs, cephalosporins, phenytoin, warfarin, 5-fluorouracil, thymidine, folic acid, and omeprazole.

Leucovorin _____ 25-mg/m^2 IV or PO every 6 hours for 12 doses beginning 24 hours after methotrexate

- Reconstitute vials with sterile water and further with NS or D5W.

Intrathecal methotrexate _____ 12-mg IT on days 1 and 10.

- Use **preservative-free** NS to dilute. **Must use immediately after reconstitution**.
- Discard unused drug.
- Available in 50- and 250-mg preservative-free vials.

Major Side Effects

- Myelosuppression: May be severe. Teach self-care measures to minimize risk of infection and bleeding.
- GI Toxicities: Nausea, vomiting, and anorexia; moderately to highly emetogenic. Mucositis and stomatitis. Constipation and paralytic ileus secondary to autonomic neuropathy.
- Chemical Arachnoidits: Severe headaches, mochal rigidity, seizures, vomiting, fever, and an inflammatory cell infiltrate in the CSF.
- Cerebral Dysfunction: Paresis, aphasia, behavioral abnormality, and seizures with high dose methotrexate. Occurs within 6 days of treatment. Resolves within 48–72 hours.
- Cardiotoxicity: Dose limit 450–550 mg/m^2. Arrhythmias and/or EKG changes, pericarditis, or myocarditis. Usually transient and asymptomatic.
- GU Toxicities: Discoloration of urine from pink to red up to 48 hours. Adequate hydration and leucovorin rescue for high-dose methotrexate to prevent acute renal tubular necrosis.
- Neurotoxicity: Peripheral neuropathy, including numbness, weakness, myalgias, and late severe motor difficulties. Jaw pain.
- Skin Alterations: Total alopecia, hyperpigmentation of nail beds and dermal crease of hands, greatest in dark-skinned individuals. Radiation recall. Sun sensitivity.

> • Reproduction: Pregnancy category D. Breastfeeding should be avoided. Discuss sperm banking.

Initiate antiemetic protocol:	Moderately to highly emetogenic protocol.
Supportive drugs:	☐ G-CSF _____ ☐ pegfilgrastim (Neulasta)
	☐ epoetin alfa (Procrit)/ ☐ Allopurinol_____
	darbepoetin alfa (Aranesp)_____
	☐ Antibiotic _____ ☐ Antifungal _____
Treatment schedule:	Repeat cycle every 21 days for three cycles.
Estimated number of visits:	Weekly chemotherapy, 16 visits.
Chair time:	Chair time of 2–3 hours.

Dose Calculation by: 1. _____   2. _____

_____

Physician   Date

_____

Patient Name   ID Number

_____   _____/_____/_____

Diagnosis   Ht   Wt   M^2

MANTLE CELL LYMPHOMA

Bortezomib (Velcade)

Baseline laboratory tests:	CBC: Chemistry, renal and liver functions
Baseline procedures or tests:	Bone marrow biopsy
Premedicate:	5-HT$_3$ and dexamethasone
Administer:	**Bortezomib** _____ 1.5-mg/m^2 IV push, followed by saline flush on days 1, 4, 8, and 11; followed by a 10-day rest period.

- Dilute powder in 3.5 mL of NS. Reconstituted product should be clear.
- Stable for 8 hours at room temperature.

Major Side Effects

- Myelosuppression: Neutropenia and thrombocytopenia.
- GI Toxicities: Nausea and vomiting, anorexia, constipation, and dehydration.
- Orthostatic hypotension.
- Fatigue: Fatigue, malaise, and generalized weakness.
- Peripheral Neuropathy: Mix of sensorimotor neuropathy. May improve and/or return to baseline with discontinuation of drug.
- Steroid Toxicities: Sodium and water retention, cushingoid changes, and behavioral changes, including emotional lability, insomnia, mood swings, and euphoria. May increase glucose and sodium levels, decrease potassium level, and affect warfarin dose.
- Musculoskeletal Changes: Muscle weakness, loss of muscle mass, osteoporosis, and pathologic fractures with prolonged use.
- Perceptual Alterations: Cataracts or glaucoma may develop.
- Reproduction: Pregnancy category D. Breast feeding should be avoided.

Initiate antiemetic protocol:	Moderately emetogenic protocol.
Supportive drugs:	☐ pegfilgrastim (Neulasta)_____ ☐ filgrastim (Neupogen) _____
	☐ epoetin alfa (Procrit)/ darbepoetin alfa (Aranesp) _____ ☐ Allopurinol_____
	☐ Antibiotic _____ ☐ Antifungal _____
Treatment schedule:	Repeat cycle every 21 days.
Chair time:	1 hour
Estimated number of visits:	Five to 6 days per cycle.

Dose Calculation by: 1. _____ 2. _____

_____
Physician

_____
Patient Name

_____
Diagnosis

_____
Date

_____
ID Number

_____/ _____/ _____
Ht   Wt   M^2

CD20$^+$, B-CELL LYMPHOMAS

CHOP + Rituxan (Rituximab)–Monoclonal Antibody (GELA Study)

Baseline laboratory tests:	CBC: Chemistry, sedimentation rate
Initiate IV:	Draw blood before each chemotherapy administration: CBC
Premedication:	5-HT$_3$ and dexamethasone

Tylenol 1000-mg PO 30 minutes and

Diphenhydramine 50 mg in 150 cc of NS over 30 minutes (or PO), may use
Cimetidine 300 mg in 100 cc NS to help reduce infusion reactions. Especially within first
treatment of Rituxan.

Administer:

Rituxan: _____ 375-mg/m^2 IV infusion on day 1

- Available in 500-mg/50-mL and 100-mg/10-mL vials. Further dilute in NS to make final concentration of 1 or 4 mg/1 mL.
- Stable for 24 hours at room temperature and an additional 24 hours refrigerated.
- Discard unused portion.
- Use infusion pump and blood pressure monitor.

First infusion: Initial rate of 50 mg/hr. Increase infusion rate in 50-mg/hr increments every 30 minutes to a maximum rate of 400 mg/hr.

- If a hypersensitivity-related event develops, the infusion should be temporarily slowed or interrupted.
- Resume infusion at 50% of previous rate after symptoms subside. May give additional cortisteroids or diphenhydramine to reduce hypersensitivity reactions.
- Monitor vital signs every 10 minutes for the first hour and then every 30 minutes thereafter.

Subsequent infusions: Initial rate of 100 mg/hr. Increase rate by 100 mg/hr every 30 minutes to a maximum rate of 400 mg/hr as tolerated. Do NOT give IV push.

Cyclophosphamide: _____ 750-mg/m^2 IV over 1 hour on day 1

- Dilute with sterile water or bacteriostatic water for injection (paraben preserved only); shake well until solution is clear.
- Final concentration equals 20 mg/mL.
- Further dilute into NS or D5W 250–500 mL.

Doxorubicin: _____ 50-mg/m^2 IV on day 1

- Vesicant
- Available as 2 mg/mL. Refrigerated. Given IV push through a free-flowing IV.

Vincristine: _____ 1.4-mg/m^2 IV push on day 1 (maximum dose 2 mg)

- Vesicant
- Available in 1-, 2-, and 5-mg vial.
- Refrigerated.
- Given IV push through a free-flowing IV.

Prednisone: _____ 40-mg PO on days 1 through 5 and then taper to 0

- Take with breakfast.

Supportive drugs:

☐ pegfilgrastim (Neulasta)_____   ☐ filgrastim (Neupogen) _____

☐ epoetin alfa (Procrit)/   ☐ Allopurinol_____
   darbepoetin alfa (Aranesp) _____

☐ Antibiotic _____   ☐ Antifungal _____

Major Side Effects

- Myelosuppression: Moderate to severe. Potential for infection with B-lymphocytes reduced, resulting in bacterial infections not related to neutropenia.
- GI Toxicities: Nausea and vomiting, anorexia; mucositis, diarrhea.
- GU Toxicities: Discoloration of urine from pink to red up to 48 hours. Hemorrhagic cystitis or irritation of bladder wall capillaries; preventable with appropriate hydration.

- Neurotoxicity: Peripheral neuropathy, including numbness, weakness, myalgias, and late severe motor difficulties. Jaw pain.

- Steroid Toxicities: Sodium and water retention, cushingoid changes, hyperglycemia, hypokalemia, and increased sodium level. Warfarin and insulin doses may need to be increased. Muscle weakness, loss of muscle mass, osteoporosis, and pathologic fractures with prolonged use. Mood changes, euphoria, headache, insomnia, depression, and psychosis. Cataracts or glaucoma may develop.

- Hypersensitivity Reactions: Infusion-related reactions occur within 30 minutes to 2 hours after the beginning of the first infusion. Fever, chills, and rigors most common. Bronchospasm, dyspnea, pruritus, hypotension, back pain, and angioedema may also be seen. Will resolve when the infusion is stopped and/or symptomatic treatment (acetaminophen, diphenhydramine, and IV NS) is given. Have emergency hypersensitivity/anaphylaxis medications available (e.g., epinephrine, antihistamines, bronchodilators, and corticosteroids).

- Skin Reactions: Rare and include paraneoplastic pemphigus, Stevens-Johnson syndrome, lichenoid dermatitis, vesiculobullous dermatitis, and toxic epidermal necrolysis. Drug therapy should be discontinued, and skin biopsy should be obtained to determine cause.

- Tumor lysis syndrome: Patients with high tumor burden or high white blood cell count at risk. Occurs in first 5 days after infusion. Treat/prevent with hydration and allopurinol.

- Reproduction: Pregnancy category D. Breast feeding should be avoided. Discuss contraception and sperm banking.

Treatment schedule: Repeat cycle every 21 days. Rituximab is to be administered first, followed by cyclophosphamide, doxorubicin, and vincristine.

Estimated number of visits: Two visits per cycle. Request 4–6 worth of visits.

Chair time: First cycle 6–8 hours, 2nd cycle 4–6 hours.

Dose Calculation by: 1. _____ 2. _____

_____

Physician

_____

Patient Name

_____

Diagnosis

Date _____

ID Number _____

_____/_____/_____
Ht   Wt   M²

CHOP + Rituxan (Rituximab)–Monoclonal Antibody (Vose or Nebraska Regimen)

Baseline laboratory tests: CBC: Chemistry and sedimentation rate

Initiate IV: Draw blood before each chemotherapy administration: CBC

Premedication: 5-HT$_3$ and dexamethasone (for nausea and may be used to prevent or treat infusion-related reactions)

Tylenol 1000-mg PO 30 minutes and

Diphenhydramine 50-mg in 150 cc of NS over 30 minutes (or PO) may use

Cimetidine 300 mg in 100cc NS to help reduce infusion reactions. Especially within first treatment of Rituxan.

Administer: **Rituxan:** _____ 375-mg/m^2 IV infusion on day 1

- Available in 500-mg/50 mL and 100-mg/10-mL vials. Further dilute in NS to make final concentration of 1 or 4 mg/1 mL.
- Stable for 24 hours at room temperature and an additional 24 hours refrigerated.
- Discard unused portion.
- Use infusion pump and blood pressure monitor.

First infusion: Initial rate of 50 mg/hr. Increase infusion rate in 50-mg/hr increments every 30 minutes to a maximum rate of 400 mg/hr.

- If a hypersensitivity-related event develops, the infusion should be temporarily slowed or interrupted. May give additional corticosteroids and/or diphenhydramine to help alleviate hypersentivity reactions.
- Resume infusion at 50% of previous rate after symptoms subside.
- Monitor vital signs every 10 minutes for the first hour and then every 30 minutes thereafter.

Subsequent infusions: Initial rate of 100 mg/hr. Increase rate by 100 mg/hr every 30 minutes to a maximum rate of 400 mg/hr as tolerated. Do NOT give IV push.

Cyclophosphamide: _____ 750-mg/m^2 IV over 1 hour on day 3

- Dilute with sterile water or bacteriostatic water for injection (paraben preserved only); shake well until solution is clear.
- Final concentration 20 mg/mL.
- Further dilute into NS or D5W 250–500 mL.

Doxorubicin: _____ 50-mg/m^2 IV on day 3

- **Vesicant**
- Available as 2 mg/mL.
- Refrigerated.
- Given IV push through a free-flowing IV.

Vincristine: _____1.4 mg/m^2 IV push on day 3 (maximum dose 2 mg)

- **Vesicant.**
- Available in 1-, 2-, and 5-mg vial.
- Refrigerated.
- Given IV push through a free-flowing IV.

Prednisone: _____ 100-mg PO on days 3–7; then taper to 0

- Take with breakfast.

Supportive drugs: □ pegfilgrastim (Neulasta)_____ □ filgrastim (Neupogen) _____

□ epoetin alfa (Procrit)/ □ Allopurinol_____
darbepoetin alfa (Aranesp) _____

□ Antibiotic _____ □ Antifungal _____

Major Side Effects
- Myelosuppression: Moderate to severe. Potential for infection with B-lymphocytes reduced, resulting in bacterial infections not related to neutropenia.
- GI Toxicities: Nausea and vomiting, anorexia; mucositis, diarrhea.
- GU Toxicities: Discoloration of urine from pink to red up to 48 hours. Hemorrhagic cystitis or irritation of bladder wall capillaries; preventable with appropriate hydration.

- Neurotoxicity: Peripheral neuropathy, including numbness, weakness, myalgias, and late severe motor difficulties. Jaw pain.
- Steroid Toxicities: Sodium and water retention, cushingoid changes, hyperglycemia, hypokalemia, and increased sodium level. Warfarin and insulin doses may need to be increased. Muscle weakness, loss of muscle mass, osteoporosis, and pathologic fractures with prolonged use. Mood changes, euphoria, headache, insomnia, depression, and psychosis. Cataracts or glaucoma may develop.
- Hypersensitivity Reactions: Infusion-related reactions occur within 30 minutes to 2 hours of the beginning of the first infusion. Fever, chills, and rigors most common. Bronchospasm, dyspnea, pruritus, hypotension, back pain, and angiodema may also be seen. Will resolve when the infusion is stopped and/or symptomatic treatment (acetaminophen, diphenhydramine, and IV saline) is given. Have emergency hypersensitivity/anaphylaxis medications available (e.g., epinephrine, antihistamines, bronchodilators, and corticosteroids).
- Skin Reactions: Rare and include paraneoplastic pemphigus, Stevens-Johnson syndrome, lichenoid dermatitis, vesiculobullous dermatitis, and toxic epidermal necrolysis. Drug therapy should be discontinued and skin biopsy should be obtained to determine cause.
- Tumor lysis syndrome: Patients with high tumor burden or high white blood cell count at risk. Occurs in first 5 days after infusion. Treat/prevent with hydration and allopurinol.
- Reproduction: Pregnancy category D. Breast feeding should be avoided. Discuss contraception and sperm banking.

Treatment schedule: Repeat cycle every 21 days. Rituximab is to be administered first, followed by cyclophosphamide, doxorubicin, and vincristine.

Estimated number of visits: Two visits per cycle. Request 4–6 worth of visits.

Chair time: Six to 8 hours day 1; 2–3 hours day 3; 4–6 hours day 1 cycles 2–6.

Dose Calculation by: 1. _____ 2. _____

_____

Physician   Date

_____

Patient Name   ID Number

_____

Diagnosis   Ht _____ / Wt _____ / M²

Salvage Regimens

Etoposide (VP-16), Cytarabine, Cisplatin (ESHAP)

Baseline laboratory tests:	CBC: Chemistry, sedimentation rate, and Mg
Perform laboratory tests monthly:	CBC: Chemistry, Mg^{2+} (Draw CBC: Chemistry, Mg^{2+} at nadir, 10 days) Access central venous catheter.
Premedicate:	5-HT_3 and dexamethasone
Administer:	

Etoposide _____ 40-mg/m^2 IV infusion on days 1–4

- Available in 500- and 1000-mg vials, 20 mg/mL.
- Further dilute with NS or D5W to 0.1-mg/mL final concentration.
- Give over 30–60 minutes to minimize risk of hypotension.
- Stable for 48 hours at room temperature.
- Enhances warfarin action by increasing PT.
- Dose modification for increased bilirubin level or creatinine clearance.

Methylprednisolone (Solu-Medrol): 500-mg IV on days 1–4

Cisplatin _____ 2000 mg/m^2 continuous infusion on days 1–4

- Available in 100-mg vials, 1-mg/mL concentration.
- Further dilute to 100–1000 mL with NS.
- Do NOT mix with D5W.
- Avoid aluminum needles.
- Stable for 24 hours at room.
- Reduces renal clearance of etoposide, and decreases effect of phenytoin.
- Cisplatin is inactivated in the presence of alkaline solutions containing sodium bicarbonate.
- May add Mg^{2+}.

Cytarabine: _____ 2000 mg/m^2 IV on day 5 over 2 hours after cisplatin and etoposide

- Reconstitute with water with benzyl alcohol, then dilute with 0.9% sodium chloride or D5W.
- Reconstituted drug is stable for 48 hours at room temperature and 7 days refrigerated.

Major Side Effects

- Myelosuppression: Moderate to severe.
- Hypersensitivity Reactions: Characterized by hypotension, bronchospasms, or wheezing may occur with etoposide. Hypersensitivity reactions can occur with cisplatin.
- GI Toxicities: Nausea and vomiting, anorexia, and metallic taste of foods; moderate to highly emetogenic; mucositis, diarrhea.
- Potential Renal Damage: Dose-limiting toxicity with cisplatin. Can be prevented by adequate hydration and diuresis.
- Neurotoxicity: Peripheral neuropathy, including numbness, weakness, myalgias, and late severe motor difficulties. Jaw pain. Neurotoxicity dose limiting. Effects on renal function dose related and seen 10–20 days after therapy. Peripheral neuropathy, including numbness, weakness, myalgias, and late severe motor difficulties. High-dose cytarabine includes cerebellar toxicity, including nystagmus, dysarthria, ataxia, slurred speech, difficulty with fine motor coordination, lethargy, or somnolence. Assess baseline neurologic status and cerebellar function (coordinated movements, such as handwriting and gait).
- Ototoxicity: High-frequency hearing loss and tinnitus.
- Steroid Toxicities: Sodium and water retention, cushingoid changes, hyperglycemia, hypokalemia, and increased sodium level. Warfarin and insulin doses may need to be increased. Muscle weakness, loss of muscle mass, osteoporosis, and pathologic fractures with prolonged use. Mood changes, euphoria, headache, insomnia, depression, and psychosis. Cataracts or glaucoma may develop.
- Reproduction: Pregnancy category D. Breast feeding should be avoided. Discuss sperm banking.

Supportive drugs:

☐ pegfilgrastim (Neulasta)_____   ☐ filgrastim (Neupogen) _____

☐ epoetin alfa (Procrit)/   ☐ Allopurinol_____
darbepoetin alfa (Aranesp) _____

☐ Antibiotic _____   ☐ Antifungal _____

**Initiate antiemetic protocol
after chemotherapy:**   Moderately emetogenic.

Treatment schedule: Repeat cycle every 21 days.

Estimated number of visits: 10 to 15 visits every 3 weeks.

Chair time: Three hours days 1–5. Mix levels and CBC as indicated by doctor.

Dose Calculation by: 1. _____   2. _____

_____

Physician   Date

_____

Patient Name   ID Number

_____   / _____ / _____

Diagnosis   Ht   Wt   M²

Dexamethasone, High-Dose Cytarabine, Cisplatin (DHAP)

Baseline laboratory tests:	CBC: Chemistry, renal and LFTs
Baseline procedures or tests:	Bone marrow biopsy, central line placement
Initiate IV:	NS
Premedicate:	5-HT$_3$ and dexamethasone IV
Administer:	

Cytarabine _____ 2000-mg/m^2/day IV over 2 hours q 12 hours for 2 doses on day 1

- Dilute in sterile water with benzyl alcohol, then further dilute with 50–100 mL of 0.9% sodium chloride or D5W.
- IV hydration at 150/mL per hour with or without alkalinization, should give oral allopurinol, strict intake and output recording, and daily weights.
- Stable for 48 hours at room temperature and 7 days refrigerated.

Cisplatin _____ 100-mg/m^2 IV on day 1

- Available in 100-mg vials, 1-mg/mL concentration.
- Further dilute to 100–1000 mL with NS.
- Do NOT mix with D5W.
- Avoid aluminum needles.
- Stable for 24 hours at room temperature.
- Reduces renal clearance of etoposide and decreases effect of phenytoin.
- Cisplatin is inactivated in the presence of alkaline solutions containing sodium bicarbonate.

Dexamethasone: _____ 40-mg PO on days 1–14

- Repeat cycle every 3–4 weeks.

Drug interactions: Decreases efficacy of gentamicin and digoxin

Major Side Effects

- Bone Marrow Depression: Nadir biphasic and severe.
- GI Toxicities: Severe nausea and vomiting acute and delayed; anorexia and taste alterations.
- Skin Alterations: Total alopecia, impaired skin/mucosal changes, including maculopapular rash.
- Neurotoxicity: High doses of cytarabine can result in cerebellar toxicity, including nystagmus, dysarthria, ataxia, slurred speech, difficulty with fine motor coordination, lethargy, or somnolence. Assess baseline neurologic status and cerebellar function (coordinated movements, such as handwriting and gait) before and during therapy. If cerebellar toxicity develops, treatment must be discontinued. Cisplatin causes peripheral neuropathy and ototoxicity.
- Saline or steroid drops to both eyes may be indicated for 24 hours after completion of high cytarabine.
- Alteration in Urinary Elimination: Tumor lysis syndrome can occur 1–5 days after initiation of treatment; treat with hydration and allopurinol. Daily weights and intake and output recording. Monitor electrolytes, creatinine, BUN, uric acid, and phosphorus daily during treatment to evaluate tumor lysis. Discontinue therapy with rapidly increasing creatinine. Cisplatin can cause necrosis of proximal and distal renal tubules.
- Steroid Toxicities: Sodium and water retention, cushingoid changes, hyperglycemia, hypokalemia, and increased sodium level. Warfarin and insulin doses may need to be increased. Muscle weakness, loss of muscle mass, osteoporosis, and pathologic fractures with prolonged use. Mood changes, euphoria, headache, insomnia, depression, and psychosis. Cataracts or glaucoma may develop.
- Sexual Dysfunction: Mutagenic and teratogenic; discuss contraception and sperm banking.

Initiate antiemetic protocol: Highly emetogenic protocol.

Supportive drugs: ☐ G-CSF (Neupogen)_____   ☐ pegfilgrastim (Neulasta) +
                                                                                          G-CSF _____

                               ☐ epoetin alfa (Procrit)/   ☐ Allopurinol_____
                                 darbepoetin alfa (Aranesp)_____

                               ☐ Antibiotic _____   ☐ Antifungal _____

Treatment schedule: Repeat cycle every 3–4 weeks.

Estimated number of visits: May require hospitalization on day 1. Daily or every other day for blood counts; 12 visits in 4 weeks. Chair time 3 hours day.

Dose Calculation by: 1. _____   2. _____

_____   _____
Physician   Date

_____   _____
Patient Name   ID Number

_____   _____/_____/_____
Diagnosis   Ht   Wt   M^2

Ifosfamide, Etoposide, Carboplatin (ICE)

Baseline laboratory tests:	CBC: Chemistry, renal and LFTs
Baseline procedures or tests:	Bone marrow biopsy, central line placement
Initiate IV:	NS
Premedicate:	5-HT$_3$ and dexamethasone IV
Administer:	

Ifosfamide _____ 5000-mg/m^2 IV continuous infusion for 24 hours on day 2

- Available in 1- and 3-g vials.
- Reconstitute with sterile water.
- Further dilute to concentrations of 0.6–20 mg/mL in D5W or NS.
- Stable for 24 hours refrigerated.
- Phenobarbital, phenytoin, cimetidine, and allopurinol increase toxicity.
- Ifosfamide may enhance anticoagulant effects of warfarin.

Etoposide _____ 100-mg/m^2/d IV over 1–2 hours on days 1–3

- VePesid 5 cc/100 mg; etopophos reconstitute with 5–10 mL NS, D5W, sterile water, bacteriostatic sterile water, or bacteriostatic NS with benzyl alcohol to 20 mg/mL or 10 mg/mL, respectively.
- Further dilute to final concentration NS or D5W to 0.1 mg/mL.
- Stability is dose concentration dependent from 8–96 hours.

Carboplatin _____ AUC of 5.0, IV infusion over 1 hour on day 2

- Available in 50-, 150-, 450-, and 600-mg vials (lyophilized powder should be diluted with sterile water).
- Dilute further in D5W or NS.
- Stable for 24 hours.
- Dose modification for creatinine clearance < 60 cc/min or if other values are abnormal.

Mesna _____ 5000-mg/m^2 continuous IV infusion in combination with ifosfamide

- Available in 1000-mg multidose vials. Dilute with D5W or NS.
- Reconstituted solution stable for 24 hours at room temperature.

GCSF is administered at 5 µg/kg on days 5–12.

- Repeat cycle every 14 days.

Major Side Effects

- Bone Marrow Depression: Myelosuppression is dose-limiting toxicity.
- GI Toxicities: Nausea and vomiting moderately to highly emetogenic, anorexia. Monitor LFT results.
- Nephrotoxicity: Patients with renal dysfunction are at risk. Monitor electrolyte, BUN, and creatinine values.
- Potential for Hypersensitivity Reactions: Carboplatin may cause allergic reactions ranging from rash, urticaria, erythema, and pruritus to anaphylaxis; occurring within minutes of infusion.
- Altered Urinary Elimination: Hemorrhagic cystitis, hematuria; frequency preventable with uroprotection and hydration of 2–3 L per day. Monitor BUN and serum creatinine levels.
- Skin Alterations: Alopecia with total hair loss. Sterile phlebitis may occur at injection site. Hyperpigmentation, dermatitis, and nail ridging may occur.
- Sensory/perceptual Alterations: Lethargy and confusion at high doses of ifosfamide, usually lasting 1–8 hours; reversible.
- Reproduction: Pregnancy category D. Breast feeding should be avoided. Discuss contraception and sperm banking.

Initiate antiemetic protocol:	Moderately to highly emetogenic protocol.
Supportive drugs:	☐ G-CSF (Neupogen) _____ ☐ pegfilgrastim (Neulasta)
	☐ epoetin alfa (Procrit)/ darbepoetin alfa (Aranesp) _____ ☐ Allopurinol _____
	☐ Antibiotic _____ ☐ Antifungal _____
Treatment schedule:	Chair time 1–2 hours on days 1 and 3, and 2–3 hours on day 2. Repeat cycle every 14 days.

Estimated number of visits: 3 days first week. Monitor CBC.

Dose Calculation by: 1. _____   2. _____

_____   _____
Physician   Date

_____   _____
Patient Name   ID Number

_____   _____/_____/_____
Diagnosis   Ht   Wt   M²

Mesna, Ifosfamide, Mitoxantrone, Etoposide (MINE)

Baseline laboratory tests: CBC: Chemistry on day 1

Premedicate: 5-HT_3 and dexamethasone 10-mg IV

Administer: **Mesna** _____ 1330-mg/m^2 IV infusion 15 minutes before ifosfamide on days 1–3 then, 500-mg/day IV 4 hours after ifosfamide on days 1–3

- Available in 1000-mg multidose vials. Dilute with D5W or NS.
- Reconstituted solution stable for 24 hours at room temperature. Also available in 400-mg, white, oblong tablets for oral use (IV dose is 20% of ifosfamide dose; oral dose is 40% of ifosfamide dose).

Ifosfamide _____ 1330-mg/m^2 IV infusion on days 1–3

- Available in 1- and 3-g vials.
- Reconstitute with sterile water.
- Further dilute to concentrations of 0.6–20 mg/mL in D5W or NS.
- Stable for 24 hours refrigerated.
- Phenobarbital, phenytoin, cimetidine, and allopurinol increase toxicity.
- Ifosfamide may enhance anticoagulant effects of warfarin.

Mitoxantrone _____ 8-mg/m^2 IV infusion on day 1 only

- IV push over 3 minutes through the side arm of a free-flowing IV or IV infusion over 5–30 minutes.
- Available at 20 mg in 10-mL dark blue solution.
- May be diluted in D5W or NS.
- Stable at room temperature for 48 hours.
- Incompatible with heparin.

Etoposide _____ 65-mg/m^2 IV infusion on days 1–3

- Available in 500- and 1000-mg vials, 20 mg/mL.
- Further dilute with NS or D5W to 0.1-mg/mL final concentration.
- Give over 30–60 minutes to minimize risk of hypotension.
- Stable 48 hours at room temperature.
- Enhances warfarin action by increasing PT.
- Dose modification for increased bilirubin level or creatinine clearance.

Major Side Effects

- Myelosuppression: Nadir in 9–14 days.
- GI Toxicities: Nausea, vomiting, and anorexia. Monitor LFT results.
- Cardiotoxicity: CHF with decreased left ventricular ejection fraction (< 3 %), increased cardiotoxicity with cumulative dose of mitoxantrone > 180 mg/m^2.
- Hypersensitivity Reactions: Infusion-related reactions occur within 30 minutes to 2 hours after the beginning of the first infusion. Fever, chills, and rigors most common. Bronchospasms may occur with etoposide; hypotension with rapid infusion.
- Skin Alterations: Alopecia with total hair loss. Sterile phlebitis may occur at injection site. Hyperpigmentation, dermatitis, and nail ridging may occur. Radiation recall with etoposide.
- Altered Urinary Elimination: Hemorrhagic cystitis, hematuria, frequency preventable with uroprotection and hydration of 2–3 L per day. Monitor BUN and serum creatinine levels. Urine will be green-blue for 24 hours; sclera may become temporarily discolored blue.
- Sensory/perceptual alterations: Lethargy and confusion at high doses of ifosfamide, usually lasting 1–8 hours; reversible.
- Reproduction: Pregnancy category D. Breast feeding should be avoided. Discuss contraception and sperm banking.

Initiate antiemetic protocol: Highly emetogenic protocol.

Supportive drugs:
☐ pegfilgrastim (Neulasta) _____   ☐ filgrastim (Neupogen) _____
☐ epoetin alfa (Procrit)/   ☐ Allopurinol _____
   darbepoetin alfa (Aranesp) _____
☐ Antibiotic _____   ☐ Antifungal _____

Treatment schedule: Repeat cycle every 21 days.

Estimated number of visits: Chair time 6 hours day 1–3. Request 5 visits per cycle. 3–6 cycles worth of visits.

Dose Calculation by: 1. _____   2. _____

_____

Physician   Date

_____

Patient Name   ID Number

_____

Diagnosis   Ht _____ / Wt _____ / M²

NON-HODGKIN'S LYMPHOMA

Primary CNS Lymphoma

3.5-g/m² IV over 2 hours every other week for five doses

Intrathecal methotrexate: 12-mg IT weekly every other week after IV MTX

Leucovorin: 10-mg IV every 6 hours for 12 doses, starting 24 hours after IV MTX

Leucovorin: 10-mg IV every 12 hours for 8 doses, starting 24 hours after IT MTX

Vincristine: 1.4-mg/m² IV every other week along with IV MTX

Procarbazine: 100-mg/m²/day PO for 7 days on first, third, and fifth cycle of IV MTX

- After chemotherapy is completed, whole-brain radiation therapy to a total dose of 45 cGy.[304]

Single-Agent Regimens

Rituximab: 375-mg/m² IV on days 1, 8, 15, and 22

May repeat one additional cycle.[1,305]

Rituximab: 250 mg/m² IV on days 1 and 8

111In-ibritumomab tiuxetan: 5 mCi of 111In, 1.6 mg of ibritumomab tiuxetan IV on day 1

90Y-ibritumomab tiuxetan: 0.4-mCi/kg IV over 10 minutes on day 8 after the day 8 rituximab dose

The dose of 90Y-ibritumomab tiuxetan is capped at 32 mCi.[1,306]

Fludarabine: 25-mg/m² IV on days 1–5

Repeat cycle every 28 days.[1,307]

Cladribine: 0.5–0.7 mg/kg SC on days 1–5 or 0.1-mg/kg IV on days 1–7
Repeat cycle every 28 days.[1,308]

Administered in radiation oncology department.[309a]

Primary CNS Lymphoma

Methotrexate, IT Methotrexate, Leucovorin, Vincristine and Procarbazine followed by Whole Brain Irradiation

Baseline laboratory tests:	CBC and Chemistry Panel, Creatinine Clearance $\geq$ 50 mL/h
Laboratory tests:	CBC before each treatment
Baseline procedures:	Diagnostic Lumbar Puncture, Ommaya reservoir
Initiate IV:	0.9% Sodium Chloride
Premedication:	5-HT$_3$, dexamethasone
Administer:	

Methotrexate _____ 3.5 gm/m2 IV over 2 hours every other week for 5 doses

- Available in 250-mg vial.
- Further diluted in NS.
- Reconstituted solution stable for 24 hours at room temperature. High-dose methotrexate requires leucovorin rescue.
- Drug interactions include aspirin, penicillins, nonsteroidal anti-inflammatory drugs (NSAIDs), cephalosporins, phenytoin warfarin, 5-fluorouracil, thymidine, folic acid, and omeprazole. Vigorously hydrate; moderate dose of MTX

Leucovorin: _____ 10 mg IV every 6 hours for 6 doses for 12 doses, starting 24 hours after IV methotrexate

Vincristine: _____1.4 mg/m2 IV every other week along with IV methotrexate

- Maximum dose 2 mg.
- Vesicant
- Available in 1-, 2-, and 5-mg vials.
- Keep refrigerated.
- Given IV push through a free-flowing IV.

Procarbazine _____100 mg/m2/day PO for 7 days on 1st, 3rd and 5th cycle of IV methotrexate

- Available in 50-mg tablets.

Intratecal Methotrexate _____ 12 mg IT weekly on alternate weeks after systemic IV methotrexate

Leucovorin _____10 mg IV every 12 hours for 8 doses starting 24 hours after IT methotrexate.

Major Side Effects

- Myelosuppression: Dose-limiting toxicity. Nadir at days 4–7.
- GI Toxicities: Nausea, vomiting, and anorexia; moderately to highly emetogenic. Mucositis and stomatitis can be severe and dose limiting. Constipation and paralytic ileus secondary to autonomic neuropathy.
- GU Toxicities: Acute renal failure, azotemia, urinary retention and uric acid nephropathy. Provide adequate hydration.
- Pulmonary Toxicities: Poorly defined Pneumonitis characterized by fever, cough and interstial infiltrates.
- Flulike Syndrome: Fever, chills, sweating, lethargy, myalgias, and arthralgias common.
- Hemorrhagic cystitis or irritation of bladder wall capillaries; preventable with appropriate hydration. Acute renal failure, azotemia, urinary retention, and uric acid nephropathy.
- Neurotoxicity: Peripheral neuropathy, including numbness, weakness, myalgias, and late severe motor difficulties. Jaw pain. CNS toxicity with paresthesias, neuropathies, ataxia, lethargy, headache, confusion, and/or seizures. Usually occurs within 6 days of high dose Methotrexate and resolves within 48-72 hours.
- Skin Alterations: Total alopecia, hyper pigmentation of nail beds and dermal crease of hands, greatest in dark-skinned individuals. Radiation recall. Sun sensitivity.
- Reproduction: Pregnancy category D. Breast feeding should be avoided.

Initiate antiemetic protocol: Moderately to highly emetogenic protocol.

Supportive drugs: ☐ G-CSF (Neupogen) _____ ☐ Peg-G-CSF _____

☐ epoetin alfa ☐ Allopurinol _____
(Procrit)/darbepoetin alfa
(Aranesp)_____

☐ Antibiotic _____ ☐ Antifungal _____

Treatment schedule: Administer one cycle.

Estimated number of visits: Weekly for 12 weeks.

Chair time: Chair time 2–3 hours every other week for Methotrexate and 1 hour of IT Methotrexate.

Dose Calculation by: 1. _____ 2. _____

_____ _____

Physician Date

_____ _____

Patient Name ID Number

_____ _____/_____/_____

Diagnosis Ht Wt M²

Single-Agent Regimens

Rituxan (Rituximab): Monoclonal Antibody; CD 20 Positive, B-Cell Non-Hodgkin's Lymphoma

Baseline laboratory tests:	CBC: Chemistry and sedimentation rate
Laboratory tests:	Perform before each chemotherapy administration: CBC
Initiate IV:	NS
Premedication:	Dexamethasone may be used for patients to prevent or treat infusion-related reactions
	Tylenol 1000-mg PO 30 minutes before infusion
	Benadryl 50 mg in 150 cc of NS over 30 minutes (or PO)

Administer: **Rituxan** _____ 375-mg/m^2 IV infusion

- Available in 500-mg/50 mL and 100-mg/10-mL vials. Further dilute in NS to make final concentration of 1 or 4 mg/1 mL.
- Stable for 24 hours at room temperature and an additional 24 hours refrigerated.
- Discard unused portion.
- Use infusion pump and blood pressure monitor.

First infusion: Initial rate of 50 mg/hr. Increase infusion rate in 50-mg/hr increments every 30 minutes to a maximum rate of 400 mg/hr. If a hypersensitivity-related event develops, the infusion should be temporarily slowed or interrupted. Resume infusion at 50% of previous rate after symptoms subside. Monitor vital signs every 10 minutes for the first hour, then every 30 minutes thereafter.

Subsequent infusions: Initial rate of 100 mg/hr. Increase rate by 100 mg/hr every 30 minutes to a maximum rate of 400 mg/hr as tolerated. Do NOT give IV push.

Major Side Effects

- Hypersensitivity Reactions: Infusion-related reactions occur within 30 minutes to 2 hours of the beginning of the first infusion. Fever, chills, and rigors most common. Bronchospasm, dyspnea, pruritus, hypotension, back pain, and angioedema may also be seen. Will resolve when the infusion is stopped and/or symptomatic treatment (acetaminophen, diphenhydramine, and IV NS) is given. Have emergency hypersensitivity/anaphylaxis medications available (e.g., epinephrine, antihistamines, bronchodilators, and corticosteroids).
- Potential for Infection: B-lymphocytes reduced, resulting in bacterial infections not related to neutropenia.
- Skin Reactions: Rare and include paraneoplastic pemphigus, Stevens-Johnson syndrome, lichenoid dermatitis, vesiculobullous dermatitis, and toxic epidermal necrolysis. Drug therapy should be discontinued and skin biopsy should be obtained to determine cause.
- Tumor Lysis Syndrome: Patients with high tumor burden or high white blood cell count at risk. Occurs in first 5 days after infusion. Treat/prevent with hydration and allopurinol.
- Reproduction: Pregnancy category C. Breast feeding should be avoided.

Treatment schedule:	Repeat cycle weekly for four doses.
	May be repeated upon relapse.
	Maintenance therapy of one infusion every 2 months or every 6 months.
Estimated number of visits:	Four for single therapy.
Chair time:	6–8 hours with first dose. 4–6 hours in weeks 2–4.

Dose Calculation by: 1. _____   2. _____

_____
Physician

_____
Date

_____
Patient Name

_____
ID Number

_____
Diagnosis

_____ / _____ / _____
Ht   Wt   M^2

Ibritumomab Tiuxetan (Zevalin) Regimen

Baseline laboratory tests: CBC: Chemistry, renal, and LFTs

Baseline procedures or tests: Bone marrow biopsy, central line placement

Initiate IV: NS

Premedicate: Diphenhydramine, acetaminophen, dexamethasone

Administer:

Rituximab _____ 250-mg/m^2 IV, days 1 and 8

- Dilute with NS or D5W to final concentration of 1–4 mg/mL.
- Infusion rates easier to calculate if solution is 1:1 concentration.
- Antibodies are fragile; do not shake vial or bag.
- Do not use a filter.
- Stable at room temperature for 24 hours.

Given in Radiation Oncology Department

^{111}In-ibritumomab tiuxetan _____ 5 mCi of ^{111}In and _____ 1.6 mg of ibritumomab tiuxetan IV on day 1

^{90}Y-ibritumomab tiuxetan _____ 0.4-mCi/kg IV over 10 minutes on day 8 after the day 8 rituximab dose. Dose of ^{90}Y-ibritumomab tiuxetan is capped at 32 mCi.

See package insert for drug preparation.

Day 1: ^{111}In IV over 10 minutes using 0.22-micron filter, followed by rituximab IV within 4 hours, initially at 50 mg/hr and gradually increasing the rate in 50-mg increments if no infusion reaction occurs to a maximum of 400 mg/hr.

Biodistribution imaging 1: 2–24 hours after ^{111}In injection; image 2: 48–72 hours later. Optional image 3; at 90–120 hours.

If biodistribution acceptable, on day 7–9, rituximab 250-mg/m^2 IV, and within 4 hours, ^{90}Y-ibritumomab tiuxetan IV over 10 minutes. Avoid extravasation.

Major Side Effects

- Myelosuppression: Severe and prolonged.
- Hypersensitivity Reactions: Occur within 30 minutes to 2 hours, most commonly seen with first infusion and patients with high tumor burden and characterized by fever, chills, rigors, back pain, flushing, bronchospasms, angioedema, and hypotension. Usually resolves when infused stopped. Premedicate with acetaminophen, diphenhydramine, and corticosteroids. Ensure that emergency medications are available (antihistamines, corticosteroids, epinephrine, and bronchodilators). When symptoms resolve, resume infusion at 50% of the previous infusion rate. Monitor vital signs frequently.
- Tumor lysis syndrome can occur if white blood cell count is elevated or large tumor burden present. Prevent with allopurinol and hydration 150 mL/hr with or without alkalinization.
- Skin Alterations: Severe mucocutaneous reactions are rare but require discontinuation of rituximab.
- Alterations in Comfort: Asthenia, headache, pruritus, myalgias, dizziness, and fatigue.
- Neurotoxicity: Agitation, confusion, visual disturbances have occurred.
- GI Toxicities: Nausea and vomiting, anorexia; mucositis, diarrhea.
- Radiation Exposure: ^{90}Y is a beta-emitter, and thus, patients should protect others from exposure to their body secretions (saliva, stool, blood, and urine).
- Reproduction: Pregnancy category D. Breast feeding should be avoided.

Initiate antiemetic protocol: Mildly emetogenic protocol.

Supportive drugs:

☐ G-CSF (Neupogen)_____   ☐ pegfilgrastim (Neulasta)

☐ epoetin alfa (Procrit)/   ☐ Allopurinol_____
darbepoetin alfa (Aranesp)_____

☐ Antibiotic _____   ☐ Antifungal _____

Treatment schedule: One cycle only, 6–8 hours days 1 and 8 for Rituximab.

Estimated number of visits: Weekly for CBCs until bone marrow recovery.

Dose Calculation by: 1. _____   2. _____

_____   _____
Physician   Date

_____   _____
Patient Name   ID Number

_____   _____ / _____   _____ / _____
Diagnosis   Ht   Wt   M²

Fludarabine

Baseline laboratory tests:	CBC: Chemistry, renal, and LFTs
Baseline procedures or tests:	Bone marrow biopsy, central line placement
Initiate IV:	NS
Premedicate:	5-HT$_3$ IV
Administer:	**Fludarabine** _____ 25-mg/m^2/d IV on days 1–5

- Dilute with 2 mL of sterile water for final concentration of 25 mg/mL.
- Further dilute in 100 mL of NS or D5W. Drug should be used within 8 hours.

Major Side Effects

- Myelosuppression: Severe and cumulative, nadir day 13.
- Fatigue: Secondary to anemia.
- Neurotoxicity: Agitation, confusion, and visual disturbances have occurred.
- Pulmonary Toxicities: Pneumonia occurs in 16%–22% of patients. Pulmonary hypersensitivity reaction characterized by dyspnea, cough, interstitial pulmonary infiltrates.
- GI Toxicities: Nausea and vomiting, anorexia; mucositis, diarrhea.
- Reproduction: Pregnancy category D. Breast feeding should be avoided. Discuss contraception and sperm banking.

Initiate antiemetic protocol:	Mildly emetogenic protocol.
Supportive drugs:	☐ G-CSF (Neupogen) _____ ☐ pegfilgrastim (Neulasta)
	☐ epoetin alfa (Procrit)/ darbepoetin alfa (Aranesp)_____ ☐ Allopurinol_____
	☐ Antibiotic _____ ☐ Antifungal _____
Treatment schedule:	Chair time 1 hour on days 1–5
Estimated number of visits:	Daily for 5 days and then weekly. Request 3–4 cycles worth of visits.
	Repeat schedule every 28 days.

Dose Calculation by: 1. _____ 2. _____

_____
Physician

_____
Date

_____
Patient Name

_____
ID Number

_____
Diagnosis

_____/ _____/ _____
Ht   Wt   M^2

Cladribine (Leustatin)

Baseline laboratory tests:	CBC: Chemistry, renal, and LFTs
Baseline procedures or tests:	Bone marrow biopsy, central line placement
Administer:	**Cladribine** _____0.5–0.7 mg/kg/day SC or 0.1 mg/kg IV on days 1–7

- Dilute 1:1 concentrated liquid in 500 mL of 0.9% NS per day.
- Unstable in D5W.
- Use 22-μm filter when preparing solution.
- Stable when diluted for 24 hours and 8 hours refrigerated.

Major Side Effects

- Bone marrow depression: Nadir at 7–14 days; neutropenia is more common than anemia or thrombocytopenia. Increased risk for opportunistic infections, including fungal, herpes, and *Pneumocystis carinii*. Teach self-care measures to minimize risk of infection and bleeding.
- Fever: >100° due to infection or release of endogenous pyrogen from lysed lymphocytes. Symptoms include chills, daiphoresis, malaise, myalgia, and arthralgias.
- GI Toxicities: Nausea and vomiting mildly emetogenic and usually controlled with phenothiazines. Diarrhea in 10% and constipation in 9% of patients.
- Neurotoxicity: Headache, insomnia, and dizziness.
- Tumor lysis syndrome rare, even with high tumor burden.
- Reproduction: Pregnancy category D. Breast feeding should be avoided. Discuss contraception and sperm banking.

Initiate antiemetic protocol:	Mildly emetogenic protocol.
Supportive drugs:	☐ G-CSF _____ ☐ pegfilgrastim (Neulasta)
	☐ epoetin alfa (Procrit)/ ☐ Allopurinol_____
	darbepoetin alfa (Aranesp)_____
	☐ Antibiotic _____ ☐ Antifungal _____
Treatment schedule:	Chair time 1 hour on days 1–5, 30 minutes for IV dose.
	Repeat cycle until remission (usually two to three cycles).
Estimated number of visits:	Seven days first week and then daily or every other day for blood counts.

Dose Calculation by: 1. _____   2. _____

_____

Physician   Date

_____

Patient Name   ID Number

_____   _____/_____/_____

Diagnosis   Ht   Wt   M^2

I 131-tositumomab (Bexxar)

Baseline laboratory tests:	TSH, CBC: Platelets $\geq$ 100,000; Neutrophil count $\geq$ 1,500; Chemistry, renal function tests, pregnancy test, (if applicable), HAMA (human anti-murine antibodies) if patient has had previous exposure to murine antibodies
Baseline procedures:	Bone marrow biopsy $\leq$ 25% lymphoma of the intratrabecular space; referral to Nuclear Medicine/ Radiation Oncology Department
Laboratory tests:	CBC weekly for 10 weeks or until bone marrow recovery; TSH at least annually

The BEXXAR therapeutic regimen consists of four components administered in two discrete steps: the dosimetric step, followed 7–14 days later by a therapeutic step.

Premedication: Day 1

- Thyroid Protection initiated 24 hours prior to administration of Iodine I 131 Tositumomab dosimetric dose and continued until 2 weeks after Iodine I 131 Tositumomab therapeutic dose.
  - SSKI—saturated solution of potassium idodide 4 drops orally t.i.d.; or potassium iodide tablets 130 mg orally

Premedication: Day 0

- Tylenol 1000 mg and Benadryl 50 mg PO 30 minutes prior to Dosimetric and Therapeutic steps

Dosimetric step

Tositumomab 450 mg intravenously in 50 ml 0.9% Sodium Chloride over 60 minutes.

- Reduce the rate of infusion by 50% for mild to moderate infusional toxicity; interrupt infusion for severe infusional toxicity. After complete resolution of severe infusional toxicity, infusion may be resumed with a 50% reduction in the rate of infusion.
- 22 micron in-line filter
- The same IV tubing set and filter must be used throughout the entire Dosimetric or Therapeutic Step. A change in filter can result in loss of drug

Followed by:

Iodine I 131 Tositumomab (containing 5.0 mCi Iodine-131 and 35 mg Tositumomab) intravenously in 30 ml 0.9% Sodium Chloride over 20 minutes.

- Reduce the rate of infusion by 50% for mild to moderate infusional toxicity; interrupt infusion for severe infusional toxicity. After complete resolution of severe infusional toxicity, infusion may be resumed with a 50% reduction in the rate of infusion.

Day 0	Whole Body Dosimetry and Biodistribution
Day 2, 3, or 4	Whole Body Dosimetry and Biodistribution
Day 6 or 7	Whole Body dosimetry and Biodistribution

If biodistribution is acceptable begin Therapeutic Step. Note: Do not administer the therapeutic step if biodistribution is altered (see **Assessment of Biodistribution of Iodine I 131 Tositumomab**).

Premedication: Tylenol 1000 mg and Benadryl 50 mg PO 30 minutes before treatment

Therapeutic step

Tositumomab 450 mg intravenously in 50 ml 0.9% Sodium Chloride over 1 hour.

- Reduce the rate of infusion by 50% for mild to moderate infusional toxicity; interrupt infusion for severe infusional toxicity. After complete resolution of severe infusional toxicity, infusion may be resumed with a 50% reduction in the rate of infusion.

Followed by:

Iodine I 131 Tositumomab (see **CALCULATION OF IODINE-131 ACTIVITY FOR THE THERAPEUTIC DOSE**).

- Reduce the rate of infusion by 50% for mild to moderate infusional toxicity; interrupt infusion for severe infusional toxicity. After complete resolution of severe infusional toxicity, infusion may be resumed with a 50% reduction in the rate of infusion.
- Patients with $\geq$150,000 platelets/mm^3: The recommended dose is the activity of Iodine-131 calculated to deliver 75 cGy total body irradiation and 35 mg Tositumomab, administered intravenously over 20 minutes.

- Patients with NCI Grade 1 thrombocytopenia (platelet counts $\geq$100,000 but < 150,000 platelets/mm^3): The recommended dose is the activity of Iodine-131 calculated to deliver 65 cGy total body irradiation and 35 mg Tositumomab, administered intravenously over 20 minutes.

ADMINISTRATION IS DONE BY A NUCLEAR MEDICINE PHYSICIAN/RADIAITON ONCOLOGIST.

SEE PACKAGE INSERT FOR DIRECTIONS FOR COMPLETE PREPARATION AND ADMINISTRATION

Major Side Effects

- Hypersensitivity Reactions: Symptoms include fever, rigors, chills, sweating, hypotension, dyspnea, bronchospasms, and nausea during the infusion or up to 48 hours after the infusion. Rare but potentially life threatening. May treat with Tylenol and/or diphendydramine.
- Bone Marrow Depression: Neutropenia, thrombocytopenia, and anemia that are prolonged and severe. Intervention with G-csf and epoetin alfa is recommended. Transfusions of RBC's and platelets were not uncommon
- GI Toxicities: Nausea (61%), anorexia (21%) and diarrhea (32%). Dehydration and hypokalemia were also seen.
- Neurotoxicity: Central neurotoxicity may occur, as well as neuropathy and optic neuritis.
- Radiation Precautions: Patients may receive outpatient treatment as long as total dose to an individual at 1 meter is < 500 millirem. Remain at distance of > 3 feet from other people for at least 2 days. Infants and pregnant women should not visit the patient, and if necessary visits should be brief and at a distance of at least 9 feet. Do not travel by commercial transportation or go on a prolonged automobile trip with others for at least the first 2 days. Have sole use of the bathroom for at least two days and drink up to 3 + quarts water per day for at least two days to prevent dehydration.
- Reproductive: Pregnancy category D. Breast feeding should be avoided.

Initiate antiemetic protocol: Moderately to highly emetogenic protocol.

Supportive drugs:

☐ G-CSF Neupogen_____   ☐ Neulasta _____

☐ epoetin alfa (Procrit)/   ☐ Allopurinol_____
darbepoetin alfa
(Aranesp)_____

☐ Antibiotic _____   ☐ Antifungal _____

Treatment schedule: Chair time 2 hours on day 0, Body scans day 0, (2, 3, or 4) and day 6 or 7. Therapeutic Step days 7–14 (one dose within that time frame). Chair time 2 hours.

Estimated number of visits: Four visits at Radiation Therapy Department for treatment. Monitor CBC at least weekly for 10 weeks or until counts stabilize.

Dose Calculation by: 1. _____   2. _____

_____

Physician   Date

_____

Patient Name   ID Number

_____ _____/ _____/ _____

Diagnosis   Ht   Wt   M^2

MALIGNANT MELANOMA

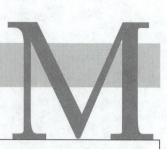

Adjuvant Therapy

Interferon-α-2b: 20-MU/m^2 IV, 5 times weekly for 4 weeks,
  then 10 MU/m^2 SC, 3 times weekly for 48 weeks

Treat for a total of 1 year.[1,309]

METASTATIC DISEASE
Combination Regimens

Dacarbazine: 220-mg/m^2 IV on days 1–3

Carmustine: 150-mg/m^2 IV on day 1

Cisplatin: 25-mg/m^2 IV on days 1–3

Repeat cycle with dacarbazine and cisplatin every 21 days and carmustine
  every 42 days.[1,310]

Dacarbazine: 220-mg/m^2 IV on days 1–3 and 22–24

Cisplatin: 25-mg/m^2 IV on days 1–3 and 22–24

Carmustine: 150-mg/m^2 IV on day 1

Tamoxifen: 10-mg PO bid starting on day 4

Repeat cycle every 6 weeks.[1,311]

Cisplatin: 20-mg/m^2 IV on days 1–5

Vinblastine: 1.6-mg/m^2 IV on days 1–5

Dacarbazine: 800-mg/m^2 IV on day 1

Repeat cycle every 21–28 days.[1,312]

Interferon-α-2b: 15-MU/m^2 IV on days 1–5, 8–12, and 15–19 as induction
  therapy

Interferon-α-2b: 10-MU/m^2 SC 3 times weekly after induction therapy

Dacarbazine: 200-mg/m^2 IV on days 22–26

Repeat cycle every 28 days.[1,313]

Cisplatin + Vinblastine + DTIC + IL-2 + IFN 510

Cisplatin: 20-mg/m^2 IV on days 1–4 and 22–25

Vinblastine: 1.5-mg/m^2 IV on days 1–4 and 22–25

Dacarbazine: 800-mg/m^2 IV on days 1 and 22

Interleukin-2: 9-MU/m^2 IV as a 24-hour continuous infusion on days 5–8 and 17–20

Interferon-α-2b: 5-MU/m^2 SC on days 5–9, 17–21, and 26–30.

Repeat cycle every 6 weeks.[1,314]

Temozolomide + Thalidomide 512

Temozolomide: 75 mg/m^2/day PO for 6 weeks

Thalidomide: 200–400 mg/m^2/day PO for 6 weeks

Repeat cycle every 10 weeks.[1,315]

Single-Agent Regimens

Dacarbazine 513

Dacarbazine: 250-mg/m^2 IV on days 1–5

Repeat cycle every 21 days.[1,316]

OR

Dacarbazine: 850-mg/m^2 IV on day 1

Repeat cycle every 3–6 weeks.[1,317]

Interferon-α-2b 514

Interferon-α-2b: 20-MU/m^2 IM, 3 × weekly for 12 weeks[1,318]

Aldesleukin 515

Aldesleukin (IL-2): 100,000 IU/kg IV on days 1–5 and 15–19

Repeat cycle every 28 days.[1,319]

Temozolomide 516

Temozolomide: 150-mg/m^2 PO on days 1–5

Repeat cycle every 28 days.[1,320]

If well tolerated, can increase dose to 200-mg/m^2 PO on days 1–5.

Adjuvant Therapy

Interferon-α-2b (Intron A, IFN-α-2b Recombinant, α-2-Interferon, rIFN-α-2)

Baseline laboratory tests:	CBC: Chemistry (including liver function tests [LFTs])
Baseline procedures or tests:	Central line
Initiate IV:	Normal saline (NS)
Premedicate:	5-HT$_3$ for IV therapy
	Acetaminophen 650 mg 30 minutes before treatment and every 4 hours
	may alternate with
	Ibuprofen 400-mg PO every 4 hours
Administer:	**Interferon-α-2b**_____MU(20×10^6 IU/m^2) IV on days 1–5 × 4 weeks

- Use only Intron A powder (interferon-α-2b) because of the amount of preservative in the premixed solution.
- **Do not use 5% dextrose and water (D5W).**
- May require increased hydration as treatment progresses.

Then

Maintenance therapy

Interferon-α-2b _____MU/m^2 SQ TIW × 48 weeks

- Available in multidose pens with 6 doses of 3 MU (18 MU) or 5 MU (30 MU) or 10 MU (60 MU).
- Keep refrigerated.

Major Side Effects	

- Flulike Symptoms: Fever, chills, headache, myalgias, and arthralgias. Occurs in 80%–90% of patients. Onset 3–4 hours after injection and lasting for up to 8–9 hours. Incidence decreases with subsequent injections. Symptoms can be managed with acetaminophen and increased oral fluid intake. Symptoms may be more pronounced during IV induction therapy.
- Bone Marrow Depression: Myelosuppression with mild leukopenia and thrombocytopenia. Cumulative effect, dose-limiting thrombocytopenia; reversible.
- Gastrointestinal (GI) Toxicities: Nausea and diarrhea are mild; vomiting is rare. Anorexia is seen in 46%–65% of patients and is cumulative and dose limiting. Taste alteration and xerostomia may occur.
- Renal/hepatic: Renal toxicity is uncommon and is manifested by mild proteinuria and hypocalcemia. Acute renal failure and nephrotic syndrome have been reported in rare instances. Mild transient elevations in serum transaminase levels. Dose-dependent toxicity observed more frequently in the presence of pre-existing liver abnormalities.
- CNS Effects: Dizziness (21–41%), confusion, decreased mental status and depression. Somnolence, irritability and poor concentration.
- Cardiotoxicity: Chest pain, arrhythmias, and congestive heart failure (CHF) are rare.
- Skin: Alopecia is partial. Dry skin, pruritus, and irritation at injection site occur.
- Reproductive: Pregnancy category C. Breast feeding should be avoided.

Initiate antiemetic protocol:	Mildly emetogenic protocol.
Supportive drugs:	☐ pegfilgrastim (Neulasta) ☐ filgrastim (Neupogen)
	☐ epoetin alfa (Procrit) ☐ darbepoetin alfa (Aranesp)
Treatment schedule:	Chair time 1 hour on days 1–5 for 4 weeks, and 1 hour on day 1 of week 5 for self-injection teaching.
Estimated number of visits:	20 visits first month, and once every 1–2 weeks for remainder of year.

Dose Calculation by: 1. _____   2. _____

_____
Physician

_____
Date

_____
Patient Name

_____
ID Number

_____
Diagnosis

_____ / _____ / _____
Ht   Wt   M^2

METASTATIC DISEASE
Combination Regimens

Dacarbazine/Carmustine/Cisplatin

Baseline laboratory tests:	CBC: Chemistry (including Mg^{2+}) and LFTs
Baseline procedures or tests:	Pulmonary function tests, central line placement
Initiate IV:	NS
Premedicate:	5-HT$_3$ and dexamethasone 20 mg in 100 cc of NS
Administer:	**Dacarbazine (DTIC)**_____mg (220 mg/m^2) IV over 1 hour on days 1–3.

- Available in 100- and 200-mg vials 10 mg/mL or
- Reconstitute with 9.9 mL sterile water, NS, or D5W to a final concentration of 10 mg/mL. Further dilute in D5W or NS 250-500 mL.
- **Vesicant**
- May cause vein burning/irritation if infused too rapidly. Reconstituted solution stable for 8 hours at room temperature, and 72 hours if refrigerated. If further diluted, solution is stable for 8 hours at room temperature and 24 hours refrigerated.

Carmustine (BCNU) _____mg (150 mg/m^2) IV in 500–1000 cc of NS over 1–2 hours on day 1

- Reconstitute with 3 mL of sterile diluent (dehydrated alcohol injection) supplied by the manufacturer.
- Further dilute with 27 mL of sterile water to a final concentration of 3.3 mg/mL.
- Further dilute with D5W for administration.
- Stable for 8 hours at room temperature.

Cisplatin _____ mg (25 mg/m^2) IV in 1000 cc of NS over 1–2 hours on days 1–3

- Available in 1-mg/1-mL solution. Multidose vial stable for 28 days under protected light or 7 days under fluorescent light.
- Do not use aluminum needles, because precipitate will form.
- Further dilute in 250 cc or more of D5W.

Major Side Effects

- Flulike Symptoms: Fever, chills, headache, myalgias, and arthralgias. Occur in 80%–90% of patients. May last for seveeral days after treatment.
- Bone Marrow Depression: Myelosuppression involving all blood elements. Delayed nadir with BCNU lasting 1–3 weeks..
- GI Toxicities: Nausea and vomiting can be severe with dacarbazine. Anorexia occurs in 46%–65% of patients and is cumulative and dose limiting. Taste alteration and xerostomia may occur. Diarrhea is rare.
- Renal/hepatic: Renal toxicity is uncommon and is manifested by mild proteinuria and hypocalcemia. Acute renal failure and nephrotic syndrome have been reported in rare instances. Mild transient elevations in serum transaminase levels. Dose-dependent toxicity observed more frequently in the presence of pre-existing liver abnormalities. Nephrotoxicity; can be prevented with vigorous hydration.
- Skin: Alopecia in 90% of patients taking DTIC. Dry skin, flushing, pruritus, photosensitivity, and irritation at injection site seen. Pain at injection site during dacarbazine infusion; phlebitis.
- Pulmonary Fibrosis: Patients receiving carmustine at cummaltive doses 1400 mg/m^2 are at higher risk.
- Neurotoxicity: Peripheral neuropathy (sensory/motor). Dose/duration dependent and progresses with continued therapy. Paresthesias and numbness in classic "stocking glove" pattern.
- Ototoxicity: Occurs in 10%–30% of patients.
- Reproductive: Pregnancy category D. Impotence and infertility can occur.

Initiate antiemetic protocol: Moderately to highly emetogenic protocol.

Supportive drugs:
☐ pegfilgrastim (Neulasta)   ☐ filgrastim (Neupogen)
☐ epoetin alfa (Procrit)   ☐ darbepoetin alfa (Aranesp)

Treatment schedule: Chair time 4 hours on day 1, and 3 hours on days 2–3. Repeat cycle for dacarbazine and cisplatin every 21 days, carmustine every 42 days.

Estimated number of visits: Four visits every 21-day cycle. Request four cycles worth of visits.

Dose Calculation by: 1. _____   2. _____

_____   _____
Physician   Date

_____   _____
Patient Name   ID Number

_____   _____/_____/_____   _____
Diagnosis   Ht   Wt   M²

DTIC + Cisplatin + BCNU + Tamoxifen

Baseline laboratory tests:	CBC: Chemistry (including Mg^{2+}) and LFTs
Baseline procedures or tests:	Pulmonary function tests, central line
Initiate IV:	NS
Premedicate:	5-HT3 and dexamethasone 20 mg in 100 cc of NS
Administer:	**Dacarbazine** _____ mg (220 mg/m^2) IV over 1 hour on days 1–3 and 22–24

- Available in 100- and 200-mg vials 10 mg/mL or
- Reconstitute with 9.9 mL sterile water, NS, or D5W to a final concentration of 10 mg/mL. Further dilute in D5W or NS 250–500 mL.
- **Vesicant**
- May cause vein burning/irritation if infused too rapidly.
- Reconstituted solution stable for 8 hours at room temperature, and 72 hours if refrigerated. If further diluted, solution is stable for 8 hours at room temperature and 24 hours refrigerated.

Cisplatin _____ mg (25 mg/m^2) IV in 1000 cc of NS over 1–2 hours on days 1–3 and 22–24.

- Available in 1-mg/1-mL solution. Multidose vial stable for 28 days under protected light or 7 days under fluorescent light.
- Do not use aluminum needles, because precipitate will form.
- Further dilute in 250 cc or more of NS.

Carmustine (BCNU) _____ mg (150 mg/m^2) IV on day 1

- Reconstitute with 3 mL of sterile diluent (dehydrated alcohol injection) supplied by the manufacturer.
- Further dilute with 27 mL of sterile water to a final concentration of 3.3 mg/mL.
- Further dilute with D5W for administraton.
- Stable for 8 hours at room temperature.

Tamoxifen 10-mg PO bid starting on day 4

Major Side Effects

- Flulike Symptoms: Fever, chills, headache, myalgias, and arthralgias. May last for several days after treatment.
- Bone Marrow Depression: Myelosuppression involving all blood elements. Delayed nadir with BCNU lasting 1–3 weeks.
- GI Toxicities: Nausea and vomiting can be severe with dacarbazine. Anorexia occurs in 46%–65% of patients and is cumulative and dose limiting. Taste alteration and xerostomia may occur. Diarrhea is rare.
- Renal/hepatic: Renal toxicity is uncommon and is manifested by mild proteinuria and hypocalcemia. Acute renal failure and nephrotic syndrome have been reported in rare instances. Mild transient elevations in serum transaminase levels. Dose-dependent toxicity observed more frequently in the presence of pre-existing liver abnormalities. Nephrotoxicity; can be prevented with vigorous hydration.
- Skin: Alopecia in 90% of patients taking DTIC. Dry skin, flushing, pruritus, photosensitivity, and irritation at injection site seen. Pain at injection site during dacarbazine infusion; phlebitis.
- Pulmonary Fibrosis: Patients receiving carmustine at cumulative doses 1400 mg/m^2 are at higher risk.
- Neurotoxicity: Peripheral neuropathy (sensory/motor) with cisplatin. Dose/duration dependent and progresses with continued therapy. Paresthesias and numbness in classic "stocking glove" pattern.
- Ototoxicity: Occurs in 10%–30% of patients.
- Hot Flashes: Occur in about 10% of patients and are usually not severe enough to discontinue therapy.
- Reproductive: Pregnancy category D. Impotence and infertility can occur.

Initiate antiemetic protocol: Moderately to highly emetogenic protocol.

Supportive drugs: ☐ pegfilgrastim (Neulasta)   ☐ filgrastim (Neupogen)
☐ epoetin alfa (Procrit)   ☐ darbepoetin alfa (Aranesp)

Treatment schedule: Chair time 4 hours on day 1, and 3 hours on days 2–3 and 22–24. Repeat cycle every 6 weeks.

Estimated number of visits: Seven visits per cycle. Request four cycles worth of visits.

Dose Calculation by: 1. _____   2. _____

_____

Physician   Date

_____

Patient Name   ID Number

_____

Diagnosis   Ht _____/ Wt _____/ M²

Cisplatin + Vinblastine + Dacarbazine (CVD)

Baseline laboratory tests:	CBC: Chemistry panel (including Mg^{2+})
Baseline procedures:	Central line placement
Premedicate:	5-HT_3 and dexamethasone 20 mg in 100 cc of NS.
Initiate IV:	NS

Cisplatin_____ mg (20 mg/m^2) IV in 1000 cc of NS over 1–2 hours days 1–5

- Available in 1-mg/1-mL solution. Multidose vial stable for 28 days under protected light or 7 days under fluorescent light.
- Do not use aluminum needles, because precipitate will form.
- Further dilute in 250 cc or more of NS

Vinblastine _____ mg (1.6 mg/m^2) IV on days 1–5

- Vesicant
- Available in 10-mg vials. 1 mg/mL. Store in refrigerator until use.

Dacarbazine (DTIC)_____ mg (800 mg/m^2) IV on day 1

- Available in 100- and 200-mg vials 10 mg/mL or
- Reconstitute with 9.9 mL sterile water, NS, or D5W to a final concentration of 10 mg/mL. Further dilute in D5W or NS 250–500 mL.
- Vesicant
- May cause vein burning/irritation if infused too rapidly. Reconstituted solution stable for 8 hours at room temperature, and 72 hours if refrigerated. If further diluted, solution is stable for 8 hours at room temperature and 24 hours refrigerated.

Major Side Effects

- Flulike Symptoms: Fever, chills, headache, myalgias, and arthralgias.
- Bone Marrow Depression: Dose limiting toxicity, nadir at 21–25 days with DTIC, days 4–6 with vinblastine.
- GI Toxicities: Nausea and vomiting can be severe with dacarbazine. Anorexia occurs in 46%–65% of patients and is cumulative and dose limiting. Taste alteration and xerostomia may occur. Diarrhea is rare.
- Renal/hepatic: Renal toxicity is uncommon and is manifested by mild proteinuria and hypocalcemia. Acute renal failure and nephrotic syndrome have been reported in rare instances. Mild transient elevations in serum transaminase levels. Dose-dependent toxicity observed more frequently in the presence of pre-existing liver abnormalities. Nephrotoxicity; can be prevented with vigorous hydration.
- Skin: Alopecia in 90% of patients taking DTIC. Dry skin, flushing, pruritus, photosensitivity, and irritation at injection site seen. Pain at injection site during dacarbazine infusion; phlebitis.
- CNS Toxicity: Peripheral neuropathy (paresthesias, paralysis, and loss of deep tendon reflexes and constipation). Paralytic ileus and urinary retention.
- Neurotoxicity: Peripheral neuropathy (sensory/motor). Dose/duration dependent and progresses with continued therapy.
- Ototoxicity: Occurs in 10%–30% of patients.
- Reproductive: Pregnancy category D. Impotence and infertility can occur.

Initiate antiemetic protocol:	Moderately to highly emetogenic protocol
Supportive drugs:	☐ pegfilgrastim (Neulasta) ☐ filgrastim (Neupogen)
	☐ epoetin alfa (Procrit) ☐ darbepoetin alfa (Aranesp)
Treatment schedule:	Chair time 5 hours on day 1, and 3 hours on days 2–5. Repeat cycle every 21–28 days.
Estimated number of visits:	Five visits per cycle. Request four cycles worth of visits.

Dose Calculation by: 1. _____   2. _____

_____

Physician   Date

_____

Patient Name   ID Number

_____   _____/_____/_____   _____

Diagnosis   Ht   Wt   M^2

Interferon (IFN) + DTIC

Baseline laboratory tests:	CBC: Chemistry panel and LFTs
Baseline procedures:	Central line placement
Initiate IV:	NS
Premedicate:	5-HT$_3$ in 100 cc of NS (add dexamethasone if indicated)
	Acetaminophen 650 mg 30 minute before treatment and q 4 hours **may alternate with** Ibuprofen 400-mg PO q 4 hours

Administer:

Induction: **Interferon-α-2b** _____ MU (15 MU/m^2) IV on days 1–5, 8–12, and 15–19

- **DO NOT USE D5W.**
- Use only Intron A powder (interferon-α-2b). Premixed solutions should not be used because of the amount of preservative in the premixed solution.
- More hydration and additional antiemetics may be needed toward the end of the patient's therapy or if they are having difficulty taking fluids.

Then

Maintenance therapy

Interferon-α-2b _____ MU (10 MU/m^2) SC (TIW—three times per week) after induction therapy

- Available in multidose pens with 6 doses of 3 MU (18 MU) or 5 MU (30 MU) or 10 MU (60 MU). Keep refrigerated.

Dacarbazine (DTIC) _____ mg (200 mg/m^2) IV on days 22–26

- Available in 100- and 200-mg vials 10 mg/mL or
- Reconstitute with 9.9 mL sterile water, NS, or D5W to a final concentration of 10 mg/mL. Further dilute in D5W or NS 250–500 mL.
- **Vesicant**
- May cause vein burning/irritation if infused too rapidly.
- Reconstituted solution stable for 8 hours at room temperature, and 72 hours if refrigerated. If further diluted, solution is stable for 8 hours at room temperature and 24 hours refrigerated.

Major Side Effects

- Flulike Symptoms: Fever, chills, headache, myalgias, and arthralgias. Occur in 80%–90% of patients. Onset 3–4 hours after injection and lasting for up to 8–9 hours. Incidence decreases with subsequent injections. Symptoms can be managed with acetaminophen and increased PO fluid intake.
- Bone Marrow Depression: Dose limiting toxicity, nadir at 21–25 days with DTIC, days 4–6 with vinblastine.
- GI Toxicities: Nausea and diarrhea are mild, vomiting is rare with interferon. Moderate to severe with dacarbazine. Anorexia occurs in 46%–65% of patients and is cumulative and dose limiting. Taste alteration and xerostomia may occur.
- Renal/hepatic: Renal toxicity is uncommon and is manifested by mild proteinuria and hypocalcemia. Acute renal failure and nephrotic syndrome have been reported in rare instances. Mild transient elevations in serum transaminase levels. Dose-dependent toxicity observed more frequently in the presence of pre-existing liver abnormalities.
- Skin: Alopecia in 90% of patients taking DTIC. Dry skin, flushing, pruritus, photosensitivity, and irritation at injection site seen. Pain at injection site during dacarbazine infusion; phlebitis.
- Reproductive: Pregnancy category D. Breast feeding should be avoided.

Initiate antiemetic protocol:	Mildly emetogenic protocol.
Supportive drugs:	☐ pegfilgrastim (Neulasta) ☐ filgrastim (Neupogen)
	☐ epoetin alfa (Procrit) ☐ darbepoetin alfa (Aranesp)
Treatment schedule:	1 hour on days 1–5, 8–12, and 15–19; 2 hours on days 22–26. Repeat cycle every 28 days.
Estimated number of visits:	20 visits first month, and every 1–2 weeks after.

Dose Calculation by: 1. _____   2. _____

_____   _____
Physician   Date

_____   _____
Patient Name   ID Number

_____   _____/_____/_____
Diagnosis   Ht   Wt   M^2

Cisplatin + Vinblastine + Dacarbazine + IL-2 + Interferon

Baseline laboratory tests:	CBC: Chemistry panel (including Mg^{2+})
Baseline procedures or tests:	Central line placement for continuous infusion
Premedicate:	5-HT$_3$ and dexamethasone 20 mg in 100 cc of NS over 30 minutes.
Initiate IV:	NS

Administer:

Cisplatin_____ mg (20 mg/m^2) IV in 1000 cc of NS over 1–2 hours on days 1–4 and 22–25

- Available in 1-mg/1-mL solution. Multidose vial stable for 28 days under protected light or 7 days under fluorescent light.
- Do not use aluminum needles, because precipitate will form.
- Further dilute in 250 cc or more of NS.

Vinblastine _____ mg (1.5 mg/m^2) IV on days 1–4 and 22–25

- Vesicant
- Available in 10-mg vials. 1-mg/1-mL concentration.
- Store in refrigerator until use.

Dacarbazine (DTIC)_____ mg (800 mg/m^2) IV in 500 mL of NS over 1–2 hours on days 1 and 22

- Vesicant
- Reconstitute with sterile water, NS, or D5W to a final concentration of 10 mg/mL. (May cause vein burning/irritation if infused too rapidly.)
- Reconstituted solution stable for 8 hours at room temperature, and 72 hours if refrigerated. If further diluted, solution is stable for 8 hours at room temperature and 24 hours refrigerated.

Interleukin-2 _____MU (9 MU/m^2) IV as a 24-hour continuous infusion on days 5–8 and 17–20

- Available in 22 MU single dose vials; discard unused portion.
- Reconstituted solution stable for 48 hours refrigerated.

IL-2 will be administered in the hospital—high dose.

Interferon-α-2b _____MU (5 MU/m^2) SC on days 5–9, 17–21, and 26–30

- Available in multidose pens with 6 doses of 3 MU (18 MU) or 5 MU (30 MU) or 10 MU (60 MU). Keep refrigerated.

Major Side Effects

- Flulike Syndrome: Chills, rigor, fever, and headache. Myalgia and arthralgias
- Myelosuppression: Dose-limiting toxicity, nadir day 4–6 with vinblastine and day 21–25 with DTIC.
- GI Toxicities: Moderate-to-severe nausea and vomiting. Can be acute or delayed with severity and intensity decreasing with subsequent doses.
- Neurotoxicity: Peripheral neuropathy (sensory/motor). Dose/duration dependent and progresses with continued therapy.
- Renal: Nephrotoxicity, can be prevented with vigorous hydration. Oliguria, proteinuria, elevated creatinine, tubular cell injury, and decreased renal blood flow with IL-2.
- Hepatic: Hepatomegaly and hypoalbuminemia and elevated LFT results may occur. Hold drug for signs of hepatic failure including encephalopathy, increasing ascites, liver pain, or hypoglycemia
- Capillary Leak Syndrome: Peripheral edema, CHF, pleural effusions, and pericardial effusions. Decreased systemic vascular resistance and hypotension, which can cause decreased renal perfusion. Extravasation of protein and fluid into extravascular space. Strict I & O, vital signs every 2–4 hours.
- Ototoxicity: Occurs in 10%–30% of patients.
- Skin: Diffuse erythematous rash, which may desquamate. Pruritus and alopecia.
- Reproductive: Pregnancy category D. Breast feeding should be avoided.

Initiate antiemetic protocol: Moderately to highly emetogenic protocol.

Supportive drugs: ☐ pegfilgrastim (Neulasta) ☐ filgrastim (Neupogen)
 ☐ epoetin alfa (Procrit) ☐ darbepoetin alfa (Aranesp)

Treatment schedule: Chair time 5 hours on days 1 and 22, and 3 hours on days 2–4 and 23–25. Repeat cycle every 6 weeks.

Estimated number of visits: Ten visits per cycle. Request four cycles worth of visits. Preauthorize prn hospital admission.

Dose Calculation by: 1. _____ 2. _____

_____ _____

Physician Date

_____ _____

Patient Name ID Number

_____ / _____ / _____

Diagnosis Ht Wt M^2

Temozolomide + Thalidomide

Baseline laboratory tests:	CBC: Chemistry and LFTs
Baseline procedures or tests:	N/A
Initiate IV:	N/A
Premedicate:	Oral phenothiazine or 5-HT$_3$
	Warfarin 2-mg PO qd to decrease risk of thromboembolic complications (if physician orders)

Administer:

Temozolomide _____ mg (75 mg/m^2/day) PO for six weeks

- Available in 5-, 20-, 100-, and 250-mg capsules for oral use.
- Store at room temperature; protect from light and moisture.

Thalidomide _____ mg (200–400 mg/m^2/day) PO for 6 weeks

- Requires registration with Celgene (Summit, NJ) STEPS program and authorization number for each 28-day prescription.
- Available in 50-, 100-, and 200-mg capsules.
- Store in a cool, dry place and protect from light.

Major Side Effects

- Teratogenic Effect: Most serious toxicity of thalidomide. Severe birth defects or death to an unborn fetus. Manifested as absent or defective limbs, hypoplasia or absence of bones, facial palsy, absent or small ears, absent or shrunken eyes, congenital heart defects, and gastrointestinal and renal abnormalities.
- Bone Marrow Depression: Myelosuppression is dose-limiting toxicity with leukopenia more frequent than thrombocytopenia. Nadir day 28–29. Anemia may also occur. Does not usually require granulocyte colony stimulating factor (G-CSF) administration.
- GI Toxicities: Nausea and vomiting occur in 75% of patients, usually mild to moderate, occurring on day 1. Diarrhea, constipation, and/or anorexia may affect up to 40% of patients. Constipation is primary GI toxicity with thalidomide.
- Cardiovascular Toxicities: Increase risk of thromboembolic complications, including deep vein thrombosis and pulmonary embolism. See earlier warfarin recommendation.
- Neurotoxicities: Fatigue, orthostatic hypotension, and dizziness. Peripheral neuropathy in the form of numbness, tingling, and pain in the feet or hands. Does not appear to be dose or duration related. Daytime sedation.
- Skin: Maculopapular skin rash, urticaria, and dry skin. Stevens-Johnson syndrome reported. Thalidomide should be discontinued if patients develop a skin rash. Therapy can be restarted with caution if the rash was not exfoliative, purpuric, bullous, or otherwise suggestive of a serious skin condition.

Initiate antiemetic protocol:	Mildly to moderately emetogenic protocol.
Supportive drugs:	☐ pegfilgrastim (Neulasta) ☐ filgrastim (Neupogen)
	☐ loperamide (Imodium) ☐ epoetin alfa (Procrit)
	☐ darbepoetin alfa (Aranesp) ☐ diphenoxylate/atropine sulfate (Lomotil)
Treatment schedule:	No chair time. Repeat cycle every 10 weeks until disease progression.
Estimated number of visits:	One visit per month.

Dose Calculation by: 1. _____   2. _____

_____
Physician

_____
Patient Name

_____
Diagnosis

_____
Date

_____
ID Number

_____/ _____/ _____
Ht   Wt   M^2

Single-Agent Regimens

Dacarbazine (DTIC)

Baseline laboratory tests:	CBC: Chemistry panel and LFTs
Baseline procedures or tests:	N/A
Initiate IV:	0.9% sodium chloride
Premedicate:	5-HT$_3$ and dexamethasone 10–20 mg in 100 cc of NS

Administer:

Dacarbazine _____ mg (250 mg/m^2) IV on days 1–5
Repeat cycle every 21 days.
OR
Dacarbazine _____ mg (850 mg/m^2) IV on day 1
Repeat cycle every 3–6 weeks

- Available in 100- and 200-mg vials 10 mg/mL or
- Reconstitute with 9.9 mL sterile water, NS, or D5W to a final concentration of 10 mg/mL. Further dilute in D5W or NS 250–500 mL.
- **Vesicant**
- May cause vein burning/irritation if infused too rapidly.
- Stable for 8 hours at room temperature, and 72 hours if refrigerated.

Major Side Effects

- Bone Marrow Suppression: Myelosuppression is a dose-limiting toxicity. Leukopenia and thrombocytopenia are equally affected, with nadir occurring at 21–25 days.
- GI Toxicities: Nausea and vomiting are moderate to severe. Onset is usually 1–3 hours after treatment and lasts for up to 12 hours. Decreases with each consecutive day of therapy. Diarrhea is uncommon. Anorexia is common.
- Hepatic: Hepatotoxicity is rare, but hepatic veno-occlusive disease has been described.
- Central Nervous System (CNS) Toxicity: Paresthesias, neuropathies, ataxia, lethargy, headache, confusion, and seizures have all been observed.
- Flulike Syndrome: Malaise, headache, myalgia, hypotension. May occur up to 7 days after first dose, lasts 7–21 days, and may recur with subsequent dosing.
- Skin: Pain at injection site during infusion, erythema and urticaria, phlebitis. Alopecia likely. Photosensitization may occur.
- Reproductive: Drug is teratogenic, mutagenic, and carcinogenic.

Initiate antiemetic protocol:	Moderately to highly emetogenic protocol.
Supportive drugs:	☐ pegfilgrastim (Neulasta) ☐ filgrastim (Neupogen)
	☐ epoetin alfa (Procrit) ☐ darbepoetin alfa (Aranesp)
Treatment schedule:	Chair time 2 hours on days 1–5. Repeat cycle every 21 days.
	OR
	Chair time 3 hours on day 2. Repeat cycle every 3–6 weeks.
Estimated number of visits:	Five visits per cycle. Request three cycles worth of visits.
	OR
	One visit per cycle. Request three cycles worth of visits.

Dose Calculation by: 1. _____   2. _____

_____
Physician

_____
Date

_____
Patient Name

_____
ID Number

_____
Diagnosis

_____ / _____ / _____
Ht   Wt   M^2

Interferon (Melanoma)

Baseline laboratory tests:	CBC: Chemistry (including LFTs)
Baseline procedures or tests:	N/A
Initiate IV:	NS
Premedicate:	Oral phenothiazine or 5-HT$_3$
	Acetaminophen 650 mg 30 minutes before treatment and q 4 hours
	may alternate with
	Ibuprofen 400-mg PO q 4 hours

Administer: **Interferon-α-2b** _____MU (20 MU/m^2) IM three times per week × 12 weeks

- Available in solution form in single-dose vials of 3, 6, 9, and 36 MU.
- DO NOT freeze or shake vials.
- Stable for 1 month under refrigeration.

Major Side Effects

- Flulike Symptoms: Fever, chills, headache, myalgias, and arthralgias. Occurs in 80%–90% of patients. Onset 3–4 hours after injection and lasting for up to 8–9 hours. Incidence decreases with subsequent injections. Symptoms can be managed with acetaminophen, ibuprofen, and/or indomethacin and increased oral fluid intake.
- Bone Marrow Depression: Myelosuppression with mild leukopenia and thrombocytopenia. Cumulative effect, dose-limiting thrombocytopenia; reversible.
- GI Toxicities: Nausea and diarrhea are mild, and vomiting is rare. Anorexia occurs in 46%–65% of patients and is cumulative and dose limiting. Taste alteration and xerostomia may occur.
- Renal/hepatic: Renal toxicity is uncommon and is manifested by mild proteinuria and hypocalcemia. Acute renal failure and nephrotic syndrome have been reported in rare instances. Mild transient elevations in serum transaminase levels. Dose-dependent toxicity observed more frequently in the presence of pre-existing liver abnormalities.
- Cardiotoxicity: Chest pain, arrhythmias, and CHF are rare.
- Skin: Alopecia is partial. Dry skin, pruritus, and irritation at injection site seen.
- Reproductive: Pregnancy category D. Breast feeding should be avoided.

Initiate antiemetic protocol:	Mildly emetogenic protocol.
Supportive drugs:	☐ pegfilgrastim (Neulasta) ☐ filgrastim (Neupogen)
	☐ epoetin alfa (Procrit) ☐ darbepoetin alfa (Aranesp)
Treatment schedule:	Chair time 1 hour on day 1 for injection teaching. Cycle is TIW × 12 weeks.
Estimated number of visits:	One visit weekly if doing own injection (total 12 visits); 36 visits if not.

Dose Calculation by: 1. _____   2. _____

_____   _____

Physician   Date

_____   _____

Patient Name   ID Number

_____   _____/ _____/ _____

Diagnosis   Ht   Wt   M^2

Aldesleukin (IL-2)

Baseline laboratory tests:	CBC: Chemistry (including LFTs)
Baseline procedures or tests:	Pulmonary function tests
Initiate IV:	NS
Premedicate:	5-HT$_3$ in 100 cc of NS

Acetaminophen 650 mg 30 minutes before treatment and q 4 hours

may alternate with

Ibuprofen 400-mg PO q 4 hours

Administer: **Aldesleukin** _____ IU (100,000 IU/kg) IV over 15 minutes on days 1–5 and 15–19

- Available in vials containing 22 MU (1.3 mg).
- Reconstituted with 1.2 mL of sterile water for injection so that each mL contains 18 IU.
- DO NOT SHAKE.
- Further dilute in 50 mL of D5W.
- Refrigerate and use within 48 hours.

Major Side Effects

- Flulike Symptoms: Chills, rigors, fever (102°–104°) and headache. Myalgia and arthralgias may occur at high doses because of accumulation of cytokine deposits/lymphocytes in joint spaces.
- CNS Toxicities: Confusion, irritability, disorientation, impaired memory, expressive aphasia, sleep disturbances, depression, hallucinations, and psychoses may occur, resolving within 24–48 hours after last drug dose.
- Capillary Leak Syndrome: Peripheral edema, CHF, pleural effusions, and pericardial effusions may occur and are reversible once treatment is stopped. IL-2 causes peripheral vasodilation, decreased systemic vascular resistance, and hypotension that may lead to decreased renal perfusion. A decrease in systolic blood pressure occurs 2–12 hours after start of therapy and typically progresses to significant hypotension with hypoperfusion. In addition, protein and fluid extravasate into the extravascular space, forming edema and new effusions. Strict I and O, vital signs 2–4 hours.
- GI Toxicities: Nausea and vomiting are mild. Diarrhea is common, can be severe, and may require bicarbonate replacement. Stomatitis is common but mild.
- Renal/hepatic Toxicity: IL-2 causes direct tubular cell injury and decreased renal blood flow with cumulative doses. Oliguria, proteinuria, increased creatinine, and LFTs. Anuria occurs in 38% of patients; is reversible after drug discontinuance. Hepatomegaly and hypoalbuminemia may occur.
- Bone Marrow Toxicity: Severe anemia, requiring transfusion. Thrombocytopenia common but rarely requires transfusion.
- Skin: Diffuse erythematous rash which may desquamate. Pruritus.
- Reproductive: Pregnancy category D. Breast feeding should be avoided.

Initiate antiemetic protocol:	Mildly emetogenic protocol.
Supportive drugs:	☐ pegfilgrastim (Neulasta) ☐ filgrastim (Neupogen)
	☐ epoetin alfa (Procrit) ☐ darbepoetin alfa (Aranesp)
Treatment schedule:	Usually administered in hospital setting. Chair time 1 hour on days 1–5 and 15–19. Repeat cycle every 28 days.
Estimated number of visits:	Ten visits every cycle. Request four cycles worth of visits.

Dose Calculation by: 1. _____   2. _____

_____   _____
Physician   Date

_____   _____
Patient Name   ID Number

_____   _____/ _____/ _____
Diagnosis   Ht   Wt   M^2

Temozolomide

Baseline laboratory tests:	CBC: Chemistry and LFTs
Baseline procedures or tests:	N/A
Initiate IV:	N/A
Premedicate:	Oral phenothiazine or 5-HT$_3$
Administer:	**Temozolomide** _____ mg (150 mg/m^2) PO on days 1–5

- If well tolerated, can increase dose to 200-mg/m^2 PO on days 1–5.
- Available in 5-, 20-, 100-, and 250-mg capsules for oral use.
- Store at room temperature; protect from light and moisture.

Major Side Effects

- Bone Marrow Depression: Myelosuppression is dose-limiting toxicity, with leukopenia more frequent than thrombocytopenia. Nadir day 28–29. Anemia may also occur. Does not usually require G-CSF administration.
- GI Toxicities: Nausea and vomiting occur in 75% of patients, usually mild to moderate and occurring on day 1. Diarrhea, constipation, and/or anorexia may affect up to 40% of patients.
- Skin: Photosensitivity. Rash, itching, and mild alopecia may occur and are mild.

Initiate antiemetic protocol:	Mildly to moderately emetogenic protocol.
Supportive drugs:	☐ pegfilgrastim (Neulasta)　　☐ filgrastim (Neupogen)
	☐ loperamide (Imodium)　　☐ epoetin alfa (Procrit)
	☐ darbepoetin alfa (Aranesp)　　☐ diphenoxylate/atropine sulfate (Lomotil)
Treatment schedule:	No chair time. Repeat cycle every 28 days until disease progression.
Estimated number of visits:	One to 2 visits per month.

Dose Calculation by:　1. _____　2. _____

_____

Physician _____　　　　Date _____

_____

Patient Name _____　　ID Number _____

_____

Diagnosis _____　　Ht _____/ Wt _____/ M^2 _____

MALIGNANT MESOTHELIOMA

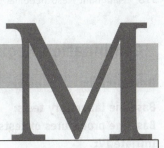

Combination Regimens

Doxorubicin + Cisplatin 518

Doxorubicin: 60-mg/m^2 IV on day 1
Cisplatin: 60-mg/m^2 IV on day 1
Repeat cycle every 21–28 days.[1,321]

CAP 519

Cyclophosphamide: 500-mg/m^2 IV on day 1
Doxorubicin: 50-mg/m^2 IV on day 1
Cisplatin: 80-mg/m^2 IV on day 1
Repeat cycle every 21 days.[1,322]

Gemcitabine + Cisplatin 520

Gemcitabine: 1000-mg/m^2 IV on days 1, 8, and 15
Cisplatin: 100-mg/m^2 IV on day 1
Repeat cycle every 28 days.[1,323]

Gemcitabine + Carboplatin...521

Gemcitabine: 1000-mg/m^2 IV on days 1, 8, and 15
Carboplatin: AUC of 5, IV on day 1
Repeat cycle every 28 days.[1,324]

Pemetrexed (Alimta) + Cisplatin 522

Pemetrexed: 500 mg/m^2 IV over 10 minutes on day 1
Cisplatin: 75-mg/m^2 IV over 2 hours on day 1
Repeat every 21 days.[1,325]

Combination Regimens

Doxorubicin + Cisplatin

Baseline laboratory tests:	CBC: Chemistry (including Mg^{2+})
Baseline procedures or tests:	Multigated angiogram (MUGA) scan
Initiate IV:	0.9% sodium chloride
Premedicate:	5-HT$_3$ and dexamethasone 20 mg in 100 cc of NS.
Administer:	**Doxorubicin** _____ mg (60 mg/m^2) IV on day 1

- **Potent vesicant**
- Available as a 2-mg/mL solution.
- Doxorubicin will form a precipitate if it is mixed with heparin or 5-FU.

Cisplatin _____ mg (60 mg/m^2) IV on day 1

- Do not use aluminum needles, because precipitate will form.
- Available in solution as 1 mg/mL.
- Further dilute solution with 250 cc or more of NS.

Major Side Effects

- Bone Marrow Depression: Leukopenia, thrombocytopenia, and anemia all can occur; may be severe.
- GI Toxicities: Nausea and vomiting are moderate to severe and can be acute or delayed. Stomatitis occurs in 10% of patients but is not dose limiting.
- Cardiac: Acutely, pericarditis-myocarditis syndrome may occur. With high cumulative doses > 550 mg/m^2, cardiomyopathy may occur.
- Renal: Nephrotoxicity is dose related with cisplatin and presents at 10–20 days. Risk may be reduced with adequate hydration.
- Electrolyte Imbalance: Decreased Mg^{2+}, K, Ca^{2+}, Na^+, and P.
- Skin: Extravasation of doxorubicin causes severe tissue destruction. Hyperpigmentation, photosensitivity, and radiation recall occur. Complete alopecia occurs with doses > 50 mg/m^2.
- Neurotoxicity: Dose-limiting toxicity, usually in the form of peripheral sensory neuropathy. Paresthesias and numbness in a classic "stocking glove" pattern. Risk increases with cumulative doses.
- Ototoxicity: High-frequency hearing loss and tinnitus with cisplatin.
- Reproductive: Pregnancy category D. Breast feeding should be avoided.

Initiate antiemetic protocol:	Moderately to highly emetogenic protocol.
Supportive drugs:	☐ pegfilgrastim (Neulasta) ☐ filgrastim (Neupogen)
	☐ epoetin alfa (Procrit) ☐ darbepoetin alfa (Aranesp)
Treatment schedule:	Chair time 3 hours on day 1. Repeat cycle every 21–28 days.
Estimated number of visits:	One per cycle. Request four cycles worth of visits.

Dose Calculation by: 1. _____   2. _____

_____
Physician

_____
Patient Name

_____
Diagnosis

_____
Date

_____
ID Number

_____ / _____ / _____
Ht   Wt   M^2

Cyclophosphamide + Doxorubicin + Cisplatin (CAP) Mesothelioma

Baseline laboratory tests:	CBC: Chemistry (including Mg^{2+})
Baseline procedures or tests:	N/A
Initiate IV:	0.9% sodium chloride
Premedicate:	5-HT$_3$ and dexamethasone 10–20 mg in 100 cc of NS
Administer:	**Cyclophosphamide** _____ mg (500 mg/m^2) IV on day 1

- Available in 100-, 200-, 500-, 1000-, and 2000-mg vials.
- Dilute with sterile water. Shake well to ensure that all particles completely dissolve.
- Reconstituted solution is stable for 24 hours at room temperature and for 6 days refrigerated.

Doxorubicin _____ mg (50 mg/m^2) IV on day 1

- **Potent vesicant**
- Available as a 2-mg/mL solution.
- Doxorubicin will form a precipitate if it is mixed with heparin or 5-FU.

Cisplatin _____ mg (80 mg/m^2) IV over 1–3 hours on day 1

- Do not use aluminum needles, because precipitate will form.
- Available in solution as 1 mg/mL.
- Further dilute solution with 250 cc or more of NS.

Major Side Effects

- Bone Marrow Depression: Neutropenia, thrombocytopenia, and anemia occur equally in 25%–30% of patients. Leukopenia and thrombocytopenia are dose related.
- GI Toxicities: Moderate-to-severe nausea and vomiting. May be acute (first 24 hours) or delayed (> 24 hours). Mucositis can occur.
- GU Toxicities: Nephrotoxicity is dose related with cisplatin and presents at 10–20 days. Bladder toxicity in the form of hemorrhagic cystitis, dysuria, and increased urinary frequency. Provide adequate hydration. Red-orange discoloration of urine for up to 48 hours.
- Electrolyte Imbalance: Decreased Mg^{2+}, K, Ca^{2+}, Na^+, and P.
- Cardiotoxicity: Acutely, pericarditis or myocarditis may occur. Later, cardiomyopathy in the form of CHF may occur.
- Neurotoxicity: Dose-limiting toxicity, usually in the form of peripheral sensory neuropathy. Paresthesias and numbness in a classic "stocking glove" pattern.
- Ototoxicity: High-frequency hearing loss and tinnitus.
- Skin: Extravasation of doxorubicin causes severe tissue damage. Hyperpigmentation, photosensitivity, and radiation recall occur. Alopecia.
- Reproductive: Pregnancy category D. Breast feeding should be avoided.

Initiate antiemetic protocol:	Moderately to highly emetogenic protocol.
Supportive drugs:	☐ pegfilgrastim (Neulasta) ☐ filgrastim (Neupogen)
	☐ epoetin alfa (Procrit) ☐ darbepoetin alfa (Aranesp)
Treatment schedule:	Chair time 3 hours on day 1. Repeat cycle every 28 days.
Estimated number of visits:	One visit per cycle. Request six cycles worth of visits.

Dose Calculation by: 1. _____   2. _____

_____   _____

Physician   Date

_____   _____

Patient Name   ID Number

_____   _____/ _____/ _____

Diagnosis   Ht   Wt M^2

Gemcitabine + Cisplatin

Baseline laboratory tests:	CBC: Chemistry panel (including Mg^{2+}) and LFTs
Baseline procedures or tests:	N/A
Initiate IV:	0.9% sodium chloride
Premedicate:	5-HT_3 and dexamethasone 10–20 mg in 100 cc of NS
Administer:	**Gemcitabine** _____ mg (1000 mg/m^2) IV on days 1, 8, and 15

Available in 1-g or 200-mg vials; reconstitute with 0.9% sodium chloride USP (5 cc for 200 mg, 25 cc for 1 g). Further dilute in 0.9% sodium chloride.

- Reconstituted solution is stable 24 hours at room temperature. DO NOT refrigerate, because precipitate will form.

Cisplatin _____ mg (100 mg/m^2) IV on day 1

- Do not use aluminum needles, because precipitate will form.
- Further dilute solution with 250 cc or more of 0.9% sodium chloride.

Major Side Effects

- Hematologic: Leukopenia (63%), thrombocytopenia (36%), and anemia (73%), with grades 3 and 4 thrombocytopenia more common in elderly patients. Myelosuppression is dose limiting. Nadir occurs in 10–14 days, with recovery at 21 days. Prolonged infusion time of gemcitabine (> 60 minutes) is associated with higher toxicities.

- GI Symptoms: Moderate to severe nausea and vomiting; may be acute or delayed. Diarrhea and/or mucositis (15%–20%).

- Flulike Syndrome (20%) with fever in absence of infection 6–12 hours after treatment (40%).

- Renal: Nephrotoxicity is dose related with cisplatin and occurs at 10–20 days. Can be avoided with adequate hydration, diuresis, as well as slower infusion time.

- Neurotoxicity: Severe neuropathy with numbness, tingling, and sensory loss in classic "stocking glove" distribution. Risk increases with cumulative doses. Proprioception, vibrating sense, and motor function can occur. Ototoxicity occurs in 30% beginning with high frequency hearing.

- Electrolyte Imbalance: Decreased Mg^{2+}, K, Ca^{2+}, Na^+, and P.

- Hepatic: Elevation of serum transaminase and bilirubin levels.

- Skin: Pruritic, maculopapular skin rash, usually involving trunk and extremities. Edema occurs in 30% of patients. Alopecia.

- Reproduction: Pregnancy category D. Breast feeding should be avoided.

Initiate antiemetic protocol:	Moderately to highly emetogenic protocol.
Supportive drugs:	☐ pegfilgrastim (Neulasta) ☐ filgrastim (Neupogen)
	☐ epoetin alfa (Procrit) ☐ darbepoetin alfa (Aranesp)
Treatment schedule:	Chair time 3 hours on day 1, and 1 hour on days 8 and 15. Repeat cycle every 28 days.
Estimated number of visits:	Three visits per cycle. Request three cycles worth of visits.

Dose Calculation by: 1. _____ 2. _____

_____

Physician

_____

Patient Name

_____

Diagnosis

_____

Date

_____

ID Number

_____ / _____ / _____
Ht   Wt   M^2

Gemcitabine + Carboplatin

Baseline laboratory tests:	CBC: Chemistry panel (with LFTs)
Baseline procedures or tests:	N/A
Initiate IV:	0.9% sodium chloride
Premedicate:	5-HT$_3$ and dexamethasone 10–20 mg in 100 cc of NS
	Diphenhydramine 25–50 mg and cimetidine 300 mg in 100 cc of NS

Administer:

Gemcitabine _____ mg (1000 mg/m^2) IV on days 1, 8, and 15

- Available in 1-g or 200-mg vials; reconstitute with 0.9% sodium chloride (5 cc for 200 mg and 25 cc for 1 g). Further dilute in 0.9% sodium chloride.
- Reconstituted solution is stable 24 hours at room temperature.
- Do not refrigerate, because precipitate will form.

Carboplatin _____ mg (area under the curve [AUC] 5) IV on day 1.

- Do not use aluminum needles, because precipitate will form.
- Available in powder or solution. Discard reconstituted powder after 8 hours.

Major Side Effects

- Hypersensitivity Reaction: Rash, urticaria, erythema, and pruritus. Bronchospasm and hypotension are uncommon, but risk increases in patients receiving more than seven courses of carboplatin therapy.
- Bone Marrow Depression: Neutropenia, thrombocytopenia, and anemia are cumulative and dose related. Can be dose limiting. G-CSF recommended.
- GI Toxicities: Moderate to severe nausea and vomiting, acute or delayed. Mucositis and diarrhea seen. Elevation of serum transaminase and bilirubin levels.
- Flulike Syndrome: Flulike symptoms with fever in absence of infection 6–12 hours after treatment.
- Renal: Nephrotoxicity less common than with cisplatin and rarely symptomatic.
- Electrolyte Imbalance: Decreases Mg^{2+}, K+, Ca^{2+}, Na$^+$ and PO^4
- Neurotoxicity: Sensory neuropathy with numbness and paresthesias.
- Skin: Pruritic, maculopapular skin rash, usually involving trunk and extremities. Edema occurs in 30% of patients. Alopecia.
- Reproductive: Pregnancy category D. Breast feeding should be avoided.

Initiate antiemetic protocol:	Moderately to highly emetogenic protocol.
Supportive drugs:	☐ pegfilgrastim (Neulasta) ☐ filgrastim (Neupogen)
	☐ epoetin alfa (Procrit) ☐ darbepoetin alfa (Aranesp)
Treatment schedule:	Chair time 2 hours on day 1, and 1 hour on days 8 and 15. Repeat cycle every 28 days.
Estimated number of visits:	Two visits per cycle. Request four cycles worth of visits.

Dose Calculation by: 1. _____   2. _____

Physician _____   Date _____

Patient Name _____   ID Number _____

Diagnosis _____   Ht _____ / Wt _____ / M^2 _____

Pemetrexed + Cisplatin

Baseline laboratory tests:	CBC: Chemistry (including Mg^{2+}) and carcinoembryonic antigen (CEA)
Baseline procedures or tests:	N/A
Initiate IV:	0.9% sodium chloride
Premedicate:	5-HT_3 in 100 cc of NS

Dexamethasone 4-mg PO bid for 3 days, starting the day before treatment

Folic acid 1-mg PO qd, starting 5 days before the first treatment ending 21 days after the last dose of pemetrexed.

Vitamin B^{12} 1000 mcg IM during the week preceding the first dose and every three cycles thereafter (may be given the same day as pemetrexed from second dose on)

Administer:

Pemetrexed _____ mg (500 mg/m²) IV in 100 cc of NS over 10 minutes on day 1

- Available in 500-mg single-use vials for reconstitution.
- Reconstitute with 20 mL of 0.9% sodium chloride (preservative free) for a final concentration of 25 mg/mL.
- Further dilute in 100 cc of NS.
- Discard any unused portion.

Cisplatin _____ mg (75 mg/m²) IV over 2 hours on day 1, approximately 30 minutes after the end of pemetrexed administration

- Do not use aluminum needles, because precipitate will form.
- Available in solution as 1 mg/mL.
- Further dilute solution with 250 cc or more of NS.

Major Side Effects

- Bone Marrow Toxicities: Myelosuppression is dose-limiting toxicity. Dose reductions or treatment delay may be necessary for subsequent doses. Administer vitamin B12 and folic acid supplements to minimize hematologic toxicities.
- GI Toxicities: Moderate to severe nausea and vomiting. May be acute (first 24 hours) or delayed (> 24 hours). Anorexia, stomatitis, and pharyngitis may occur. Instruct patient to take vitamin B12 and folic acid supplements to minimize GI toxicities. Patients with hepatic impairment may require dose adjustments.
- Renal: Nephrotoxicity is dose related with cisplatin and presents at 10–20 days. Patients with renal impairment may require dose adjustments. Can be avoided with adequate hydration, diuresis, as well as slower infusion time.
- Electrolyte Imbalance: Decreases Mg^{2+}, K+, Ca^{2+}, Na^+, and P.
- Neurotoxicity: Severe neuropathy with numbness, tingling, and sensory loss is classic "stocking glove" distribution. Risk increases with cumulative doses. Proprioception, vibrating sense, and motor function can occur. Ototoxicity occurs in 30% beginning with high frequency hearing.
- Ototoxicity: High-frequency hearing loss and tinnitus.
- Skin: Alopecia. Pruritus and rash may occur with pemetrexed. Premedication with dexamethasone is effective in preventing or minimizing symptoms of rash and pruritis.
- Reproductive: Pregnancy category D. Breast feeding should be avoided.

Initiate antiemetic protocol:	Moderately to highly emetogenic protocol.
Supportive drugs:	☐ pegfilgrastim (Neulasta) ☐ filgrastim (Neupogen) ☐ epoetin alfa (Procrit) ☐ darbepoetin alfa (Aranesp)
Treatment schedule:	Chair time 3 hours day 1. Repeat cycle every 21 days.
Estimated number of visits:	Two visits per cycle. Request 6 cycles worth of visits.

Dose Calculation by: 1. _____   2. _____

_____

Physician

_____

Patient Name

_____

Diagnosis

_____

Date

_____

ID Number

_____/_____/_____

Ht   Wt   M^2

MULTIPLE MYELOMA

M

Combination Regimens

Melphalan: 8–10 mg/m^2 PO on days 1–4

Prednisone 60 mg/m^2 on days 1–4

Repeat cycle every 42 days.[1,326]

Vincristine: 0.4-mg/day IV continuous infusion on days 1–4

Doxorubicin: 9-mg/m^2/day IV continuous infusion on days 1–4

Dexamethasone: 40-mg PO on days 1–4, 9–12, and 17–20

Repeat cycle every 28 days.[1,327]

Thalidomide: 200-mg/day PO

Dexamethasone: 40-mg/day PO on days 1–4, 9–12, and 17–20 (odd cycles)

40-mg/day PO on days 1–4 (even cycles).

Repeat cycle every 28 days.[1,328]

Vincristine: 0.03-mg/kg IV on day 1

Carmustine: 0.5-mg/kg IV on day 1

Melphalan: 0.25-mg/kg PO on days 1–4

Cyclophosphamide: 10-mg/kg IV on day 1

Prednisone: 1-mg/kg PO on days 1–7, taper after first week, discontinue on day 21

Repeat cycle every 35 days.[1,329]

Vincristine: 1.2-mg/m^2 IV on day 1

Carmustine: 20-mg/m^2 IV on day 1

Melphalan: 8-mg/m^2 PO on days 1–4

Cyclophosphamide: 400-mg/m^2 IV on day 1

Prednisone: 40-mg/m^2 PO on days 1–7, all cycles, then 20 mg/m^2 PO on day 8–14 first three cycles only

Repeat cycle every 35 days for 10 cycles (induction), then every 42 days for three cycles, then every 56 days until relapse.[1,330]

Dose Calculation by: 1. _____   2. _____

_____

Physician

_____

Date

_____

Patient Name

_____

ID Number

_____

Diagnosis

_____ /   _____ /   _____

Ht   Wt   M^2

MULTIPLE MYELOMA

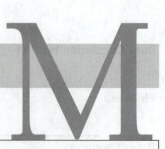

Combination Regimens

Melphalan: 8–10 mg/m^2 PO on days 1–4
Prednisone 60 mg/m^2 on days 1–4
Repeat cycle every 42 days.[1,326]

Vincristine: 0.4-mg/day IV continuous infusion on days 1–4
Doxorubicin: 9-mg/m^2/day IV continuous infusion on days 1–4
Dexamethasone: 40-mg PO on days 1–4, 9–12, and 17–20
Repeat cycle every 28 days.[1,327]

Thalidomide: 200-mg/day PO
Dexamethasone: 40-mg/day PO on days 1–4, 9–12, and 17–20 (odd cycles)
40-mg/day PO on days 1–4 (even cycles).
Repeat cycle every 28 days.[1,328]

Vincristine: 0.03-mg/kg IV on day 1
Carmustine: 0.5-mg/kg IV on day 1
Melphalan: 0.25-mg/kg PO on days 1–4
Cyclophosphamide: 10-mg/kg IV on day 1
Prednisone: 1-mg/kg PO on days 1–7, taper after first week, discontinue on day 21
Repeat cycle every 35 days.[1,329]

Vincristine: 1.2-mg/m^2 IV on day 1
Carmustine: 20-mg/m^2 IV on day 1
Melphalan: 8-mg/m^2 PO on days 1–4
Cyclophosphamide: 400-mg/m^2 IV on day 1
Prednisone: 40-mg/m^2 PO on days 1–7, all cycles, then 20 mg/m^2 PO on day 8–14 first three cycles only
Repeat cycle every 35 days for 10 cycles (induction), then every 42 days for three cycles, then every 56 days until relapse.[1,330]

Single-Agent Regimens

Dexamethasone: 40-mg IV or PO on days 1–4, 9–12, and 17–20
Repeat cycle every 21 days.[1,331]

Melphalan: 90–140 mg/m^2 IV on day 1
Repeat cycle every 28–42 days.[1,332]

Thalidomide: 200–800 mg PO daily
Continue treatment until disease progression or undue toxicity.[1,328]

Bortezomib: 1.3-mg/m^2 IV on days 1, 4, 8, and 11.
Repeat cycle every 21 days.[1,334]

If disease is progressive after two cycles or stable after four cycles, may
  add dexamethasone 20-mg PO daily on the day of and the day after
  bortezomib.

Interferon-α-2b: 2 MU SC or IM, 3 times weekly

Use as maintenance therapy in patients with significant response to induction chemotherapy.[1,335]

10-mg PO daily[1,336]

Combination Regimens

Melphalan + Prednisone

Baseline laboratory tests: CBC: Chemistry, renal and liver functions

Baseline procedures or tests: Bone marrow biopsy

Administer: **Melphalan:** _____ 8–10 mg/m^2 PO on days 1–4

Prednisone: _____ 60-mg/m^2 PO on days 1–4

Repeat every 42 days.

OR

Melphalan: _____ 9-mg/m^2 PO on days 1–4

Prednisone: _____ 40-mg/m^2 PO tid on days 1–4

Repeat every 28 days.

Melphalan (2-mg tablets) should be taken on an empty stomach, and prednisone should be taken with food.

Major Side Effects

- Myelosuppression: Dose limiting, with leukopenia and thrombocytopenia equally affected. Effect may be prolonged and cumulative. Nadir 4–6 weeks.
- GI Toxicities: Gastric irritation, increased appetite. Nausea and vomiting minimal, but severe with high doses.
- Steroid Toxicities: Sodium and water retention, cushingoid changes, behavioral changes, including emotional lability, insomnia, mood swings, and euphoria. May increase glucose and sodium levels, decrease potassium level, and affect warfarin dose.
- Musculoskeletal Changes: Muscle weakness, loss of muscle mass, osteoporosis, and pathological fractures with prolonged use of steroids.
- Perceptual Alterations: Cataracts or glaucoma may develop.
- Reproductive: Pregnancy category D. Breast feeding should be avoided.

Chair time: None

Estimated number of visits: Weekly or every other week for CBC.

Dose Calculation by: 1. _____   2. _____

_____
Physician

_____
Date

_____
Patient Name

_____
ID Number

_____
Diagnosis

_____/ _____/ _____
Ht   Wt   M^2

VAD

Baseline laboratory tests:	CBC: Chemistry, renal and liver functions
Baseline procedures or tests:	Bone marrow biopsy, MUGA, central line placement
Administer:	**Vincristine** _____0.4-mg/day IV continuous infusion on days 1–4

- Vesicant
- Available in 1-, 2-, and 5-mg vials. 1mg/mL.

Doxorubicin _____ 9-mg/m2 IV continuous infusion on days 1–4

- Potent vesicant
- Available in 2 mg/mL solution.
- Doxorubicin will form precipitant with heparin.

Dexamethasone: 40-mg PO on days 1–4, 9–12, and 17–20

Mix vincristine and doxorubicin in 50–100 mL to run over 4 days

Major Side Effects

- Myelosuppression: Dose limiting toxicity, nadir usually occurs at days 10–14.
- GI Toxicities: Mild nausea and vomiting. Constipation and paralytic ileus secondary to autonomic neuropathy. Gastric irritation, increased appetite.
- Cardiotoxicity: Dosage 550 mg/m^2. May result in cardiomyopathy. Acutely, pericarditic-myocarditis syndrome may occur and can be acute or delayed.
- GU Toxicities: Discoloration of urine from pink to red up to 48 hours.
- Neurotoxicity: Peripheral neuropathy including numbness, weakness, myalgias, and late severe motor difficulties. Jaw pain.
- Skin alterations: Alopecia.
- Elevated white blood cell secondary to demargination.
- Steroid Toxicities: Sodium and water retention, cushingoid changes, hyperglycemia, hypokalemia, increased sodium. Warfarin and insulin doses may need to be increased. Muscle weakness, loss of muscle mass, osteoporosis, and pathological fractures with prolonged use; mood changes, euphoria, headache, insomnia, depression and psychosis; cataracts or glaucoma may develop.
- Reproductive: Pregnancy category D. Breast feeding should be avoided.

Initiate antiemetic protocol:	Mildly to moderately emetogenic protocol.
Supportive drugs:	

☐ pegfilgrastim (Neulasta)_____   ☐ filgrastim (Neupogen) _____

☐ epoetin alfa (Procrit)/darbepoetin alfa (Aranesp) _____   ☐ Allopurinol_____

☐ Antibiotic _____   ☐ Antifungal _____

Treatment schedule:	Repeat cycle every 28 days.
Chair time:	30 minutes on day 1, and 30 minutes for pump discontinuation
Estimated number of visits:	Days 1 and 4, weekly to monitor blood counts

Dose Calculation by: 1. _____   2. _____

_____

Physician

_____

Date

_____

Patient Name

_____

ID Number

_____

Diagnosis

_____/ _____/ _____

Ht   Wt   M^2

Thalidomide + Dexamethasone

Baseline laboratory tests:	CBC: Chemistry, renal and liver functions
Baseline procedures or tests:	Bone marrow biopsy
Administer:	**Thalidomide:** _____ 200-mg day PO daily

- Available in 50- and 100-mg tablets. Take at bedtime.

Dexamethasone: 40-mg PO on days 1–4, 9–12, and 17–20 (odd cycles)

40-mg PO on days 1–4 (even cycles). Should be taken with food.

Major Side Effects

- Reproductive: ABSOLUTE CONTRAINDICATION IN PREGNANCY. Teratogenic. Patients must be using birth control. Negative pregnancy test required for women of childbearing age. Must complete registration with Celgene (STEPS program, Summit, NJ) to dispense.
- Neurologic: Drowsiness, fatigue, peripheral neuropathy. Increased sedation with barbiturates, alcohol, chlorampromazine, and reserpine
- GI Toxicity: Constipation; can be severe and should be treated with prophylaxis. Gastric irritation with dexamethasone; increased appetite.
- Skin Integrity: Maculopapular skin rash, urticaria, and dry skin. Serious reactions, including Stevens-Johnson syndrome, have been reported. Discontinue if patient develops rash.
- Elevated white blood cell secondary to demargination.
- Steroid Toxicities: Sodium and water retention, cushingoid changes, hyperglycemia, hypokalemia, increased sodium level. Warfarin and insulin doses may need to be increased.
- Musculoskeletal Changes: Muscle weakness, loss of muscle mass, osteoporosis, and pathological fractures with prolonged use.
- Neuropsychiatric Effects: Mood changes, euphoria, headache, insomnia, depression, and psychosis.
- Perceptual Alterations: Cataracts or glaucoma may develop.

Treatment schedule:	Repeat cycles every 28 days.
Estimated number of visits:	Monthly

Dose Calculation by: 1. _____   2. _____

_____
Physician

_____
Date

_____
Patient Name

_____
ID Number

_____
Diagnosis

_____ / _____ / _____
Ht   Wt   M²

M2 Protocol

Baseline laboratory tests:	CBC: Chemistry, renal and liver functions
Baseline procedures or tests:	Bone marrow biopsy, pulmonary function tests
Premedicate:	5-HT$_3$ and dexamethasone
Administer:	**Vincristine** _____0.03-mg/kg IV through side port of free-flowing IV on day 1

- Vesicant
- Available in 1-, 2-, and 5-mg vials. 1mg/mL.

Carmustine (BCNU): _____ 0.5-mg/kg IV on day 1

- Available in 100 mg powder, add 3 mL sterile diluent and add sterile water.
- Stable for 8 hours at room temperature or 24 hours when refrigerated.

Melphalan: _____ 0.25-mg/kg PO on days 1–4

- Available in 2 mg tablets.

Cyclophosphamide: _____10-mg/kg IV on day 1

- Available 100-, 200-, 500-, 1000-, and 2000-mg vials.
- Reconstituted solution stable for 24 hours at room temperature and 6 days if refrigerated.
- Dilute with sterile water or bacteriostatic water for injection (paraben preserved only); shake well until solution is clear. Final concentration equals 20 mg/mL. Further dilute into 250–500 mL of NS or D5W.

Prednisone: _____ 1-mg/kg PO on days 1–7; taper after first week; discontinue on day 21

Repeat cycle every 35 days.

Major Side Effects

- Myelosuppression: Dose limiting. Involving all blood elements, delayed and cumulative. Double nadir days 7–14 and 4–6 weeks after tx.
- GI Toxicities: Severe nausea with carmustine; otherwise nausea and vomiting are mild. Constipation and paralytic ileus secondary to autonomic neuropathy. Gastric irritation, increased appetite with prednisone.
- Hemorrhagic Cystitis: Irritation of bladder wall capillaries; preventable with appropriate hydration.
- Pulmonary toxicity with carmustine doses >1400 mg.
- Neurotoxicity: Peripheral neuropathy, including numbness, weakness, myalgias, and late severe motor difficulties. Jaw pain.
- Skin Alterations: Alopecia.
- Elevated white blood cell count secondary to demargination.
- Steroid Toxicities: Sodium and water retention, cushingoid changes, hyperglycemia, hypokalemia, increased sodium level. Warfarin and insulin doses may need to be increased. Muscle weakness, loss of muscle mass, osteoporosis, and pathological fractures with prolonged use; mood changes, euphoria, headache, insomnia, depression, and psychosis; cataracts or glaucoma may develop.
- Reproductive: Pregnancy category D. Breast feeding should be avoided.

Initiate antiemetic protocol:	Moderately emetogenic protocol.
Supportive drugs:	☐ pegfilgrastim (Neulasta)_____ ☐ filgrastim (Neupogen) _____
	☐ epoetin alfa (Procrit)/ darbepoetin alfa (Aranesp) _____ ☐ Allopurinol_____
	☐ Antibiotic _____ ☐ Antifungal _____
Treatment Schedule:	Chair time 3 hours on day 1.
Estimated number of visits:	Day 1, then weekly to monitor blood counts.

Dose Calculation by: 1. _____   2. _____

Physician _____   Date _____

Patient Name _____   ID Number _____

Diagnosis _____   Ht _____ / Wt _____ / M^2 _____

VBMCP (Vincristine, Carmustine, Melphalan, Cyclophosphamide, Prednisone)

Baseline laboratory tests: CBC: Chemistry, renal and liver functions

Baseline procedures or tests: Bone marrow biopsy, pulmonary function tests

Premedicate: 5-HT$_3$ and dexamethasone

Administer:

Vincristine _____ 1.2-mg/m^2 IV through side port of free-flowing IV on day 1

Carmustine: _____ 20-mg/m^2 IV on day 1

Add sterile alcohol (provided with drug), then add sterile water. May be further diluted in 100–250 mL D5W or NS.

Melphalan: _____ 8-mg/m2 PO on days 1–4

Cyclophosphamide: _____ 400-mg/m^2 IV on day 1 dilute with sterile water or bacterio-static water for injection (paraben preserved only); shake well until solution is clear. Final concentration equals 20 mg/mL. Further dilute into NS or D5W 250–500 mL.

Prednisone: _____ 40-mg/m^2/d PO on days 1–7 (all cycles), and _____ 20-mg/m^2/d PO, on days 8–14 (first three cycles only)

Major Side Effects

- Myelosuppression: Teach self care measures to minimize risk of infection and bleeding.
- GI Toxicities: Severe nausea with carmustine, otherwise nausea and vomiting is mild. Constipation and paralytic ileus secondary to autonomic neuropathy. Gastric irritation, increased appetite with prednisone.
- Hemorrhagic Cystitis: Irritation of bladder wall capillaries; preventable with appropriate hydration.
- Pulmonary toxicity with Carmustine doses > 1400 mg.
- Neurotoxicity: Peripheral neuropathy including numbness, weakness, myalgias, and late severe motor difficulties. Jaw pain.
- Skin Alterations: Alopecia
- Elevated white blood cell count secondary to demargination.
- Steroid Toxicities: Sodium and water retention, cushingoid changes, hyperglycemia, hypokalemia, increased sodium. Warfarin and insulin doses may need to be increased; muscle weakness, loss of muscle mass, osteoporosis, and pathological fractures with prolonged use; mood changes, euphoria, headache, insomnia, depression and psychosis; cataracts or glaucoma may develop.
- Reproductive: Mutagenic and potentially teratogenic, impotence secondary to neuropathy.

Initiate antiemetic protocol: Moderately emetogenic protocol.

Supportive drugs:
☐ pegfilgrastim (Neulasta)_____   ☐ filgrastim (Neupogen) _____
☐ epoetin alfa (Procrit)/   ☐ Allopurinol_____
   darbepoetin alfa (Aranesp) _____
☐ Antibiotic _____   ☐ Antifungal _____

Treatment schedule: Repeat cycle every 35 days for 10 cycles (induction), then every 42 days for 3 cycles, then every 56 days until relapse.

Chair time: 30 minutes on day 1, and 30 minutes for pump discontinuation.

Estimated number of visits: Days 1 and 4, then weekly to monitor blood counts.

Dose Calculation by: 1. _____   2. _____

_____
Physician

_____
Date

_____
Patient Name

_____
ID Number

_____
Diagnosis

_____/_____/_____
Ht   Wt   M^2

Single-Agent Regimens

Dexamethasone

Baseline laboratory tests:	CBC: Chemistry, renal and liver functions
Baseline procedures or tests:	Bone marrow biopsy
Administer:	**Dexamethasone:** _____ 40-mg IV or PO on days 1–4, 9–12, and 17–20
	Repeat every 21 days.
	Take with food.

Major Side Effects

- Elevated white blood cell count secondary to demargination.
- GI Toxicities: Gastric irritation, increased appetite
- Steroid toxicities: Sodium and water retention, cushingoid changes, hyperglycemia, hypokalemia, increased sodium level. Warfarin and insulin doses may need to be increased.
- Musculoskeletal Changes: Muscle weakness, loss of muscle mass, osteoporosis, and pathological fractures with prolonged use.
- Neuropsychiatric Effects: Mood changes, euphoria, headache, insomnia, depression, and psychosis.
- Perceptual Alterations: Cataracts or glaucoma may develop.

Chair time:	None
Estimated number of visits:	Weekly or every other week for CBC

Dose Calculation by: 1. _____ 2. _____

_____

Physician

_____

Patient Name

_____

Diagnosis

Date

ID Number

_____ / _____ / _____
Ht   Wt   M^2

Melphalan

Baseline laboratory tests:	CBC: Chemistry, renal and liver functions
Baseline procedures or tests:	Bone marrow biopsy
Premedicate:	5-HT$_3$ and dexamethasone
Administer:	**Melphalan:** _____ 90–140 mg/m^2 IV on day 1

- Available in 50 mg vial. Add 10 mL of supplied diluent, shake until clear.
- Further dilute in NS to concentration not greater than 0.45 mg/mL.
- Administer over a minimum of 15 minutes, within 60 minutes.
- Stability, must be used within 60 minutes after dilution. Do Not Refrigerate.

Repeat every 28–42 days

Major Side Effects

- Myelosuppression: Dose limiting with leukopenia and thrombocytopenia equally affected. Effect may be prolonged and cumulative. Nadir 4–6 weeks.
- Hypersensitivity Reaction: Observed in 10% of patients treated with IV melphalan. Characterized by diaphuresis, usticaria, skin rashes, bronchospasm, dyspnea, tachycardia, and hypotension.
- Skin: Alopecia rare. Skin ulcerations at injection site rare.
- GI Toxicities: Severe nausea and vomiting with IV therapy.
- Reproductive: Pregnancy category D. Breast feeding should be avoided.

Chair time:	1 hour
Estimated number of visits:	Weekly or every other week for CBC.

Dose Calculation by: 1. _____ 2. _____

Physician _____ Date _____

Patient Name _____ ID Number _____

Diagnosis _____ Ht _____/ Wt _____/ M^2 _____

Thalidomide

Baseline laboratory tests: CBC: Chemistry, renal and liver functions

Baseline procedures or tests: Bone marrow biopsy

Administer: **Thalidomide:** _____ 200–800 mg/m^2/day PO daily

Available in 50- and 100-mg tablets. Take at bedtime.

Major Side Effects

- Alteration in Sexuality/Reproductive: ABSOLUTE CONTRAINDICATION IN PREGNANCY. Teratogenic. Patients must be taking birth control. Negative pregnancy test required for women of childbearing age. Must complete registration with Celgene (STEPS program; Summit, NY) to dispense.

- Neurologic: Drowsiness, fatigue, peripheral neuropathy. Increased sedation with barbiturates, alcohol, chlorampromazine, and reserpine.

- GI Toxicity: Constipation; can be severe and should be treated with prophylaxis.

- Skin Integrity: Maculopapular skin rash, urticaria, and dry skin. Serious reactions, including Stevens-Johnson syndrome, have been reported. Discontinue if patient develops rash.

Chair time: None

Estimated number of visits: Monthly

Dose Calculation by: 1. _____   2. _____

_____   _____

Physician   Date

_____   _____

Patient Name   ID Number

_____   _____/_____/_____

Diagnosis   Ht   Wt   M^2

Bortezomib (Velcade)

Baseline laboratory tests:	CBC: Chemistry, renal and liver functions
Baseline procedures or tests:	Bone marrow biopsy
Premedicate:	5-HT$_3$ and dexamethasone
Administer:	**Bortezomib:** _____ 1.3-mg/m^2 IV push followed by saline flush on days 1, 4, 8, and 11; followed by a 10-day rest period.

- Dilute powder in 3.5 mL of NS.
- Reconstituted product should be clear.
- Stable for 8 hours at room temperature.

If disease is progressive after two cycles, may add:

Dexamethasone at 20-mg PO daily on the day of and the day after borteximib.

- Available in 10 mg vial. 3.5 mg of bortezomib cake or powder.

Major Side Effects

- Myelosuppression: Neutropenia and thrombocytopenia
- GI Toxicities: Nausea and vomiting, anorexia, constipation, and dehydration. Orthostatic hypotension.
- Fatigue: Fatigue, malaise, and generalized weakness
- Peripheral Neuropathy: Mix of sensorimotor neuropathy. May improve and or return to baseline with discontinuation of drug.
- Steroid Toxicities: Sodium and water retention, cushingoid changes, behavioral changes, including emotional lability, insomnia, mood swings, and euphoria. May increase glucose and sodium levels, decrease potassium level, and affect warfarin dose.
- Musculoskeletal Changes: Muscle weakness, loss of muscle mass, osteoporosis, and pathological fractures with prolonged use.
- Perceptual Alterations: Cataracts or glaucoma may develop.
- Reproductive: Pregnancy category D. Breast feeding should be avoided.

Initiate antiemetic protocol:	Moderately emetogenic protocol.
Supportive drugs:	☐ pegfilgrastim (Neulasta)_____ ☐ filgrastim (Neupogen) _____ ☐ epoetin alfa (Procrit)/ darbepoetin alfa (Aranesp) _____ ☐ Allopurinol_____ ☐ Antibiotic _____ ☐ Antifungal _____
Treatment schedule:	Repeat cycle every 21 days.
Chair time:	1 hour day 1–4, 8–11.
Estimated number of visits:	5 visits per cycle. Request 4 cycles worth of visits.

Dose Calculation by: 1. _____ 2. _____

_____

Physician

_____

Patient Name

_____

Diagnosis

_____

Date

_____

ID Number

_____/ _____/ _____

Ht   Wt   M^2

Interferon-α-2b

Baseline laboratory tests:	CBC: Chemistry, renal and liver functions
Baseline procedures or tests:	Bone marrow biopsy
Administer:	**Interferon-α-2b** _____ 2 MU SQ or IM 3 times per week

- Available in multidose pens with 6 doses of 3 MU (18 MU) or 5 MU (30 MU) or 10 MU (60 MU). Keep refrigerated.

Major Side Effects

- Flulike Symptoms: Fever, chills, headache, myalgias, and arthralgias. Occurs in 80%–90% of patients. Onset 3–4 hours after injection and lasting for up to 8–9 hours. Incidence decreases with subsequent injections. Symptoms can be managed with acetaminophen, ibuprofen, and/or indomethacin and increased oral fluid intake.
- Bone Marrow Depression: Myelosuppression with mild leukopenia and thrombocytopenia. Cumulative effect, dose-limiting thrombocytopenia; reversible.
- GI Toxicities: Nausea and diarrhea are mild, and vomiting is rare. Anorexia occurs in 46%–65% of patients and is cumulative and dose limiting. Taste alteration and xerostomia may occur.
- Renal/hepatic: Renal toxicity is uncommon and is manifested by mild proteinuria and hypocalcemia. Acute renal failure and nephrotic syndrome have been reported in rare instances. Mild transient elevations in serum transaminase levels. Dose-dependent toxicity observed more frequently in the presence of pre-existing liver abnormalities.
- Cardiotoxicity: Chest pain, arrhythmias, and CHF are rare.
- Skin: Alopecia is partial. Dry skin, pruritus, and irritation at injection site seen.
- Reproductive: Pregnancy category D. Breast feeding should be avoided.

Initiate antiemetic protocol:	Mildly to moderately emetogenic protocol.
Supportive drugs:	☐ G-CSF _____ ☐ Peg-G-CSF _____
	☐ epoetin alfa/ ☐ Allopurinol _____
	darbepoetin alfa _____
	☐ Antibiotic _____ ☐ Antifungal _____
Treatment schedule:	Use as a maintenance therapy in patients with significant response to induction therapy.
Estimated number of visits:	Weekly or every other week for CBC

Dose Calculation by: 1. _____   2. _____

_____   _____
Physician   Date

_____   _____
Patient Name   ID Number

_____   _____ / _____ / _____
Diagnosis   Ht   Wt   M²

Lenalidomide (Revlimid)

Baseline laboratory tests: CBC, Chemistry Panel, LFTs, and pregnancy test for females of childbearing potential

Baseline procedures or tests: Bone marrow biopsy to establish myelodysplastic syndrome associated with a deletion 5q cytogenetic abnormality with or without additional cytogenetic abnormalities.

Initiate IV: N/A

Premedicate: Oral 5-HT$_3$ if nausea occurs.

Administer: **Lenalidomide** _____10 mg by mouth daily

- Available in 5-mg (pale yellow opaque) and 10-mg (blue/green) capsules for oral use.
- Take with water. Do not break, chew, or open capsules.
- Store at 25° C (77° F), excursions permitted to 15–30°C (59–86°F).
- Drug is only available under a special restricted distribution program called the Revassist program.

Major Side Effects:

- Reproductive: Teratogenic. Pregnancy category X. Lenalidomide is an analogue of thalidomide. Thalidomide is a known human teratogen that causes life-threatening human defects. If lenalidomide is taken during pregnancy, it may cause birth defects or death to an unborn baby. All patients on lenalidomide must participate in telephone surveys and patient registry (Revassist program). Under this program, all female patients of childbearing potential must have a negative pregnancy test done by their doctors within 10–14 days and 24 hours before lenalidomide therapy, then weekly during the first 4 weeks of lenalidomide therapy. Thereafter, the patient must have a pregnancy test every 4 weeks if she has regular menstrual cycles, or every 2 weeks if her cycles are irregular while she is taking lenalidomide. Two forms of birth control, one highly effective and an additional effective method, must be used simultaneously at least 4 weeks before beginning lenalidomide therapy, during therapy, during therapy interruption, and for 4 weeks following discontinuation of lenalidomide therapy. Male patients must never have unprotected sexual contact with a female who can become pregnant. Call 1-888-423-5436 for information/assistance with Revassist program and enrollment.
- Hematologic Toxicities: Neutropenia and thrombobytopenia. Grade 3 and 4 hematologic toxicity was seen in 80% of patients studied. Eighty percent of patients had to have a dose delay/reduction during the major study. Thirty-four percent of patients had to have a second dose delay/reduction. Patients may require use of blood product support and/or growth factors. See package insert for delays/reductions.
- Thromboembolic Events: Increased risk of deep venous thrombois (DVT) and pulmonary embolism (PE) in patients with multiple myeloma who were treated with lenalidomide combination therapy. It is not known whether prophylactic anticoagulation or antiplatelet therapy prescribed in conjunction with lenalidomide may lessen the potential for venous thromboembolic events. Instruct patients to seek medical attention if they develop symptoms such as shortness of breath, chest pain, or arm or leg swelling.
- Renal Toxicities: Drug is known to be substantially excreted by the kidney, and the risk of toxic reactions to this drug is expected to be greater in patients with impaired renal function. Care should be taken in patients with impaired renal function.
- GI Toxicities: Diarrhea common. Constipation also seen. Nausea occurs, sometimes with vomiting and stomach pain. Dry mouth reported in many patients. Anorexia.
- Hepato Toxicities: Hyperbilirubinemia, cholecystitis, and hepatic failure uncommon.
- Respiratory Toxicities: Nasopharyngitis, cough dyspnea, pharyngitis, epistaxis, dyspnea on exertion, rhinitis, and bronchitis all reported (listed by frequency of occurrence).
- Musculoskeletal: Arthralgia, back pain, muscle cramps, and myalgias can occur.
- Neurosensory Effects: Fatigue is common. Dizziness, vertigo, headache, hypoesthesia, insomnia, depression, and peripheral neuropathy can occur.
- Skin: Pruritus, rash, and dry skin commonly occur. Edema in extremities with or without pain.

Initiate antiemetic protocol: Mildly emetogenic protocol.

Supportive drugs:
- ☐ Neulasta
- ☐ Imodium
- ☐ Aranesp
- ☐ Neupoge
- ☐ Procrit
- ☐ Lomotil

Treatment schedule: No chair time. Weekly visits for CBC first 8 weeks of therapy, then monthly thereafter.

Estimated number of visits: Ten visits first three months of therapy.

Dose Calculation by: 1. _____   2. _____

_____

Physician

_____

Patient Name

_____

Diagnosis

_____

Date

_____

ID Number

_____ / _____ / _____

Ht   Wt   M^2

MYELODYSPLASTIC SYNDROME

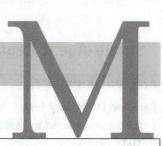

Single-Agent Regimens

75-mg/m^2 SQ days 1–7
Repeat cycle every 28 days.[410]

0.3-mg/kg IV days 1–5, then twice weekly for 11 more weeks.
May repeat cycle if response is seen.[411]

10-mg PO daily.[412]

Dacogen 15 mg/m^2 IV over 3 hours every 8 hours, for 3 days
OR
Dacogen 20 mg/m^2 IV over 1 hour daily for 5 days
OR
Dacogen 10 mg/m^2 IV over 1 hour daily for 10 days
OR
Dacogen 10 mg/m^2 Subcutaneously BID for 5 days[413,414]

Single-Agent Regimens

Azacitidine (Vidaza)

Baseline laboratory tests:	CBC, Chemistry Panel, and LFTs
Baseline procedures or tests:	N/A
Initiate IV:	N/A
Premedicate:	Oral 5-HT$_3$ or phenothiazine orally 30 minutes prior to daily dosing.
Administer:	**Azacitidine** _____ mg (75 mg/m^2) subcutaneously, daily for 7 days. Give a minimum of 4 cycles, therapeutic effects may not be seen until 5 or more cycles completed.

- Dose may be increased to 100 mg/m^2 if no beneficial effect is seen after two treatment cycles and if no toxicity other than nausea and vomiting has occurred.
- Available as lyophilized powder in 100-mg vials for subcutaneous injection.
- Reconstitute drug with 4 mL sterile water for injection. Inject diluent slowly into the vial. Invert 2–3 times and gently rotate until a uniform suspension is achieved. Suspension will be cloudy.
- The resulting suspension will contain azacitidine 25 mg/mL.
- Doses greater than 4 mL should be divided equally into two syringes.
- Must be administered within 1 hour after reconstitution.

Major Side Effects

- Myelotoxicities: Neutropenia and thrombocytopenia may require dose reductions as follows: Baseline (start of treatment) WBC $\geq 3.0 \times 10^9$/L, ANC $\geq 1.5 \times 10^9$/L, and platelets $\geq 75 \times 10^9$/L:

Nadir Counts		Percentage Dose in the
ANC ($\times 10^9$/L)	Platelets ($\times 10^9$/L)	Next Course
<0.5	<25.0	50%
0.5–1.5	25.0–50.0	67%
>1.5	>50.0	100%

See package insert for dose reductions for patients whose counts are less than those stated above. Dose adjustments should then be based on nadir counts and bone marrow biopsy cellularity at the time of the nadir. Anemia may occur or be exacerbated.

- GI Toxicities: Nausea is common. Vomiting, diarrhea, constipation, stomatitis, and tongue ulceration also occur. Dysphagia, dyspepsia, and abdominal distension were also reported.
- Renal Toxicities: Patients with renal impairment should be closely monitored. Elevated serum creatinine, renal failure, renal tubular acidosis seen. If unexplained reductions in serum bicarbonate levels (< 20 mEq/L) occur, the dose should be reduced by 50% on the next course. If unexplained elevations of BUN or serum creatinine occur, the next cycle should be delayed until values return to normal or baseline, and the dose should be reduced by 50% on the next treatment course.
- Respiratory Toxicities: Decreased breath sounds, pleural effusion, rhonchi atelectasis, exacerbation of dyspnea, postnasal drip, and chest wall pain seen in study.
- Cardiovascular Toxicities: Hypotension, syncope, and chest pain can occur.
- Sensory/neurotoxicities: Lethargy, increased fatigue, malaise, and hypoesthesia reported.
- **Skin:** Injection site reactions (erythema, pruritus, swelling, pain, bruising, injection site granuloma, and injection site pigmentation changes) can occur. Rotate injection sites; give at least one inch from an old site and never into areas where the site is tender, bruised, red, or hard. Peripheral edema, urticaria, and dry skin reported.
- Reproductive: Pregnancy Category D. Breast feeding should be avoided.

Initiate antiemetic protocol: Mildly to moderately emetogenic protocol.

Supportive drugs: ☐ Neulasta   ☐ Neupogen
                               ☐ Imodium   ☐ Procrit
                               ☐ Aranesp   ☐ Lomotil

Treatment schedule: Thirty minutes for injection days 1–7. Repeat cycle every 28 days as tolerated.

Estimated number of visits: Ten visits per month. Request 5 months worth of visits.

Dose Calculation by: 1. _____   2. _____

_____

Physician   Date

_____

Patient Name   ID Number

_____   / _____ / _____

Diagnosis   Ht   Wt   M^2

Arsenic Trioxide (Trisenox)

Baseline laboratory tests:	CBC, Chemistry Panel (including Mg^{2+}), and LFTs
Baseline procedures or tests:	12-lead EKG
Initiate IV:	Normal saline
Premedicate:	Oral 5-HT$_3$ or phenothiazine if nausea occurs.
Administer:	**Arsenic trioxide** _____ mg (0.3 mg/kg) IV days 1–5, then twice weekly for 11 weeks.

- Available in 10-mL, single-use ampules containing 10 mg of arsenic trioxide, at a concentration of 1 mg/mL.
- Further dilute in 100–250 cc D5W or 0.9% sodium chloride injection, USP.
- Give IV over 1–2 hours (or up to 4 hours if acute vasomotor reactions occur).
- Drug is chemically and physically stable for 24 hours at room temperature and 48 hours when refrigerated. However, does not contain any preservatives, so unused portions should be discarded.

Major Side Effects

- Vasomotor Reactions: Symptoms include flushing, tachycardia, dizziness, and lightheadedness. Increasing the infusion time to 4 hours usually resolves these symptoms. Stop infusion for tachycardia and/or hypotension. Resume at decreased rate after resolution. Headaches can also occur; treat with acetaminophen as needed.
- APL Differentiation Syndrome: Characterized by fever, dyspnea, weight gain, pulmonary infiltrates, and pleural or pericardial effusions, with or without leukocytosis. Can be fatal. At the first suggestion, high-dose steroids should be instituted (dexamethasone 10-mg IV bid) for at least 3 days or longer until signs and symptoms abate. Most patients do not require termination of arsenic trioxide therapy during treatment of the syndrome.
- Cardiotoxicities: Drug can cause QT interval prolongation and complete atrioventricular block. Prolonged QT interval can progress to a torsade de pointes-type fatal ventricular arrhythmia. Patients with history of QT prolongation, concomitant administration of drugs that prolong the QT interval, CHF, administration of potassium-wasting diuretics, and conditions resulting in hypokalemia or hypomagnesemia such as concurrent administration of amphotericin B. EKGs should be done weekly, more often if abnormal.
- Fluid/electrolyte Imbalance: Hypokalemia occurs in about 50% of patients. Hypomagnesemia and hyperglycemia also commonly occur. Edema seen in 40% of patients. Less commonly, hyperkalemia, hypocalcemia, hypoglycemia, and acidosis occur. Potassium levels should be kept > 4.0 mEq/dL and magnesium > 1.8 mg/dL during arsenic trioxide therapy.
- Hematologic Effects: Leukocytosis seen in 50%–60% of patients with a gradual increase in WBC that peaks between 2 and 3 weeks after starting therapy. Usually resolves spontaneously without treatment and/or complications. Anemia (14%), thrombocytopenia (19%) and neutropenia (10%). Disseminated intravascular coagulation (DIC) occurred in 8% of patients.
- GI Toxicities: Nausea is most common (75%) and is usually mild, followed by vomiting (58%), abdominal pain (58%), diarrhea (53%), constipation (28%), anorexia (23%), dyspepsia (10%), abdominal tenderness or distention (8%), and dry mouth (8%).
- Hepatic Toxicities: Increased hepatic transaminases ALT and AST seen.
- Renal Toxicities: Use with caution in patients with renal impairment. Kidney is the main route of elimination of arsenic.
- Respiratory Toxicities: Cough is common. Other symptoms include dyspnea, epistaxis, hypoxia, pleural effusion, postnasal drip, wheezing, decreased breath sounds, crepitations, rales/crackles, hemoptysis, tachypnea, and rhonchi.
- Musculoskeletal: Arthralgias (33%), myalgias (25%), bone pain (23%), back pain (18%), neck pain, and pain in limbs (13%).
- Sensory/perception: Fatigue was reported by 63% of patients. Headache, insomnia, and pareshtesias common. Dizziness, tremors, seizures, somnolence, and (rarely) coma can occur.

- Skin: Dermatitis common. Pruritis, ecchymosis, dry skin, erythema, hyperpigmentation, and urticaria also reported. Injection site reactions (pain, erythema, and edema) can occur.
- Reproductive: Pregnancy category D. Breast feeding should be avoided.

Initiate antiemetic protocol:	Mildly emetogenic protocol.

Supportive drugs:

☐ Neulasta ☐ Neupogen
☐ Imodium ☐ Procrit
☐ Aranesp ☐ Lomotil

Treatment schedule: Chair time 2 hours days 1–5 then, twice weekly for 11 weeks. May repeat cycle if response is seen.

Estimated number of visits: Twenty-seven visits per cycle.

Dose Calculation by: 1. _____ 2. _____

_____
Physician

_____
Date

_____
Patient Name

_____
ID Number

_____
Diagnosis

_____/_____/_____
Ht   Wt   M^2

Lenalidomide (Revlimid)

Baseline laboratory tests:	CBC, Chemistry Panel, LFTs, and pregnancy test for females of childbearing potential
Baseline procedures or tests:	Bone marrow biopsy to establish myelodysplastic syndrome associated with a deletion 5q cytogenetic abnormality with or without additional cytogenetic abnormalities.
Initiate IV:	N/A
Premedicate:	Oral 5-HT$_3$ if nausea occurs.
Administer:	**Lenalidomide** 10 mg by mouth daily

- Available in 5-mg (pale yellow opaque) and 10-mg (blue/green) capsules for oral use.
- Take with water. Do not break, chew, or open capsules.
- Store at 25° C (77° F), excursions permitted to 15–30°C (59–86°F)
- Drug is only available under a special restricted distribution program called the Revassist program.

Major Side Effects

- Reproductive: Teratogenic. Pregnancy category X. Lenalidomide is an analogue of thalidomide. Thalidomide is a known human teratogen that causes life-threatening human defects. If lenalidomide is taken during pregnancy, it may cause birth defects or death to an unborn baby. All patients on lenalidomide must participate in telephone surveys and patient registry (Revassist program). Under this program, all female patients of childbearing potential must have a negative pregnancy test done by her doctor within 10–14 days and 24 hours before lenalidomide therapy, then weekly during the first 4 weeks of lenalidomide therapy. Thereafter, the patient must have a pregnancy test every 4 weeks if she has regular menstrual cycles, or every 2 weeks if her cycles are irregular while she is taking lenalidomide. Two forms of birth control, one highly effective and an additional effective method, must be used simultaneously at least 4 weeks before beginning lenalidomide therapy, during therapy, during therapy interruption, and for 4 weeks following discontinuation of lenalidomide therapy. Male patients must **never** have unprotected sexual contact with a female who can become pregnant. Call 1-888-423-5436 for information/assistance with Revassist program and enrollment.
- Hematologic Toxicities: Neutropenia and thrombobytopenia. Grade 3 and 4 hematologic toxicity was seen in 80% of patients studied. Eighty percent of patients had to have a dose delay/reduction during the major study. Thirty-four percent of patients had to have a second dose delay/reduction. Patients may require use of blood product support and/or growth factors. See package insert for delays/reductions.
- Thromboembolic Events: Increased risk of deep venous thrombois (DVT) and pulmonary embolism (PE) in patients with multiple myeloma who were treated with lenalidomide combination therapy. It is not known whether prophylactic anticoagulation or antiplatelet therapy prescribed in conjunction with lenalidomide may lessen the potential for venous thromboembolic events. Instruct patient to seek medical attention if they develop symptoms such as shortness of breath, chest pain, or arm or leg swelling.
- Renal Toxicities: Drug is known to be substantially excreted by the kidney and the risk of toxic reactions to this drug is expected to be greater in patients with impaired renal function. Care should be taken in patients with impaired renal function.
- GI Toxicities: Diarrhea common. Constipation also seen. Nausea occurs, sometimes with vomiting and stomach pain. Dry mouth reported in many patients. Anorexia.
- Hepatotoxicities: Hyperbilirubinemia, cholecystitis, and hepatic failure uncommon.
- Respiratory Toxicities: Nasopharyngitis, cough dyspnea, pharyngitis, epistaxis, dyspnea on exertion, rhinitis and bronchitis all reported (listed by frequency of occurrence).
- Musculoskeletal: Arthralgia, back pain, muscle cramps, and myalgias can occur.
- Neurosensory Effects: Fatigue is common. Dizziness, vertigo, headache, hypoesthesia, insomnia, depression, and peripheral neuropathy can occur.
- Skin: Pruritus, rash, and dry skin commonly occur. Edema in extremities with or without pain.

Initiate antiemetic protocol:	Mildly emetogenic protocol.

Supportive drugs: ☐ Neulasta ☐ Neupogen
☐ Imodium ☐ Procrit
☐ Aranesp ☐ Lomotil

Treatment schedule: No chair time. Weekly visits for CBC first 8 weeks of therapy, then monthly thereafter.

Estimated number of visits: Ten visits first three months of therapy.

Dose Calculation by: 1. _____ 2. _____

_____ _____
Physician Date

_____ _____
Patient Name ID Number

_____ _____/_____/_____
Diagnosis Ht Wt M^2

Decitabine (Dacogen)

Baseline laboratory tests:	CBC, Chemistry
Monitor:	CBC
Baseline procedures or tests:	Bone marrow biopsy
Administer:	**Dacogen** _____ 15 mg/m^2 IV over 3 hours every 8 hours, for 3 days

OR

Dacogen _____ 20 mg/m^2 IV over 1 hour daily for 5 days

OR

Dacogen _____ 10 mg/m^2 IV over 1 hour daily for 10 days

OR

Dacogen _____ 10 mg/m^2 Subcutaneously BID for 5 days

- Available in 50 mg single dose vials. Dilute with 10 mL Sterile Water for injection resulting in 5mg/mL
- Further dilute in Sodium Chloride, D5W, or Lactated Ringer's Solution within 15 minutes of preparation to a final concentration of 0.1–1.0 mg/mL (250 mL is a safe volume for most doses).
- Final solution should be used infused within 15 minutes and infusion should be completed within 3 hours or it must be refrigerated at 2° C and is stable for a maximum of 7 hours until administration.

Major Side Effects

- Bone Marrow Depression: Neutropenia, febrile neutropenia, thrombocytopenia and anemia are the most common side effects. Growth factors and prophylactic antibiotics are recommended. Transfusions as indicated.
- Flulike Symptoms: Fatigue with pyrexia, arthralgias, myalgias, bone, and back pain may be present but mild.
- GI Toxicities: Mild nausea and vomiting, anorexia; stomatitis is usually minimal; constipation and diarrhea infrequent and mild.
- Skin Integrity: Ecchymosis, rash, and petechaie are usually mild.
- Reproduction: Pregnancy Category D. Breast feeding should be avoided.

Initiate antiemetic protocol:	Mildly emetogenic protocol
Supportive drugs:	☐ G-CSF (neupogen) ☐ Peg-G-CSF (neulasta)
	☐ epoetin alfas (Procrit) ☐ darbepoeitn alfa (Aranesp)
	☐ Antibiotic _____ ☐ Antifungal _____
Treatment schedule:	Chair time 4 hours, for 3 day protocol; 2 hours for 3 or 5 day protocol. 30 minutes for subcutaneous dosing.
Estimated number of visits:	3–5 days the week of treatment and weekly CBC; Repeat cycle every 6 weeks for a minimum of 4 cycles; however, a complete or partial response may take longer than 4 cycles. Continue as long as the patient continues to benefit.

Dose Calculation by: 1. _____ 2. _____

_____
Physician

_____
Date

_____
Patient Name

_____
ID Number

_____
Diagnosis

_____/ _____/ _____
Ht   Wt   M^2

OVARIAN CANCER

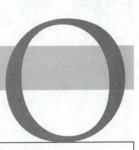

Combination Regimens

Carboplatin: 300-mg/m^2 IV on day 1
Cyclophosphamide: 600-mg/m^2 IV on day 1
Repeat cycle every 28 days.[1,337]

Cisplatin: 100-mg/m^2 IV on day 1
Cyclophosphamide: 600-mg/m^2 IV on day 1
Repeat cycle every 28 days.[1,338]

Cisplatin: 75-mg/m^2 IV on day 2
Paclitaxel: 135-mg/m^2 IV over 24 hours on day 1
Repeat cycle every 21 days.[1,339]
Paclitaxel must be administered first, followed by cisplatin.

Carboplatin: AUC of 6–7.5, IV on day 1
Paclitaxel: 175-mg/m^2 IV over 3 hours on day 1
Repeat cycle every 21 days.[1,340]
Paclitaxel must be administered first, followed by carboplatin.

Carboplatin: AUC of 6, IV on day 1
Docetaxel: 60-mg/m^2 IV on day 1
Repeat cycle every 21 days.[1,341]

Gemcitiabine: 1,000-mg/m^2 IV on days 1 and 8
Doxil: 30-mg/m^2 IV on day 1
Repeat cycle every 21 days.[1,342]

Gemcitiabine: 800–1,000 mg/m^2 IV on days 1 and 8
Cisplatin: 30 mg/m^2 IV on days 1 and 8
Repeat cycle every 21 days.[1,343]

Single-Agent Regimens

Altretamine: 260-mg/m^2/day PO in four divided doses after meals and at
  bedtime
Repeat cycle every 14–21 days.[1,344]

Liposomal doxorubicin: 50-mg/m^2 IV over 1 hour on day 1
Repeat cycle every 28 days.[1,345]

Paclitaxel: 135-mg/m^2 IV over 3 hours on day 1
Repeat cycle every 21 days.[1,346]

Topotecan: 1.5-mg/m^2 IV on days 1–5
Repeat cycle every 21 days.[1,347]

Gemcitabine: 800-mg/m^2 IV weekly for 3 weeks
Repeat cycle every 4 weeks.[1,348]

Etoposide: 50-mg/m^2/day PO on days 1–21
Repeat cycle every 28 days.[1,349]

Combination Regimens

Carboplatin + Cyclophosphamide (CC)

Baseline laboratory tests:	CBC: Chemistry (including Mg^{2+}) and LFTs, CA 125
Baseline procedures or tests:	N/A
Initiate IV:	0.9% sodium chloride
Premedicate:	5-HT$_3$ and dexamethasone 10–20 mg in 100 cc of NS
Administer:	**Carboplatin** _____ mg (300 mg/m²) IV on day 1

- Do not use aluminum needles, because precipitate will form.
- Available in 50, 150, and 450 lyopholized powder or 50, 150, 450, and 600 mg solution.
- Discard reconstituted powder after 8 hours.
- Multidose vial stable for 15 days after first use.

Cyclophosphamide _____ mg (600 mg/m²) IV on day 1

- Available in 100-, 200-, 500-, 1000-, and 2000-mg vials.
- Dilute with sterile water and shake well to ensure that solution is completely dissolved.
- Reconstituted solution stable for 24 hours at room temperature, and 6 days refrigerated.

Major Side Effects

- Hypersensitivity Reactions: Rash, urticaria, erythema, and pruritus. Bronchospasm and hypotension are uncommon, but risk increases from 1%–27% in patients receiving more than seven courses of carboplatin-based therapy.
- Bone Marrow Depression: Dose-limiting myelosuppression
- GI Toxicities: Moderate-to-severe nausea and vomiting within first 24 hours.
- Hepatic Toxicity: Reversible hepatic dysfunction is mild to moderate; increased LFTs and bilirubin.
- Renal: Nephrotoxicity less common than with cisplatin and rarely symptomatic.
- GU: Hemorrhagic cystitis, dysuria, and increased urinary frequency occurs in 5%–10% of patients. Usually reversible on discontinuation of drug.
- Electrolyte Imbalance: Decreased Mg^{2+}, K, Ca^{2+}, Na^+, and P.
- Skin: Hyperpigmentation of skin and nails may occur. Alopecia likely.
- Reproduction: Pregnancy category D. Breast feeding should be avoided.

Initiate antiemetic protocol:	Moderately to highly emetogenic protocol.
Supportive drugs:	☐ pegfilgrastim (Neulasta) ☐ filgrastim (Neupogen)
	☐ epoetin alfa (Procrit) ☐ darbepoetin alfa (Aranesp)
Treatment schedule:	Chair time 3 hours on day 1. Repeat cycle every 28 days.
Estimated number of visits:	One visit per cycle. Request three cycles worth of visits.

Dose Calculation by: 1. _____   2. _____

_____   _____
Physician   Date

_____   _____
Patient Name   ID Number

_____   _____/_____/_____
Diagnosis   Ht   Wt   M²

Cisplatin + Cyclophosphamide (CP)

Baseline laboratory tests:	CBC: Chemistry (including Mg^{2+}), CA 125
Baseline procedures or tests:	N/A
Initiate IV:	0.9% sodium chloride
Premedicate:	5-HT_3 and dexamethasone 20 mg in 100 cc of NS.
Administer:	

Cisplatin _____ mg (100 mg/m^2) IV on day 1

- Do not use aluminum needles, because precipitate will form.
- Available in 1-mg/mL solution.
- Further dilute in 250 cc or more of NS.

Cyclophosphamide _____ mg (600 mg/m^2) IV on day 1

- Available in 100-, 200-, 500-, 1000-, and 2000-mg vials.
- Dilute with sterile water and shake well to ensure that solution is completely dissolved.
- Reconstituted solution stable for 24 hours at room temperature, and 6 days refrigerated.

Major Side Effects

- Bone Marrow Depression: Leukopenia, thrombocytopenia, and anemia all seen; may be severe and dose limiting.
- GI Toxicities: Nausea and vomiting is moderate to severe and can be acute or delayed.
- Renal/bladder Toxicities: Nephrotoxicity is dose related with cisplatin and presents at 10–20 days. Hemorrhagic cystitis, dysuria, and urinary frequency.
- Electrolyte Imbalance: Decreased Mg^{2+}, K, Ca^{2+}, Na^+, and P.
- Skin: Hyperpigmentation of skin and nails. Complete alopecia.
- Neurotoxicity: Dose-limiting toxicity, usually in the form of peripheral sensory neuropathy. Paresthesias and numbness in a classic "stocking glove" pattern. Increased risk with cumulative dosing.
- Ototoxicity: High-frequency hearing loss and tinnitus with cisplatin.
- Reproductive: Drugs are teratogenic and mutagenic. Sterility may be permanent.

Initiate antiemetic protocol:	Moderately to highly emetogenic protocol.
Supportive drugs:	☐ pegfilgrastim (Neulasta) ☐ filgrastim (Neupogen)
	☐ epoetin alfa (Procrit) ☐ darbepoetin alfa (Aranesp)
Treatment schedule:	Chair time 4 hours on day 1. Repeat cycle every 28 days.
Estimated number of visits:	Two visits per cycle. Request three cycles worth of visits.

Dose Calculation by: 1. _____   2. _____

_____

Physician

_____

Patient Name

_____

Diagnosis

_____

Date

_____

ID Number

_____ / _____ / _____
Ht   Wt   M^2

Cisplatin + Paclitaxel (CT)

Baseline laboratory tests:	CBC: Chemistry (including Mg^{2+}) and CA 125
Baseline procedures or tests:	Central line placement
Initiate IV:	0.9% sodium chloride
Premedicate:	5-HT$_3$ and dexamethasone 10–20 mg in 100 cc of NS (days 1 and 2)
	Diphenhydramine 25–50 mg and cimetidine 300 mg in 100 cc of NS (day 1 only)
Administer:	**Paclitaxel** _____ mg (135 mg/m^2) IV over 24 hours on day 1

- Available in 30 mg and 300 mg vials (6 mg/mL) or 100 mg (16.7 mg/mL).
- Final concentration is $\leq$ 1.2 mg/mL.
- **Use non-PVC containers and tubing with 0.22-micron inline filter for administration.**

Cisplatin _____ mg (75 mg/m^2) IV on day 2

- Available in 1 mg/mL solution.
- Do not use aluminum needles, because precipitate will form.
- Further dilute solution with 250 cc or more of NS.

Repeat cycle every 21 days.

Paclitaxel must be administered first, followed by carboplatin.

Major Side Effects

- Hypersensitivity Reaction: Paclitaxel (30%–40%). Premedicate as described.
- Bone Marrow Depression: Neutropenia, thrombocytopenia, and anemia are cumulative and dose related. Can be dose limiting. G-CSF support recommended.
- GI Toxicities: Moderate-to-severe nausea and vomiting may be acute or delayed.
- Renal: Nephrotoxicity is dose related with cisplatin and presents at 10–20 days. Risk may be reduced with adequate hydration.
- Electrolyte Imbalance: Decreases MG^{2+}, K^+, Ca^{2+}, Na^+, and P.
- Neurotoxicity: Severe neuropathy with numbness, tingling, and sensory loss in classic "stocking and glove" distribution. Proprioception, vibrating sense, and loss of motor function can occur. Increased risk with cumulative dose, more frequent with longer infusions.
- Alopecia: Total loss of body hair occurs in nearly all patients.
- Reproduction: Pregnancy category D. Breast feeding should be avoided.

Initiate antiemetic protocol:	Moderate to highly emetogenic protocol.
Supportive drugs:	☐ pegfilgrastim (Neulasta) ☐ filgrastim (Neupogen)
	☐ epoetin alfa (Procrit) ☐ darbepoetin alfa (Aranesp)
Treatment schedule:	Chair time 1 hour on day 1, and 3 hours on day 2. Repeat every 21 days as tolerated or until disease progression.
Estimated number of visits:	Two visits per cycle. Request three cycles worth of visits.

Dose Calculation by: 1. _____   2. _____

_____

Physician

_____

Patient Name

_____

Diagnosis

_____

Date

_____

ID Number

_____ / _____ / _____

Ht   Wt   M^2

Carboplatin + Paclitaxel

Baseline laboratory tests:	CBC: Chemistry, CA 125
Baseline procedures or tests:	N/A
Initiate IV:	0.9% sodium chloride
Premedicate:	5-HT$_3$ and dexamethasone 10–20 mg in 100 cc of NS
	Diphenhydramine 25–50 mg and cimetidine 300 mg in 100 cc of NS

Administer:

Paclitaxel _____ mg (175 mg/m^2) IV over 3 hours day 1

- Available in 30 mg and 300 mg vials (6 mg/mL) or 100 mg vial (16.7 mg/mL).
- Final concentration is ≤ 1.2 mg/mL.
- **Use non-PVC containers and tubing with 0.22-micron inline filter to administer.**

Carboplatin _____ mg (AUC 6–7.5) IV on day 1

- Available in 50-, 150-, and 450-mg lyopholized powder or 50-, 150-, 450-, and 600-mg solution (10 mg/mL).
- Multidose vial stable for 15 days after first use.
- Do not use aluminum needles, because precipitate will form.
- Give carboplatin **after** paclitaxel to decrease toxicities.

Major Side Effects

- Hypersensitivity Reaction: Paclitaxel (30%–40%). Characterized by rash, urticaria, erythema, and pruritis. Bronchospasms and hypotension uncommon but may occur 1–4% of patients. Premedicate as described. Increased risk of hypersensitivity reactions in patients receiving more than seven courses of carboplatin therapy.
- Bone Marrow Depression: Neutropenia, thrombocytopenia, and anemia are cumulative and dose related. Can be dose limiting. G-CSF support recommended.
- GI Toxicities: Moderate to severe nausea and vomiting may be acute or delayed. Mucositis and/or diarrhea occurs in 30%–40% of patients.
- Renal: Nephrotoxicity less common than with cisplatin and rarely symptomatic.
- Electrolyte imbalance: Decreases Mg^{2+}, K$^+$, Ca^{2+}, Na$^+$, and P.
- Neurotoxicity: Severe neuropathy with numbness and tingling in classic "stocking and glove" distribution. Proprioception, vibrating sense, and motor function loss can occur. Increased risk with cumulative dosing and longer infusions.
- Alopecia: Total loss of body hair occurs in nearly all patients.
- Reproduction: Pregnancy category D. Breast feeding should be avoided.

Initiate antiemetic protocol:	Moderately to highly emetogenic protocol.
Supportive drugs:	☐ pegfilgrastim (Neulasta) ☐ filgrastim (Neupogen)
	☐ epoetin alfa (Procrit) ☐ darbepoetin alfa (Aranesp)
Treatment schedule:	Chair time 5 hours on day 1. Repeat cycle every 21 days until disease progression.
Estimated number of visits:	Two visits per cycle. Request three cycles worth of visits.

Dose Calculation by: 1. _____ 2. _____

_____

Physician

_____

Patient Name

_____

Diagnosis

_____

Date

_____

ID Number

_____ / _____ / _____

Ht   Wt   M^2

Carboplatin + Docetaxel

Baseline laboratory tests:	CBC: Chemistry (including Mg^{2+}) and CA 125
Baseline procedures or tests:	N/A
Initiate IV:	0.9% sodium chloride
Premedicate:	Dexamethasone 8-mg PO bid for 3 days, starting the day before treatment
	5-HT$_3$ and dexamethasone 10–20 mg in 100 cc of NS day of treatment
Administer:	**Carboplatin** _____ mg (AUC 6) IV on day 1

- Available in 50-, 150-, and 450-mg lyopolized powder or 50-, 150-, 450-, and 600-mg solution (10 mg/mL).
- Multidose vial stable for 15 days after first use.
- Do not use aluminum needle, because precipitate will form.
- Available in powder or solution. Discard reconstituted powder after 8 hours.

Docetaxel _____ mg (60 mg/m^2) IV on day 1

- Available in 20- or 80-mg doses; comes with own diluent. Do not shake.
- Reconstituted vials stable at room temperature or if refrigerated for 8 hours.
- Further dilute in 250 cc of D5W or 0.9% sodium chloride.
- **Use non-PVC containers and tubings to administer.**

Major Side Effects

- Hypersensitivity Reaction: Severe hypersensitivity reactions with docetaxel in 2%–3% of patients. Premedication with dexamethasone recommended. Carboplatin can cause rash, urticaria, erythema, and pruritus. Bronchospasm and hypotension are uncommon, but risk increases from 1% to 27% in patients receiving more than seven courses of carboplatin-based therapy.
- Bone Marrow Depression: Neutropenia, thrombocytopenia, and anemia are dose related and can be dose limiting.
- GI Toxicities: Moderate-to-severe nausea and vomiting within first 24 hours.
- Renal: Nephrotoxicity less common than with cisplatin and rarely symptomatic.
- Electrolyte Imbalance: Decreased Mg^{2+}, K, Ca^{2+}, and Na^+
- Neuropathy: Neurologic dysfunction is infrequent, but there is increased risk in patients > 65 years old or those previously treated with cisplatin and receiving prolonged carboplatin treatment.
- Skin: Alopecia is common and pruritic rash may occur with docetaxel. Nail changes, occurring in 11–40% of patients may include onycholysis (loss of nail). Keep nails clean, use nail hardeners, tea tree oil. Lotrimin if indicated.
- Reproductive: Pregnancy category D. Breast feeding should be avoided.

Initiate antiemetic protocol:	Moderately to highly emetogenic protocol.
Supportive drugs:	☐ pegfilgrastim (Neulasta) ☐ filgrastim (Neupogen)
	☐ epoetin alfa (Procrit) ☐ darbepoetin alfa (Aranesp)
Treatment schedule:	Chair time 4 hours on day 1. Repeat cycle every 21 days.
Estimated number of visits:	Two visits per cycle. Request 6 months worth of visits.

Dose Calculation by: 1. _____   2. _____

Physician _____   Date _____

Patient Name _____   ID Number _____

Diagnosis _____   Ht _____ / Wt _____ / M^2 _____

Gemcitabine + Liposomal Doxorubicin

Baseline laboratory tests: CBC: Chemistry panel, LFTs, and CA 125
Baseline procedures or tests: N/A
Initiate IV: 0.9% sodium chloride
Premedicate: Oral 5-HT$_3$ or IV 5-HT$_3$ and dexamethasone 10 mg in 100 cc of NS
Administer: **Gemcitabine** _____ mg (1000 mg/m2) IV on days 1 and 8

- Available in 1-g or 200-mg vials, reconstitute with 0.9% sodium chloride.
- USP (5 cc for 200 mg, 25 cc for 1 g). Further dilute in 0.9% sodium chloride.
- Reconstituted solution is stable 24 hours at room temperature. DO NOT refrigerate, because precipitate will form.

Liposomal doxorubicin _____ mg (30 mg/m2) IV over 1 hour on day 1

- Available as a 2-mg/mL solution in 20- or 50-mg vials.
- Further dilute drug (doses up to 90 mg) in 250 cc of D5W.

Major Side Effects

- Infusion Reaction: Flushing, dyspnea, facial swelling, headache, back pain, tightness in the chest and throat, and/or hypotension with liposomal doxorubicin. Usually occurs during first treatment and is seen in 5%–10% of patients. Resolves quickly after infusion stopped.
- Bone Marrow Depression: Leukopenia occurs in 63–91% of patients, with anemia (73%), with grades 3 and 4 thrombocytopenia more common in elderly patients. Myelosuppression is dose limiting. Nadir occurs in 10–14 days with recovery at 21 days. Prolonged infusion time of gemcitabine (> 60 minutes) is associated with higher toxicities.
- GI Toxicities: Nausea and vomiting are usually mild to moderate (70%). Stomatitis occurs in 7% of patients and diarrhea in 8%; both are usually mild.
- Cardiac: Acutely, pericarditis and/or myocarditis, electrocardiographic changes, or arrhythmias. Not dose related. With high cumulative doses > 550 mg/m2, cardiomyopathy may occur. Increased risk of cardiotoxicity when liposomal doxorubicin is given with trastuzumab (Herceptin) or mitomycin.
- Skin: Manifested as hand-foot syndrome with skin rash, swelling, erythema, pain, and/or desquamation. Occurs in 3.4% of patients and is dose related. Edema occurs in 30% of patients. Alopecia is rare. Hyperpigmentation of nails, urticaria, and radiation recall can occur.
- Flulike Syndrome (20%) with fever in absence of infection 6–12 hours after treatment (40%).
- Hepatic: Elevation of serum transaminase and bilirubin levels.
- Reproduction: Pregnancy category D. Breast feeding should be avoided.

Initiate antiemetic protocol: Mildly to moderately emetogenic protocol.
Supportive drugs:
☐ pegfilgrastim (Neulasta)   ☐ filgrastim (Neupogen)
☐ epoetin alfa (Procrit)   ☐ darbepoetin alfa (Aranesp)
Treatment schedule: Chair time 1 hour weekly for 3 weeks. Repeat cycle every 4 weeks.
Estimated number of visits: Three visits per cycle. Request three cycles worth of visits.

Dose Calculation by: 1. _____   2. _____

_____
Physician

_____
Date

_____
Patient Name

_____
ID Number

_____
Diagnosis

_____ / _____ / _____
Ht   Wt   M^2

Gemcitabine + Cisplatin

Baseline laboratory tests:	CBC: Chemistry panel, LFTs, and CA 19-9
Baseline procedures or tests:	N/A
Initiate IV:	0.9% sodium chloride
Premedicate:	5-HT$_3$ and dexamethasone 10–20 mg in 100 cc of NS

Administer:

Gemcitabine _____ mg (800–1000 mg/m^2) IV on days 1 and 8

- Available in 1-g or 200-mg vials; reconstitute with 0.9% sodium chloride USP (5 cc for 200 mg, 25 cc for 1 g). Further dilute in 0.9% sodium chloride.
- Reconstituted solution is stable for 24 hours at room temperature. DO NOT refrigerate, because precipitate will form.

Cisplatin _____ mg (30 mg/m^2) IV on days 1 and 8

- Available in 1 mg/mL.
- Do not use aluminum needles, because precipitate will form.
- Further dilute solution with 250 cc or more 0.9% sodium chloride.

Major Side Effects

- Hematologic: Leukopenia (63%), thrombocytopenia (36%), and anemia (73%), with grade 3 and 4 thrombocytopenia more common in elderly patients. Myelosuppression is dose limiting. Nadir occurs in 10–14 days, with recovery at 21 days. Prolonged infusion time (> 60 minutes) is associated with higher toxicities.
- GI Symptoms: Moderate-to-severe nausea and vomiting; may be acute or delayed. Diarrhea and/or mucositis (15%–20%).
- Flulike Syndrome (20%) with fever in absence of infection 6–12 hours after treatment (40%).
- Renal: Nephrotoxicity is dose related with cisplatin and occurs at 10–20 days. Risk may be reduced with adequate hydration.
- Neurotoxicity: Neuropathy with numbness, tingling, and sensory loss in classic "stocking and glove" distribution. Proprioception, vibrating sense, and motor function loss can occur. Increased risk with cumulative doses and more frequent in longer infusions.
- Electrolyte Imbalance: Decreased Mg^{2+}, K, Ca^{2+}, Na$^+$, and P.
- Hepatic: Elevation of serum transaminase and bilirubin levels.
- Skin: Pruritic, maculopapular skin rash, usually involving trunk and extremities. Edema occurs in 30% of patients. Alopecia.
- Reproduction: Pregnancy category D. Breast feeding should be avoided.

Initiate antiemetic protocol:	Moderately to highly emetogenic protocol.

Supportive drugs:

☐ pegfilgrastim (Neulasta)   ☐ filgrastim (Neupogen)

☐ epoetin alfa (Procrit)   ☐ darbepoetin alfa (Aranesp)

Treatment schedule:	Chair time 3 hours on days 1 and 15, and 1 hour on day 8. Repeat cycle every 21 days.
Estimated number of visits:	Three visits per cycle. Request three cycles worth of visits.

Dose Calculation by: 1. _____   2. _____

_____
Physician

Date _____

_____
Patient Name

ID Number _____

_____
Diagnosis

_____ / _____ / _____
Ht   Wt   M^2

Single-Agent Regimens

Altretamine (Hexalen)

Baseline laboratory tests:	CBC: Chemistry, CA 125
Baseline procedures or tests:	N/A
Initiate IV:	N/A
Premedicate:	Oral phenothiazine or 5-HT$_3$
Administer:	**Altretamine** _____ mg (260 mg/m^2/day) PO in four divided doses (after meals and at bed time)

- Available in 50-mg gelatin capsules for oral use.

Major Side Effects

- Bone Marrow Suppression: Dose limiting toxicity; nadir occurs at 21–28 days and rapid recovery within 1 week of cessation of drug.
- GI Toxicities: Nausea and vomiting in 30% of patients; is usually mild to moderate. Worsens with increasing cumulative doses of drug. Usual dose-limiting toxicity. Diarrhea and cramps may also be dose limiting.
- Neurotoxicities. Peripheral sensory neuropathy occurs in 31% of patients and is moderate to severe in 9% of patients.
- CNS: Agitation, confusion, hallucinations, depression, mood disorders, and Parkinson-like symptoms may occur and are usually reversible. Neurological effects are more common with continuous dosing > 3 months rather than pulse dosing.
- Skin: Rashes, pruritus, eczematous skin lesions may occur but are rare.
- Renal: Elevations in blood urea nitrogen (BUN) (9%) or creatinine (7%) can occur.
- Reproductive: Pregnancy category D. Breat feeding should be avoided.

Initiate antiemetic protocol:	Mildly to moderately emetogenic protocol.
Supportive drugs:	☐ pegfilgrastim (Neulasta) ☐ filgrastim (Neupogen)
	☐ loperamide (Imodium) ☐ epoetin alfa (Procrit)
	☐ darbepoetin alfa (Aranesp) ☐ diphenoxylate/atropine sulfate (Lomotil)
Treatment schedule:	No chair time. Repeat cycle every 14–21 days.
Estimated number of visits:	One per cycle.

Dose Calculation by: 1. _____ 2. _____

_____

Physician

_____

Date

_____

Patient Name

_____

ID Number

_____

Diagnosis

_____ / _____ / _____
Ht   Wt   M^2

Liposomal Doxorubicin (Doxil)

Baseline laboratory tests:	CBC: Chemistry, CA 125
Baseline procedures or tests:	MUGA scan
Initiate IV:	0.9% sodium chloride
Premedicate:	5-HT$_3$ and dexamethasone 10–20 mg in 100 cc of NS.
Administer:	**Liposomal doxorubicin** _____ mg (50 mg/m^2) IV over 1 hour on day 1

- Available as a 2-mg/mL solution in 20- or 50-mg vials
- Further dilute drug (doses up to 90 mg) in 250 cc of D5W.

Major Side Effects

- Infusion Reaction: Flushing, dyspnea, facial swelling, headache, back pain, tightness in the chest and throat, and/or hypotension. Usually occurs during first treatment and is seen in 5%–10% of patients. Resolves quickly after infusion stopped.
- Bone Marrow Depression: Dose-limiting toxicity in the treatment of HIV-infected patients. Leukopenia occurs in 91% of patients, with anemia and thrombocytopenia less common.
- GI Toxicities: Nausea and vomiting are usually mild to moderate. Stomatitis occurs in 7% of patients and diarrhea in 8%; both are usually mild.
- Cardiac: Acutely, pericarditis and/or myocarditis, electrocardiographic changes, or arrhythmias. Not dose related. With high cumulative doses > 550 mg/m^2, cardiomyopathy may occur. Increased risk of cardiotoxicity when liposomal doxorubicin is given with trastuzumab (Herceptin) or mitomycin.
- Skin: Skin toxicity manifested as hand-foot syndrome with skin rash, swelling, erythema, pain, and/or desquamation. Occurs in 3.4% of patients and is dose related. Hyperpigmentation of nails, skin rash, urticaria, and radiation recall occur. Alopecia occurs in 9% of patients with Kaposi's sarcoma.
- Reproductive: Pregnancy category D. Breast feeding should be avoided.

Initiate antiemetic protocol:	Moderately to highly emetogenic protocol.
Supportive drugs:	☐ pegfilgrastim (Neulasta) ☐ filgrastim (Neupogen) ☐ epoetin alfa (Procrit) ☐ darbepoetin alfa (Aranesp)
Treatment schedule:	Chair time 2 hours on day 1. Repeat cycle every 28 days.
Estimated number of visits:	Two visits per cycle. Request four cycles worth of visits.

Dose Calculation by: 1. _____ 2. _____

Physician _____ Date _____

Patient Name _____ ID Number _____

Diagnosis _____ _____/_____/_____
Ht   Wt   M^2

Paclitaxel

Baseline laboratory tests:	CBC: Chemistry (including Mg2+) and CA 125
Baseline procedures or tests:	N/A
Initiate IV:	0.9% sodium chloride
Premedicate:	5-HT$_3$ and dexamethasone 10–20 mg in 100 cc of NS
	Diphenhydramine 25–50 mg and cimetidine 300 mg in 100 cc of NS
Administer:	**Paclitaxel _____ mg (135 mg/m^2) IV over 3 hours on day 1**

- Final concentration is $\leq$ 1.2 mg/mL.
- **Use non-PVC containers and tubing with 0.22-micron inline filter for administration.**

Major Side Effects

- Hypersensitivity Reaction: Occurs in 20%–40% of patients. Characterized by generalized skin rash, flushing, erythema, hypotension, dyspnea, and/or bronchospasm. Usually occurs within the first 2–3 minutes of infusion and almost always within the first 10 minutes. Premedicate as described.
- Bone Marrow Depression: Dose-limiting neutropenia with nadir at days 8–10 and recovery by days 15–21. Decreased incidence of neutropenia with 3-hour schedule when compared with 24-hour schedule. G-CSF support recommended.
- GI Toxicity: Nausea and vomiting occur in 52% of patients, mild and preventable with anitemetics. Diarrhea in 38% of patients and stomatitis in 31%.
- Neurotoxicity: Severe neuropathy with numbness, tingling, and sensory loss in arms and legs. Proprioception and vibratory sense and loss of motor function can occur. Paresthesias are dose related and can be severe, requiring pain medication or neurontin. More frequent with longer infusions and at doses > 175 mg/m^2.
- Ototoxicity occurs in > 30% beginning with high-frequency hearing.
- Alopecia: Total loss of body hair occurs in nearly all patients.
- Reproduction: Pregnancy category D. Breast feeding should be avoided.

Initiate antiemetic protocol:	Mildly emetogenic protocol.
Supportive drugs:	☐ pegfilgrastim (Neulasta) ☐ filgrastim (Neupogen)
	☐ epoetin alfa (Procrit) ☐ darbepoetin alfa (Aranesp)
Treatment schedule:	Chair time 4 hours on day 1. Repeat every 21 days as tolerated or until disease progression
Estimated number of visits:	Two visits per cycle. Request three cycles worth of visits.

Dose Calculation by: 1. _____   2. _____

_____   _____
Physician   Date

_____   _____
Patient Name   ID Number

_____   _____/ _____/ _____
Diagnosis   Ht   Wt   M^2

Topotecan

Baseline laboratory tests:	CBC: Chemistry panel, LFTs, and CA 125
Baseline procedures or tests:	N/A
Initiate IV:	0.9% sodium chloride
Premedicate:	5-HT$_3$ and dexamethasone 10 mg in 100 cc of NS
Administer:	**Topotecan** _____ mg (1.5 mg/m^2) IV on days 1–5

- Available as a 4-mg vial.
- Reconstitute vial with 4 mL of sterile water for injection.
- Further dilute in 0.9% sodium chloride or D5W.
- Use immediately.

Major Side Effects

- Hematologic: Severe grade 4 myelosuppression occurs during the first course of therapy in 60% of patients. Dose-limiting toxicity. Typical nadir occurs at days 7–10 with full recovery by days 21–28. If severe neutropenia occurs, reduce dose by 0.25 mg/m^2 for subsequent doses, or may use G-CSF to prevent neutropenia 24 hours after last day of topotecan therapy.
- GI Toxicities: Nausea and vomiting, mild to moderate and dose related. Occurs in 60%–80% of patients. Diarrhea occurs in 42% of patients, and constipation occurs in 39%. Abdominal pain may occur in 33% of patients.
- Hepatic Toxicity: Evidence of increased drug toxicity in patients with low protein levels and hepatic dysfunction. Dose reductions may be necessary.
- Renal: Use with caution in patients with abnormal renal function. Dose reduction is necessary in this setting. Microscopic hematuria occurs in 10% of patients.
- Skin: Alopecia.
- Reproduction: Pregnancy category D. Breast feeding should be avoided.

Initiate antiemetic protocol:	Mildly to moderately emetogenic protocol.	
Supportive drugs:	☐ pegfilgrastim (Neulasta)	☐ filgrastim (Neupogen)
	☐ epoetin alfa (Procrit)	☐ darbepoetin alfa (Aranesp)
Treatment schedule:	Chair time 1 hour on days 1–5. Repeat every 21 days until disease progression.	
Estimated number of visits:	Six visits per cycle. Request three cycles.	

Dose Calculation by: 1. _____   2. _____

_____

Physician

Date _____

_____

Patient Name

ID Number _____

_____

Diagnosis

Ht _____ / Wt _____ / M^2 _____

Gemcitabine

Baseline laboratory tests:	CBC: Chemistry panel, LFTs, and CA 125
Baseline procedures or tests:	N/A
Initiate IV:	0.9% sodium chloride
Premedicate:	Oral phenothiazine
	OR
	5-HT$_3$ and dexamethasone 10 mg in 100 cc of NS
Administer:	**Gemcitabine** _____ mg (800 mg/m^2) IV weekly for 3 weeks

- Available in 1-g or 200-mg vials, reconstitute with 0.9% sodium chloride USP (5 cc for 200 mg, 25 cc for 1 g). Further dilute in 0.9% sodium chloride.
- Reconstituted solution is stable 24 hours at room temperature. DO NOT refrigerate, because precipitate will form.

Major Side Effects

- Infusion Reactions: Characterized by flushing, facial swelling, headache, dyspnea and/or hypotension. Usually related to rate of infusion and resolves with discontinuation of infusion.
- Hematologic: Leukopenia (63%), thrombocytopenia (36%), and anemia (73%), with grades 3 and 4 thrombocytopenia more common in elderly patients. Myelosuppression is dose limiting. Nadir occurs in 10–14 days with recovery at 21 days. Prolonged infusion time (> 60 minutes) is associated with higher toxicities.
- GI Symptoms: Mild to moderate nausea and vomiting (70%), diarrhea, and/or mucositis (15%–20%).
- Flulike Syndrome (20%) with fever in absence of infection 6–12 hours after treatment (40%).
- Hepatic: Elevation of serum transaminase and bilirubin levels.
- Pulmonary Toxicities: Mild dyspnea or drug induced pneumonitis may occur.
- Skin: Pruritic, maculopapular skin rash, usually involving trunk and extremities. Edema occurs in 30% of patients. Alopecia is rare.
- Reproduction: Pregnancy category D. Breast feeding should be avoided.

Initiate antiemetic protocol:	Mildly to moderately emetogenic protocol.
Supportive drugs:	☐ pegfilgrastim (Neulasta) ☐ filgrastim (Neupogen)
	☐ epoetin alfa (Procrit) ☐ darbepoetin alfa (Aranesp)
Treatment schedule:	Chair time 1 hour weekly for 3 weeks. Repeat cycle every 4 weeks.
Estimated number of visits:	Six visits per cycle. Request three cycles worth of visits.

Dose Calculation by: 1. _____   2. _____

_____

Physician

_____

Patient Name

_____

Diagnosis

_____

Date

_____

ID Number

_____ / _____ / _____

Ht   Wt   M^2

Etoposide

Baseline laboratory tests:	CBC: Chemistry, LFTs, and CA 125
Baseline procedures or tests:	N/A
Initiate IV:	0.9% sodium chloride
Premedicate:	Oral phenothiazine or 5-HT$_3$.
Administer:	**Etoposide** _____ mg (50 mg/m^2/day) PO days 1–21

- Available in 50- or 100-mg capsules for oral use
- May give as a single dose up to 400 mg; > 400 mg, divide dose into 2–4 doses.
- Store in refrigerator.

Major Side Effects

- Bone Marrow Depression: Nadir 10–14 days after drug dose, with recovery on days 21–22. Neutropenia may be severe.
- GI Toxicities: Nausea and vomiting and anoxeria occur in 30%–40% of patients and is generally mild to moderate. More commonly observed with oral administration.
- Skin: Alopecia observed in nearly two thirds of patients.
- Neurotoxicities: Peripheral neuropathies may occur but are rare and mild.
- Reproductive: Pregnancy category D. Breast feeding should be avoided.

Initiate antiemetic protocol:	Mildly emetogenic protocol.
Supportive drugs:	☐ pegfilgrastim (Neulasta) ☐ filgrastim (Neupogen) ☐ epoetin alfa (Procrit) ☐ darbepoetin alfa (Aranesp)
Treatment schedule:	No chair time. Repeat cycle every 28 days as tolerated or until disease progression.
Estimated number of visits:	One to two visits per cycle. Request three cycles worth of visits.

Dose Calculation by: 1. _____ 2. _____

_____   _____

Physician   Date

_____   _____

Patient Name   ID Number

_____   _____/ _____/ _____

Diagnosis   Ht   Wt   M^2

OVARIAN CANCER

(Germ Cell)

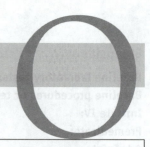

Combination Regimens

Bleomycin: 30 U IV on days 2, 9, and 16
Etoposide: 100 mg/m²/day IV on days 1–5
Cisplatin: 20 mg/m²/day IV on days 1–5
Repeat cycle every 21 days.[1,350]

Combination Regimens

Etoposide + Bleomycin + Cisplatin (BEP)

Baseline laboratory tests:	CBC: Chemistry (including Mg^{2+})
Baseline procedures or tests:	PFTs and chest x-ray study at baseline and before each cycle of therapy
Initiate IV:	0.9% sodium chloride
Premedicate:	5-HT$_3$ and dexamethasone 10–20 mg in 100 cc of NS
	Acetaminophen 30 minutes before bleomycin

Administer:

Bleomycin 30 units IV push or infusion over 15 minutes on days 2, 9, and 16

- A test dose of 2 units is recommended before the first dose to detect hypersensitivity.
- Available as a powder in 15- or 30-unit sizes. Dilute powder in 0.9% sodium chloride or sterile water.
- Reconstituted solution is stable for 24 hours at room temperature.

Etoposide _____ mg (100 mg/m^2) IV infusion over 1 hour on days 1–5

- Available in 100-mg vials; when reconstituted with 5 or 10 mL of NS, D5W or sterile water with benzyl alcohol makes a 20- or 10-mg/mL solution. Also available in solution as a 20-mg/mL concentration.
- May be further diluted in NS or D5W to final concentration of 0.1 mg/mL

Cisplatin _____ mg (20 mg/m^2) IV infusion over 1–2 hours on days 1–5

- Do not use aluminum needles, because precipitate will form.
- Available in solution as 1 mg/mL.
- Further dilute solution with 250 cc or more of NS.

Major Side Effects

- Allergic Reaction: Bleomycin—fever and chills observed in up to 25% of patients. True anaphylactic reactions are rare. Etoposide—bronchospasm, with or without fever, chills. Hypotension may occur during rapid infusion. Anaphylaxis may occur but is rare.
- Bone Marrow Depression: Myelosuppression can be a dose-limiting toxicity.
- GI Toxicities: Moderate-to-severe nausea and vomiting. May be acute (first 24 hours) or delayed (> 24 hours). Mucositis and diarrhea are rare.
- Pulmonary Toxicities: Pulmonary toxicity is dose limiting in bleomycin. Seen more frequently cumulative with bleomycin dose > 400 units.
- Renal: Nephrotoxicity is dose related with cisplatin and presents at 10–20 days. Risk may be reduced with adequate hydration
- Electrolyte Imbalance: Decreased Mg^{2+}, K, Ca^{2+}, Na^+, and P.
- Neurotoxicity: Dose-limiting toxicity, usually in the form of peripheral sensory neuropathy. Paresthesias and numbness in a classic "stocking glove" pattern.
- Ototoxicity: High-frequency hearing loss and tinnitus.
- Skin: Alopecia
- Reproductive: Pregnancy category D. Breast feeding should be avoided.

Initiate antiemetic protocol:	Moderately to highly emetogenic protocol.
Supportive drugs:	☐ pegfilgrastim (Neulasta) ☐ filgrastim (Neupogen)
	☐ epoetin alfa (Procrit) ☐ darbepoetin alfa (Aranesp)
Treatment schedule:	Chair time 3 hours on days 1, 1–5, and 1 hour on days 9 and 16. Repeat every 21 days.
Estimated number of visits:	Seven visits per cycle. Request three cycles worth of visits.

Dose Calculation by: 1. _____ 2. _____

_____
Physician

_____
Date

_____
Patient Name

_____
ID Number

_____
Diagnosis

_____/_____/_____
Ht   Wt   M^2

PANCREATIC CANCER

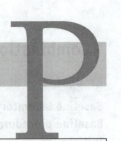

LOCALLY ADVANCED DISEASE

5-Fluorouracil + Radiation Therapy
(Gastrointestinal Tumor Study) 567

Group [GITSG] Regimen)

5-Fluorouracil: 500-mg/m^2/day IV on days 1–3 and 29–31, then weekly
  beginning on day 71

Radiation therapy: Total dose, 4000 cGy

Chemotherapy and radiation therapy started on the same day and given
  concurrently.[1,351]

METASTATIC DISEASE
Combination Regimens

5-Fluorouracil + Leucovorin 568

5-Fluorouracil: 425-mg/m^2 IV on days 1–5

Leucovorin: 20-mg/m^2 IV on days 1–5

Repeat cycle every 28 days.[1,352]

Gemcitabine + Capecitabine...569

Gemcitabine: 1000-mg/m^2 IV on days 1 and 8

Capecitabine: 650-mg/m^2 PO bid on days 1–14

Repeat cycle every 21 days.[1,353]

Gemcitabine + Docetaxel + Capecitabine (GTX) 570

Gemcitabine: 750-mg/m^2 IV over 75 minutes on days 4 and 11

Docetaxel: 30-mg/m^2 IV on days 4 and 11

Capecitabine: 1000–1500 mg/m^2 PO bid on days 1–14

Repeat cycle every 2 weeks.[1,354]

Gemcitabine + Cisplatin..572

Gemcitabine: 1000-mg/m^2 IV on days 1, 8, and 15

Cisplatin: 50-mg/m^2 IV on days 1 and 15

Repeat cycle every 28 days.[1,355]

Gemcitabine + Cisplatin (Modified) **573**

Gemcitabine: 600–750 mg/m^2 IV on days 1 and 15
Cisplatin: 25-mg/m^2 IV on days 1 and 15
Repeat cycle every 28 days.[1,356]

Gemcitabine + Cisplatin (Fixed Dose Rate) **574**

Gemcitabine: 1000-mg/m^2 IV on days 1 and 8
Cisplatin: 20-mg/m^2 IV on days 1 and 8
Repeat cycle every 28 days[1,357,358]

Gemcitabine + Oxaliplatin **575**

Gemcitabine: 1000-mg/m^2 IV over 100 minutes at 10 mg/m^2/min on day 1
Oxaliplatin: 100-mg/m^2 over 2 hours on day 2.
Repeat cycle every 2 weeks.[1,359]

Gemcitabine + Irinotecan **576**

Gemcitabine: 1000-mg/m^2 IV over 30 minutes on days 1 and 8
Irinotecan: 100-mg/m^2 IV over 90 minutes on days 1 and 8
Repeat cycle every 21 days.[1,360]

FAM **577**

5-Fluorouracil: 600-mg/m^2 IV on days 1, 8, 29, and 36
Doxorubicin: 30-mg/m^2 IV on days 1 and 29
Mitomycin: 10-mg/m^2 IV on day 1
Repeat cycle every 56 days.[1,361]

Gemcitabine + Erlotinib (Tarcera) **578**

Gemcitabine: 1000-mg/m^2 IV weekly for 7 weeks, then 1 week rest,
  subsequent cycles
1000-mg/m^2 IV weekly for 3 weeks with 1 week rest
Erlotinib: 100-mg PO daily
Repeat 3-week cycles every 28 days.[1,362]

5-Fluorouracil + Streptozocin + Mitomycin **580**

5-Fluorouracil: 600-mg/m^2 IV on days 1, 8, 29, and 36
Streptozocin: 1000-mg/m^2 IV over 1 hour on days 1, 8, 29, and 36
Mitomycin: 10-mg/m^2 IV bolus on day 1
Repeat cycle every 72 days.[1,363]

Single-Agent Regimens

Gemcitabine: 1000-mg/m^2 IV weekly for 7 weeks, then 1-week rest
Subsequent cycles 1000-mg/m^2 IV weekly for 3 weeks with 1-week rest
Repeat 3-week cycle every 28 days.[1,364]

OR

Gemcitabine: 1000-mg/m^2 IV over 100 minutes at 10 mg/m^2/min on days
 1, 8, and 15
Repeat cycle every 28 days.[1,365]

Capecitabine: 1250-mg/m^2 PO bid on days 1–14
Repeat cycle every 21 days.[1,366]

LOCALLY ADVANCED DISEASE

5-Fluorouracil + Radiation Therapy (GITSG)

Baseline laboratory tests:	CBC: Chemistry and CA 19-9
Baseline procedures or tests:	N/A
Initiate IV:	0.9% sodium chloride
Premedicate:	Oral phenothiazine or 5-HT$_3$
Administer:	**Fluorouracil** _____ mg (500 mg/m^2/day) IV on days 1–3 and 29–31, then weekly beginning on day 71

- Available 500 mg/10mL.
- No dilution required. Can be further diluted with 0.9% sodium chloride or D5W.

Radiation therapy:	Total dose, 4000 cGy

Chemotherapy and radiation therapy are started on the same day and given concurrently.

Major Side Effects

- Bone Marrow Depression: Nadir 10–14 days. Neutropenia, thrombocytopenia are dose related. Can be dose limiting for daily for 5 or weekly regimens.
- GI Toxicities: Nausea and vomiting occur in 30%–50% of patients but is usually mild. Nausea and vomiting and dehydration may worsen thoughout treatment may require IV hydration and additional antiemetics. Mucositis and diarrhea can be severe and dose limiting.
- Skin: Local tissue irritation in radiation field progressing to desquamation can occur. Do not use oil-based lotions or creams in radiation field. Hyperpigmentation, photosensitivity, and nail changes may occur with 5-fluorouracil as well as hand-foot syndrome can be dose limiting.
- Ocular: Photophobia, increased lacrimation, conjunctivitis, and blurred vision may occur with 5-fluorouracil.
- Reproduction: Pregnancy category D. Breast feeding should be avoided.

Initiate antiemetic protocol:	Mildly emetogenic protocol.
Supportive drugs:	☐ pegfilgrastim (Neulasta) ☐ filgrastim (Neupogen)
	☐ epoetin alfa (Procrit) ☐ darbepoetin alfa (Aranesp)
Treatment schedule:	Chair time 1 hour on days 1–3 and 29–31, then weekly beginning on day 71.
Estimated number of visits:	Six visits first month. One visit weekly beginning week 10 and through the end of radiation therapy.

Dose Calculation by: 1. _____   2. _____

_____   _____
Physician   Date

_____   _____
Patient Name   ID Number

_____   _____ / _____ / _____
Diagnosis   Ht   Wt   M^2

METASTATIC DISEASE
Combination Regimens

5-Fluorouracil+Leucovorin (Mayo Clinic Regimen)

Baseline laboratory tests:	CBC: Chemistry and CA 19-9
Baseline procedures or tests:	N/A
Initiate IV:	0.9% sodium chloride
Premedicate:	Oral phenothiazine or 5-HT$_3$
Administer:	**Leucovorin** _____ mg (20 mg/m^2/day) IV bolus on days 1–5

- Available in solution or powder. Reconstitute solution with sterile water. May further dilute with 0.9% sodium chloride or D5W.
- Do not mix in same solution with 5-FU, because a precipitate will form.

5-FU_____ mg (425 mg/m^2/day) IV bolus 1 hour after start of leucovorin, days 1–5.

- Available 500 mg/10mL.
- No dilution required. Can be further diluted with 0.9% sodium chloride or D5W.

Major Side Effects

- Bone Marrow Depression: Nadir 10–14 days. Neutropenia, thrombocytopenia are dose related. Can be dose limiting for daily for 5 or weekly regimens.
- GI Toxicities: Nausea and vomiting occur in 30%–50% of patients but is usually mild. Mucositis and diarrhea can be severe and dose limiting.
- Skin: Alopecia is more common in the 5-day course and results in diffuse thinning of hair. Hyperpigmentation, photosensitivity, and nail changes may occur. Hand-foot syndrome can be dose limiting.
- Ocular: Photophobia, increased lacrimation, conjunctivitis, and blurred vision.
- Reproduction: Pregnancy category D. Breast feeding should be avoided.

Initiate antiemetic protocol:	Mildly emetogenic protocol.
Supportive drugs:	☐ pegfilgrastim (Neulasta) ☐ filgrastim (Neupogen)
	☐ epoetin alfa (Procrit) ☐ darbepoetin alfa (Aranesp)
Treatment schedule:	Chair time 1 hour on days 1–5. Repeat cycle every 28 days for six cycles.
Estimated number of visits:	Six visits per cycle. 36 per treatment course.

Dose Calculation by: 1. _____   2. _____

_____
Physician

_____
Date

_____
Patient Name

_____
ID Number

_____
Diagnosis

_____ / _____ / _____
Ht   Wt   M^2

Gemcitabine + Capecitabine (Xeloda)

Baseline laboratory tests:	CBC: Chemistry panel, LFTs, CA 19-9, and creatinine clearance
Baseline procedures or tests:	N/A
Initiate IV:	0.9% sodium chloride
Premedicate:	Oral phenothiazine or 5-HT$_3$ and dexamethasone 10 mg
Administer:	**Gemcitabine** _____ mg (1000 mg/m^2) IV on days 1 and 8

- Available in 1-g or 200-mg vials, reconstitute with 0.9% sodium chloride USP (5 cc for 200 mg, 25 cc for 1 g). Further dilute in 0.9% sodium chloride.
- Reconstituted solution is stable for 24 hours at room temperature. DO NOT refrigerate, because precipitate will form.

Capecitabine _____ mg (650 mg/m^2) PO bid on days 1–14

- Available in 150 mg and 500 mg tablets. Do not cut tablets.
- Administer within 30 minutes of a meal with plenty of water.
- Monitor international normalized ratios (INRs) closely in patients taking warfarin; may increase INR.

Major Side Effects	

- Hematologic: Leukopenia (63%), thrombocytopenia (36%), and anemia (73%), with grades 3 and 4 thrombocytopenia more common in elderly patients. Myelosuppression is dose limiting. Nadir occurs in 10–14 days with recovery at 21 days. Prolonged infusion time (> 60 minutes) is associated with higher toxicities.
- GI Symptoms: Mild-to-moderate nausea and vomiting (70%), diarrhea and/or mucositis (15%–20%). Diarrhea occurs in up to 40% with 12% being grade 3–4. Stomatitis is common, 3% of which is severe.
- Flulike Syndrome: (20%) with fever in absence of infection 6–12 hours after treatment (40%).
- Renal Insufficiency: Xeloda is contraindicated in patients with creatinine clearance < 30 mL/min. CRCL 30–50 mL/min at baseline should be dose reduced to 75% of total xeloda dose.
- Hepatic: Elevation of serum transaminase and bilirubin levels. Dose modifications may be required if hyperbilirubinemia occurs.
- Skin: Hand-foot syndrome (15%–20%). Pruritic, maculopapular skin rash, usually involving trunk and extremities. Edema occurs in 30% of patients. Alopecia is rare.
- Reproduction: Pregnancy category D. Breast feeding should be avoided.

Initiate antiemetic protocol:	Mildly to moderately emetogenic protocol.
Supportive drugs:	☐ pegfilgrastim (Neulasta) ☐ filgrastim (Neupogen)
	☐ epoetin alfa (Procrit) ☐ darbepoetin alfa (Aranesp)
	☐ loperamide (Imodium) ☐ diphenoxylate/atropine sulfate (Lomotil)
Treatment schedule:	Chair time 1 hour. Repeat weekly for 7 weeks, then 1-week rest. Then weekly for 3 weeks with 1 week off.
	Repeat every 21 days until disease progression.
Estimated number of visits:	Ten visits initial course (3 months). Three visits per month subsequent courses.

Dose Calculation by: 1. _____   2. _____

_____
Physician

_____
Patient Name

_____
Diagnosis

_____
Date

_____
ID Number

_____ / _____ / _____
Ht   Wt   M^2

Gemcitabine + Docetaxel + Capecitabine (GTX)

Baseline laboratory tests:	CBC: Chemistry panel, LFTs, and CA 19-9
Baseline procedures or tests:	N/A
Initiate IV:	0.9% sodium chloride
Premedicate:	Oral phenothiazine

OR

5-HT$_3$ and dexamethasone 10 mg in 100 cc of NS and dexamethasone 8-mg PO bid for 3 days, starting the day before treatment

Administer:

Gemcitabine _____ mg (750 mg/m^2) IV over 75 minutes days 4 and 11

- Available in 1-g or 200-mg vials; reconstitute with 0.9% sodium chloride USP (5 cc for 200 mg, 25 cc for 1 g). Further dilute in 0.9% sodium chloride.
- Reconstituted solution is stable for 24 hours at room temperature. DO NOT refrigerate, because precipitate will form.

Docetaxel _____ mg (30 mg/m^2) IV on days 4 and 11

- Available in 20- or 80-mg doses; comes with own diluent. Do not shake. Reconstituted drug stable at room temperature or if refrigerated for 8 hours.
- Further dilute in 250 cc of D5W or 0.9% sodium chloride.
- Use non-PVC containers and tubings to administer.

Capecitabine _____ mg (1000–1250 mg/m^2) PO bid on days 1–14

- Available in 150 and 500 mg tablets. Do not cut tablets.
- Administer within 30 minutes of a meal with plenty of water.
- Monitor INRs closely in patients taking warfarin; may increase INR

Major Side Effects

- Hypersensitivity: Severe hypersensitivity reactions with docetaxel in 2%–3% of patients. Characterized by skin rash, erythema, hypotension, dyspnea and /or bronchospasm. Usually occurs within first 2–3 minutes, usually after first dose. May be prevented with premedication with steroid and addition of diphenhydramine 50 mg IV and/or cimetidine 300 mg IV. Premedication with dexamethasone recommended.
- Hematologic: Myelosuppression is dose limiting.
- GI Symptoms: Mild to moderate nausea and vomiting, diarrhea, and mucositis. May require additional antiemetics and IV hydration.
- Sensory Neuropathy: Peripheral paresthesias and numbness (49%).
- Flulike Syndrome: (20%) with fever 6–12 hours after treatment.
- Hepatic: Elevation of serum transaminase and bilirubin levels.
- Skin: Pruritic rash and nail changes. Nail changes may include brown discoloration of nail beds and/or onycholysis (loss of nail). Keep nails clean. Use nail hardeners and tea tree oil. Lotrimin if indicated.
- Reproduction: Pregnancy category D. Breast feeding shoud be avoided.

Initiate antiemetic protocol:	Mildly to moderately emetogenic protocol.
Supportive drugs:	

- ☐ pegfilgrastim (Neulasta)   ☐ filgrastim (Neupogen)
- ☐ epoetin alfa (Procrit)   ☐ darbepoetin alfa (Aranesp)
- ☐ loperamide (Imodium)   ☐ diphenoxylate/atropine sulfate (Lomotil)

Treatment schedule:	Chair time 3 hours on days 4 and 11. Repeat cycle every 21–28 days until disease progression.
Estimated number of visits:	Three visits per cycle. Request three cycles worth of visits.

Dose Calculation by: 1. _____   2. _____

_____   _____

Physician   Date

_____   _____

Patient Name   ID Number

_____   _____/_____/_____

Diagnosis   Ht   Wt   M^2

Gemcitabine + Cisplatin

Baseline laboratory tests:	CBC: Chemistry panel, LFTs, and CA 19-9
Baseline procedures or tests:	N/A
Initiate IV:	0.9% sodium chloride
Premedicate:	5-HT$_3$ and dexamethasone 10–20 mg in 100 cc of NS
Administer:	**Gemcitabine** _____ mg (1000 mg/m^2) IV on days 1, 8, and 15

- Available in 1-g or 200-mg vials; reconstitute with 0.9% sodium chloride USP (5 cc for 200 mg, 25 cc for 1 g). Further dilute in 0.9% sodium chloride.
- Reconstituted solution is stable for 24 hours at room temperature. DO NOT refrigerate, because precipitate will form.

Cisplatin _____ mg (50 mg/m^2) IV on days 1 and 15

- Available 1 mg/mL.
- Do not use aluminum needles, because precipitate will form.
- Further dilute solution with 250 cc or more 0.9% sodium chloride.

Major Side Effects

- Hematologic: Leukopenia (63%), thrombocytopenia (36%), and anemia (73%), with grade 3 and 4 thrombocytopenia more common in elderly patients. Myelosuppression is dose limiting. Nadir occurs in 10–14 days, with recovery at 21 days. Prolonged infusion time (> 60 minutes) is associated with higher toxicities.
- GI Symptoms: Moderate-to-severe nausea and vomiting; may be acute or delayed. Diarrhea and/or mucositis (15%–20%).
- Flulike Syndrome (20%) with fever in absence of infection 6–12 hours after treatment (40%).
- Renal: Nephrotoxicity is dose related with cisplatin and occurs at 10–20 days. Risk may be reduced with adequate hydration.
- Neurotoxicity: Sensory neuropathy; dose related. Neuropathy with numbness, tingling, and sensory loss in classic "stocking and glove" distribution. Proprioception, vibrating sense, and motor function loss can occur. Increased risk with cumulative doses and more frequent in longer infusions.
- Electrolyte Imbalance: Decreased Mg^{2+}, K, Ca^{2+}, Na$^+$, and P.
- Hepatic: Elevation of serum transaminase and bilirubin levels.
- Skin: Pruritic, maculopapular skin rash, usually involving trunk and extremities. Edema occurs in 30% of patients. Alopecia.
- Reproduction: Pregnancy category D. Breast feeding should be avoided.

Initiate antiemetic protocol:	Moderately to highly emetogenic protocol.
Supportive drugs:	☐ pegfilgrastim (Neulasta) ☐ filgrastim (Neupogen)
	☐ epoetin alfa (Procrit) ☐ darbepoetin alfa (Aranesp)
Treatment schedule:	Chair time 3 hours on days 1 and 15, and 1 hour on day 8. Repeat cycle every 28 days.
Estimated number of visits:	Four visits per cycle. Request three cycles worth of visits.

Dose Calculation by: 1. _____ 2. _____

_____
Physician

_____
Date

_____
Patient Name

_____
ID Number

_____
Diagnosis

_____ / _____ / _____
Ht   Wt   M^2

Gemcitabine + Cisplatin (Modified)

Baseline laboratory tests:	CBC: Chemistry panel, LFTs, and CA 19-9
Baseline procedures or tests:	N/A
Initiate IV:	0.9% sodium chloride
Premedicate:	5-HT$_3$ and dexamethasone 10–20 mg in 100 cc of NS
Administer:	**Gemcitabine** _____ mg (600–750 mg/m^2) IV on days 1 and 15

- Available in 1-g or 200-mg vials; reconstitute with 0.9% sodium chloride USP (5 cc for 200 mg, 25 cc for 1 g). Further dilute in 0.9% sodium chloride.
- Reconstituted solution is stable 24 hours at room temperature. DO NOT refrigerate, because precipitate will form.

Cisplatin _____ mg (25–30 mg/m^2) IV on days 1 and 15

- Available in 1 mg/mL.
- Do not use aluminum needles, because precipitate will form.
- Further dilute solution with 250 cc or more 0.9% sodium chloride.

Major Side Effects

- Hematologic: Leukopenia (63%), thrombocytopenia (36%), and anemia (73%), with grade 3 and 4 thrombocytopenia more common in elderly patients. Myelosuppression is dose limiting. Nadir occurs in 10–14 days, with recovery at 21 days. Prolonged infusion time (> 60 minutes) is associated with higher toxicities.
- GI Symptoms: Moderate-to-severe nausea and vomiting; may be acute or delayed. Diarrhea and/or mucositis (15%–20%).
- Flulike Syndrome (20%) with fever in absence of infection 6–12 hours after treatment (40%).
- Renal: Nephrotoxicity is dose related with cisplatin and occurs at 10–20 days. Risk may be reduced with adequate hydration.
- Neurotoxicity: Sensory neuropathy; dose related. Neuropathy with numbness, tingling, and sensory loss in classic "stocking and glove" distribution. Proprioception, vibrating sense, and motor function loss can occur. Increased risk with cumulative doses and more frequent in longer infusions.
- Electrolyte Imbalance: Decreased Mg^{2+}, K, Ca^{2+}, Na$^+$, and P.
- Hepatic: Elevation of serum transaminase and bilirubin levels.
- Skin: Pruritic, maculopapular skin rash, usually involving trunk and extremities. Edema occurs in 30% of patients. Alopecia.
- Reproduction: Pregnancy category D. Breast feeding should be avoided.

Initiate antiemetic protocol:	Moderately to highly emetogenic protocol.
Supportive drugs:	☐ pegfilgrastim (Neulasta) ☐ filgrastim (Neupogen) ☐ epoetin alfa (Procrit) ☐ darbepoetin alfa (Aranesp)
Treatment schedule:	Chair time 3 hours. Repeat cycle every 28 days.
Estimated number of visits:	Three visits per cycle. Request three cycles worth of visits.

Dose Calculation by: 1. _____ 2. _____

_____
Physician

_____
Date

_____
Patient Name

_____
ID Number

_____
Diagnosis

____/____/____
Ht   Wt   M^2

Gemcitabine + Cisplatin (Fixed Dose Rate)

Baseline laboratory tests:	CBC: Chemistry panel, LFTs, and CA 19-9
Baseline procedures or tests:	N/A
Initiate IV:	0.9% sodium chloride
Premedicate:	5-HT$_3$ and dexamethasone 10–20 mg in 100 cc of NS
Administer:	**Gemcitabine** _____ mg (1000 mg/m^2) IV on days 1 and 8

- Available in 1-g or 200-mg vials; reconstitute with 0.9% sodium chloride USP (5 cc for 200 mg, 25 cc for 1 g). Further dilute in 0.9% sodium chloride.
- Reconstituted solution is stable for 24 hours at room temperature. DO NOT refrigerate, because precipitate will form.

Cisplatin _____ mg (20 mg/m^2) IV on days 1 and 8

- Available 1 mg/mL.
- Do not use aluminum needles, because precipitate will form.
- Further dilute solution with 250 cc or more 0.9% sodium chloride.

Major Side Effects

- Hematologic: Leukopenia (63%), thrombocytopenia (36%), and anemia (73%), with grade 3 and 4 thrombocytopenia more common in elderly patients. Myelosuppression is dose limiting. Nadir occurs in 10–14 days, with recovery at 21 days. Prolonged infusion time (> 60 minutes) is associated with higher toxicities.
- GI Symptoms: Moderate-to-severe nausea and vomiting; may be acute or delayed. Diarrhea and/or mucositis (15%–20%).
- Flulike Syndrome (20%) with fever in absence of infection 6–12 hours after treatment (40%).
- Renal: Nephrotoxicity is dose related with cisplatin and occurs at 10–20 days. Risk may be reduced with adequate hydration.
- Neurotoxicity: Sensory neuropathy; dose related. Neuropathy with numbness, tingling, and sensory loss in classic "stocking and glove" distribution. Proprioception, vibrating sense, and motor function loss can occur. Increased risk with cumulative doses and more frequent in longer infusions.
- Electrolyte Imbalance: Decreased Mg^{2+}, K, Ca^{2+}, Na^+, and P.
- Hepatic: Elevation of serum transaminase and bilirubin levels.
- Skin: Pruritic, maculopapular skin rash, usually involving trunk and extremities. Edema occurs in 30% of patients. Alopecia.
- Reproduction: Pregnancy category D. Breast feeding should be avoided.

Initiate antiemetic protocol:	Moderately to highly emetogenic protocol.
Supportive drugs:	☐ pegfilgrastim (Neulasta) ☐ filgrastim (Neupogen)
	☐ epoetin alfa (Procrit) ☐ darbepoetin alfa (Aranesp)
Treatment schedule:	Chair time 3 hours. Repeat cycle every 21 days
Estimated number of visits:	Three visits per cycle. Request three cycles worth of visits.

Dose Calculation by: 1. _____   2. _____

_____   _____
Physician   Date

_____   _____
Patient Name   ID Number

_____   _____ / _____ / _____
Diagnosis   Ht   Wt   M^2

Gemcitabine + Oxaliplatin (GemOx)

Baseline laboratory tests:	CBC: Chemistry panel, LFTs, and CA 19-9
Baseline procedures or tests:	N/A
Initiate IV:	0.9% sodium chloride
Premedicate:	5-HT$_3$ and dexamethasone 10–20 mg in 100 cc of NS
Administer:	**Gemcitabine** _____ mg (1000 mg/m^2) IV over 100 minutes (10 mg/m^2/min) on day 1

- Available in 1-g or 200-mg vials; reconstitute with 0.9% sodium chloride USP (5 cc for 200 mg, 25 cc for 1 g). Further dilute in 0.9% sodium chloride.
- Reconstituted solution is stable for 24 hours at room temperature. DO NOT refrigerate, because precipitate will form.

Oxaliplatin _____ mg (100 mg/m^2) IV over 2 hours on day 2

- Available in 50- and 100-mg vials.
- **Do not use** aluminum needles or chloride solutions.
- Reconstitute powder with bacteriostatic water for injection or D5W injection (10-cc 50-mg vial and 20-cc 100-mg vial); then further dilute in 250–500 cc of D5W.

Major Side Effects

- Hematologic: Leukopenia (63%), thrombocytopenia (36%), and anemia (73%), with grade 3 and 4 thrombocytopenia more common in elderly patients. Myelosuppression is dose limiting. Nadir occurs in 10–14 days, with recovery at 21 days. Prolonged infusion time (> 60 minutes) is associated with higher toxicities.
- GI Symptoms: Moderate-to-severe nausea and vomiting (70%). Diarrhea in 80%–90% of patients, mucositis in 15%–20%.
- Neurotoxicity: Peripheral sensory neuropathy with distal paresthesias can be dose-limiting. Acute dysesthesias in the laryngopharyngeal region can occur within hours or 1–3 days after therapy. Exposure to cold can exacerbate these symptoms. **AVOID** cold beverages and food as well as cold air.
- Flulike Syndrome: (20%) with fever in absence of infection 6–12 hours after treatment (40%).
- Hepatic: Elevation of serum transaminase and bilirubin levels.
- Skin: Pruritic, maculopapular skin rash, usually involving trunk and extremities. Edema occurs in 30% of patients. Alopecia is rare.
- Delayed Hypersensitivity: May occur after 10–12 cycles. Symptoms range from mild symptoms to anaphylaxis and severe hypersensitivity (characterized by dyspnea, hypotension, angioedema, and generalized urticaria).
- Reproduction: Pregnancy category D. Breast feeding should be avoided.

Initiate antiemetic protocol:	Moderately to highly emetogenic protocol.
Supportive drugs:	☐ pegfilgrastim (Neulasta) ☐ filgrastim (Neupogen) ☐ epoetin alfa (Procrit) ☐ darbepoetin alfa (Aranesp)
Treatment schedule:	Chair time 2 hours on day 1, and 3 hours on day 2. Repeat every 2 weeks until disease progression.
Estimated number of visits:	Three visits per cycle. Request six cycles worth of visits.

Dose Calculation by: 1. _____   2. _____

_____   _____
Physician   Date

_____   _____
Patient Name   ID Number

_____   _____ / _____ / _____
Diagnosis   Ht   Wt   M^2

Gemcitabine + Irinotecan (Gemiri)

Baseline laboratory tests:	CBC: Chemistry panel, LFTs, and CA 19-9
Baseline procedures or tests:	N/A
Initiate IV:	0.9% sodium chloride
Premedicate:	5-HT$_3$ and dexamethasone 10 mg in 100 cc of NS
	Atropine 0.5–1.0 mg IV unless contraindicated.

Administer:

Gemcitabine _____ mg (1000 mg/m^2) IV over 30 minutes on days 1 and 8

- Available in 1-g or 200-mg vials; reconstitute with 0.9% sodium chloride USP (5 cc for 200 mg, 25 cc for 1 g). Further dilute in 0.9% sodium chloride.
- Reconstituted solution is stable for 24 hours at room temperature. DO NOT refrigerate, because precipitate will form.

Irinotecan _____ mg (100 mg/m^2) IV on days 1 and 8

- Available in 2- and 5-mL vials (20 mg/mL).
- May dilute in 500 cc of D5W (preferred) or 0.9% sodium chloride.
- Administer over 90 minutes.

Major Side Effects

- Hematologic: Myelosuppression is dose limiting. Nadir occurs at days 7–10, recovery by days 21–28. GCSF reccommended.
- GI Symptoms: Moderate-to-severe nausea and vomiting. Diarrhea, acute (cholinergic effect) or delayed, can be severe and should be aggressively treated and may be dose limiting. Mucositis (15%–20%).
- Flulike Syndrome (20%) with fever in absence of infection 6–12 hours after treatment (40%).
- Hepatic: Elevation of serum transaminase and bilirubin levels.
- Skin: Pruritic, maculopapular skin rash, usually involving trunk and extremities. Edema occurs in 30% of patients. Alopecia is mild.
- Reproduction: Pregnancy category D. Breast feeding should be avoided.

Initiate antiemetic protocol:	Moderately to highly emetogenic protocol.

Supportive drugs:

☐ pegfilgrastim (Neulasta)	☐ filgrastim (Neupogen)
☐ epoetin alfa (Procrit)	☐ darbepoetin alfa (Aranesp)
☐ loperamide (Imodium)	☐ diphenoxylate/atropine sulfate (Lomotil)

Treatment schedule:	Chair time 3 hours on days 1 and 8. Repeat cycle every 21 days until disease progression.
Estimated number of visits:	Three visits per cycle. Request three cycles worth of visits.

Dose Calculation by: 1. _____ 2. _____

_____ _____
Physician   Date

_____ _____
Patient Name   ID Number

_____ _____/_____/_____
Diagnosis   Ht   Wt   M^2

5-Fluorouracil + Doxorubicin + Mitomycin (FAM)

Baseline laboratory tests:	CBC: Chemistry and CA 19-9
Baseline procedures or tests:	MUGA scan
Initiate IV:	0.9% sodium chloride
Premedicate:	5-HT$_3$ and dexamethasone 10–20 mg in 100 cc of NS

Administer: **Fluorouracil** _____ mg (600 mg/m^2/day) IV on days 1, 8, 29, and 36

- Available 500 mg/10mL.
- No dilution required. Can be further diluted with 0.9% sodium chloride or D5W.

Doxorubicin _____ mg (30 mg/m^2) IV on days 1 and 29

- Available 2 mg/mL.
- **Potent vesicant**
- Drug will form a precipitate if it is mixed with heparin or 5-FU.

Mitomycin _____ mg (10 mg/m^2) IV bolus on day 1

- Available 5 mg (2 mg/mL) vial, 20- and 40-mg vials.
- **Potent vesicant**
- Dilute with sterile water to give a final concentration of 0.5 mg/mL. Reconstituted solution stable for 14 days is refrigerated or 7 days at room temperature

Major Side Effects

- Bone Marrow Depression: Dose-limiting and cumulative toxicity with leukopenia being more common than thrombocytopenia. Nadir counts are delayed at 4–6 weeks with mitomycin but occur at 10–14 days with doxorubicin.
- GI Toxicities: Nausea and vomiting in 50% of patients and are moderate to severe. Mucositis and diarrhea can be severe and dose limiting.
- Skin: Vesicants cause tissue necrosis if extravasated. Hyperpigmentation, photosensitivity, radiation recall, and nail changes may occur. Hand-foot syndrome can be dose limiting.
- Cardiac Toxicity: Acutely, pericarditis, myocarditis syndrome may occur. Later, cardiomyopathy in the form of CHF may occur (dose limit 550 mg/m^2).
- Ocular: Photophobia, increased lacrimation, conjunctivitis, and blurred vision.
- GU: Hemolytic-uremic syndrome: Hematocrit<25%, platelets<100K, and renal failure (serum creatinine >1.6 mg/dL). Rare event (< 2%). Red-orange discoloration of urine for up to 48 hours after infusion of doxorubicin.
- Reproduction: Pregnancy category D. Breast feeding should be avoided.

Initiate antiemetic protocol:	Moderately to highly emetogenic protocol.

Supportive drugs:

☐ pegfilgrastim (Neulasta)	☐ filgrastim (Neupogen)
☐ epoetin alfa (Procrit)	☐ darbepoetin alfa (Aranesp)
☐ loperamide (Imodium)	☐ diphenoxylate/atropine sulfate (Lomotil)

Treatment schedule:	Chair time 1 to 2 hours on days 1, 8, 29, and 36. Repeat every 56 days until progression.
Estimated number of visits:	Five visits per treatment course, CBC weekly.

Dose Calculation by: 1. _____   2. _____

_____
Physician

_____
Date

_____
Patient Name

_____
ID Number

_____
Diagnosis

_____ / _____ / _____
Ht   Wt   M^2

Gemcitabine + Erlotinib (Tarceva)

Baseline laboratory tests:	CBC: Chemistry panel, LFTs
Baseline procedures or tests:	N/A
Initiate IV:	0.9% sodium chloride
Premedicate:	Oral phenothiazine or $5HT_3$ oral or IV
Administer:	**Gemcitabine:** 1000-mg/m^2 IV weekly for 7 weeks, then 1 week rest, subsequent cycles: 1000 mg/m^2 IV weekly for 3 weeks with 1 week rest

- Available in 1-g or 200-mg vials; reconstitute with 0.9% sodium chloride USP (5 cc for 200 mg, 25 cc for 1 g). Further dilute in 0.9% sodium chloride.
- Reconstituted solution is stable for 24 hours at room temperature. DO NOT refrigerate, because precipitate will form.

Erlotinib: 100-mg PO daily

- Available in 25-, 100-, and 150-mg tablets.
- Taken 1 hour prior to eating or 2 hours after eating.
- Dose reductions should be considered with hepatic and renal impairments.
- Dose modification: Decrease in 50 mg increments.

Major Side Effects

- Hematologic: Leukopenia (63%), thrombocytopenia (36%), and anemia (73%), with grade 3 and 4 thrombocytopenia more common in elderly patients. Myelosuppression is dose limiting. Nadir occurs in 10–14 days, with recovery at 21 days. Prolonged infusion time (> 60 minutes) is associated with higher toxicities.
- GI Symptoms: Mild-to-moderate nausea and vomiting (70%), mucositis (15%–20%). Diarrhea is seen in 54% of patients, and is mild to moderate, only 6% grade 3.
- Flulike Syndrome (20%) with fever in the absence of infection 6–12 hours after treatment (40%).
- Hepatic: Elevation of serum transaminase and bilirubin levels.
- Skin Alterations: Rash with tarceva, from maculopapular to pustular on the face, neck, chest, back, and arms affecting up to 75% of patients. Most rashes are mild to moderate beginning on day 8-10, maximizing in intensity by week 2, and gradually resolving by week 2. Use of skin treatments such as corticorsteriods, topical clindamycin or minocycline have been used with varying results.
- Visual Alterations: Conjuctivitis and dry eyes may occur and are mild to moderate (grade 1–2).
- Interstitial Lung Disease: Seen in 1% of patients with 33% mortality. Symptoms include dyspnea, sometimes with cough or low grade fever, rapidly becoming more severe. This is a class effect. Drug should be stopped immediately in patients with worsening or unexplained pulmonary symptoms.
- Drug Interactions: Inducers of the CYP3A4 pathway may increase metabolism of erlotinib and decrease plasma concentrations; and inhibitors of the CYP3A4 pathway may increase the metabolism of erlogitnib and increase plasma concentrations.
- Reproduction: Pregnancy category D. Breast feeding should be avoided.

Initiate antiemetic protocol:	Mildly to moderately emetogenic protocol.
Supportive drugs:	☐ pegfilgrastim (Neulasta) ☐ filgrastim (Neupogen) ☐ epoetin alfa (Procrit) ☐ darbepoetin alfa (Aranesp)
Treatment schedule:	Chair time 1 hour. Weekly for 7 weeks with 1 week rest, then weekly for 3-week increments, one week off. Repeat 3 week cycles every 28 days.
Estimated number of visits:	Weekly appointments throughout therapy, for treatment or blood counts. Request 6 months worth of visits.

Dose Calculation by: 1. _____   2. _____

_____

Physician   Date

_____

Patient Name   ID Number

_____   _____/_____/_____

Diagnosis   Ht   Wt   M²

5-Fluorouracil + Streptozocin + Mitomycin (SMF)

Baseline laboratory tests:	CBC: Chemistry and CA 19-9
Baseline procedures or tests:	N/A
Initiate IV:	0.9% sodium chloride
Premedicate:	5-HT$_3$ and dexamethasone 10–20 mg in 100 cc of NS
Administer:	

Fluorouracil _____ mg (600 mg/m²/day) IV on days 1, 8, 29, and 36

- Available 500 mg/10mL.
- No dilution required. Can be further diluted with 0.9% sodium chloride or D5W.

Streptozocin _____ mg (1000 mg/m²) IV over 1 hour on days 1, 8, 29, and 36

- 1-g vial; reconstitute with sterile water or 0.9% sodium chloride
- Irritant; avoid contact with skin or extravasation.
- Administer with 1–2 L of hydration to avoid renal toxicity.

Mitomycin _____ mg (10 mg/m²) IV bolus on day 1

- Available 5 mg/10 mL. 20- and 40-mg vials.
- **Potent vesicant**
- Dilute with sterile water to give a final concentration of 0.5 mg/mL. Reconstituted solution stable for 14 days if refrigerated or 7 days at room temperature

Major Side Effects

- Renal: Renal dysfunction occurs in 60% of patients receiving streptozocin. Usually transient proteinuria and azotemia, but may progress to permanent renal failure. Dose limiting.
- Bone Marrow Depression: Dose-limiting and cumulative toxicity, with leukopenia being more common than thrombocytopenia. Nadir counts are delayed at 4–6 weeks with mitomycin but occur at 7–14 days with streptozocin.
- GI Toxicities: Nausea and vomiting occur in up to 90% of patients and are moderate to severe. Mucositis and diarrhea can be severe and dose limiting.
- Skin: Vesicants cause tissue necrosis if extravasated. Hyperpigmentation, photosensitivity, and nail changes may occur. Hand-foot syndrome can be dose limiting.
- Blood Glucose Levels: Hypoglycemia (20%) or hyperglycemia may occur.
- Ocular: Photophobia, increased lacrimation, conjunctivitis, and blurred vision.
- Hemolytic-uremic Syndrome: Hematocrit< 25%, platelets < 100K, and renal failure (serum creatinine > 1.6 mg/dL). Rare event (< 2%). Hydrate with 1–2 liters of fluid.
- Reproduction: Pregnancy category D. Breast feeding should be avoided.

Initiate antiemetic protocol:	Moderately to highly emetogenic protocol.
Supportive drugs:	☐ pegfilgrastim (Neulasta)　　☐ filgrastim (Neupogen)
	☐ epoetin alfa (Procrit)　　☐ darbepoetin alfa (Aranesp)
	☐ loperamide (Imodium)　　☐ diphenoxylate/atropine sulfate (Lomotil)
Treatment schedule:	Chair time 3 hours on days 1, 8, 29, and 36. Repeat every 72 days until disease progression.
Estimated number of visits:	Four visits per treatment course.

Dose Calculation by:　1. _____　2. _____

_____
Physician

_____
Patient Name

_____
Diagnosis

_____
Date

_____
ID Number

_____/_____/_____
Ht　　　　　　Wt　　　　　　M²

Single-Agent Regimens

Gemcitabine

Baseline laboratory tests:	CBC: Chemistry panel, LFTs
Baseline procedures or tests:	N/A
Initiate IV:	0.9% sodium chloride
Premedicate:	Oral phenothiazine

OR

5-HT$_3$ and dexamethasone 10 mg in 100 cc of NS

Administer: **Gemcitabine** _____ mg (1000 mg/m^2) IV over 30 minutes weekly for 7 days, then 1-week rest.

Subsequent cycles:

Gemcitabine _____ mg (1000 mg/m^2) IV weekly for 3 weeks with 1-week rest. Repeat 3 week cycle every 28 days

- Available in 1-g or 200-mg vials; reconstitute with 0.9% sodium chloride USP (5 cc for 200 mg, 25 cc for 1 g). Further dilute in 0.9% sodium chloride.
- Reconstituted solution is stable for 24 hours at room temperature. DO NOT refrigerate, because precipitate will form.

Major Side Effects

- Infusion Reactions: Characterized by flushing, facial swelling, headache, dyspnea and/or hypotension. Usually related to rate of infusion and resolves with discontinuation of infusion.
- Hematologic: Leukopenia (63%), thrombocytopenia (36%), and anemia (73%), with grades 3 and 4 thrombocytopenia more common in elderly patients. Myelosuppression is dose limiting. Nadir occurs in 10–14 days with recovery at 21 days. Prolonged infusion time (> 60 minutes) is associated with higher toxicities.
- GI Symptoms: Mild to moderate nausea and vomiting (70%), diarrhea, and/or mucositis (15%–20%).
- Flulike Syndrome (20%) with fever in absence of infection 6–12 hours after treatment (40%).
- Hepatic: Elevation of serum transaminase and bilirubin levels.
- Pulmonary Toxicities: Mild dyspnea or drug induced pneumonitis may occur.
- Skin: Pruritic, maculopapular skin rash, usually involving trunk and extremities. Edema occurs in 30% of patients. Alopecia is rare.
- Reproduction: Pregnancy category D. Breast feeding should be avoided.

Initiate antiemetic protocol:	Mildly to moderately emetogenic protocol.
Supportive drugs:	☐ pegfilgrastim (Neulasta) ☐ filgrastim (Neupogen)
	☐ epoetin alfa (Procrit) ☐ darbepoetin alfa (Aranesp)
Treatment schedule:	Chair time 1 hour. (See schedules above.)
Estimated number of visits:	Weekly. Request 2–3 months worth of visits.

Dose Calculation by: 1. _____   2. _____

_____   _____

Physician   Date

_____   _____

Patient Name   ID Number

_____   _____/ _____/ _____

Diagnosis   Ht   Wt   M^2

Capecitabine (Xeloda)

Baseline laboratory tests:	CBC: Chemistry, bilirubin, LFTs, and CEA
Baseline procedures or tests:	N/A
Initiate IV:	N/A
Premedicate:	Oral phenothiazine or 5-HT$_3$
Administer:	**Capecitabine** _____ mg (1250 mg/m^2) PO bid on days 1–14

- Available in 150- and 500-mg tablets. Do not cut tablets.
- Administer within 30 minutes of a meal with plenty of water.
- Monitor INRs closely in patients taking warfarin; may increase INR

Major Side Effects

- GI Toxicities: Nausea and vomiting, in 30%–50% of patients, is usually mild to moderate. Diarrhea occurs in up to 40%, with 15% being grade 3–4. Stomatitis is common, 3% of which is severe.
- Bone Marrow Suppression: Less than 5-FU.
- Renal Insufficiency: Contraindicated in patients with creatinine clearance < 30 mL/min, CrCl 30–50 mL/min at baseline should have dose reduction to 75% of total dose.
- Skin: Hand-foot syndrome (palmar-plantar erythrodysesthesia) seen in 15%–20% of patients. Characterized by tingling, numbness, pain, erythema, dryness, rash, swelling, increased pigmentation, and/or pruritus of the hands and feet. Less frequent in reduced doses.
- Ocular: Blepharitis, tear-duct stenosis, acute and chronic conjunctivitis.
- Hepatic: Elevations in serum bilirubin (20%–40%), alkaline phosphatase, and hepatic transaminase (SGOT, SGPT) levels. Dose modifications may be required if hyperbilirubinemia occurs.
- Reproductive: Pregnancy category D. Breast feeding should be avoided.

Initiate antiemetic protocol:	Mildly to moderately emetogenic protocol.
Supportive drugs:	☐ pegfilgrastim (Neulasta) ☐ filgrastim (Neupogen)
	☐ loperamide (Imodium) ☐ epoetin alfa (Procrit)
	☐ darbepoetin alfa (Aranesp) ☐ diphenoxylate/atropine sulfate (Lomotil)
Treatment schedule:	No chair time, treatment days 1–14. Repeat cycle every 21 days.
Estimated number of visits:	Two visits per cycle.

Dose Calculation by: 1. _____   2. _____

Physician _____   Date _____

Patient Name _____   ID Number _____

Diagnosis _____   _____/_____/_____
Ht   Wt   M^2

PROSTATE CANCER

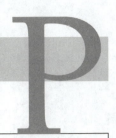

Combination Regimens

Flutamide: 250-mg PO tid
Leuprolide: 7.5-mg IM every 28 days or 22.5-mg IM every 12 weeks

Flutamide: 250-mg PO tid
Goserelin: 10.8-mg SC every 12 weeks

Estramustine: 15-mg/kg/day PO in four divided doses on days 1–21
Etoposide: 50-mg/m^2/day PO in two divided doses on days 1–21
Repeat cycle every 28 days.[1,369]

Estramustine: 600-mg/m^2 PO daily on days 1–42
Vinblastine: 4-mg/m^2 IV weekly for 6 weeks
Repeat cycle every 8 weeks.[1,370]

Paclitaxel: 120-mg/m^2 IV continuous infusion on days 1–4
Estramustine: 600-mg/m^2 PO daily, starting 24 hours before paclitaxel
  therapy
Repeat cycle every 21 days.[1,371]

Mitoxantrone: 12-mg/m^2 IV on day 1
Prednisone: 5-mg PO bid daily
Repeat cycle every 21 days.[1,372]

Docetaxel: 35-mg/m^2 IV on day 2 of weeks 1 and 2

Estramustine: 420-mg PO for the first four doses and 280-mg PO for the
next five doses on days 1–3 of weeks 1 and 2

Repeat cycle every 21 days.[1,373]

Dexamethasone (Decadron) 4-mg PO bid on days 1–3 of weeks 1 and 2.

Docetaxel: 75-mg/m^2 IV on day

Prednisone: 5-mg PO daily

Repeat cycle every 21 days for up to a total of 10 cycles.[1,374]

Single-Agent Regimens

Paclitaxel: 135–170 mg/m^2 IV as a 24-hour infusion on day 1
Repeat cycle every 3 weeks.[1,375]
OR
Paclitaxel: 150-mg/m^2 IV as a 1-hour infusion weekly for 6 weeks
Repeat cycle every 8 weeks.[1,376]

Docetaxel: 75-mg/m^2 IV on day 1
Repeat cycle every 21 days.[1,377]
OR
Docetaxel: 20–40 mg/m^2 weekly for 3 weeks
Repeat cycle every 4 weeks.[1,377]

Estramustine: 14-mg/kg/day PO in three to four divided doses[1,378]

Goserelin: 3.6-mg SC on day 1; repeat cycle every 28 days.[1,379]
OR
Goserelin: 10.8-mg SC on day 1; repeat cycle every 12 weeks.[1,379]

Leuprolide: 7.5-mg IM on day 1; repeat cycle every 28 days.[1,380]
OR
Leuprolide: 22.5-mg IM on day 1; repeat cycle every 12 weeks. [11,381]

Bicalutamide **601**

Bicalutamide: 50-mg PO bid

In patients who do not respond to other antiandrogen agents, may start
with a higher dose of 150-mg PO daily.[1, 382]

Flutamide **602**

Flutamide: 250-mg PO tid.[1,383]

Nilutamide **603**

Nilutamide: 300-mg PO on days 1–30; then 150-mg PO daily.[1,384]

Prednisone **604**

Prednisone: 5-mg PO bid.[1,372]

Ketoconazole **605**

Ketoconazole: 1200-mg PO daily.[1,385]

Aminoglutethimide **606**

Aminoglutethimide: 250-mg PO qid; if tolerated, may increase to 500-mg
PO qid.[1,386]

Combination Regimens

Flutamide + Leuprolide

Baseline laboratory tests: CBC: Chemistry, LFTs, and prostate-specific antigen (PSA)

Baseline procedures or tests: None

Initiate IV: N/A

Premedicate: Oral phenothiazine or 5-HT$_3$ if nausea occurs

Administer: **Flutamide** 250-mg PO tid (three times per day)

- Available in 125-mg capsules for oral use
- Monitor patients taking warfarin carefully; increased anticoagulant effect may occur.

Leuprolide 7.5-mg IM every 28 days or 22.5-mg IM every 12 weeks

- Use syringes, diluent, kit provided by manufacturer.

Major Side Effects

- GI Toxicities: Nausea and vomiting occur in 10% of patients. Diarrhea occurs in 10% of patients, and if it is severe, flutamide may need to be discontinued.
- Sexual Function: Decreased libido and impotence in 33% of patients. Gynecomastia occurs in 10% of patients.
- Tumor Flare: May occur in up to 20% of patients, usually within the first 2 weeks of starting therapy. May observe increased bone pain, urinary retention, or back pain with spinal cord compression. May be prevented by pretreating with an antiandrogen agent such as flutamide. High-risk patients (those with painful bone metastases or those with impending ureteral obstruction and/or spinal cord compression) start flutamide at least 2 weeks before starting leuprolide.
- Hot Flashes: Occur in 60% of patients. Clonidine 0.1–0.2 mg PO daily, megestrol acetate (Megace) 20-mg PO bid, or soy tablets 1 PO tid may be successful in treatment or prevention.
- Hepatic Toxicity: Transient elevations in serum transaminase levels are rare but may necessitate discontinuation of therapy.
- Renal: Use with caution in patients with abnormal renal function. Leuprolide can increase BUN and creatinine levels. Peripheral edema secondary to sodium retention.
- Lab Values: Elevated serum cholesterol levels.
- GU Effects: Yellow-green discoloration of urine with flutamide.
- Reproduction: Pregnancy category D. Breast feeding should be avoided.

Initiate antiemetic protocol: Mildly emetogenic protocol.

Treatment schedule: Office visits every 4 or 12 weeks for leuprolide injections

Estimated number of visits: Monthly while taking treatment

Dose Calculation by: 1. _____ 2. _____

_____
Physician

_____
Date

_____
Patient Name

_____
ID Number

_____
Diagnosis

_____/_____/_____
Ht   Wt   M^2

Flutamide + Goserelin

Baseline laboratory tests:	CBC: Chemistry, LFTs, and PSA
Baseline procedures or tests:	None
Initiate IV:	N/A
Premedicate:	Oral phenothiazine or 5-HT$_3$ if nausea occurs
Administer:	**Flutamide** 250-mg PO tid (three times per day)

- Available in 125-mg capsules for oral use.
- Monitor patients taking warfarin carefully increased anticoagulant effect may occur.

Goserelin 10.8-mg SQ every 12 weeks

- Inject into upper abdomen parallel to the abdominal wall.
- May use lidocaine before injection if ordered.

Major Side Effects

- GI Toxicities: Nausea and vomiting occur in 10% of patients. Diarrhea occurs in 10% of patients, and if it is severe, flutamide may need to be discontinued.
- Sexual Function: Decreased libido and impotence in 33% of patients. Gynecomastia occurs in 10% of patients.
- Tumor Flare: May occur in up to 20% of patients, usually within the first 2 weeks of starting therapy. May observe increased bone pain, urinary retention, or back pain with spinal cord compression. May be prevented by pretreating with an antiandrogen agent, such as flutamide. High-risk patients (those with painful bone metastases or those with impending ureteral obstruction and/or spinal cord compression) should start flutamide at least 2 weeks before starting leuprolide.
- Hot Flashes: Occur in 50% of patients. Clonidine 0.1–0.2 mg PO daily, megestrol acetate (Megace) 20-mg PO bid, or soy tablets 1 PO tid may be successful in treatment or prevention.
- Hepatic Toxicity: Transient elevations in serum transaminases are rare but may necessitate discontinuation of therapy.
- Renal: Use with caution in patients with abnormal renal function. Leuprolide can increase BUN and creatinine levels.
- Laboratory Values: Elevated serum cholesterol levels.
- Genitourinary Effects: Yellow-green discoloration of urine with flutamide.

Initiate antiemetic protocol:	Mildly emetogenic protocol.
Supportive drugs:	☐ loperamide (Imodium) ☐ diphenoxylate/atropine sulfate (Lomotil)
Treatment schedule:	Office visits every 12 weeks for leuprolide injections
Estimated number of visits:	Monthly during treatment.

Dose Calculation by: 1. _____   2. _____

Physician _____   Date _____

Patient Name _____   ID Number _____

Diagnosis _____   Ht _____ / Wt _____ / M^2 _____

Estramustine + Etoposide

Baseline laboratory tests:	CBC: Chemistry, LFTs, and PSA
Baseline procedures or tests:	None
Initiate IV:	N/A
Premedicate:	Oral phenothiazine or 5-HT$_3$.

Administer:

Estramustine _____ mg (15 mg/kg/day) PO in four divided doses on days 1–21

- Available in 140-mg capsules.
- Store in refrigerator; may be stored at room temperature for 24–48 hours.
- Take at least 1 hour before or 2 hours after meals.
- Milk products and calcium-rich foods may impair absorption of drug.
- Contraindicated in patients with thrombophlebitis or thromboembolic disorder.

Etoposide _____ mg (50 mg/m^2/day) PO in two divided doses on days 1–21

- Available in 50- or 100-mg capsules for oral use.
- Store capsules in refrigerator.
- Monitor patients on warfarin closely, may prolong PT/INR.

Major Side Effects

- GI Toxicities: Nausea and vomiting occur within 2 hours of ingestion; are usually mild to moderate. Intractable vomiting may occur after prolonged therapy (6–8 weeks). Diarrhea occurs in 10%–25% of patients.
- Sexual Function: Gynecomastia occurs in 50% of patients. Breast tenderness may occur.
- Myelosuppression: Nadir 10–14 days after treatment. Dose-limiting toxicity with leukopenia more common than thrombocytopenia.
- Hot Flashes: Occur in 60% of patients. Clonidine 0.1–0.2 mg PO daily, megestrol acetate (Megace) 20-mg PO bid, or soy tablets 1 PO tid may be successful in treatment or prevention.
- Hepatic Toxicity: Mild abnormalities in liver function test results may occur (elevations in lactate dehydrogenase, SGOT, bilirubin levels) with or without jaundice but are usually self-limiting.
- Renal Toxicity: Use with caution in patients with abnormal renal function; dose reduction recommended. Renal status should be closely monitored during therapy.
- Skin: Rash, pruritus, dry skin, peeling skin of fingertips, thinning hair, and night sweats.
- Reproductive: Pregnancy category D. Breast feeding should be avoided.

Initiate antiemetic protocol:	Mildly emetogenic protocol.

Supportive drugs:

- ☐ pegfilgrastim (Neulasta)
- ☐ filgrastim (Neupogen)
- ☐ loperamide (Imodium)
- ☐ epoetin alfa (Procrit)
- ☐ darbepoetin alfa (Aranesp)
- ☐ diphenoxylate/atropine sulfate (Lomotil)

Treatment schedule:	Office visits weekly for CBC. Repeat cycle every 28 days.
Estimated number of visits:	Four visits per cycle. Request three cycles worth.

Dose Calculation by: 1. _____ 2. _____

_____

Physician

_____

Date

_____

Patient Name

_____

ID Number

_____

Diagnosis

_____ / _____ / _____

Ht   Wt   M^2

Estramustine + Vinblastine

Baseline laboratory tests:	CBC: Chemistry, LFTs, and PSA
Baseline procedures or tests:	None
Initiate IV:	N/A
Premedicate:	Oral phenothiazine or 5-HT$_3$.
Administer:	**Estramustine** _____ mg (600 mg/m^2) PO daily on days 1–42

- Available in 140-mg capsules.
- Store in refrigerator; may be stored at room temperature for 24–48 hours.
- Take at least 1 hour before or 2 hours after meals.
- Milk products and calcium-rich foods may impair absorption of drug.
- Contraindicated in patients with thrombophlebitis or thromboembolic disorder

Vinblastine _____ mg (4 mg/m^2) IV weekly for 6 weeks

- **Vesicant**
- Available in 10-mg vials for IV use.
- Reduces blood levels of phenytoin; monitor patients for therapeutic dosing.

Major Side Effects	• GI Toxicities: Nausea and vomiting occur within 2 hours of ingestion; are usually mild. Intractable vomiting may occur after prolonged therapy (6–8 weeks). Diarrhea occurs in 15%–25% of patients. However, abdominal pain, constipation, or adynamic ileus may occur. Stomatitis is uncommon but can be severe.

- Sexual Function: Gynecomastia occurs in 50% of patients. Breast tenderness may occur.
- Myelosuppression: Nadir 4–10 days after treatment. Neutrophils greatly affected. Thrombocytopenia may be severe in patients who have undergone prior XRT or chemotherapy.
- Cardiovascular: CHF, cardiac ischemia, and thromboembolism have occurred but are rare.
- Hepatic Toxicity: Contraindicated in patients with severe liver disease. Dose reduction may be necessary in the presence of hepatic failure.
- Skin: Rash, pruritus, dry skin, peeling skin of fingertips, and night sweats. Alopecia is mild and reversible in 45%–50% of patients.
- Reproductive: Likely to cause azoospermia. Pregnancy category D. Breast feeding should be avoided.

Initiate antiemetic protocol:	Mildly emetogenic protocol.
Supportive drugs:	☐ pegfilgrastim (Neulasta) ☐ filgrastim (Neupogen)
	☐ loperamide (Imodium) ☐ epoetin alfa (Procrit)
	☐ darbepoetin alfa (Aranesp) ☐ diphenoxylate/atropine sulfate (Lomotil)
Treatment schedule:	Chair time 1 hour weekly for 6 weeks. Repeat cycle every 8 weeks.
Estimated number of visits:	Weekly. Request three cycles worth.

Dose Calculation by: 1. _____ 2. _____

_____

Physician

_____

Patient Name

_____

Diagnosis

Date

ID Number

_____ / _____ / _____

Ht   Wt   M^2

Paclitaxel + Estramustine

Baseline laboratory tests:	CBC: Chemistry (including Mg^{2+}) and PSA
Baseline procedures or tests:	Central line placement
Initiate IV:	0.9% sodium chloride
Premedicate:	5-HT$_3$ and dexamethasone 10–20 mg in 100 cc of NS

AND

Diphenhydramine 25–50 mg and cimetidine 300 mg in 100 cc of NS before paclitaxel day 1

Oral phenothiazine or 5-HT$_3$ before estramustine on subsequent days

Administer: **Paclitaxel** _____ mg (120 mg/m^2) IV continuous infusion days 1–4

- Available in 30- and 300-mg (6 mg/mL) and 100-mg (16.7mg/mL) vials.
- Final concentration is $\leq$ 1.2 mg/mL
- Use non-PVC containers and tubing with 0.22-micron inline filter for administration.

Estramustine _____ mg (600 mg/m^2) PO daily; start 24 hours before paclitaxel

- Available in 140-mg capsules.
- Store in refrigerator; may be stored at room temperature for 24–48 hours
- Take at least 1 hour before or 2 hours after meals.
- Milk products and calcium-rich foods may impair absorption of drug.

Major Side Effects

- Hypersensitivity Reaction: Occurs in 20%–40% of patients. Characterized by generalized skin rash, flushing, erythema, hypotension, dyspnea, and/or bronchospasm. Usually occurs within the first 2–3 minutes of infusion and almost always within the first 10 minutes. Premedicate as described.
- GI Toxicities: Nausea and vomiting occur within 2 hours of ingestion; usually mild to moderate. Intractable vomiting may occur after prolonged therapy. Diarrhea occurs in 15%–25% of patients.
- Bone Marrow Depression: Dose-limiting neutropenia with nadir at days 8–10 and recovery by days 15–21. Decreased incidence of neutropenia with 3-hour schedule when compared with 24-hour schedule. G-CSF support recommended.
- Neurotoxicity: Sensory neuropathy with numbness and paresthesias in classic "stocking and glove" distribution. Proprioception, vibrating sense, and motor function loss may occur. More frequent with longer infusions and at doses > 175 mg/m^2.
- Sexual Function: Gynecomastia occurs in 50% of patients. Breast tenderness.
- Hepatic toxicity: Mild abnormalities (elevations) in LFT results with or without jaundice.
- Skin: Alopecia in nearly all patients. Rash, pruritus, dry skin, peeling skin of fingertips, and night sweats.
- Reproductive: Pregnancy category D. Breast feeding should be avoided.

Initiate antiemetic protocol: Mildly emetogenic protocol.

Supportive drugs:

☐ pegfilgrastim (Neulasta) ☐ filgrastim (Neupogen)

☐ epoetin alfa (Procrit) ☐ darbepoetin alfa (Aranesp)

☐ loperamide (Imodium) ☐ diphenoxylate/atropine sulfate (Lomotil)

Treatment schedule: Chair time 2 hours. Repeat every 21 days as tolerated or until disease progression.

Estimated number of visits: Three visits per cycle. Request three cycles worth of visits.

Dose Calculation by: 1. _____   2. _____

_____   _____

Physician   Date

_____   _____

Patient Name   ID Number

_____   _____ / _____ / _____

Diagnosis   Ht   Wt   M^2

Mitoxantrone + Prednisone

Baseline laboratory tests:	CBC: Chemistry, LFTs, and PSA
Baseline procedures or tests:	MUGA scan
Initiate IV:	N/A
Premedicate:	Oral phenothiazine or 5-HT$_3$ if nausea occurs
Administer:	**Mitoxantrone** _____ mg (12 mg/m^2) IV on day 1

- **Vesicant**
- Available as a dark blue solution in multidose 2-mg/mL vials.
- Store at room temperature; precipitate forms when refrigerated. Precipitate can be dissolved when vial is warmed to room temperature.
- May be diluted in at least 50 mL of D5W or 0.9% sodium chloride
- Solution is stable at room temperature for at least 48 hours.

Prednisone 5-mg PO bid daily

- Available in 5-mg tablet.
- Administer with meals or an antacid.

Major Side Effects	

- Bone Marrow Suppression: Myelosuppression is a dose-limiting toxicity. Nadir at 10–14 days; greater in elderly or pretreated patients.
- GI Toxicities: Gastric irritation. May increase appetite and cause weight gain. Nausea and vomiting frequent, usually mild. Mucositis and diarrhea common, not severe. Use with caution in patients with abnormal liver function. Dose modification should be considered for mitoxantrone.
- Infection: Increased susceptibility to infections; may mask infections.
- Cardiotoxicity: Cardiomyopathy in cumulative doses greater than 140 mg/m^2 similar to but less severe than those of doxorubicin.
- Fluid/electrolyte Imbalance: CHF, hypertension, and edema. Hypokalemia and hypocalcemia may occur because of increased excretion of potassium and calcium.
- Musculoskeletal: Osteoporosis, loss of muscle mass, muscle weakness, tendon rupture, pathological fractures, and aseptic necrosis of the heads of the humerus and femur can occur. However, usually occurs with long-term, high-dose therapy.
- Adrenal: Rapid cessation of therapy leads to adrenal insufficiency.
- Optic Toxicities: Cataracts or glaucoma may develop with prolonged use.
- Behavioral: Emotional lability, insomnia, mood swings, euphoria, and psychosis
- Skin: Tissue necrosis with extravasation. Alopecia observed in 40% of patients. Blue discoloration of fingernails, sclera, and urine for 1–2 days after treatment.
- Reproduction: Pregnancy category D. Breast feeding should be avoided.

Initiate antiemetic protocol:	Mildly emetogenic protocol.
Supportive drugs:	☐ pegfilgrastim (Neulasta) ☐ filgrastim (Neupogen)
	☐ loperamide (Imodium) ☐ epoetin alfa (Procrit)
	☐ darbepoetin alfa (Aranesp) ☐ diphenoxylate/atropine sulfate (Lomotil)
Treatment schedule:	Chair time 1 hour on day 1. Repeat cycle every 21 days.
Estimated number of visits:	Two visits per cycle. Request four cycles worth of visits. Note: Need weekly CBCs.

Dose Calculation by: 1. _____   2. _____

_____

Physician   Date

_____

Patient Name   ID Number

_____ / _____ / _____

Diagnosis   Ht   Wt   M^2

Docetaxel + Estramustine

Baseline laboratory tests:	CBC: Chemistry (including Mg^{2+}) and PSA
Baseline procedures or tests:	N/A
Initiate IV:	0.9% sodium chloride
Premedicate:	**Dexamethasone** 4-mg PO bid on days 1–3 of weeks 1 and 2
	Oral phenothiazine or 5-HT_3 days 1–3 of weeks 1 and 2
Administer:	**Docetaxel** _____ mg (35 mg/m^2) IV on day 2 of weeks 1 and 2

- Comes in 20 or 80 mg blister packs with own diluent. Do not shake. Reconstituted vials stable at room temperature or if refrigerated for 8 hours.
- Further dilute in 250 cc of D5W or 0.9% sodium chloride.
- **Use non-PVC containers and tubing to administer**

Estramustine PO tid (three times per day) on days 1–3 weeks 1 and 2 (420 mg first four doses, 280 mg next five doses)

- Available in 140-mg capsules.
- Store in refrigerator; may be stored at room temperature for 24–48 hours.
- Take at least 1 hour before or 2 hours after meals.
- Milk products and calcium-rich foods may impair absorption of drug.

Major Side Effects	

- Hypersensitivity Reactions: Severe hypersensitivity reactions with docetaxel in 2%–3% of patients. Characterized by generalized skin rash, erythema, hypotension, dyspnea, and/or bronchospasm. Usually occurs in the first 10 minutes of infusion with first or second treatment. Treat with hydrocortisone IV, dipheahydrum 50 mg IV and/or cimetidine 300 mg IV. Premedication with dexamethasone recommended.
- Bone Marrow Depression: Neutropenia is dose limiting, with nadir at days 7–10 and recovery by day 14. Thrombocytopenia and anemia also occur.
- GI Toxicities: Nausea and vomiting occur within 2 hours of ingestion and are usually mild to moderate. Intractable vomiting may occur after prolonged therapy. Diarrhea occurs in 15%–25% of patients.
- Neuropathy: Peripheral neuropathy may affect up to 49% of patients. Sensory alterations are paresthesias in a glove and stocking distribution and numbness.
- Fluid Balance: Fluid retention syndrome. Symptoms include weight gain, peripheral and/or generalized edema, pleural effusion, and ascites. Occurs in about 50% of patients. Premedication with dexamethasone effective in preventing or minimizing occurrences.
- Sexual Function: Gynecomastia occurs in 50% of patients. Breast tenderness.
- Hepatic Toxicity: Mild abnormalities (elevations) in LFT results may occur with or without jaundice.
- Laboratory Tests: Abnormal Ca^{2+} and P levels may occur.
- Skin: Alopecia occurs in 80% of patients. Nail changes, rash, and dry, pruritic skin seen. Nail changes may include brown discoloration of nail beds, onycholysis (loss of nail) may occur. Keep nails clean, use tea tree oil and nail hardener. Lotromin if indicated. Hand-foot syndrome has also been reported.
- Reproductive: Pregnancy category D. Breast feeding should be avoided.

Initiate antiemetic protocol:	Mildly to moderately emetogenic protocol.	
Supportive drugs:	☐ pegfilgrastim (Neulasta)	☐ filgrastim (Neupogen)
	☐ epoetin alfa (Procrit)	☐ darbepoetin alfa (Aranesp)
Treatment schedule:	Chair time hour on day 2 weeks 1 and 2. Repeat cycle every 21 days.	
Estimated number of visits:	Three visits per cycle. Request four cycles worth of visits.	

Dose Calculation by: 1. _____ 2. _____

_____

Physician   Date

_____   _____

Patient Name   ID Number

_____   _____/_____/_____

Diagnosis   Ht   Wt   M^2

Docetaxel + Prednisone

Baseline laboratory tests:	CBC: Chemistry (including Mg^{2+}) and PSA
Baseline procedures or tests:	Central line placement
Initiate IV:	0.9% sodium chloride
Premedicate:	5-HT$_3$ or oral phenothiazine
Administer:	

Docetaxel _____ 75 mg/m^2 IV on day 1

Comes in 20- or 80-mg blister packs with own diluent. Do not shake. Reconstituted vials stable at room temperature, refrigerated for 8 hours

- Further dilute in 250 cc of D5W or 0.9% sodium chloride.
- Use non-PVC containers and tubing to administer.

Prednisone 5-mg PO bid

- Available in 5-mg tablet.
- Administer with meals or an antacid.

Major Side Effects

- GI Toxicities: Gastric irritation due to increased secretion of hydrochloric acid and decreased secretion of protective gastric mucus. May increase appetite and cause weight gain.
- Infection: Steroids increase susceptibility to infections and tuberculosis, may mask or aggravate infection, and may prolong or delay healing of injuries.
- Fluid/electrolyte Imbalance: Sodium and water retention may occur and lead to CHF, hypertension, and edema in susceptible patients. Hypokalemia and hypocalcemia may occur because of increased excretion of potassium and calcium.
- Fluid Retention Syndrome: Symptoms include weight gain, peripheral and/or generalized edema, pleural effusion, and ascites. Occurs in about 50% of patients. Concurrent administration with oral prednisone in this protocol may be effective in preventing or minimizing occurrences.
- Musculoskeletal: Osteoporosis may occur with long-term use. Loss of muscle mass, muscle weakness (steroid myopathy), tendon rupture, pathological fractures, and aseptic necrosis of the heads of the humerus and femur can occur. However, usually occurs with long-term, high-dose therapy.
- Adrenal: Long-term therapy leads to suppression of normal adrenal function. Rapid cessation of therapy leads to adrenal insufficiency.
- Optic Toxicities: Cataracts or glaucoma may develop with prolonged used. Risk of ocular infections from virus or fungi is increased.
- Behavioral: Emotional lability, insomnia, mood swings, euphoria, and psychosis may occur, causing ineffective coping and role-relationship problems.
- Hypersensitivity Reactions: Severe hypersensitivity reactions with docetaxel in 2%–3% of patients. Characterized by generalized skin rash, erythema, hypotension, dyspnea, and/or bronchospasm. Usually occurs in the first 10 minutes of infusion with first or second treatment. Treat with hydrocortisone IV, dipheahydrum 50 mg IV and/or cimetidine 300 mg IV. Premedication with dexamethasone recommended.
- Bone Marrow Depression: Neutropenia is dose-limiting, with nadir at days 7–10 and recovery by day 14. Thrombocytopenia and anemia also occur.
- GI Toxicities: Nausea and vomiting are mild to moderate. Mucositis and diarrhea occur in 40% of patients.
- Neuropathy: Peripheral neuropathy may affect up to 49% of patients. Sensory alterations are paresthesias in a glove and stocking distribution and numbness.
- Skin: Alopecia occurs in 80% of patients. Nail changes, rash, and dry, pruritic skin seen. Nail changes may include brown discoloration of nail beds, onycholysis (loss of nail) may occur. Keep nails clean, use tea tree oil and nail hardener. Lotromin if indicated. Hand-foot syndrome has also been reported.
- Reproduction: Pregnancy category D. Breast feeding should be avoided.

Initiate antiemetic protocol: Mildly to moderately emetogenic protocol.

Supportive drugs: ☐ pegfilgrastim (Neulasta)   ☐ filgrastim (Neupogen)
                        ☐ epoetin alfa (Procrit)   ☐ darbepoetin alfa (Aranesp)

Treatment schedule: Chair time 2 hours on day 1. Repeat cycle every 21 days **OR** every 4 weeks.

Estimated number of visits: Weekly. Request three cycles worth of visits.

Dose Calculation by: 1. _____   2. _____

_____

Physician   Date

_____

Patient Name   ID Number

_____

Diagnosis   Ht _____ / Wt _____ / M² _____

Single-Agent Regimens

Paclitaxel

Baseline laboratory tests:	CBC: Chemistry (including Mg^{2+}) and PSA
Baseline procedures or tests:	Central line placement
Initiate IV:	0.9% sodium chloride
Premedicate:	5-HT$_3$ and dexamethasone 10–20 mg in 100 cc of NS
	Diphenhydramine 25–50 mg and cimetidine 300 mg in 100 cc of NS

Administer:

Paclitaxel _____ mg (135–170 mg/m^2) IV over 24 hours on day 1 every 3 weeks

- Available in 30- and 300-mg (6 mg/mL) or 100-mg (16.7 mg/mL) vials.
- Final concentration is $\leq$ 1.2 mg/mL.
- **Use non-PVC containers and tubing with 0.22-micron inline filter for administration.**

OR

Paclitaxel _____ mg (150 mg/m^2) IV over 1 hour on day 1 weekly for 6 weeks

- Final concentration is $\leq$ 1.2 mg/mL.
- **Use non-PVC containers and tubing with 0.22-micron inline filter for administration.**

Major Side Effects

- Hypersensitivity reaction: Occurs in 20%–40% of patients. Characterized by generalized skin rash, flushing, erythema, hypotension, dyspnea, and/or bronchospasm. Usually occurs within the first 2–3 minutes of infusion and almost always within the first 10 minutes. Premedicate as described.
- Bone Marrow Depression: Dose-limiting neutropenia with nadir at days 8–10 and recovery by days 15–21. Decreased incidence of neutropenia with 3-hour schedule when compared with 24-hour schedule. G-CSF support recommended.
- Neurotoxicity: Severe neuropathy with numbness and tingling in classic "stocking and glove" distribution. Proprioception, vibrating sense, and motor function loss can occur. Increased risk with cumulative dosing and longer infusions.
- GI Toxictiy: Mucositis and/or diarrhea seen in 30–40% of patients. Nausea and vomiting is mild to moderate.
- Alopecia: Total loss of body hair occurs in nearly all patients.
- Reproduction: Pregnancy category D. Breast feeding should be avoided.

Initiate antiemetic protocol:	Mildly to moderately emetogenic protocol.
Supportive drugs:	☐ pegfilgrastim (Neulasta) ☐ filgrastim (Neupogen)
	☐ epoetin alfa (Procrit) ☐ darbepoetin alfa (Aranesp)
Treatment schedule:	Chair time 2 hours. Repeat every 21 days as tolerated or every 8 weeks for hourly dosing until disease progression
Estimated number of visits:	Two visits per cycle. Request three cycles worth of visits.

Dose Calculation by: 1. _____   2. _____

_____
Physician

_____
Date

_____
Patient Name

_____
ID Number

_____
Diagnosis

_____ / _____ / _____
Ht   Wt   M^2

Docetaxel

Baseline laboratory tests:	CBC: Chemistry (including Mg^{2+}) and PSA
Baseline procedures or tests:	Central line placement
Initiate IV:	0.9% sodium chloride
Premedicate:	Dexamethasone 8-mg bid for 3 days, starting the day before treatment
	Oral phenothiazine or 5-HT$_3$

Administer: Docetaxel _____ mg (75 mg/m^2) IV on day 1 every 21 days

OR

Docetaxel _____mg (20–40 mg/m^2) IV weekly × 3 weeks, repeat every 4 weeks

- Comes in 20- or 80-mg blister packs with own diluent. Do not shake. Reconstituted vials stable at room temperature or if refrigerated for 8 hours
- Further dilute in 250 cc of D5W or 0.9% sodium chloride.
- Use non-PVC containers and tubing to administer.

Major Side Effects

- Hypersensitivity: Severe hypersensitivity reactions with docetaxel in 2%–3% of patients. Characterized by skin rash, erythema, hypotension, dyspnea and /or bronchospasm. Usually occurs within first 2–3 minutes, usually after first dose. May be prevented with premedication with steroid and addition of diphenhydramine 50 mg IV and/or cimetidine 300 mg. IV. Premedication with dexamethasone recommended.
- Bone Marrow Depression: Neutropenia is dose-limiting, with nadir at days 7–10 and recovery by day 14. Thrombocytopenia and anemia also occur.
- GI Toxicities: Nausea and vomiting are mild to moderate. Mucositis and diarrhea occur in 40% of patients.
- Neuropathy: Peripheral neuropathy may affect up to 49% of patients. Sensory alterations are paresthesias in a glove and stocking distribution and numbness. Risk increases with cumulative doses.
- Fluid Balance: Fluid retention syndrome. Symptoms include weight gain, peripheral and/or generalized edema, pleural effusion, and ascites. Occurs in about 50% of patients. Premedication with dexamethasone effective in preventing or minimizing occurrences.
- Skin: Pruritic rash and nail changes. Nail changes may include brown discoloration of nail beds and/or onycholysis (loss of nail). Keep nails clean. Use nail hardeners and tea tree oil. Lotrimin if indicated.
- Reproduction: Pregnancy category D. Breast feeding should be avoided.

Initiate antiemetic protocol:	Mildly to moderately emetogenic protocol.
Supportive drugs:	☐ pegfilgrastim (Neulasta) ☐ filgrastim (Neupogen)
	☐ epoetin alfa (Procrit) ☐ darbepoetin alfa (Aranesp)
Treatment schedule:	Chair time 2 hours on day 1. Repeat cycle every 21 days OR every 4 weeks.
Estimated number of visits:	Two OR four visits per cycle. Request three cycles worth of visits.

Dose Calculation by: 1. _____   2. _____

_____

Physician

_____

Patient Name

_____

Diagnosis

_____

Date

_____

ID Number

_____/ _____/ _____

Ht   Wt   M^2

Estramustine

Baseline laboratory tests:	CBC: Chemistry, LFTs, and PSA
Baseline procedures or tests:	None
Initiate IV:	N/A
Premedicate:	Oral phenothiazine or 5-HT$_3$.
Administer:	**Estramustine** _____ mg (14 mg/kg/day) PO in three to four divided doses

- Available in 140-mg capsules.
- Store in refrigerator; may be stored at room temperature for 24–48 hours
- Take at least 1 hour before or 2 hours after meals.
- Milk products and calcium-rich foods may impair absorption of drug.
- Contraindicated in patients with thrombophlebitis or thromboembolic disorder

Major Side Effects

- GI Toxicities: Nausea and vomiting occur within 2 hours of ingestion; are usually mild to moderate. Intractable vomiting may occur after prolonged therapy (6–8 weeks). Diarrhea occurs in 15%–25% of patients.
- Sexual Function: Gynecomastia occurs in 50% of patients. Breast tenderness.
- Myelosuppression: Rare.
- Hepatic Toxicity: Mild abnormalities in liver function tests may occur (elevations in lactate dehydrogenase, SGOT, bilirubin levels) with or without jaundice, but are usually self-limiting.
- Laboratory Values: Abnormal Ca and P levels may occur.
- Skin: Rash, pruritus, dry skin, peeling skin of fingertips, thinning hair, and night sweats.
- Reproductive: Pregnancy category D. Breast feeding should be avoided.

Initiate antiemetic protocol:	Mildly emetogenic protocol.
Supportive drugs:	☐ pegfilgrastim (Neulasta) ☐ filgrastim (Neupogen)
	☐ loperamide (Imodium) ☐ epoetin alfa (Procrit)
	☐ darbepoetin alfa (Aranesp) ☐ diphenoxylate/atropine sulfate (Lomotil)
Treatment schedule:	Office visits every 1–2 weeks for evaluation by physician.
Estimated number of visits:	Two visits per month. Request 3 months worth of visits.

Dose Calculation by: 1. _____ 2. _____

_____   _____
Physician   Date

_____   _____
Patient Name   ID Number

_____   _____ / _____ / _____
Diagnosis   Ht   Wt   M^2

Goserelin (Zoladex)

Baseline laboratory tests:	CBC: Chemistry, LFTs, and PSA
Baseline procedures or tests:	None
Initiate IV:	N/A
Premedicate:	Oral phenothiazine or 5-HT$_3$ if nausea occurs
Administer:	**Goserelin** 3.6-mg SC every 28 days
	OR
	Goserelin 10.8-mg SQ every 12 weeks

- Inject into upper abdomen parallel to the abdominal wall.
- May use lidocaine before injection if ordered.

Major Side Effects

- GI Toxicities: Nausea and vomiting rarely occur and are usually mild. Constipation or diarrhea occurs in < 5% of patients.
- Sexual Function: Decreased libido and impotence in 33% of patients. Gynecomastia occurs in 10% of patients.
- Tumor Flare: May occur in up to 20% of patients, usually within the first 2 weeks of start of therapy. May observe increased bone pain, urinary retention, or back pain with spinal cord compression. May be prevented by pretreating with an antiandrogen agent. High-risk patients (those with painful bone metastases or those with impending ureteral obstruction and/or spinal cord compression) should start antiandrogen therapy at least 2 weeks before starting drug.
- Hot Flashes: Occur in 50% of patients. Clonidine 0.1–0.2 mg PO daily, megestrol acetate (Megace) 20-mg PO bid, or soy tablets 1 PO tid may be successful in treatment or prevention.
- Hepatic Toxicity: Transient elevations in serum transaminases are rare but may necessitate discontinuation of therapy.
- Renal: Use with caution in patients with abnormal renal function.
- Laboratory Values: Elevated serum cholesterol levels.
- Reproduciton: Pregnancy category D. Breast feeding should be avoided.

Initiate antiemetic protocol:	Mildly emetogenic protocol.
Supportive drugs:	☐ loperamide (Imodium) ☐ epoetin alfa (Procrit)
	☐ darbepoetin alfa (Aranesp) ☐ diphenoxylate/atropine sulfate (Lomotil)
Treatment schedule:	Office visits every 28 days **OR** every 12 weeks for injections.
Estimated number of visits:	Monthly during treatment.

Dose Calculation by: 1. _____   2. _____

_____   _____
Physician   Date

_____   _____
Patient Name   ID Number

_____   _____/_____/_____
Diagnosis   Ht   Wt   M^2

Leuprolide (lupron)

Baseline laboratory tests:	CBC: Chemistry, LFTs, and PSA
Baseline procedures or tests:	None
Initiate IV:	N/A
Premedicate:	Oral phenothiazine or 5-HT$_3$ if nausea occurs
Administer:	**Leuprolide** 7.5-mg IM every 28 days
	OR
	Leuprolide 22.5-mg IM every 12 weeks

- Use syringes, diluent, kit provided by manufacturer

Major Side Effects

- GI Toxicities: Nausea and vomiting rarely observed
- Sexual function: Decreased libido and impotence. Gynecomastia occurs in 3%–6.9% of patients.
- Tumor Flare: May occur in up to 20% of patients, usually within the first 2 weeks of start of therapy. May observe increased bone pain, urinary retention, or back pain with spinal cord compression. May be prevented by pretreating with an antiandrogen agent. High-risk patients (those with painful bone metastases or those with impending ureteral obstruction and/or spinal cord compression) should start antiandrogen therapy at least 2 weeks before starting leuprolide.
- Hot Flashes: Occur in 67.9% of patients. Clonidine 0.1–0.2 mg PO daily, megestrol acetate (Megace) 20-mg PO bid, or soy tablets 1 PO tid may be successful in treatment or prevention.
- Myelosuppression: Rare
- Renal: Use with caution in patients with abnormal renal function. Leuprolide can increase BUN and creatinine levels.
- Laboratory Values: Elevated serum cholesterol levels.

Initiate antiemetic protocol:	Mildly emetogenic protocol.
Supportive drugs:	☐ loperamide (Imodium) ☐ epoetin alfa (Procrit)
	☐ darbepoetin alfa (Aranesp) ☐ diphenoxylate/atropine sulfate (Lomotil)
Treatment schedule:	Office visits every 4 or 12 weeks for leuprolide injections.
Estimated number of visits:	Monthly during treatment.

Dose Calculation by: 1. _____   2. _____

_____
Physician

_____
Patient Name

_____
Diagnosis

_____
Date

_____
ID Number

_____ / _____ / _____
Ht   Wt   M^2

Bicalutamide

Baseline laboratory tests:	CBC: Chemistry, LFTs, and PSA
Baseline procedures or tests:	None
Initiate IV:	N/A
Premedicate:	Oral phenothiazine or 5-HT$_3$ if nausea occurs
Administer:	**Bicalutamide** 50-mg PO bid

- In patients who do not respond to other antiandrogen agents, may start with a higher dose of 150-mg PO daily.
- Available as a 50-mg white, film-coated tablet for oral use.
- Monitor patients taking warfarin carefully; can increase anticoagulant effect.

Major Side Effects

- GI Toxicities: Nausea, vomiting, and diarrhea are rarely observed. Constipation observed in 10% of patients.
- Sexual Function: Decreased libido, impotence, gynecomastia, nipple pain, and galactorrhea occur in 50% of patients.
- Hot Flashes: Occur in 67.9% of patients. Clonidine 0.1–0.2 mg PO daily, megestrol acetate (Megace) 20-mg PO bid, or soy tablets 1 PO tid may be successful in treatment or prevention.
- Myelosuppression: Rare.
- Hepatic: Use with caution in patients with abnormal liver function. Monitor LF at baseline and throughout treatment.
- Renal: No dose modification needed for renal dysfunction.
- Reproduction: Pregnancy category D. Breast feeding should be avoided.

Initiate antiemetic protocol:	Mildly emetogenic protocol.
Supportive drugs:	☐ loperamide (Imodium) ☐ epoetin alfa (Procrit)
	☐ darbepoetin alfa (Aranesp) ☐ diphenoxylate/atropine sulfate (Lomotil)
Treatment schedule:	Daily until disease progression.
Estimated number of visits:	Monthly during treatment.

Dose Calculation by: 1. _____   2. _____

_____

Physician   Date

_____

Patient Name   ID Number

_____   _____/_____/_____

Diagnosis   Ht   Wt   M^2

Flutamide

Baseline laboratory tests:	CBC: Chemistry, LFTs, and PSA
Baseline procedures or tests:	None
Initiate IV:	N/A
Premedicate:	Oral phenothiazine or 5-HT$_3$
Administer:	**Flutamide** 250-mg PO tid (three times per day)

- Available in 125-mg capsules for oral use.
- Use with caution in patients taking warfarin; may increase anticoagulation effect.

Major Side Effects

- GI Toxicities: Nausea, vomiting, and diarrhea observed in 10% of patients. If severe diarrhea occurs, flutamide may need to be discontinued.
- Sexual Function: Decreased libido and impotence in 33% of patients. Gynecomastia occurs in 10% of patients.
- Hot Flashes: Occur in 60% of patients. Clonidine 0.1–0.2 mg PO daily, megestrol acetate (Megace) 20-mg PO bid, or soy tablets 1 PO tid may be successful in treatment or prevention.
- Myelosuppression: Rare
- Hepatic: Transient elevations in serum transaminase levels are rare but may necessitate discontinuation of therapy if levels are two to three times the upper limit of normal.
- Renal: Increased BUN and creatinine levels. Yellow-green discoloration of urine.
- Reproduciton: Pregnancy category D. Breast feeding should be avoided.

Initiate antiemetic protocol:	Mildly emetogenic protocol.
Supportive drugs:	☐ loperamide (Imodium) ☐ epoetin alfa (Procrit)
	☐ darbepoetin alfa (Aranesp) ☐ diphenoxylate/atropine sulfate (Lomotil)
Treatment schedule:	Daily until disease progression.
Estimated number of visits:	Monthly during treatment.

Dose Calculation by: 1. _____   2. _____

_____
Physician

_____
Date

_____
Patient Name

_____
ID Number

_____
Diagnosis

_____ / _____ / _____
Ht   Wt   M^2

Nilutamide

Baseline laboratory tests:	CBC: Chemistry, LFTs, and PSA
Baseline procedures or tests:	None
Initiate IV:	N/A
Premedicate:	Oral phenothiazine or 5-HT$_3$
Administer:	**Nilutamide** 300-mg PO on days 1–30; then 150-mg PO daily

- Available in 50- and 150-mg tablets for oral use.
- Use with caution in patients taking warfarin; may cause increased anticoagulation effects.
- Treatment should begin the day of or the day after surgical castration.

Major Side Effects

- GI Toxicities: Nausea and anorexia occur infrequently. Constipation.
- Sexual Function: Decreased libido, impotence, gynecomastia, nipple pain, and galactorrhea
- Hot Flashes: Occur in 28% of patients and are the most common side effect. Clonidine 0.1–0.2 mg PO daily, megestrol acetate (Megace) 20-mg PO bid, or soy tablets 1 PO tid may be successful in treatment or prevention.
- Alcohol: Patients should be advised to abstain from alcohol while taking nilutamide because of increased risk of intolerance.
- Hepatic: Use with caution in patients with abnormal liver function. Contraindicated in patients with severe liver impairment.
- Respiratory: Contraindicated in patients with severe respiratory insufficiency. Dyspnea is rare but is related to interstitial pneumonitis, a serious side effect of the drug. Pneumonitis usually observed within the first 3 months of treatment; incidence may be higher in patients of Asian descent.
- Vision: Impaired adaptation to dark, abnormal vision, and alterations in color vision occur in up to 57% of patients.
- Reproduction: Pregnancy category C.

Initiate antiemetic protocol:	Mildly emetogenic protocol.
Supportive drugs:	☐ loperamide (Imodium) ☐ epoetin alfa (Procrit)
	☐ darbepoetin alfa (Aranesp) ☐ diphenoxylate/atropine sulfate (Lomotil)
Treatment schedule:	Daily until disease progression.
Estimated number of visits:	Monthly during treatment.

Dose Calculation by: 1. _____   2. _____

Physician _____   Date _____

Patient Name _____   ID Number _____

Diagnosis _____   Ht _____ / Wt _____ / M^2 _____

Prednisone

Baseline laboratory tests:	CBC: Chemistry, LFTs, and PSA
Baseline procedures or tests:	None
Initiate IV:	N/A
Premedicate:	N/A
Administer:	**Prednisone** 5-mg PO bid

- Available in 5-mg tablet.
- Administer with meals or an antacid.

Major Side Effects

- GI Toxicities: Gastric irritation due to increased secretion of hydrochloric acid and decreased secretion of protective gastric mucus. May increase appetite and cause weight gain.
- Infection: Steroids increase susceptibility to infections and tuberculosis, may mask or aggravate infection, and may prolong or delay healing of injuries.
- Fluid/electrolyte Imbalance: Sodium and water retention may occur and lead to CHF, hypertension, and edema in susceptible patients. Hypokalemia and hypocalcemia may occur because of increased excretion of potassium and calcium.
- Musculoskeletal: Osteoporosis may occur with long-term use. Loss of muscle mass, muscle weakness (steroid myopathy), tendon rupture, pathological fractures, and aseptic necrosis of the heads of the humerus and femur can occur. However, usually occurs with long-term, high-dose therapy.
- Adrenal: Long-term therapy leads to suppression of normal adrenal function. Rapid cessation of therapy leads to adrenal insufficiency.
- Optic Toxicities: Cataracts or glaucoma may develop with prolonged used. Risk of ocular infections from virus or fungi is increased.
- Behavioral: Emotional lability, insomnia, mood swings, euphoria, and psychosis may occur, causing ineffective coping and role-relationship problems.

Initiate antiemetic protocol:	Mildly emetogenic protocol.
Supportive drugs:	☐ loperamide (Imodium) ☐ epoetin alfa (Procrit)
	☐ darbepoetin alfa (Aranesp) ☐ diphenoxylate/atropine sulfate (Lomotil)
Treatment schedule:	No chair time. Treatment daily as tolerated or until disease progression.
Estimated number of visits:	Monthly during treatment.

Dose Calculation by: 1. _____ 2. _____

_____   _____
Physician   Date

_____   _____
Patient Name   ID Number

_____   _____ / _____ / _____
Diagnosis   Ht   Wt   M^2

Ketoconazole

Baseline laboratory tests:	CBC: Chemistry, LFTs, and PSA
Baseline procedures or tests:	None
Initiate IV:	N/A
Premedicate:	Oral phenothiazine or 5-HT$_3$ if nausea occurs
Administer:	**Ketoconazole** 1200-mg PO daily

- Store in tightly closed container at < 40°C (104°F).
- May take with meals to decrease GI side effects.
- Do not give antacids, cimetidine, ranitidine, famotidine, sucralfate, or other drugs that increase gastric pH for at least 2 hours after taking ketoconazole.

Major Side Effects

- Sexual Function: Breast enlargement and tenderness may occur in some men, lasting weeks to duration of therapy. Oligospermia, azoospermia, decreased libido, and impotence may also occur.
- GI Side Effects: Nausea and vomiting occur in 3%–10% of patients. Anorexia affects about 10% of patients. Diarrhea, abdominal pain, flatulence, and constipation may occur less frequently.
- Hepatic Toxicities: Abnormalities (elevations) in LFT results may occur. Hepatotoxicity is less common, is usually reversible, and is rarely fatal.
- Skin: Rash, dermatitis, purpura, urticaria occur in 1% of patients.
- CNS Effects: Dizziness, headache, nervousness, insomnia, lethargy, somnolence, and paresthesia have occurred in about 1% of patients.

Initiate antiemetic protocol:	Mildly emetogenic protocol.
Supportive drugs:	☐ loperamide (Imodium) ☐ epoetin alfa (Procrit)
	☐ darbepoetin alfa (Aranesp) ☐ diphenoxylate/atropine sulfate (Lomotil)
Treatment schedule:	No chair time. Treatment is daily as tolerated or until disease progression.
Estimated number of visits:	Monthly during treatment.

Dose Calculation by: 1. _____   2. _____

Physician _____   Date _____

Patient Name _____   ID Number _____

Diagnosis _____   Ht _____ / Wt _____ / M^2 _____

Aminoglutethimide (Cytadren)

Baseline laboratory tests:	CBC: Chemistry, LFTs, thyroid function tests, and PSA
Baseline procedures or tests:	None
Initiate IV:	N/A
Premedicate:	Oral phenothiazine or 5-HT$_3$ if nausea occurs
Administer:	**Aminoglutethimide** 250-mg PO qid
	OR
	Aminoglutethimide 500 mg PO qid

- If tolerated, may increase to 500-mg PO qid.
- Available as 250-mg tablets for oral use.
- Decreases levels of warfarin, phenytoin, phenobarbital, theophylline, medroxyprogesterone, digoxin, and dexamethasone (Decadron) by enhancing their metabolism.
- **Administer hydrocortisone along with drug to prevent adrenal insufficiency.** Usual dose is 40-mg PO qd, although higher doses (100 mg) are sometimes used during the initial 2 weeks of therapy to reduce frequency of adverse events.

Major Side Effects

- Skin: Maculopapular skin rash, usually occurring in the first week of therapy. Self-limited with resolution in 5–7 days, and discontinuation of therapy is not necessary. May be accompanied by malaise and low-grade fever.
- Sensory: Fatigue, lethargy, and somnolence. Occurs in 40% of patients, and onset is within the first week of therapy. Dizziness, nystagmus, and ataxia are less common.
- GI Toxicities: Mild nausea and vomiting occur in 10%–13% of patients.
- Hypothyroidism: Monitor thyroid function.
- Adrenal Insufficiency: Occurs in the absence of hydrocortisone replacement. Presents as postural hypotension, hyponatremia, and hyperkalemia.
- Myelosuppression: Leukopenia and thrombocytopenia rarely occur.
- Reproduction: Pregnancy category D. Breast feeding should be avoided.

Initiate antiemetic protocol:	Mildly emetogenic protocol.
Supportive drugs:	☐ pegfilgrastim (Neulasta) ☐ filgrastim (Neupogen)
	☐ loperamide (Imodium) ☐ epoetin alfa (Procrit)
	☐ darbepoetin alfa (Aranesp) ☐ diphenoxylate/atropine sulfate (Lomotil)
Treatment schedule:	No chair time. Treatment is daily as tolerated or until disease progression.
Estimated number of visits:	Biweekly during treatment

Dose Calculation by: 1. _____   2. _____

_____
Physician

_____
Date

_____
Patient Name

_____
ID Number

_____
Diagnosis

_____/_____/_____
Ht   Wt   M^2

RENAL CELL CANCER

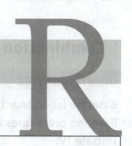

Combination Regimens

Interferon-α-2a + IL-2

Baseline laboratory tests:	CBC: Chemistry (including LFTs)
Baseline procedures or tests:	N/A
Initiate IV:	N/A
Premedicate:	Oral phenothiazine or 5-HT$_3$
	Acetaminophen 325 or 500 mg 2 tablets PO
Administer:	**Interferon-α-2a** 9 MU SC on days 1–4, weeks 1–4

- Available in multidose pens 6 doses of 3 MU (18 MU) or 5 MU (30 MU) or 10 MU (60 MU).
- Keep refrigerated.

AND

Interleukin-2 12 MU SC on days 1–4, weeks 1–4

- Available in lyophilized vials containing 22 MU.
- Reconstitute with 1.2 mL sterile water to final concentration of 18 MU/mL.
- Stable for 48 hours refrigerated.

Major Side Effects	

- Flulike Symptoms: Fever, chills, headache, myalgias, and arthralgias. Occurs in 80%–90% of patients. Symptoms can be managed with acetaminophen, nonsteroidal anti-inflammatory drugs, and increased oral fluid intake.
- Bone Marrow Depression: Myelosuppression with anemia, mild leukopenia, and thrombocytopenia.
- GI Toxicities: Nausea and diarrhea are mild, vomiting is rare. Diarrhea is common, can be severe, and may require bicarbonate replacement. Anorexia occurs in 46%–65% of patients and is cumulative and dose limiting. Taste alteration and xerostomia may occur. Stomatitis is common but mild.
- Renal/hepatic: Renal toxicity is uncommon and is manifested by mild proteinuria and hypocalcemia. Direct tubular cell injury and decreased renal blood flow occur with cumulative doses of IL-2. Acute renal failure and nephrotic syndrome have been reported in rare instances. Mild transient elevations in serum transaminase levels. Dose-dependent toxicity observed more frequently in the presence of pre-existing liver abnormalities.
- Vascular Leak Syndrome: Characterized by weight gain, arrythmias, and/or tachycentias, hypotension, edema, oliguria, and renal insufficiency, pleural effusions and pulmonary congestion.
- Neuro: Somnolence, delirium, and confusion are common but usually resolve after interleukin-2 is stopped. More common with continuous infusion.
- Cardiotoxicity: Chest pain, arrhythmias, and CHF are rare.
- Skin: Alopecia is partial. Diffuse erythematous rash, which may desquamate. Pruritus (with or without rash) and irritation at injection site.
- Reproductive: Pregnancy category C.

Initiate antiemetic protocol:	Mildly emetogenic protocol.
Supportive drugs:	☐ pegfilgrastim (Neulasta) ☐ filgrastim (Neupogen)
	☐ epoetin alfa (Procrit) ☐ darbepoetin alfa (Aranesp)
Treatment schedule:	Chair time 1 hour on day 1 for self-injection teaching. Repeat every 6 weeks.
Estimated number of visits:	One per week for laboratory tests. Request 12 weeks worth of visits. May require extra visits for hydration.

Dose Calculation by: 1. _____   2. _____

_____   _____
Physician   Date

_____   _____
Patient Name   ID Number

_____   _____ / _____ / _____
Diagnosis   Ht   Wt   M^2

5-Fluorouracil + Gemcitabine

Baseline laboratory tests:	CBC: Chemistry and CEA
Baseline procedures or tests:	Central line placement
Initiate IV:	0.9% sodium chloride
Premedicate:	Oral phenothiazine or 5-HT$_3$
Administer:	**5-Fluorouracil** _____ mg (150 mg/m^2/day) IV continuous infusion on days 1–21

- Available 500 mg/mL
- No dilution required. Can be further diluted with 0.9% sodium chloride or D5W.

Gemcitabine _____ mg (600 mg/m^2) IV on days 1, 8, and 15

- Available in 1-g or 200-mg vials; reconstitute with 0.9% sodium chloride USP (5 cc for 200 mg, 25 cc for 1 g). Further dilute in 0.9% sodium chloride.
- Reconstituted solution is stable 24 hours at room temperature. DO NOT refrigerate, because precipitate will form.

Major Side Effects

- Hematologic: Leukopenia, thrombocytopenia, and anemia, with grades 3 and 4 thrombocytopenia more common in elderly patients. Myelosuppression is dose limiting. Nadir occurs in 10–14 days with recovery at 21 days. Prolonged infusion time of Gemcitabine (> 60 minutes) is associated with higher toxicities.
- GI Symptoms: Mild to moderate nausea and vomiting, diarrhea, and/or mucositis, and diarrhea can be severe and dose limiting.
- Flulike Syndrome with fever in absence of infection 6–12 hours after treatment.
- Hepatic: Elevation of serum transaminase and bilirubin levels.
- Skin: Pruritic, maculopapular skin rash, usually involving trunk and extremities. Edema can occur. Alopecia is rare, but diffuse thinning of hair may occur. Hyperpigmentation, photosensitivity, and nail changes may occur. Hand-foot syndrome can be dose limiting.
- Ocular: Photophobia, increased lacrimation, conjunctivitis, and blurred vision.
- Reproduction: Pregnancy category D. Breast feeding should be avoided.

Initiate antiemetic protocol:	Mildly emetogenic protocol.
Supportive drugs:	☐ pegfilgrastim (Neulasta) ☐ filgrastim (Neupogen)
	☐ epoetin alfa (Procrit) ☐ darbepoetin alfa (Aranesp)
	☐ loperamide (Imodium) ☐ diphenoxylate/atropine sulfate (Lomotil)
Treatment schedule:	Chair time 1 hour days 1, 8, and 15. Repeat cycle every 28 days until disease progression.
Estimated number of visits:	Four visits per cycle. Request three to four cycles worth of visits.

Dose Calculation by: 1. _____ 2. _____

_____

Physician

_____

Patient Name

_____

Diagnosis

_____

Date

_____

ID Number

_____/ _____/ _____

Ht   Wt   M^2

Single-Agent Regimens

Low-Dose IL-2 (Aldesleukin)

Baseline laboratory tests:	CBC: Chemistry (including LFTs)
Baseline procedures or tests:	Central line placement
Initiate IV:	0.9% sodium chloride
Premedicate:	Oral phenothiazine or 5-HT$_3$
	DO NOT USE corticosteroids
	Acetaminophen 325 or 500 mg 2 tablets PO
Administer:	**Interleukin-2** 3 MU/day IV continuous infusion on days 1–5

- Available in lyophilized vials containing 22 MU.
- Reconstitute with 1.2 mL of sterile water to a final concentration of 18 MU/mL.
- For IV use, further dilute drug with D5W; aggregation of IL-2 occurs in 0.9% sodium chloride or bacteriostatic water.
- Reconstituted solution is stable for 48 hours on refrigeration.

Major Side Effects

- Flulike Symptoms: Fever, chills, headache, malaise, myalgias, and arthralgias. Occurs in all patients. Symptoms can be managed with acetaminophen, nonsteroidal anti-inflammatory drugs, and increased oral fluid intake.
- Capillary Leak Syndrome: Peripheral edema, CHF, pleural effusions, and pericardial effusions may occur and are reversible once treatment is stopped. Peripheral vasodilation, decreased systemic vascular resistance, and hypotension may lead to decreased renal perfusion. A decrease in systolic blood pressure occurs 2–12 hours after the start of therapy and progresses to significant hypotension with hypoperfusion. **Syndrome seen in high-dose therapy.**
- Pulmonary Toxicities: Dyspnea, tachypnea. Pulmonary edema may occur with hypoxia, as a result of fluid shifts.
- Bone Marrow Depression: Myelosuppression with anemia, thrombocytopenia, and neutropenia. Severe anemia occurs in 70% of patients, requiring transfusion. Thrombocytopenia common but rarely requires transfusion.
- GI Toxicities: Nausea and vomiting are mild. Diarrhea is common, can be severe, and may require bicarbonate replacement. Stomatitis is common but mild.
- Renal Toxicities: Direct tubular cell injury and decreased renal blood flow with cumulative doses. Oliguria, proteinuria, and increased serum creatinine and BUN levels. Anuria occurs in 38% of patients: renal dysfunction is reversible after drug discontinuation.
- Hepatic Toxicities: Abnormal (elevations) LFT results. Hepatomegaly and hypoalbuminemia.
- Skin: All patients develop diffuse erythematous rash, which may desquamate. Pruritus may occur with or without rash.
- Reproduction: Pregnancy category C.

Initiate antiemetic protocol:	Mildly emetogenic protocol.
Supportive drugs:	☐ pegfilgrastim (Neulasta) ☐ filgrastim (Neupogen)
	☐ epoetin alfa (Procrit) ☐ darbepoetin alfa (Aranesp)
Treatment schedule:	Chair time 1 hour on day 1. Repeat cycle every 14 days for 1 month.
Estimated number of visits:	One visit per cycle. Two for course.

Dose Calculation by: 1. _____ 2. _____

_____

Physician   Date

_____   _____

Patient Name   ID Number

_____   _____/_____/_____

Diagnosis   Ht   Wt   M²

Interferon-α-2a

Baseline laboratory tests: CBC: Chemistry (including LFTs)
Baseline procedures or tests: N/A
Initiate IV: N/A
Premedicate: Oral phenothiazine or 5-HT$_3$
Acetaminophen 325 or 500 mg 2 tablets PO

Administer: **Interferon-α-2a** _____ MU (5–15 MU) SC daily or three to five times per week
- Available in multidose pens 6 doses of 3 MU (18 MU) or 5 MU (30 MU) or 10 MU (60 MU).
- Keep refrigerated.

Major Side Effects
- Flulike Symptoms: Fever, chills, headache, myalgias, and arthralgias. Occur in 80%–90% of patients. Onset 3–4 hours after injection and lasting for up to 8–9 hours. Incidence decreases with subsequent injections. Symptoms can be managed with acetaminophen and increased oral fluid intake.
- Bone Marrow Depression: Myelosuppression with mild leukopenia and thrombocytopenia.
- GI Toxicities: Nausea and diarrhea are mild; vomiting is rare. Anorexia occurs in 46%–65% of patients and is cumulative and dose limiting. Taste alteration and xerostomia may occur.
- Renal/hepatic: Renal toxicity is uncommon and is manifested by mild proteinuria and hypocalcemia. Acute renal failure and nephrotic syndrome have been reported in rare instances. Mild transient elevations in serum transaminase levels. Dose-dependent toxicity observed more frequently in the presence of pre-existing liver abnormalities.
- Cardiotoxicity: Chest pain, arrhythmias, and CHF are rare.
- Skin: Alopecia is partial. Dry skin, pruritus, and irritation at injection site.
- Reproductive: Pregnancy category C.

Initiate antiemetic protocol: Mildly emetogenic protocol.
Supportive drugs:
☐ pegfilgrastim (Neulasta)   ☐ filgrastim (Neupogen)
☐ epoetin alfa (Procrit)   ☐ darbepoetin alfa (Aranesp)

Treatment schedule: Chair time 1 hour on day 1 for self-injection teaching
Estimated number of visits: One visit per week for laboratory tests. Request 12 weeks worth of visits. May require extra visits for hydration.

Dose Calculation by: 1. _____ 2. _____

Physician _____   Date _____

Patient Name _____   ID Number _____

Diagnosis _____   Ht _____ / Wt _____ / M^2 _____

Nexavar (Sorafenib)

Baseline laboratory tests:	CBC: Chemistry with P, LFT
Premedicate:	Oral phenothiazine
Administer:	**Nexavar** 400 mg (2 × 200-mg tab) PO BID

- Available in 200-mg tablets.
- Must be taken without food (at least one hour before or two hours after administration).
- Dose modification: Decrease to 400 mg (2 tablets) one time per day.

Major Side Effects

- Skin Reaction: Rash on trunk and neck, red raised rash with pruritis and can resolve after first 6 weeks of therapy. There is no correlation between developing a rash and response rates.
- Hand- and Foot Skin Reaction: May start with hardened calluses and turn into blisters with moist desquamation, ulceration with severe pain and sloughing of skin. Grade 3 hand and foot requires interruption/discontinuation of drug therapy. Resume at 50% of the dose when symptom resolve. May be able to increase dose if tolerated.
- Gastrointestinal: Diarrhea 43%, nausea and vomiting 23%–16%, (5HT$_3$'s were not used in clinical trials), constipation 15% all grades 1 and 2. Mucositis, stomatitis, dyspepsia, and dysphagia are common.
- Cardiac: Hypertension: 15%, grade 3 only 3% (20% increase in systolic blood pressure). Monitor blood pressure weekly for 6 weeks. May resolve on its own after 6 weeks, or treat for hypertension as necessary.
- Hemorrhagic Events: Most common is splinter hemorrhages of the nails.
- Multiple Drug Interactions: CYP2B6 and CYP28 pathway. INR may increase with patients on warfarin therapy.
- Reproductive: Pregnancy category D. Breast feeding should be avoided.

Initiate antiemetic protocol:	Mildly to moderately emetogenic protocol.
Supportive drugs:	☐ pegfilgrastim (Neulasta) ☐ filgrastim (Neupogen)
	☐ epoetin alfa (Procrit) ☐ darbepoetin alfa (Aranesp)
Treatment schedule:	Daily as tolerated until disease progression.
Estimated number of visits:	Monthly during treatment.

Dose Calculation by: 1. _____ 2. _____

_____ _____
Physician   Date

_____ _____
Patient Name   ID Number

_____ _____/_____/_____
Diagnosis   Ht   Wt   M^2

Sutent (Sunitinib malate)

Baseline laboratory tests:	CBC: Chemistry with P, LFT
Premedicate:	Oral phenothiazine or 5-HT$_3$
Administer:	**Sutent** 50-mg PO per day, 4 weeks on 2 weeks off.

- Available in 12.5-, 25- and 50-mg capsules.
- May be taken with or without food.
- Dose modification: Increase or decrease by 12.5 mg based on individual safety and tolerance.

Major Side Effects

- Bone Marrow Depression: Neutropenia occurs in 39–45%, anemia 25–37%, and thrombocytopermia in 18–19% af patients.
- Potential Activity Intolerance: Fatigue occurs in 22–38% of patients.
- Skin Alterations: Skin discoloration, dryness, thickness or cracking of the skin, blister or rash on palms of hands and soles of feet.
- Gastrointestinal: Diarrhea 81%, nausea and vomiting 49%–63%, stomatitis 58%, constipation 41%, and abdominal pain 57%.
- Cardiac: 15% of patients had decreases in Left Ventricular Ejection Fraction Dysfunction (LVEF). Monitor for signs and symptoms of congestive heart failure (CHF). Patients with cardiac history should have a baseline LVEF.
- Hypertension: 15%, grade 3, 4%
- Hemorrhagic Events: Epistaxis is the most common hemorrhagic event, bleeding from all sites 37%.
- Musculoskeletal: Arthalgia 24%, back pain 23%, and myalgias 28%.
- Multiple Drug Interacations: CYP3A4 pathway.
- Reproductive: Pregnancy category D. Breast feeding should be avoided.

Initiate antiemetic protocol:	Mildly to moderately emetogenic protocol.
Supportive drugs:	☐ loperamide (Imodium) ☐ diphenoxylate/atropine sulfate (Lomotil)
Treatment schedule:	Daily as tolerated until disease progression.
Estimated number of visits:	Monthly during treatment.

Dose Calculation by: 1. _____ 2. _____

Physician _____   Date _____

Patient Name _____   ID Number _____

Diagnosis _____   Ht _____ / Wt _____ / M^2 _____

SOFT TISSUE SARCOMAS

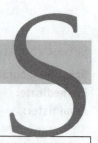

Combination Regimens

Doxorubicin: 15-mg/m^2/day IV continuous infusion on days 1–4
Dacarbazine: 250-mg/m^2/day IV continuous infusion on days 1–4
Repeat cycle every 21 days.[1,393]

Mesna: 2500-mg/m^2/day IV continuous infusion on days 1–4
Doxorubicin: 20-mg/m^2/day IV continuous infusion on days 1–3
Ifosfamide: 2500-mg/m^2/day IV continuous infusion on days 1–3
Dacarbazine: 300-mg/m^2/day IV continuous infusion on days 1–3
Repeat cycle every 21 days.[1,394]

Cyclophosphamide: 500-mg/m^2 IV on day 1
Vincristine: 1.5-mg/m^2 IV on day 1 (maximum, 2 mg)
Doxorubicin: 50-mg/m^2 IV on day 1
Dacarbazine: 750-mg/m^2 IV on day 1
Repeat cycle every 21 days.[1,395]

Cyclophosphamide: 1200-mg/m^2 IV on day 1
Doxorubicin: 75-mg/m^2 IV on day 1
Vincristine: 2-mg IV on day 1
AND
Ifosfamide: 1800-mg/m^2 IV on days 1–5
Etoposide: 100-mg/m^2 IV on days 1–5
Alternate CAV with IE every 21 days for a total of 17 cycles.[1, 396]

Single-Agent Regimens

Doxorubicin: 75-mg/m^2 IV on day 1
Repeat cycle every 21 days.[1,395]

Gemcitabine: 1000-mg/m^2 IV weekly for 7 weeks, then 1-week rest
Subsequent cycles 1000-mg/m^2 IV weekly for 3 weeks with 1-week rest
Repeat 3-week cycle every 28 days.[1,397]

Imatinib: 400-mg/day PO
Continue treatment until disease progression.[1,398]

Combination Regimens

Doxorubicin + Dacarbazine (AD)

Baseline laboratory tests: CBC: Chemistry
Baseline procedures or tests: Central line placement, MUGA scan
Initiate IV: 0.9% sodium chloride
Premedicate: 5-HT$_3$ and dexamethasone 20 mg in 100 cc of NS.
Administer: **Doxorubicin** _____ mg (15 mg/m^2) IV continuous infusion days 1–4

- Potent vesicant
- Available as a 2-mg/mL solution
- Doxorubicin will form a precipitate if it is mixed with heparin or 5-FU.

Dacarbazine _____ mg (250 mg/m^2) IV continuous infusion on days 1–4

- Potent vesicant
- Available in 100- and 200-mg vials for IV use. Reconstitute with sterile water or 0.9% sodium chloride. Solution should be yellow; discard if it turns pink or red.
- Stable for 8 hours at room temperature, 72 hours if refrigerated

Major Side Effects
- Bone Marrow Depression: Myelosuppression is a dose-limiting toxicity.
- GI Toxicities: Nausea and vomiting can be severe; aggressive antiemetic therapy is strongly recommended.
- Flulike Syndrome: Fever, chills malaise, myalgias, and arthralgias.
- GU Toxicities: Discoloration of urine from pink to red for up to 48 hours after doxorubicin.
- Cardiac: Acutely, pericarditis-myocarditis syndrome may occur. With high cumulative doses > 550 mg/m^2, cardiomyopathy may occur.
- Skin: Extravasation of either drug causes severe tissue destruction. Hyperpigmentation, photosensitivity, and radiation recall occur. Complete alopecia likely.
- CNS: Paresthesias, neuropathies, ataxia, lethargy, headache, confusion, and seizures have been observed.
- Reproductive: Pregnancy category D. Breast feeding should be avoided.

Initiate antiemetic protocol: Highly emetogenic protocol.
Supportive drugs:
☐ pegfilgrastim (Neulasta)   ☐ filgrastim (Neupogen)
☐ epoetin alfa (Procrit)   ☐ darbepoetin alfa (Aranesp)

Treatment schedule: Chair time 1 hour on day 1. Repeat cycle every 21 days.
Estimated number of visits: One visit per cycle. Request three cycles worth of visits.

Dose Calculation by: 1. _____   2. _____

_____
Physician

_____
Date

_____
Patient Name

_____
ID Number

_____
Diagnosis

_____/_____/_____
Ht   Wt   M^2

Mesna + Doxorubicin + Ifosfamide + Dacarbazine (MAID)

Baseline laboratory tests:	CBC: Chemistry (including Mg^{2+})
Baseline procedures or tests:	Central line placement, MUGA scan
Initiate IV:	0.9% sodium chloride
Premedicate:	5-HT$_3$ and dexamethasone 10–20 mg in 100 cc of NS (days 1–4)
Administer:	**Mesna** _____ mg (2500 mg/m^2/day) IV continuous infusion days 1–4

- Available in 200 mg glass ampule, 100 mg/mL or 1000 mg multidose vial.
- Refrigerate and use reconstituted solution within 6 hours. Diluted solution is stable for 24 hours at room temperature.

Doxorubicin _____ mg (20 mg/m^2/day) IV continuous infusion on days 1–3

- Potent vesicant
- Available in a 2-mg/mL solution.
- Doxorubicin will form a precipitate if it is mixed with heparin or 5-FU.

Ifosfamide _____ mg (2500 mg/m^2) IV continuous infusion on days 1–3

- Available in 1 and 3 gram single dose vials. Use within 24 hours.
- Reconstitute powder with sterile water for injection; discard unused portion after 8 hours.
- May further dilute in D5W or 0.9% sodium chloride.

Dacarbazine _____ mg (300 mg/m^2) IV continuous infusion on days 1–3

- Potent vesicant
- Available in 100- and 200-mg vials for IV use. Reconstitute with sterile water or 0.9% sodium chloride. Solution should be yellow; discard if it turns pink or red.
- Stable for 8 hours at room temperature, 72 hours if refrigerated.

Major Side Effects	- Bone Marrow Depression: Myelosuppression can be dose limiting.

- Flulike Syndrome: Fever, chills, malaise, myalgias, and arthralgias. That may last several days after treatment.
- GI Toxicities: Moderate-to-severe nausea and vomiting. Mucositis and/or diarrhea occurs in 30%–40% of patients.
- GU Toxicities: Bladder irritation--hemorrhagic cystitis with hematuria, dysuria, urinary frequency. Renal toxicity--increased BUN and serum creatinine levels, decreased urine creatinine clearance, acute tubular necrosis, pyelonephritis, glomerular dysfunction, and metabolic acidosis. Risk may be reduced with adequate hydration.
- Neurotoxicity: Lethargy, confusion, seizure, cerebellar ataxia, weakness, hallucinations, and cranial nerve dysfunction.
- CNS: Somnolence, confusion, depressive psychosis, or hallucinations (12%)
- Skin Alterations: Alopecia with photosensitivity and radiation recall. Total loss of body hair occurs in nearly all patients.
- Reproductive: Pregnancy category D. Breast feeding should be avoided.

Initiate antiemetic protocol:	Moderately to highly emetogenic protocol.
Supportive drugs:	☐ pegfilgrastim (Neulasta) ☐ filgrastim (Neupogen)
	☐ epoetin alfa (Procrit) ☐ darbepoetin alfa (Aranesp)
Treatment schedule:	Refill/mix infusion daily. 1 hour daily for four days. Weekly CBCS. Repeat every 21 days.
Estimated number of visits:	Five visits per cycle. Request three cycles worth of visits.

Dose Calculation by: 1. _____ 2. _____

_____
Physician

_____
Date

_____
Patient Name

_____
ID Number

_____
Diagnosis

_____ / _____ / _____
Ht   Wt   M^2

Cyclophosphamide + Vincristine + Doxorubicin + Dacarbazine (CYVADIC)

Baseline laboratory tests:	CBC: Chemistry
Baseline procedures or tests:	MUGA scan
Initiate IV:	0.9% sodium chloride
Premedicate:	5-HT$_3$ and dexamethasone 20 mg in 100 cc of NS.

Administer:

Cyclophosphamide _____ mg (500 mg/m^2) IV on day 1

- Available in 100-, 200-, 500-, 1000-, and 2000-mg vials.
- Dilute with sterile water. Shake well to ensure that all particles completely dissolve.
- Reconstituted solution is stable for 24 hours at room temperature and for 6 days if refrigerated.

Vincristine _____ mg (1.5 mg/m^2) IV on day 1. **Maximum dose is 2 mg.**

- Vesicant
- Available in 1-, 2-, or 5-mg vials. Refrigerate until use.

Doxorubicin _____ mg (50 mg/m^2) IV on day 1

- Potent vesicant
- Available as a 2-mg/mL solution.
- Doxorubicin will form a precipitate if it is mixed with heparin or 5-FU.

Dacarbazine _____ mg (750 mg/m^2) IV on day 1

- Potent vesicant
- Available in 100- and 200-mg vials for IV use. Reconstitute with sterile water or 0.9% sodium chloride. Solution should be yellow; discard if it turns pink or red.
- Stable for 8 hours at room temperature, 72 hours if refrigerated.

Major Side Effects

- Bone Marrow Depression: Myelosuppression is a dose-limiting toxicity.
- GI Toxicities: Nausea and vomiting can be severe; aggressive antiemetic therapy is strongly recommended. Constipation, abdominal pain, or paralytic ileus. Aggressive bowel program suggested.
- Flulike Syndrome: Fever, chills malaise, myalgias, and arthralgias.
- Cardiac: Acutely, pericarditis-myocarditis syndrome may occur. With high cumulative doses of doxorubicin > 550 mg/m^2, cardiomyopathy may occur.
- GU Toxicities: Bladder toxicity in the form of hemorrhagic cystitis, dysuria, and increased urinary frequency occurs in 5%–10% of patients. Risk may be reduced with adequate hydration. Discoloration of urine from pink to red for up to 48 hours after doxorubicin.
- Skin: Extravasation of doxorubicin or vincristine causes severe tissue damage. Hyperpigmentation, photosensitivity, and radiation recall occur. Alopecia.
- Neuropathies: Peripheral neuropathies as a result of toxicity to nerve fibers. Automatic nervous system dysfunction or thostasis, sphincter problems and paralytic ileus. Bone, back, limb, jaw, and partial gland pain may occur.
- CNS: Paresthesias, neuropathies, ataxia, lethargy, headache, confusion, and seizures have been observed.
- Reproductive: Pregnancy category D. Breast feeding should be avoided.

Initiate antiemetic protocol:	Highly emetogenic protocol.

Supportive drugs:

☐ pegfilgrastim (Neulasta)   ☐ filgrastim (Neupogen)

☐ epoetin alfa (Procrit)   ☐ darbepoetin alfa (Aranesp)

Treatment schedule:	Chair time 4 hours on day 1. Repeat cycle every 21 days.
Estimated number of visits:	One visit per cycle. Request three cycles worth of visits.

Dose Calculation by: 1. _____   2. _____

_____

Physician

_____

Patient Name

_____

Diagnosis

_____

Date

_____

ID Number

_____ / _____ / _____

Ht   Wt   M²

Cyclophosphamide + Doxorubicin + Vincristine (CAV) Alternating with Ifosfamide + Etoposide (IE)

Baseline laboratory tests:	CBC: Chemistry and LFTs
Baseline procedures or tests:	MUGA scan
Initiate IV:	0.9% sodium chloride
Premedicate:	5-HT$_3$ and dexamethasone 20 mg in 100 cc of NS.
Administer: CAV	**Cyclophosphamide** _____ mg (1200 mg/m^2) IV on day 1

- Available in 100-, 200-, 500-, 1000-, and 2000-mg vials.
- Dilute with sterile water and shake well to ensure that solution completely dissolves.
- Reconstituted solution stable for 24 hours at room temperature, 6 days if refrigerated.

Doxorubicin _____ mg (75 mg/m^2) IV on day 1

- **Potent vesicant**
- Available as a 2-mg/mL solution
- Doxorubicin will form a precipitate if it is mixed with heparin or 5-FU.

Vincristine _____ 2-mg IV on day 1

- **Vesicant**
- Available in 1-, 2-, and 5-mg vials.
- Refrigerate vials until use.

Alternate every 21 days with:

Ifosfamide _____ 1800-mg/m^2 IV on days 1–5

- Available in 1- and 3-g vials.
- Reconstitute with sterile water. Further dilute to concentrations of 0.6–20 mg/mL in D5W or NS.
- Stable for 24 hours if refrigerated.
- Drug interactions phenobarbital, phenytoin, cimetidine, and allopurinol increase toxicity. Ifosfamide may enhance anticoagulant effects of warfarin.

Mesna

- 15 minutes before, 4 and 8 hours after, ifosfamide dose or Mesna tablets at 40% of ifosfamide dose at 2 and 6 hours after ifosfamide.

Etoposide _____ 100-mg/m^2/day IV over 1–2 hours on days 1–5

- Etoposide (VePesid) 5 cc/100 mg; etoposide phosphate diethanolate (Etopophos) reconstitute with 5–10 mL of NS, D5W, sterile water, bacteriostatic sterile water, or bacteriostatic NS with benzyl alcohol to 20 mg/mL or 10 mg/mL, respectively. Further dilute to final concentration NS or to final concentration of 0.1 mg/mL.

Major Side Effects

- Bone Marrow Depression: Leukopenia, thrombocytopenia, and anemia all seen; may be severe.
- GI Toxicities: Nausea and vomiting are moderate to severe and can be acute or delayed. Stomatitis and diarrhea (10%); not dose limiting. Constipation, abdominal pain, or paralytic ileus as a result of nerve toxicity.
- Cardiac: Acutely, pericarditis-myocarditis syndrome may occur. With high cumulative doses of doxorubicin > 550 mg/m^2, cardiomyopathy may occur. Cyclophosphamide may increase the risk of doxorubicin-induced cardiotoxicity.
- Neurotoxicities: Peripheral neuropathies as a result of toxicity to nerve fibers. Cranial nerve dysfunction may occur (rare), as well as jaw pain, diplopia, vocal cord paresis, mental depression, and metallic taste.
- Altered Urinary Elimination: Hemorrhagic cystitis, hematuria; occurance preventable with uroprotection and hydration with 2–3 L per day. Monitor BUN and serum creatinine levels. Uroprotection with mesna 20% of ifosfamide dose and hydration to prevent bladder toxicity. Risk may be reduced with adequate hydration.
- Hepatic: Use with caution in patients with abnormal liver function. Dose reduction is required in the presence of liver dysfunction.
- Bladder Toxicities: Hemorrhagic cystitis, dysuria, and urinary frequency. Red-orange discoloration of urine; resolves by 24–48 hours.

- Skin: Extravasation of vesicants causes severe tissue destruction. Hyperpigmentation, photosensitivity, and radiation recall occur. Complete alopecia.
- Sensory/perceptual Alterations: Lethargy and confusion at high doses of ifosfamide, usually lasting 1–8 hours and is reversible.
- Reproductive: Pregnancy category D. Breast feeding should be avoided. Impotence may occur.

Initiate antiemetic protocol: Moderately to highly emetogenic protocol.

Supportive drugs:
☐ pegfilgrastim (Neulasta)   ☐ filgrastim (Neupogen)
☐ epoetin alfa (Procrit)   ☐ darbepoetin alfa (Aranesp)

Treatment schedule: Chair time 2 hours on day 1 with CAV, 3–4 hours with IE.

Alternate CAV with IE every 21 days for a total of 17 cycles.

Estimated number of visits: Two visits for each CAV and six visits for each IE

Dose Calculation by: 1. _____   2. _____

_____

Physician   Date

_____

Patient Name   ID Number

_____ / _____ / _____

Diagnosis   Ht   Wt M^2

Single-Agent Regimens

Doxorubicin (Soft Tissue Sarcoma)

Baseline laboratory tests:	CBC: Chemistry
Baseline procedures or tests:	MUGA scan, central line placement
Initiate IV:	0.9% sodium chloride
Premedicate:	5-HT$_3$ and dexamethasone 10–20 mg in 100 cc of NS
Administer:	**Doxorubicin** _____ mg (75 mg/m^2) IV on day 1

- **Potent vesicant**
- Available as a 2-mg/mL solution.
- Doxorubicin will form a precipitate if it is mixed with heparin or 5-FU.

Major Side Effects

- Bone Marrow Depression: WBC and platelet nadir 10–14 days after drug dose, with recovery from days 15–21. Myelosuppression may be severe but is less severe with weekly dosing.
- GI Toxicities: Nausea and vomiting are moderate to severe and occur in 44% of patients. Stomatitis occurs in 10% of patients but is not dose limiting.
- GU Toxicity: Red-orange discoloration of urine, resolves in 24–48 hours.
- Cardiac: Acutely, pericarditis-myocarditis syndrome may occur. With high cumulative doses > 550 mg/m^2, cardiomyopathy may occur. Increased risk of cardiotoxicity when doxorubicin is given with trastuzumab (Herceptin) or mitomycin.
- Skin: Extravasation of doxorubicin causes severe tissue destruction. Hyperpigmentation, photosensitivity, and radiation recall occur. Complete alopecia occurs with doses > 50 mg/m^2.
- Reproductive: Pregnancy category D. Breast feeding should be avoided.

Initiate antiemetic protocol:	Moderately to highly emetogenic protocol.
Supportive drugs:	☐ pegfilgrastim (Neulasta) ☐ filgrastim (Neupogen)
	☐ epoetin alfa (Procrit) ☐ darbepoetin alfa (Aranesp)
Treatment schedule:	Chair time 1 hour on day 1. Repeat cycle every 21 days.
Estimated number of visits:	Two visits per cycle. CBC day 10–14. Request four cycles worth of visits.

Dose Calculation by: 1. _____   2. _____

_____   _____
Physician   Date

_____   _____
Patient Name   ID Number

_____   _____/ _____/ _____
Diagnosis   Ht   Wt   M^2

Gemcitabine (Soft Tissue Sarcoma)

Baseline laboratory tests:	CBC: Chemistry panel, LFTs
Baseline procedures or tests:	N/A
Initiate IV:	0.9% sodium chloride
Premedicate:	Oral phenothiazine
	OR
	5-HT$_3$ and dexamethasone 10 mg in 100 cc of NS
Administer:	**Gemcitabine** _____ mg (1000 mg/m^2) IV over 30 minutes weekly

- Available in 1-g or 200-mg vials; reconstitute with 0.9% sodium chloride USP (5 cc for 200 mg, 25 cc for 1 g). Further dilute in 0.9% sodium chloride.
- Reconstituted solution is stable 24 hours at room temperature. DO NOT refrigerate, because precipitate will form.

Major Side Effects

- Hematologic: Leukopenia (63%), thrombocytopenia (36%), and anemia (73%), with grade 3 and 4 thrombocytopenia more common in elderly patients. Myelosuppression is dose limiting. Nadir occurs in 10–14 days, with recovery at 21 days. Prolonged infusion time (> 60 minutes) is associated with higher toxicities.
- GI Symptoms: Mild-to-moderate nausea and vomiting (70%), diarrhea, and/or mucositis (15%–20%).
- Flulike Syndrome: (20%) with fever in absence of infection 6–12 hours after treatment (40%).
- Hepatic: Elevation of serum transaminase and bilirubin levels.
- Skin: Pruritic, maculopapular skin rash, usually involving trunk and extremities. Edema occurs in 30% of patients. Alopecia is rare.
- Reproduction: Pregnancy category D. Breast feeding should be avoided.

Initiate antiemetic protocol:	Mildly to moderately emetogenic protocol.
Supportive drugs:	☐ pegfilgrastim (Neulasta) ☐ filgrastim (Neupogen)
	☐ epoetin alfa (Procrit) ☐ darbepoetin alfa (Aranesp)
Treatment schedule:	Chair time 1 hour. Repeat weekly for 7 weeks, then 1-week rest; then weekly for 3 weeks with 1 week off.
	Repeat 3 weeks on, 1 week off until disease progression.
Estimated number of visits:	Weekly for 3 months. Three visits per month subsequent courses.

Dose Calculation by: 1. _____   2. _____

_____   _____
Physician   Date

_____   _____
Patient Name   ID Number

_____   _____/ _____/ _____
Diagnosis   Ht   Wt   M^2

Imatinib (Gleevec)

Baseline laboratory tests:	CBC: Chemistry and LFTs
Baseline procedures or tests:	c-kit (CD117) expression
Initiate IV:	N/A
Premedicate:	Oral phenothiazine or 5-HT_3
Administer:	**Imatinib** 400-mg PO per day

- May increase dose to 600-mg PO per day if no response.
- Available in 100- or 400-mg capsules.
- Monitor INRs closely in patients taking warfarin; inhibits metabolism of warfarin.

Major Side Effects

- GI Toxicities: Nausea and vomiting, 40%–50% of patients. Usually relieved when the drug is taken with food. Diarrhea observed in 25%–30% of patients.
- Bone Marrow Suppression: Myelosuppression, neutropenia, and thrombocytopenia common and can be dose related.
- Fluid/electrolyte Imbalance: Fluid retention is common, especially in the elderly. Periorbital and lower extremity edema primarily occurs. However, pleural effusions, ascites, rapid weight gain, and pulmonary edema may develop. Hypokalemia reported in 2%–12% of patients.
- Laboratory Values: Mild, transient elevation in serum transaminase and bilirubin levels.
- Reproductive: Pregnancy category D. Breast feeding should be avoided.

Initiate antiemetic protocol:	Mildly to moderately emetogenic protocol.
Supportive drugs:	☐ pegfilgrastim (Neulasta) ☐ filgrastim (Neupogen)
	☐ loperamide (Imodium) ☐ epoetin alfa (Procrit)
	☐ darbepoetin alfa (Aranesp) ☐ diphenoxylate/atropine sulfate (Lomotil)
Treatment schedule:	Daily as tolerated until disease progression.
Estimated number of visits:	Monthly during treatment.

Dose Calculation by: 1. _____ 2. _____

Physician _____   Date _____

Patient Name _____   ID Number _____

Diagnosis _____   _____/_____/_____
                                          Ht   Wt M^2

TESTICULAR CANCER

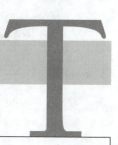

Adjuvant Therapy

Cisplatin: 20-mg/m^2 IV on days 1–5

Etoposide: 100-mg/m^2 IV on days 1–5

Bleomycin: 30 U IV on days 2, 9, and 16

Repeat cycle every 28 days for a total of two cycles.[1,399]

Adjuvant therapy for stage II testicular cancer treated with orchiectomy and retroperitoneal lymph node dissection.

Advanced Disease

Bleomycin: 30 U IV on days 2, 9, and 16

Etoposide: 100-mg/m^2 IV on days 1–5

Cisplatin: 20-mg/m^2 IV on days 1–5

Repeat cycle every 21 days.[1,400]

Etoposide: 100-mg/m^2 IV on days 1–5

Cisplatin: 20-mg/m^2 IV on days 1–5

Repeat cycle every 21 days.[1,401]

Cisplatin: 20-mg/m^2 IV on days 1–5

Vinblastine: 0.15-mg/kg IV on days 1 and 2

Bleomycin: 30 units IV on days 2, 9, and 16

Repeat cycle every 21 days.[1,402]

Vinblastine: 4-mg/m^2 IV on day 1

Dactinomycin: 1-mg/m^2 IV on day 1

Bleomycin: 30 U IV on day 1, then 20 U/m^2 continuous infusion on days 1–3

Cisplatin: 20-mg/m^2 IV on day 4

Cyclophosphamide: 600-mg/m^2 IV on day 1

Repeat cycle every 21 days.[1,403]

Salvage Regimens

Vinblastine: 0.11-mg/kg IV on days 1 and 2

Ifosfamide: 1200-mg/m^2 IV on days 1–5

Cisplatin: 20-mg/m^2 IV on days 1–5

Mesna: 400-mg/m^2 IV, given 15 minutes before first ifosfamide dose, then 1200-mg/m^2/day IV continuous infusion for 5 days

Repeat cycle every 21 days.[1,404]

Etoposide (VP-16): 75-mg/m^2 IV on days 1–5

Ifosfamide: 1200-mg/m^2 IV on days 1–5

Cisplatin: 20-mg/m^2 IV on days 1–5

Mesna: 400-mg/m^2 IV, given 15 minutes before first ifosfamide dose, then 1200-mg/m^2/day IV continuous infusion for 5 days

Repeat cycle every 21 days.[1,405]

Adjuvant Therapy

Cisplatin + Etoposide + Bleomycin (PEB)

Baseline laboratory tests:	CBC: Chemistry (including Mg^{2+})
Baseline procedures or tests:	PFTs and chest x-ray study at baseline and before each cycle of therapy
Initiate IV:	0.9% sodium chloride
Premedicate:	5-HT$_3$ and dexamethasone 10–20 mg in 100 cc of NS
	Acetaminophen 30 minutes before bleomycin

Administer:

Cisplatin _____ mg (20 mg/m^2) IV infusion over 1–2 hours on days 1–5

- Do not use aluminum needles, because precipitate will form.
- Available in solution as 1 mg/mL.
- Further dilute solution with 250 cc or more of NS.

Etoposide _____ mg (100 mg/m^2) IV infusion over 1 hour on days 1–5

- Available in 100-mg vials; when reconstituted with 5 or 10 mL of NS, D5W or sterile water with benzyl alcohol makes a 20- or 10-mg/mL solution. Also available in solution as a 20-mg/mL concentration.
- May be further diluted in NS or D5W to final concentration of 0.1 mg/mL.

Bleomycin 30 units IV push or infusion over 15 minutes on days 2, 9, and 16

- A test dose of 2 units is recommended before the first dose to detect hypersensitivity.
- Available as a powder in 15- or 30-unit sizes. Dilute powder in 0.9% sodium chloride or sterile water.
- Reconstituted solution is stable for 24 hours at room temperature.

Major Side Effects

- Allergic Reaction: Bleomycin—fever and chills observed in up to 25% of patients. True anaphylactic reactions are rare. Etoposide—bronchospasm, with or without fever, chills. Hypotension may occur during rapid infusion. Anaphylaxis may occur but is rare.
- Bone Marrow Depression: Myelosuppression can be a dose-limiting toxicity.
- GI Toxicities: Moderate-to-severe nausea and vomiting. May be acute (first 24 hours) or delayed (> 24 hours). Mucositis and diarrhea are rare.
- Pulmonary Toxicities: Pulmonary toxicity is dose limiting in bleomycin. Seen more frequently in cumulative dose > 400 units with bleomycin.
- Renal: Nephrotoxicity is dose related with cisplatin and presents at 10–20 days.
- Electrolyte Imbalance: Decreased Mg^{2+}, K, Ca^{2+}, Na^+, and P.
- Neurotoxicity: Dose-limiting toxicity, usually in the form of peripheral sensory neuropathy. Paresthesias and numbness in a classic "stocking glove" pattern.
- Ototoxicity: High-frequency hearing loss and tinnitus
- Skin: Alopecia
- Reproductive: Pregnancy category D. Breast feeding should be avoided.

Initiate antiemetic protocol:	Moderately to highly emetogenic protocol.
Supportive drugs:	☐ pegfilgrastim (Neulasta) ☐ filgrastim (Neupogen)
	☐ epoetin alfa (Procrit) ☐ darbepoetin alfa (Aranesp)
Treatment schedule:	Chair time 3 hours on days 1, 1–5, and 1 hour on days 9 and 16. Repeat every 28 days for two cycles.
Estimated number of visits:	Seven visits per cycle. Request two cycles worth of visits.

Dose Calculation by: 1. _____ 2. _____

_____
Physician

_____
Date

_____
Patient Name

_____
ID Number

_____
Diagnosis

_____/_____/_____
Ht   Wt   M^2

Advanced Disease

Etoposide + Bleomycin + Cisplatin (BEP)

Baseline laboratory tests:	CBC: Chemistry (including Mg^{2+})
Baseline procedures or tests:	PFTs and chest x-ray study at baseline and before each cycle of therapy
Initiate IV:	0.9% sodium chloride
Premedicate:	5-HT_3 and dexamethasone 10–20 mg in 100 cc of NS
	Acetaminophen 30 minutes before bleomycin

Administer: **Bleomycin** 30 units IV push or infusion over 15 minutes on days 2, 9, and 16

- A test dose of 2 units is recommended before the first dose to detect hypersensitivity.
- Available as a powder in 15- or 30-unit sizes. Dilute powder in 0.9% sodium chloride or sterile water.
- Reconstituted solution is stable for 24 hours at room temperature.

Etoposide _____ mg (100 mg/m^2) IV infusion over 1 hour on days 1–5

- Available in 100-mg vials; when reconstituted with 5 or 10 mL of NS, D5W or sterile water with benzyl alcohol makes a 20- or 10-mg/mL solution. Also available in solution as a 20-mg/mL concentration.
- May be further diluted in NS or D5W to final concentration of 0.1 mg/mL

Cisplatin _____ mg (20 mg/m^2) IV infusion over 1–2 hours on days 1–5

- Do not use aluminum needles, because precipitate will form.
- Available in solution as 1 mg/mL.
- Further dilute solution with 250 cc or more of NS.

Major Side Effects

- Allergic Reaction: Bleomycin—fever and chills observed in up to 25% of patients. True anaphylactic reactions are rare. Etoposide—bronchospasm, with or without fever, chills. Hypotension may occur during rapid infusion. Anaphylaxis may occur but is rare.
- Bone Marrow Depression: Myelosuppression can be a dose-limiting toxicity.
- GI Toxicities: Moderate-to-severe nausea and vomiting. May be acute (first 24 hours) or delayed (> 24 hours). Mucositis and diarrhea are rare.
- Pulmonary Toxicities: Pulmonary toxicity is dose limiting in bleomycin. Seen more frequently in cumulative dose > 400 units with bleomycin.
- Renal: Nephrotoxicity is dose related with cisplatin and presents at 10–20 days. Risk may be reduced with adequate hydration.
- Electrolyte Imbalance: Decreased Mg^{2+}, K, Ca^{2+}, Na^+, and P.
- Neurotoxicity: Dose-limiting toxicity, usually in the form of peripheral sensory neuropathy. Paresthesias and numbness in a classic "stocking glove" pattern.
- Ototoxicity: High-frequency hearing loss and tinnitus.
- Skin: Alopecia
- Reproductive: Pregnancy category D. Breast feeding should be avoided.

Initiate antiemetic protocol:	Moderately to highly emetogenic protocol.
Supportive drugs:	☐ pegfilgrastim (Neulasta) ☐ filgrastim (Neupogen)
	☐ epoetin alfa (Procrit) ☐ darbepoetin alfa (Aranesp)
Treatment schedule:	Chair time 3 hours on days 1, 1–5, and 1 hour on days 9 and 16. Repeat every 21 days.
Estimated number of visits:	Seven visits per cycle. Request three cycles worth of visits.

Dose Calculation by: 1. _____   2. _____

_____   _____
Physician   Date

_____   _____
Patient Name   ID Number

_____   _____/_____/_____
Diagnosis   Ht   Wt   M^2

Etoposide + Cisplatin (EP)

Baseline laboratory tests:	CBC: Chemistry (including Mg^{2+}) and CEA
Baseline procedures or tests:	N/A
Initiate IV:	0.9% sodium chloride
Premedicate:	5-HT_3 and dexamethasone 10–20 mg in 100 cc of NS
Administer:	**Etoposide** _____ mg (100 mg/m^2) IV infusion over 1 hour on days 1–5

- Available in 100-mg vials, when reconstituted with 5 or 10 mL of NS, D5W or sterile water with benzyl alcohol makes a 20- or 10-mg/mL solution. Also available in solution as a 20-mg/mL concentration.
- May be further diluted in NS or D5W to final concentration of 0.1 mg/mL.

Cisplatin _____ mg (20 mg/m^2) IV infusion over 1–2 hours on days 1–5

- Do not use aluminum needles, because precipitate will form.
- Available in solution as 1 mg/mL.
- Further dilute solution with 250 cc or more of NS.

Major Side Effects

- Allergic Reaction: Bronchospasm, with or without fever, chills. Hypotension may occur during rapid infusion. Anaphylaxis may occur but is rare.
- Bone Marrow Depression: Myelosuppression can be a dose-limiting toxicity.
- GI Toxicities: Moderate-to-severe nausea and vomiting. May be acute (first 24 hours) or delayed (> 24 hours). Mucositis and diarrhea are rare.
- Renal: Nephrotoxicity is dose related with cisplatin and presents at 10–20 days. Risk may be reduced with adequate hydration.
- Electrolyte Imbalance: Decreased Mg^{2+}, K, Ca^{2+}, Na^+, and P.
- Neurotoxicity: Dose-limiting toxicity, usually in the form of peripheral sensory neuropathy. Paresthesias and numbness in a classic "stocking glove" pattern.
- Ototoxicity: High-frequency hearing loss and tinnitus
- Skin: Alopecia
- Reproductive: Pregnancy category D. Breast feeding should be avoided.

Initiate antiemetic protocol:	Moderately to highly emetogenic protocol.
Supportive drugs:	☐ pegfilgrastim (Neulasta) ☐ filgrastim (Neupogen)
	☐ epoetin alfa (Procrit) ☐ darbepoetin alfa (Aranesp)
Treatment schedule:	Chair time 2 hours on days 1–5. Repeat cycle every 21 days.
Estimated number of visits:	Five visits per cycle. Request three cycles worth of visits.

Dose Calculation by: 1. _____   2. _____

Physician _____   Date _____

Patient Name _____   ID Number _____

Diagnosis _____   _____/ _____/ _____
                                        Ht   Wt   M^2

Cisplatin + Vinblastine + Bleomycin (PVB)

Baseline laboratory tests:	CBC: Chemistry (including Mg^{2+})
Baseline procedures or tests:	PFTs and chest x-ray study baseline and before each cycle of therapy
Initiate IV:	0.9% sodium chloride
Premedicate:	5-HT$_3$ and dexamethasone 10–20 mg in 100 cc of NS
	Acetaminophen 30 minutes before bleomycin

Administer:

Cisplatin _____ mg (20 mg/m^2) IV infusion on days 1–5

- Do not use aluminum needles, because precipitate will form.
- Available in solution as 1 mg/mL.
- Further dilute solution with 250 cc or more of NS.

Vinblastine _____ mg (0.15 mg/kg) IV push on days 1 and 2

- Vesicant
- Available in 10-mg vials.
- Store in refrigerator until use.

Bleomycin 30 units IV push or infusion on days 2, 9, and 16

- A test dose of 2 units is recommended before the first dose to detect hypersensitivity.
- Available as a powder in 15- or 30-unit sizes. Dilute powder in 0.9% sodium chloride or sterile water.
- Reconstituted solution is stable for 24 hours at room temperature.

Major Side Effects

- Allergic Reaction: Bleomycin—fever and chills observed in up to 25% of patients. True anaphylactic reactions are rare.
- Bone Marrow Depression: Myelosuppression can be a dose-limiting toxicity.
- GI Toxicities: Moderate-to-severe nausea and vomiting. May be acute (first 24 hours) or delayed (>24 hours). Mucositis and diarrhea are rare. Constipation resulting from neurotoxicity, abdominal pain, or paralytic ileus.
- Pulmonary Toxicities: Pulmonary toxicity is dose limiting in bleomycin.
- Renal: Nephrotoxicity is dose related with cisplatin and presents at 10–20 days. Risk may be reduced with adequate hydration.
- Electrolyte Imbalance: Decreases Mg^{2+}, K^+, Ca^{2+}, Na^+, and P.
- Neurotoxicity: Paresthesias, peripheral neuropathy, depression, headache, malaise, jaw pain, urinary retention, tachycardia, orthostatic hypotension, and seizures can occur in high doses or with prolonged therapy.
- Ototoxicity: High-frequency hearing loss and tinnitus.
- Skin: Alopecia
- Reproductive: Pregnancy category D. Breast feeding should be avoided.

Initiate antiemetic protocol:	Moderately to highly emetogenic protocol.
Supportive drugs:	☐ pegfilgrastim (Neulasta) ☐ filgrastim (Neupogen)
	☐ epoetin alfa (Procrit) ☐ darbepoetin alfa (Aranesp)
Treatment schedule:	Chair time 3 hours on days 1–5, and 1 hour on days 9 and 16. Repeat every 21 days.
Estimated number of visits:	Seven visits per cycle. Request three cycles worth of visits.

Dose Calculation by: 1. _____ 2. _____

_____

Physician

_____

Date

_____

Patient Name

_____

ID Number

_____

Diagnosis

_____ / _____ / _____

Ht   Wt   M^2

Vinblastine + Dactinomycin + Bleomycin (VAB-6)

Baseline laboratory tests:	CBC: Chemistry panel (including Mg^{2+})
Baseline procedures or tests:	PFTs and chest x-ray study at baseline and before each cycle of therapy.
	Central line placement for continuous infusion
Initiate IV:	0.9% sodium chloride
Premedicate:	5-HT_3 and dexamethasone 20 mg in 100 cc of NS
	Acetaminophen 30 minutes before bleomycin
Administer:	**Vinblastine** _____ mg (4 mg/m²) IV push on day 1

* Vesicant
* Available in 10-mg vials
* Store in refrigerator until use.

Dactinomycin _____ mg (1 mg/m²) IV infusion on day 1

* Vesicant
* Available as a lyophilized powder in vials containing 0.5 mg of dactinomycin and 20 mg of mannitol for IV use
* Add sterile water to give a final concentration of 500 mcg/mL. Use preservative-free water to avoid formation of a precipitate.
* Can be further diluted in D5W or NS for IV infusion or bolus

Bleomycin 30 units IV push or infusion over 15 minutes on day 1, then

Bleomycin _____units (20 units/m²) IV continuous infusion on days 1–3

* A test dose of 2 units is recommended before the first dose to detect hypersensitivity.
* Available as a powder in 15- or 30-unit sizes. Dilute powder in 0.9% sodium chloride or sterile water.
* Reconstituted solution is stable for 24 hours at room temperature.

Cisplatin _____ mg (20 mg/m²) IV infusion over 1 hour on day 4

* Do not use aluminum needles, because precipitate will form.
* Available in solution as 1 mg/mL
* Further dilute in 250 cc or more of NS.

Cyclophosphamide _____ mg (600 mg/m²) IV infusion over 1 hour on day 1

* Available in 100-, 200-, 500-, 1000-, and 2000-mg vials for IV use.
* Dilute vials with sterile water.
* Important to shake well so that the solution is completely dissolved.

Major Side Effects

* Allergic Reaction: Bleomycin—fever and chills observed in up to 25% of patients. True anaphylactic reactions are rare.
* Bone Marrow Depression: Myelosuppression can be a dose-limiting toxicity.
* GI Toxicities: Moderate-to-severe nausea and vomiting, acute or delayed. Irritation and ulceration may occur along the entire GI mucosa. Diarrhea with or without cramps. Anorexia common. Constipation, abdominal pain, or ileus.
* Pulmonary Toxicities: Pulmonary toxicity is dose limiting in bleomycin. Seen more frequently in cumulative dose > 400 units with bleomycin.
* Hepatic: Hepatotoxicity dose reduction may be necessary.
* Renal/urinary: Nephrotoxicity or hemorrhagic cystitis possible. Dose reduction may be needed for alterations in renal function. Risk may be reduced with adequate hydration.
* Electrolyte Imbalance: Decreases Mg^{2+}, K^+, Ca^{2+}, Na^+, and P.
* Neurotoxicity: Paresthesias, peripheral neuropathy, depression, headache, jaw pain, urinary retention, tachycardia, orthostatic hypotension, and seizures.
* Skin: Tissue damage if extravasation of dactinomycin occurs. Alopecia. Hyperpigmentation, radiation recall, photosensitivity, rash, and nail changes.
* Flulike Symptoms: Malaise, myalgia, fever, depression.
* Reproductive: Pregnancy category D. Breastfeeding should be avoided.

Initiate antiemetic protocol: Moderately to highly emetogenic protocol.

Supportive drugs:
☐ pegfilgrastim (Neulasta)   ☐ filgrastim (Neupogen)
☐ epoetin alfa (Procrit)   ☐ darbepoetin alfa (Aranesp)

Treatment schedule: Chair time 2 hours on day 1, and 3 hours on day 4. Repeat cycle every 21 days.

Estimated number of visits: Two visits per cycle. Request three cycles worth of visits.

Dose Calculation by: 1. _____   2. _____

_____
Physician

_____
Date

_____
Patient Name

_____
ID Number

_____
Diagnosis

_____ / _____ / _____
Ht   Wt M^2

Salvage Regimens

Vinblastine + Ifosfamide + Cisplatin + Mesna (VeIP)

Baseline laboratory tests:	CBC: Chemistry (including Mg^{2+})
Baseline procedures or tests:	Central line placement for continuous infusion
Initiate IV:	0.9% sodium chloride
Premedicate:	5-HT_3 and dexamethasone 20 mg in 100 cc of NS
Administer:	**Vinblastine** _____ mg (0.11 mg/kg) IV on days 1 and 2

- Vesicant
- Available in 10-mg vials
- Store in refrigerator until

Ifosfamide _____ mg (1200 mg/m²) IV on days 1–5

- Reconstitute powder with sterile water for injection; discard unused portion after 8 hours.
- May further dilute in D5W or 0.9% sodium chloride

Cisplatin _____ mg (20 mg/m²) IV on days 1–5

- Do not use aluminum needles, because precipitate will form.
- Further dilute solution with 250 cc or more of NS.

Mesna _____ mg (400 mg/m²) IV, given 15 minutes before first ifosfamide dose, then

Mesna _____ mg (1200 mg/m²/day) IV continuous infusion for 5 days

- Available in 200-mg ampules or 1000-mg multidose vial for IV use.
- Dilute with D5W, D5NS, or NS.
- Reconstituted solution is stable for 24 hours at room temperature.

Major Side Effects

- Bone Marrow Depression: Myelosuppression is cumulative and dose related. Can be dose limiting. G-CSF support recommended.
- GI Toxicities: Moderate-to-severe nausea and vomiting may be acute or delayed. Mucositis and/or diarrhea may occur. Constipation, abdominal pain, ileus rare.
- Renal: Nephrotoxicity and/or hemorrhagic cystitis possible. Mesna and vigorous hydration necessary to prevent.
- Electrolyte Imbalance: Decreases Mg^{2+}, K^+, Ca^{2+}, Na^+, and P.
- Neurotoxicity: Sensory neuropathy with numbness and paresthesias in classic "stocking and glove" distribution.
- CNS: Somnolence, confusion, depressive psychosis, or hallucinations with ifosfamide. Paresthesias, jaw pain, urinary retention, and tachycardia occur with vinblastine but are less frequent than with other vinca alkaloids.
- Alopecia: Total loss of body hair occurs in nearly all patients.
- Reproductive: Pregnancy category D. Breast feeding should be avoided.

Initiate antiemetic protocol:	Moderately to highly emetogenic protocol.
Supportive drugs:	☐ pegfilgrastim (Neulasta) ☐ filgrastim (Neupogen) ☐ epoetin alfa (Procrit) ☐ darbepoetin alfa (Aranesp)
Treatment schedule:	Chair time 4 hours on day 1, and 3 hours on days 2–5. Repeat cycle every 21 days.
Estimated number of visits:	Five visits per cycle. Request three cycles worth of visits.

Dose Calculation by: 1. _____   2. _____

_____

Physician

_____

Patient Name

_____

Diagnosis

_____

Date

_____

ID Number

_____ / _____ / _____

Ht   Wt   M²

Etoposide + Ifosfamide + Cisplatin + Mesna (VIP)

Baseline laboratory tests:	CBC: Chemistry (including Mg^{2+})
Baseline procedures or tests:	Central line placement for continuous infusion.
Initiate IV:	0.9% sodium chloride
Premedicate:	5-HT_3 and dexamethasone 20 mg in 100 cc of NS
Administer:	**Etoposide** _____ mg (75 mg/m²) IV over 30–60 minutes on days 1–5

- Available in solution or powder.
- May be further diluted in NS or D5W to a final concentration of 0.1 mg/mL

Ifosfamide _____ mg (1200 mg/m²) IV on days 1–5

- Reconstitute powder with sterile water for injection; discard unused portion after 8 hours.
- May further dilute in D5W or 0.9% sodium chloride.

Cisplatin _____ mg (20 mg/m²) IV over 1 hour on days 1–5

- Do not use aluminum needles, because precipitate will form.
- Further dilute solution with 250 cc or more of NS.

Mesna _____ mg (400 mg/m²) IV, given 15 minutes before first ifosfamide dose, then

Mesna _____ mg (1200 mg/m²/day) IV continuous infusion for 5 days

- Available in 200-mg ampules or 1000-mg multidose vial for IV use.
- Dilute with D5W, D5NS, or NS.
- Reconstituted solution is stable for 24 hours at room temperature.

Major Side Effects	• Bone Marrow Depression: Myelosuppression is cumulative and dose related. Can be dose limiting.

- GI Toxicities: Moderate-to-severe nausea and vomiting may be acute or delayed. Mucositis, diarrhea, and anorexia may occur. Metallic taste common.
- Hepatic: Use etoposide with caution in patients with abnormal liver function. Dose reduction is recommended in this setting.
- Cardiovascular Toxicities: Hypotension if etoposide infused too rapidly.
- Renal: Nephrotoxicity and/or hemorrhagic cystitis possible. Mesna and vigorous hydration necessary to prevent. Dose reduction may be necessary.
- Electrolyte Imbalance: Decreases MG^{2+}, K^+, Ca^{2+}, Na^+, and PO^4
- Neurotoxicity: Sensory neuropathy with numbness and paresthesias in classic "stocking and glove" distribution.
- CNS: Somnolence, confusion, depressive psychosis, or hallucinations with ifosfamide.
- Hypersensitivity reaction: Chills, fever, bronchospasm, dyspnea, tachycardia, facial and tongue swelling, and hypotension with etoposide.
- Skin: Total alopecia occurs in nearly all patients. Radiation recall, skin changes.
- Reproductive: Pregnancy category D. Breast feeding should be avoided.

Initiate antiemetic protocol:	Moderately to highly emetogenic protocol.
Supportive drugs:	☐ pegfilgrastim (Neulasta) ☐ filgrastim (Neupogen)
	☐ epoetin alfa (Procrit) ☐ darbepoetin alfa (Aranesp)
Treatment schedule:	Chair time 5 hours on day 1, and 4 hours on days 2–5. Repeat cycle every 21 days.
Estimated number of visits:	Five visits per cycle. Request three cycles worth of visits.

Dose Calculation by: 1. _____   2. _____

_____   _____

Physician   Date

_____   _____

Patient Name   ID Number

_____   _____ / _____ / _____

Diagnosis   Ht   Wt M^2

THYMOMA

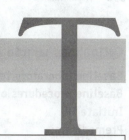

Cyclophosphamide: 500-mg/m^2 IV on day 1
Doxorubicin: 50-mg/m^2 IV on day 1
Cisplatin: 50-mg/m^2 IV on day 1
Repeat cycle every 21 days.[1,406]

Cisplatin: 60-mg/m^2 IV on day 1
Etoposide: 120-mg/m^2 IV on days 1–3
Repeat cycle every 21 days.[1,407]

Cisplatin: 50-mg/m^2 IV on day 1
Doxorubicin: 40-mg/m^2 IV on day 1
Vincristine: 0.6-mg/m^2 IV on day 3
Cyclophosphamide: 700-mg/m^2 IV on day 4
Repeat cycle every 28 days.[1,408]

Cyclophosphamide + Doxorubicin + Cisplatin (CAP)

Baseline laboratory tests:	CBC: Chemistry (including Mg^{2+})
Baseline procedures or tests:	N/A
Initiate IV:	0.9% sodium chloride
Premedicate:	5-HT_3 and dexamethasone 10–20 mg in 100 cc of NS
Administer:	**Cyclophosphamide** _____ mg (500 mg/m^2) IV over 1 hour on day 1

- Available in 100-, 200-, 500-, 1000-, and 2000-mg vials.
- Dilute with sterile water. Shake well to ensure that all particles completely dissolve.
- Reconstituted solution is stable for 24 hours at room temperature and for 6 days refrigerated.

Doxorubicin _____ mg (50 mg/m^2) IV push on day 1

- Potent vesicant
- Available as a 2-mg/mL solution.
- Doxorubicin will form a precipitate if it is mixed with heparin or 5-FU.

Cisplatin _____ mg (50/m^2) IV over 1–3 hours on day 1

- Do not use aluminum needles, because precipitate will form.
- Available in solution as 1 mg/mL.
- Further dilute solution with 250 cc or more of NS.

Major Side Effects

- Bone Marrow Depression: Neutropenia, thrombocytopenia, and anemia occur equally in 25%–30% of patients. Leukopenia and thrombocytopenia are dose related.
- GI Toxicities: Moderate-to-severe nausea and vomiting. May be acute (first 24 hours) or delayed (> 24 hours). Mucositis may occur.
- GU Toxicities: Nephrotoxicity is dose related with cisplatin and presents at 10–20 days. Bladder toxicity in the form of hemorrhagic cystitis, dysuria, and increased urinary frequency. Red-orange discoloration of urine up to 48 hours after doxurubicin.
- Electrolyte Imbalance: Decreased Mg^{2+}, K, Ca^{2+}, Na^+, and P.
- Cardiotoxicity: Acutely, pericarditis or myocarditis may occur. Later, cardiomyopathy in the form of CHF may occur.
- Neurotoxicity: Dose-limiting toxicity, usually in the form of peripheral sensory neuropathy. Paresthesias and numbness in a classic "stocking glove" pattern.
- Ototoxicity: High-frequency hearing loss and tinnitus.
- Skin: Extravasation of doxorubicin causes severe tissue damage. Hyperpigmentation, photosensitivity, and radiation recall occur. Alopecia.
- Reproductive: Pregnancy category D. Breast feeding should be avoided.

Initiate antiemetic protocol:	Moderately to highly emetogenic protocol.
Supportive drugs:	☐ pegfilgrastim (Neulasta) ☐ filgrastim (Neupogen)
	☐ epoetin alfa (Procrit) ☐ darbepoetin alfa (Aranesp)
Treatment schedule:	Chair time 3 hours on day 1. Repeat cycle every 28 days.
Estimated number of visits:	One visit per cycle. Request six cycles worth of visits.

Dose Calculation by: 1. _____   2. _____

_____   _____
Physician   Date

_____   _____
Patient Name   ID Number

_____   _____/ _____/ _____
Diagnosis   Ht   Wt   M^2

Cisplatin + Etoposide

Baseline laboratory tests:	CBC: Chemistry (including Mg^{2+}) and CEA
Baseline procedures or tests:	N/A
Initiate IV:	0.9% sodium chloride
Premedicate:	5-HT$_3$ and dexamethasone 10–20 mg in 100 cc of NS
Administer:	**Cisplatin** _____ mg (60 mg/m^2) IV over 1–2 hours on day 1

- Do not use aluminum needles, because precipitate will form.
- Available in solution as 1 mg/mL.
- Further dilute solution with 250 cc or more of NS.

Etoposide _____ mg (120 mg/m^2) IV over 1 hour on days 1–3

- Available in 100-mg vials; when reconstituted with 5 or 10 mL of NS, D5W or sterile water with benzyl alcohol makes a 20- or 10-mg/mL solution. Also available in solution as a 20-mg/mL concentration.
- May be further diluted in NS or D5W to final concentration of 0.1 mg/mL.

Major Side Effects

- Allergic Reaction: Bronchospasm, with or without fever, chills. Hypotension may occur during rapid infusion of etoposide. Anaphylaxis may occur but is rare.
- Bone Marrow Depression: Myelosuppression can be a dose-limiting toxicity.
- GI Toxicities: Moderate-to-severe nausea and vomiting. May be acute (first 24 hours) or delayed (> 24 hours). Mucositis and diarrhea are rare.
- Renal: Nephrotoxicity is dose related with cisplatin and presents at 10–20 days. Risk may be reduced with adequate hydration.
- Electrolyte Imbalance: Decreased Mg^{2+}, K, Ca^{2+}, Na^+, and P.
- Neurotoxicity: Dose-limiting toxicity, usually in the form of peripheral sensory neuropathy. Paresthesias and numbness in a classic "stocking glove" pattern.
- Ototoxicity: High-frequency hearing loss and tinnitus.
- Skin: Alopecia
- Reproductive: Pregnancy category D. Breast feeding should be avoided.

Initiate antiemetic protocol:	Moderately to highly emetogenic protocol.
Supportive drugs:	☐ pegfilgrastim (Neulasta) ☐ filgrastim (Neupogen)
	☐ epoetin alfa (Procrit) ☐ darbepoetin alfa (Aranesp)
Treatment schedule:	Chair time 3 hours on day 1, and 1 hour on days 2 and 3. Repeat cycle every 21 days.
Estimated number of visits:	Three visits per cycle. Request three cycles worth of visits.

Dose Calculation by: 1. _____   2. _____

_____   _____

Physician   Date

_____   _____

Patient Name   ID Number

_____   _____ / _____ / _____

Diagnosis   Ht   Wt   M^2

Cisplatin + Doxorubicin + Vincristine + Cyclophosphamide (ADOC)

Baseline laboratory tests:	CBC: Chemistry (including Mg^{2+})
Baseline procedures or tests:	N/A
Initiate IV:	0.9% sodium chloride
Premedicate:	5-HT$_3$ and dexamethasone 10–20 mg in 100 cc of NS
Administer:	

Cisplatin _____ mg (50 mg/m^2) IV over 1–2 hours on day 1

- Do not use aluminum needles, because precipitate will form.
- Available as a 1-mg/mL solution
- Further dilute in 250 cc or more of NS.

Doxorubicin _____ mg (40 mg/m^2) IV push on day 1

- Potent vesicant
- Available as a 2-mg/mL solution
- Doxorubicin will form a precipitate if it is mixed with heparin or 5-FU.

Vincristine _____ mg (0.6 mg/m^2) IV on day 3

- Vesicant
- Available in 1-, 2-, or 5-mg vials. Refrigerate until use.

Cyclophosphamide _____ mg (700 mg/m^2) IV over 1 hour on day 4

- Available in 100-, 200-, 500-, 1000-, or 2000- mg vials
- Dilute with sterile water. Shake well to ensure that all particles completely dissolve.
- Reconstituted solution is stable for 24 hours at room temperature, and 6 days if refrigerated.

Major Side Effects

- Bone Marrow Depression: Myelosuppression can be dose limiting.
- GI Toxicities: Moderate-to-severe nausea and vomiting. May be acute (first 24 hours) or delayed (>24 hours). Mucositis may occur. Constipation, abdominal pain, and paralytic ileus possible. Aggressive bowel protocol recommended.
- GU: Nephrotoxicity is dose related with cisplatin and presents at 10–20 days. Bladder toxicity in the form of hemorrhagic cystitis, dysuria, and increased urinary frequency. Risk may be reduced with adequate hydration.
- Electrolyte imbalance: Decreases in electrolytes expected.
- Cardiotoxicity: Acutely, pericarditis or myocarditis may occur. Later, cardiomyopathy in the form of CHF may occur.
- Neurotoxicity: Dose-limiting toxicity, usually in the form of peripheral sensory neuropathy. Paresthesias and numbness in a classic "stocking glove" pattern.
- Skin: Extravasation of doxorubicin or vincristine causes severe tissue damage. Hyperpigmentation, photosensitivity, and radiation recall occur. Alopecia.
- Reproductive: Pregnancy category D. Breast feeding should be avoided.

Initiate antiemetic protocol:	Moderately to highly emetogenic protocol.
Supportive drugs:	☐ pegfilgrastim (Neulasta) ☐ filgrastim (Neupogen)
	☐ epoetin alfa (Procrit) ☐ darbepoetin alfa (Aranesp)
Treatment schedule:	Chair time 3 hours on day 1, 1 hour on day 3, and 2 hours on day 4. Repeat cycle every 28 days.
Estimated number of visits:	Four visits per cycle. CBC day 10–14. Request three cycles worth of visits.

Dose Calculation by: 1. _____ 2. _____

_____

Physician

_____

Patient Name

_____

Diagnosis

_____

Date

_____

ID Number

_____/_____/_____
Ht   Wt   M^2

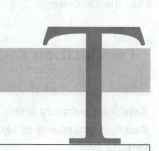

THYROID CANCER

Combination Regimen

Doxorubicin + Cisplatin 642

Doxorubicin: 60-mg/m^2 IV on day 1
Cisplatin: 40-mg/m^2 IV on day 1
Repeat cycle every 21 days.[1,409]

Single-Agent Regimen

Doxorubicin 643

Doxorubicin: 60-mg/m^2 IV on day 1
Repeat cycle every 21 days.[1, 409]

Combination Regimen

Doxorubicin + Cisplatin

Baseline laboratory tests: CBC: Chemistry (including Mg^{2+})

Baseline procedures or tests: MUGA scan

Initiate IV: 0.9% sodium chloride

Premedicate: 5-HT$_3$ and dexamethasone 20 mg in 100 cc of NS

Administer: **Doxorubicin** _____ mg (60 mg/m^2) IV push on day 1

- **Potent vesicant**
- Available as a 2-mg/mL solution.
- Doxorubicin will form a precipitate if it is mixed with heparin or 5-FU.

Cisplatin _____ mg (40 g/m^2) IV over 1–2 hours on day 1

- Do not use aluminum needles, because precipitate will form.
- Available in solution as 1 mg/mL.
- Further dilute solution with 250 cc or more of NS.

Major Side Effects

- Bone Marrow Depression: Leukopenia, thrombocytopenia, and anemia all occur; may be severe.
- GI Toxicities: Nausea and vomiting are moderate to severe and can be acute or delayed. Stomatitis occurs in 10% of patients but is not dose limiting.
- GU Toxicities: Red-orange discoloration of urine for up to 48 hours after doxorubicin.
- Cardiac: Acutely, pericarditis-myocarditis syndrome may occur. With high cumulative doses > 550 mg/m^2, cardiomyopathy may occur. Increased risk of cardiotoxicity when doxorubicin is given with trastuzumab (Herceptin) or mitomycin.
- Renal: Nephrotoxicity is dose related with cisplatin and presents at 10–20 days. Risk may be reduced with adequate hydration.
- Electrolyte Imbalance: Decreased Mg^{2+}, K, Ca^{2+}, Na^+, and P.
- Skin: Extravasation of doxorubicin causes severe tissue destruction. Hyperpigmentation, photosensitivity, and radiation recall occur. Complete alopecia occurs with doses > 50 mg/m^2.
- Neurotoxicity: Dose-limiting toxicity, usually in the form of peripheral sensory neuropathy. Paresthesias and numbness in a classic "stocking glove" pattern.
- Ototoxicity: High-frequency hearing loss and tinnitus with cisplatin.
- Reproductive: Pregnancy category D. Breast feeding should be avoided.

Initiate antiemetic protocol: Moderately to highly emetogenic protocol.

Supportive drugs:
☐ pegfilgrastim (Neulasta) ☐ filgrastim (Neupogen)
☐ epoetin alfa (Procrit) ☐ darbepoetin alfa (Aranesp)

Treatment schedule: Chair time 3 hours on day 1. Repeat cycle every 21 days.

Estimated number of visits: Two visits per cycle. CBC day 10–14. Request four cycles worth of visits.

Dose Calculation by: 1. _____ 2. _____

_____
Physician

_____
Patient Name

_____
Diagnosis

_____
Date

_____
ID Number

_____ / _____ / _____
Ht   Wt   M^2

Single-Agent Regimen

Doxorubicin

Baseline laboratory tests:	CBC: Chemistry
Baseline procedures or tests:	MUGA scan
Initiate IV:	0.9% sodium chloride
Premedicate:	5-HT$_3$ and dexamethasone 10–20 mg in 100 cc of NS
Administer:	**Doxorubicin** _____ mg (60 mg/m^2) IV on day 1

- **Potent vesicant**
- Available as a 2-mg/mL solution.
- Doxorubicin will form a precipitate if it is mixed with heparin or 5-FU.

Major Side Effects

- Bone Marrow Depression: WBC and platelet nadir 10–14 days after drug dose, with recovery from days 15–21. Myelosuppression may be severe but is less severe with weekly dosing.
- GI Toxicities: Nausea and vomiting are moderate to severe and occur in 44% of patients. Stomatitis occurs in 10% of patients but is not dose limiting.
- GU Toxicities: Red-orange discoloration of urine for up to 48 hours after doxorubicin.
- Cardiac: Acutely, pericarditis-myocarditis syndrome may occur. With high cumulative doses > 550 mg/m^2, cardiomyopathy may occur. Increased risk of cardiotoxicity when doxorubicin is given with trastuzumab (Herceptin) or mitomycin.
- Skin: Extravasation of doxorubicin causes severe tissue destruction. Hyperpigmentation, photosensitivity, and radiation recall occur. Complete alopecia occurs with doses > 50 mg/m^2.
- Reproductive: Pregnancy category D. Breast feeding should be avoided.

Initiate antiemetic protocol:	Moderately to highly emetogenic protocol.
Supportive drugs:	☐ pegfilgrastim (Neulasta) ☐ filgrastim (Neupogen)
	☐ epoetin alfa (Procrit) ☐ darbepoetin alfa (Aranesp)
Treatment schedule:	Chair time 1 hour on day 1. Repeat cycle every 21 days.
Estimated number of visits:	Two visits per cycle. CBC day 10–14. Request four cycles worth of visits.

Dose Calculation by: 1. _____ 2. _____

_____ _____

Physician   Date

_____ _____

Patient Name   ID Number

_____ _____/_____/_____

Diagnosis   Ht   Wt   M^2

Appendix A

Billing and Reimbursment

Risë Marie Cleland

Introduction

Oncology nurses have a clear understanding of their vital role in patient care. It is increasingly important that nurses help the practice to capture charges for the services they provide and to ensure that those services are being reported with the proper billing codes. The ever-changing rules and regulations make billing for cancer services especially challenging. Nurses who have an understanding of billing for these services bring additional value to their practice.

The following information is from *Oplinc's Best Practices Review* newsletter. This newsletter focuses on issues relevant to cancer centers and their mission to provide and protect patient access to quality cancer care. *Oplinc's Best Practices Review* is published by Risë Marie Cleland and Oplinc and is supported by an unrestricted educational grant provided by Genentech.

Nurses and other oncology professionals can sign up for this complimentary bi-monthly newsletter at http://oplinc.com.gravitatehosting.com/newsletter.asp.

The billing examples, using actual chemotherapy protocols, illustrate the key coding and billing rules and regulations for cancer services in 2006.

New 2006 Drug Administration Codes

The new 2006 CPT® (Current Procedural Terminology) codes for drug administration have replaced the 18 temporary G-codes that were in use for Medicare in 2005. The American Medical Association (AMA) has developed a total of two new codes for hydration infusion, nine new codes for therapeutic, prophylactic, and diagnostic injections and infusions, and 11 new codes for chemotherapy services including injections and infusions.

The descriptions for the drug administration codes previously reported to Medicare with the temporary G-codes have largely been kept intact allowing for a rather straightforward crosswalk from the temporary G-codes to the new CPT codes.

The CPT code set has been designated as the national coding standard for healthcare professional services and procedures under the Health Insurance Portability and Accountability Act (HIPAA). HIPAA mandates that all electronic transactions include only HIPAA compliant codes. Therefore healthcare providers, health plans, and other covered entities conducting financial or administrative healthcare transactions electronically must use the CPT code set.

In order to review the billing rules, we have included two sample protocols and the coding rules that apply to them. *Note: Please be aware that these examples are included for educational purposes only. Always consult your Medicare carrier and the CMS website for specific coding guidance.*

2006 CPT Coding Exercises
Sample Protocol

Drug	Dose	Start	Stop	Route
Calcium Gluconate	1 GM	09:35	10:40	IV
Magnesium	1 GM	09:35	10:40	IV (same bag as calcium gluconate)
Zofran	32 mg	10:40	11:00	IV
Decadron	10 mg	10:40	11:00	IV (same bag as Zofran)
Oxaliplatin	200 mg	11:00	13:00	IV
Leucovorin	1040 mg	11:00	13:00	IV (separate bag)
5-FU	832 mg	13:03	13:05	IV Push
5-FU	4992 mg	13:05		Ambulatory Pump

Assign the codes

Drug   Calcium Gluconate

Administration Code: 90761—Hydration each additional hour

Rule
1. Electrolytes whether pre-packaged or added to fluids are billed under hydration codes;
2. Ea. additional hour code is used because hydration is a *secondary service* in this patient encounter, the "initial" code will be used for the *primary service* chemotherapy.

Drug   Magnesium

Administration Code: Ø

Rule
1. No separate administration code because the magnesium was in the same bag as the calcium gluconate. To report the concurrent infusion code the drugs must be in separate bags.

Drug   Zofran

Administration Code: 90767—Additional sequential infusion, therapeutic
Diagnostic

Rule   Infusion time was greater than 15 minutes and drug was administered sequential to the other drugs.

Drug   Decadron

Administration Code: Ø

Rule
1. No separate administration code as this drug was in the same bag as the Zofran.

Drug   Oxaliplatin

Administration Code: 96413—chemo admin. IV single or initial
96415—each additional hour

Rule
1. Use the initial code as chemotherapy is the *primary service* for this encounter;
2. Bill one unit of **96415** for the 2nd hour of infusion.

Drug   Leucovorin

Administration Code: 90768—concurrent infusion

Rule
1. Concurrent code is used because leucovorin was administered at the same time as the oxaliplatin in a separate bag. *Note: If your carrier has instructed you to bill the leucovorin with the chemotherapy administration codes you will not be able to bill for this administration as there is no concurrent code for chemotherapy.*
2. There is no 2nd hour billed for the leucovorin as the concurrent code is only reportable once per patient per encounter.

Drug   5-FU

Administration Code: 96411—chemo IV push, ea additional substance/drug

Rule
1. Use each additional IV push code as the initial code was used with oxaliplatin; only 1 initial code is to be billed per patient per encounter.

Drug	5-FU
Administration Code:	96416—initiation of prolonged chemotherapy infusion
Rule	When a drug is administered by different administration techniques bill for each method of administration (as long as it meets medical necessity).

Sample Protocol

Drug	Dose	Start	Stop	Route
Normal Saline	1 liter	08:45	10:35	IV
Aloxi	0.25	10:35	10:45	IV
Decadron	10 mg	10:35	10:45	IV (same bag as Aloxi)
VP-16	203 mg	10:45	11:55	IV
Cisplatin	41 mg	11:55	12:55	IV
Bleomycin	30 units	12:55	13:05	IV push

Assign the codes

Drug	Normal Saline
Administration Code:	90761 × 2—hydration each additional hour
Rule	1. Hydration administered sequentially to chemo is separately billable (when medically necessary). In this encounter hydration is a *secondary service* so you would not use the initial code;
	2. NS dripped for 1 hr. 50 minutes, additional infusion time past 1st hour was greater than 30 minutes so it is reported with a 2nd unit of the additional hour code.

Drug	Aloxi
Administration Code:	90775—each additional sequential IV push
Rule	1. Infusions lasting 15 minutes or less are to be billed with the IV push codes, Aloxi dripped for 10 minutes;
	2. This is a *secondary service* in this encounter so you would not use the initial code.

Drug	Decadron
Administration Code:	Ø
Rule	1. No separate administration code as this drug was in the same bag as the Aloxi.

Drug	VP-16
Administration Code:	96413—Chemotherapy administration, IV up to 1 hr. single or initial substance/drug
Rule	1. Use the initial code as chemotherapy is the *primary service* for this encounter;
	2. The infusion ran ten minutes past the 1st hour, you would not bill for an additional hour until 31 minutes past the 1st hour.

Drug	Cisplatin
Administration Code:	96417—each additional sequential infusion up to 1 hour, chemo
Rule	1. The drug was dripped sequentially to the other drugs; the initial code was already reported with VP-16.

Drug	Bleomycin
Administration Code:	96411—chemo IV push, each additional substance/drug
Rule	1. The initial code was already reported with VP-16.

KEY MEDICARE BILLING RULES FOR 2006

The list below summarizes some of the key billing rules in 2006 but is not a complete listing. For additional Medicare guidance, access the physician page on the Medicare website at www.cms.hhs.gov.

- If used to facilitate the infusion or injection, the following procedures/services are not to be billed separately:

  —Use of local anesthesia

  —IV start: 36000 *Introduction of needle or intracatheter, vein* or 36410 *Venipuncture, age 3 years or older, necessitating physician's skill (separate procedure), for diagnostic or therapeutic purposes (not to be used for routine venipuncture)*

  —Access to indwelling IV, subcutaneous catheter or port

  —Flush before or after infusion (96523)

  —Standard tubing, syringes and supplies

- A port flush (96523) is only payable when no other service payable from the Medicare Physician Fee Schedule (MPFS) is billed on the same day by the same provider

- 96522 *Refilling and maintenance of an implantable pump or reservoir for systemic drug delivery* is to be used for pumps or reservoirs that are capable of programmed release of a drug at a prescribed rate and is not to be used for accessing or flushing a port

- 36540 *Collection of blood specimen from a completely implantable venous* access device is a bundled code and not separately payable

- Fluid administered with the sole purpose of maintaining patency of the access device is not separately billable

- Medically necessary hydration administration (for dehydration or to prevent nephrotoxicity) is separately payable when administered sequentially to chemotherapy or blood transfusion, append modifier -59 on the hydration administration code

- When a separately identifiable E&M visit is performed on the same day as hydration or drug administration append the modifier -25 on the E&M code

- 96545 (provision of chemotherapy) has been deleted

- Infusions of 15 minutes or less are to be billed with the appropriate push codes

- Only 1 initial code is to be billed (unless protocol requires two separate IV sites be used)

- Bill only 1 concurrent code per encounter

- When a bone marrow biopsy and aspiration are performed on the same site through the same skin incision on the same date of service report 38221 *Bone marrow biopsy* and G0364 *Bone marrow aspiration performed with bone marrow biopsy through the same incision on the same date of service*. CMS defines a separate site as different bones or two separate skin incisions over the same bone

- Report additional hours of infusion (90761, 90766, and 96415) for infusions lasting greater than 30 minutes beyond the initial hour

FREQUENTLY ASKED BILLING QUESTIONS

Q. We have been coding the bone marrow biopsy and aspiration as 38220-59 and 38221-50. Is this correct?

A. Modifier -50 is appended to the bone marrow biopsy code 38221 to report bilateral bone marrow biopsies. The modifier -59 is used to report that the bone marrow biopsy and aspiration were performed through separate incisions.

For Medicare patients, as of January 1, 2005 if the bone marrow biopsy and aspiration are performed through the same incision you should be billing G0364 (bone marrow aspiration performed on the same date through the same incision as a bone marrow biopsy) with the bone marrow biopsy code, 38221.

If the biopsy and aspiration are performed through different incisions or different patient encounters on the same day, then Medicare will make separate payments for each procedure. In this case, you would report both the bone marrow aspiration (38220) and bone marrow biopsy (38221) codes and append the modifier -59. It must be medically necessary to perform the procedures through two separate incisions.

Q. Is it necessary to restage the patient each time we bill for the 2006 Oncology Demonstration Project?

A. No. In the MedLearn Matters document: MM4219 2006 Oncology Demonstration Project CMS states: *"Disease status should be based on the best available data at the time of the visit, unless otherwise specified. No additional diagnostic tests or evaluations should be performed for the purposes of further determining disease status for the purposes of this Demonstration Project."*

Q. Where can I find information on billing for concurrent infusions? In particular, I am looking for guidance on drugs infused in one bag.

A. The AMA publication, CPT Changes 2006 An Insider's View states on page 253, *"An infusion consisting of three substances in a single bag is not intended to be reported as three separate infusion services, because the parenteral administration codes are intended to report the separate work of administration and IV access and not the inclusion of multiple agents in a bag prepared prior to infusion."* ASCO also addresses this in their FAQs for 2006 Drug Administration.

Q. When giving an injection and port flush on the same day, can you bill the port flush (96523)?

A. No. According to the American Medical Association CPT, a port flush 96523 is not separately billable when a drug infusion or injection is provided on the same day. For Medicare patients the port flush is only billable when no other Medicare Physician Fee Schedule service is provided.

Risë Marie Cleland holds degrees in Human Ecology and Business Management, with a concentration in the effectual aspects of business on society. Ms. Cleland was the Business Director for a cancer research and treatment center before founding Oplinc in June of 1999. Oplinc is a national organization of oncology professionals. Through Oplinc Ms. Cleland publishes the weekly *Oplinc Fax Tracts* focusing on the timely dissemination of information pertaining to billing, reimbursement and practice management in the oncology office. She also publishes *Oplinc's Best Practices Review* which provides a more in-depth look at the issues and challenges facing oncology practices.

Ms. Cleland is a nationally recognized speaker and author providing educational programs for state societies, the Oncology Nursing Society (ONS), the Medical Group Management Association's Administrators of Oncology Hematology Assembly, and through national oncology publications including the Association of Community Cancer Centers *Oncology Issues and Hematology Oncology News and Issues*. Ms. Cleland also works as a consultant and advisor for physician practices, pharmaceutical companies, and distributors.

She is the past president of the Medical Group Management Association's Administrators of Oncology Hematology Assembly, Executive Director of the Washington State Medical Oncology Society, and President of the Society of Administrators in Medical Oncology of the Northwest.

REFERENCES

1. Wilkes GM, Barton-Burke M. *Oncology Nursing Drug Handbook 2006.* Sudbury, MA: Jones and Barlett Publishers; 2006.
2. Nigro ND, Seydel HG, Considine B, Vaitkevicius VK, Leichmanl, Kinzie JJ. Combined preoperative radiation and chemotherapy for squamous cell carcinoma of the anal canal. *Cancer.* 1983;51:1826–1829.
3. Bartelink H, Roelofsen F, Eschwege F, et al. Concomitant radiotherapy and chemotherapy is superior to radiotherapy alone in the treatment of locally advanced anal cancer: results of a phase III randomized trial of the European Organization for Research and Treatment of Cancer Radiotherapy and Gastrointestinal Cooperative Groups. *J Clin Oncol.* 1997;15:2040–2049.
4. Hung A, Crane C, Delclos M, et al. Cisplatin-based combined modality therapy for anal carcinoma: a wider therapeutic index. *Cancer.* 2003;97:1195–1202.
5. Flam MS, et al. Role of mitomycin in combination with fluorouracil and radiotherapy, and of salvage chemoradiation in the definitive nonsurgical treatment of epidermoid carcinoma of the anal canal: results of a phase III randomized intergroup study. *J Clin Oncol.* 1996;16:227–253.
6. Thongprasert S, Napapan S, Charoentum C, Moonprakan S. Phase II study of gemcitabine and cisplatin as first line chemotherapy in inoperable biliary tract carcinoma. *Ann Oncol.* 2005;16:279–281.
7. Knox JJ, Hedley D, Oza A, et al. Combining gemcitabine and capecitabine in patients with advanced biliary cancer: a phase II trial. *J Clin Oncol.* 2005; 23:2332–2338.
8. Bajorin DF, McCaffrey JA, Dodd PM, et al. Ifosfamide, paclitaxel, and cisplatin for patients with advanced carcinoma of the urothelial tract: final report of a phase II trial evaluating 2 dosing schedules. *Cancer.* 2000; 88:1671–1678.
9. Kaufman D, et al. Phase II trial of gemcitabine plus cisplatin in patients with metastatic urothelial cancer. *J Clin Oncol.* 2000;18:1921–1927.
10. Sternberg CN, et al. Methotrexate, vinblastine, doxorubicin, and cisplatin for advanced transitional cell carcinoma of the urothelium. Efficacy and patterns of response and relapse. *Cancer.* 1989;64:2448–2458.
11. Harker WG, Meyers FJ, Freisha FS, et al. Cisplatin, methotrexate, and vinblastine (CMV): an effective chemotherapy regimen for metastatic transitional cell carcinoma of the urinary tract. A Northern California Oncology Group study. *J Clin Oncol.* 1985;3:1463–1470.
12. Logothetis CJ, et al. A prospective randomized trial comparing MVAC and CISCA chemotherapy for patients with metastatic urothelial tumors. *J Clin Oncol.* 1990;8:1050–1055.
13. Vaughn D, Manola J, Dreicer R, et al. Phase II study of paclitaxel plus carboplatin in patients with advanced carcinoma of the urothelium and renal dysfunction (E2896). *Cancer.* 2002;95:1022–1027.
14. Campbell M, Baker LH, Opipari M, al-Sarraf M. Phase II trial with cisplatin, doxorubicin, and cyclophosphamide (CAP) in the treatment of urothelial transitional cell carcinoma. *Cancer Treat Rep.* 1981; 65:897–899.
15. Kachnic LA, et al. Bladder preservation by combined modality therapy for invasive bladder cancer. *J Clin Oncol.* 1997;15:1022–1029.
16. Moore MJ, et al. Gemcitabine: a promising new agent in the treatment of advanced urothelial cancer. *J Clin Oncol.* 1997;15:3441–3445.
17. Roth BJ, et al. Significant activity of paclitaxel in advanced transitional-cell carcinoma of the urothelium: a phase II trial of the Eastern Cooperative Oncology Group. *J Clin Oncol.* 1994;12:2264–2270.
18. Vaughn D, et al. Phase II trial of weekly paclitaxel in patients with previously treated advanced urothelial cancer. *J Clin Oncol.* 2002;20:937–940.
19. Chu E, DeVita VT. *Physicians Cancer Chemotherapy Drug Manual 2004.* Sudbury, MA: Jones and Bartlett Publishers; 2004.
20. Wilkes G, Barton-Burke M. *Oncology Nursing Drug Handbook 2005.* Sudbury, MA: Jones and Bartlett Publishers; 2005, 94–99, 137–140, 222–226, 310–313.
21. Zometa full prescribing information. Novartis Pharmaceuticals Corporation, 2002.
22. Saad F, Gleason DM, Murray R, et al. Long-term efficacy of zoledronic acid for the prevention of skeletal complications in patients with metastatic hormonerefractory prostate cancer. *J Natl Cancer Inst.* 2004; 96(11):879–882.
23. Rosen LS, Gordon D, Kaminski M, et al. Zoledronic acid versus pamidronate in the treatment of skeletal metastases in patients with breast cancer or osteolytic lesions of multiple myeloma: a phase III, double-blind, comparative trial. *Cancer J.* 2001;7(5):377–387.
24. Kohno N, Aogi K, Minabi H, et al. Zoledronic acid significantly reduces skeletal complications compared with placebo in Japanese women with bone metastases from breast cancer: a randomized, placebocontrolled trial. *J Clin Oncol.* 2005; 23:1–8.
25. Rosen LS, Gordon D, Tchekmedyian S, et al. Zoledronic acid versus placebo in the treatment of skeletal metastases in patients with lung cancer and other solid tumors: a phase III, double-blind, randomized trial—the Zoledronic Acid Lung Cancer and Other Solid Tumors Study Group. *J Clin Oncol.* 2003; 21: 3150–3157.
26. Pamidronate full prescribing information. Novartis Pharmaceuticals Corporation, 2005.
27. Stupp R, et al. Radiotherapy plus concomitant and adjuvant temozolomide for glioblastoma. *N Engl J Med.* 2005;352:987–995.

28. Levin VA, Silver P, Hannigan J, et al. Superiority of post-radiotherapy adjuvant chemotherapy with CCNU, procarbazine, and vincristine (PCV) over BCNU for anaplastic gliomas: NCOG 6G61 final report. *Int J RadiatOncol Biol Phys.* 1990;18:321–324.

29. DeAngelis LM, et al. Malignant gliomas: who benefits from adjuvant chemotherapy? *Ann Neurol.* 1998; 44:691–695.

30. Buckner JC, et al. Phase II trial of procarbazine, lomustine, and vincristine as initial therapy for patients with low-grade oligodendroglioma or oligoastrocytoma: efficacy and associations with chromosomal abnormalities. *J Clin Oncol.* 2003;21:251–255.

31. Yung A, et al. Randomized trial of temodal (TEM) vs. Procarbazine (PCB) in glioblastoma multiforme (GBM) at first relapse. *Proc Am Soc Clin Oncol.* 1999; 18:139a.

32. Yung A, et al. Multicenter phase II trial of temozolomide in patients with anaplastic astrocytoma or anaplastic oligoastrocytoma at first relapse. *J Clin Oncol.* 1999;17:2762–2771.

33. Raymond E, et al. Multicenter phase II study and pharmacokinetic analysis of irinotecan in chemotherapy-naïve patients with glioblastoma. *Ann Oncol.* 2003;14: 603–614.

34. Friedman H, et al. Irinotecan therapy in adults with recurrent or progressive malignant glioma. *J Clin Oncol.* 1999;17:1516–1525.

35. Bear H, Anderson, S, Brown A, et al. The effect on tumor response of adding sequential preoperative docetaxel to preoperative doxorubicin and cyclophosphamide: preliminary results from National Surgical Adjuvant Breast and Bowel Project B-27. *J Clin Oncol.* 2003;21:4165-4174.

36. Fisher B, et al. Two months of doxorubicin-cyclophosphamide with and without interval reinduction therapy compared with 6 months of cyclophosphamide, methotrexate, and fluorouracil in positivenode breast cancer patients with tamoxifen-nonresponsive tumors: results from the National Surgical Adjuvant Breast and Bowel Project B-15. *J Clin Oncol.* 2000;8:1483–1496.

37. Hudis C, et al. Sequential dose-dense doxorubicin, paclitaxel, and cyclophosphamide for resectable high-risk breast cancer: feasibility and efficacy. *J Clin Oncol.* 1999;17:93–100.

38. Romond E, et al. Doxorubicin and cyclophosphamide followed by paclitaxel with or without trastuzumab as adjuvant therapy for patients with HER-2 positive operable breast cancer: combined analysis of NSABP-B31/NCCTG-N9381. http://www.asco.org/ac/1.1003, fl12-002511-00fl18-0034-00fl19-005816-00fl21-001,00 (accessed July 2005).

39. Citron M, Berry DA, Cirrincine C, et al. Randomized trial of dose-dense versus conventionally scheduled and sequential versus concurrent combination chemotherapy as postoperative adjuvant treatment of node-positive primary breast cancer: first report of intergroup trial C9741/Cancer and Leukemia Group B trial 9741. *J Clin Oncol.* 2003;21:1431–1439.

40. Martin M, Villar A, Sole-Calvo A, et al. Doxorubicin in combination with fluorouracil and cyclophosphamide (i.v. FAC regimen, day 1, 21) versus methotrexate in combination with fluorouracil and cyclophosphamide (i.v. CMF regimen, day 1, 21) as adjuvant chemotherapy for operable breast cancer: a study by the GEICAM group. *Ann Oncol.* 2003; 14:833–842.

41. Aisner J, et al. Chemotherapy versus chemoimmunotherapy (CAF v CAFVP v CMF each +/- MER) for metastatic carcinoma of the breast: a CALGB study. Cancer and Leukemia Group B. *J Clin Oncol.* 1987;5: 1523–1533.

42. Bonadonna G, et al. Combination chemotherapy as an adjuvant treatment in operable breast cancer. *N Engl J Med.* 1976;294:405–410.

43. Weiss RB, et al. Adjuvant chemotherapy after conservative surgery plus irradiation versus modified radical mastectomy. Analysis of drug dosing and toxicity. *Am J Med.* 1987;83:455–463.

44. Bonadonna G, Zambetti M, Valagussa P. Sequential or alternating doxorubicin and CMF regimens in breast cancer with more than three positive nodes. Ten-year results. *JAMA.* 1995;273:542–543.

45. Coombes RC, et al. Adjuvant cyclophosphamide, methotrexate, and fluorouracil versus fluorouracil, epirubicin, and cyclophosphamide chemotherapy in premenopausal women with axillary nodepositive operable breast cancer: results of a randomized trial. *J Clin Oncol.* 1996;14:35–45.

46. Marschke RF, et al. Randomized clinical trial of CFP versus CMFP in women with metastatic breast cancer. *Cancer.* 1989;63:1931–1937.

47. Fisher B, Dignam J, Wolmark N, et al. Tamoxifen and chemotherapy for lymph node-negative, estrogen receptor-positive breast cancer. *J Natl Cancer Inst.* 1997;89:1673–1682.

48. Howell A, et al. Results of the ATAC (Arimidex, Tamoxifen Alone or in Combination) trial after completion of 5-years' adjuvant treatment for breast cancer. *Lancet.* 2005;365:60–62.

49. Goss PE, et al. Randomized trial of letrozole following tamoxifen as extended adjuvant therapy in receptor positive breast cancer: updated findings from NCIC CTG MA.17. *J Natl Cancer Inst.* 2005; 97:1262–1271.

50. Coombes RC, et al. A randomized trial of exemestane after two to three years of tamoxifen therapy in postmenopausal women with primary breast cancer. *N Engl J Med.* 2004;350:1081–1092.

51. Sledge GE, et al. Phase III trial of doxorubicin, paclitaxel, and the combination of doxorubicin and paclitaxel as front-line chemotherapy for metastatic breast cancer: an intergroup trial (E1193). *J Clin Oncol.* 2003;21:588–592.

52. Levine MN, Bramwell VH, Pritchard KI, et al. Randomized trial of intensive cyclophosphamide, epirubicin, and fluorouracil chemotherapy compared with cyclophosphamide, methotrexate, and fluorouracil in premenopausal women with node-positive breast cancer. National Cancer Institute of Canada Clinical Trials Group. *J Clin Oncol.* 1998;16:2651–2658.

53. O'Shaughnessy J, et al. Superior survival with capecitabine plus docetaxel combination therapy in anthracycline-pretreated patients with advanced breast cancer: phase III trial results. *J Clin Oncol.* 2002;20:2812–2123.

54. Biganzoli L, et al. Moving forward with capecitabine: a glimpse of the future. *Oncologist.* 2002;7(Suppl 6): 29–35.

55. Dieras V. Review of docetaxel/doxorubicin combination in metastatic breast cancer. *Oncology.* 1997; 11:31–33.

56. Brufman G, Colajori E, Ghilezan N, et al. Doubling epirubicin dose intensity (100 mg/m² versus 50 mg/m²) in the FEC regimen significantly increases response rates. An international randomized phase III in metastatic breast cancer. The Epirubicin High Dose (HEPI 010) Study Group. *Ann Oncol.* 1997;8:155–162.

57. Acuna LR, et al. Vinorelbine and paclitaxel as first-line chemotherapy in metastatic breast cancer. *J Clin Oncol.* 1999;17:74–81.

58. Spielman M, et al. Phase II trial of vinorelbine/doxorubicin as first-line therapy of advanced breast cancer. *J Clin Oncol.* 1994;12:1764–1770.

59. Slamon DJ, Leyland-Jones B, Shak S, et al. Use of chemotherapy plus a monoclonal antibody against HER2 for metastatic breast cancer that overexpresses HER2. *N Engl J Med.* 2001;344:783–792.

60. Goldenberg MM, et al. Trastuzumab, a recombinant DNA-derived humanized monoclonal antibody, a novel agent for the treatment of metastatic breast cancer. *Clin Ther.* 1999;21:309–318.

61. Francisco E, et al. Phase II study of weekly docetaxel and trastuzumab for patients with HER-2 overexpressing metastatic breast cancer. *J Clin Oncol.* 2002;20: 1800–1808.

62. O'Shaughnessy J, et al. Gemcitabine plus paclitaxel (GT) versus paclitaxel (T) as first-line treatment for anthracycline pre-treated metastatic breast cancer (MBC): interim results of a global phase III study. *Proc Am Soc Clin Oncol.* 2003;22:7(abstract 25).

63. Perez EA, et al. A phase II study of paclitaxel plus carboplatin as first-line chemotherapy for women with metastatic breast carcinoma. *Cancer.* 2000;88:124–131.

64. Fitch V, et al. N9332: phase II cooperative group trial of docetaxel (D) and carboplatin (CBCDA) as first-line chemotherapy for metastatic breast cancer (MBC). *Proc Am Soc Clin Oncol.* 2003;22:23(abstract 90).

65. Garewal HS, et al. Treatment of advanced breast cancer with mitomycin C combined with vinblastine or vindesine. *J Clin Oncol.* 1983;1:772–775.

66. Jaiyesimi IA, et al. Use of tamoxifen for breast cancer: twenty-eight years later. *J Clin Oncol.* 1995;13: 513–529.

67. Hayes DF, Van Zyl JA, Hacking A, et al. Randomized comparison of tamoxifen and two separate doses of toremifene in postmenopausal patients with metastatic breast cancer. *J Clin Oncol.* 1995;13:2556–2566.

68. Lonning PE, et al. Activity of exemestane in metastatic breast cancer after failure of nonsteroidal aromatase inhibitors, a phase I trial. *J Clin Oncol.* 2000;18: 2234–2244.

69. Buzdar A, et al. Anastrozole, a potent and selective aromatase inhibitor, versus megestrol acetate in postmenopausal women with advanced breast cancer: results of overview analysis of two phase II trials. Arimidex Study Group. *J Clin Oncol.* 1996;14: 2000–2011.

70. Dombernowsky P, et al. Letrozole, a new oral aromatase inhibitor for advanced breast cancer: double-blind randomized trial showing a dose effect and improved efficacy and tolerability compared with megestrol acetate. *J Clin Oncol.* 1998;16:453–461.

71. Howell A. Future use of selective estrogen receptor modulators and aromatase inhibitors. *Clin Cancer Res.* 2001;7(Suppl 12):4402s–4410s.

72. Kimmick GG, Muss HB. Endocrine therapy in breast cancer. *Cancer Treat Res.* 1998;94:231–254.

73. Baselga J, et al. Phase II study of weekly intravenous trastuzumab (Herceptin) in patients with HER2/neu-overexpressing metastatic breast cancer. *Semin Oncol.* 1999;26(Suppl 12):78–83.

73a. Baselga J, Carbonell X, Castaneda-Soto NJ, et al. Phase II study of efficacy, safety, and pharmacokinetics of trastuzumab monotherapy administered on a 3-weekly schedule. *J Clin Oncol* 2005;23:2162–2171.

74. Blum JL, et al. Multicenter phase II study of capecitabine in paclitaxel-refractory metastatic breast cancer. *J Clin Oncol.* 1999;17:485–493.

75. Chan S. Docetaxel vs doxorubicin in metastatic breast cancer resistant to alkylating chemotherapy. *Oncology.* 1997;11(Suppl 8):19–24.

76. Baselga J, Tabernero JM. Weekly docetaxel in breast cancer: applying clinical data to patient therapy. *Oncologist.* 2001;6(Suppl 3):26–29.

77. Holmes FA, et al. Phase II trial of taxol, an active drug in the treatment of metastatic breast cancer. *J Natl Cancer Inst.* 1991;83:1797–1805.

78. Perez EA. Paclitaxel in breast cancer. *Oncologist.* 1998;3:373–389.

79. Fumoleau P, Delozier T, Extra JM, Canobbio L, Delgado FM, Hurteloup P. Vinorelbine (Navelbine) in the treatment of breast cancer: the European experience. *Semin Oncol.* 1995;22(Suppl 5):22–28.

80. Torti FM, et al. Reduced cardiotoxicity of doxorubicin delivered on a weekly schedule. Assessment by endomyocardial biopsy. *Ann Intern Med.* 1983;99:745–749.

81. Carmichael J, et al. Phase II activity of gemcitabine in advanced breast cancer. *Semin Oncol.* 1996;23 (Suppl 10):77–81.

82. Ranson MR, et al. Treatment of advanced breast cancer with sterically stabilized liposomal doxorubicin: results of a multicenter phase II trial. *J Clin Oncol.* 1997;15:3185–3191.

83. O'Shaughnessy J, et al. ABI-007 (ABRAXANE), a nanoparticle albumin-bound (nab) paclitaxel demonstrates superior efficacy vs Taxol in MBC: a phase III trial. *Breast Cancer Res Treat.* 2003;82:(Suppl 1) (abstract 43).

84. O'Shaughnessy JA, et al. Weekly nanoparticle albumin paclitaxel (Abraxane) results in long-term disease control in patients with taxane-refractory metastatic breast cancer. *Breast Cancer Res Treat.* 2004;88:(Suppl 1):S65(abstract 1070).

85. Hainsworth JD, et al. Carcinoma of unknown primary site: treatment with 1-hour paclitaxel, carboplatin, and extended-schedule etoposide. *J Clin Oncol.* 1997; 15:2385–2393.

86. Longeval E, Klastersky J. Combination chemotherapy with cisplatin and etoposide in bronchogenic squamous cell carcinoma and adenocarcinoma. A study by the EORTC lung cancer working party. *Cancer.* 1982;50:2751–2756.

87. Hainsworth JD, Johnson DH, Greco FA. Cisplatin-based combination chemotherapy in the treatment of poorly differentiated carcinoma and poorly differentiated adenocarcinoma of unknown primary site:

results of a 12-year experience. *J Clin Oncol.* 1992; 10:912–922.

88. Greco FA, et al. Gemcitabine, carboplatin, and paclitaxel for patients with carcinoma of unknown primary site: a Minnie Pearl Cancer Research network study. *J Clin Oncol.* 2002;20:1651–1656.

89. Moertel CG, et al. Streptozocin-doxorubicin, streptozocin-fluorouracil, or hlorozotocin in the treatment of advanced islet-cell carcinoma. *N Engl J Med.* 1992;326:519–526.

90. Moertel CG, et al. Treatment of neuroendocrine carcinomas with combined etoposide and cisplatin. *Cancer.* 1991;68:227–232.

91. Saltz L, Trochanowski B, Buckley M, et al. Octreotide as an antineoplastic agent in the treatment of functional and nonfunctional neuroendocrine tumors. *Cancer.* 1993;72:244.

92. Sandostatin LAR full prescribing information. Novartis Pharmaceuticals Corportation, February 2005.

93. Rubin J, Alani J, Schrimer W, et al. Octreotide acetate long-acting formulation versus open-label subcutaneous octreotide acetate in malignant carcinoid syndrome. *J Clin Oncol.* 1999;17:660-606.

94. Rose PG, et al. Concurrent cisplatin-based radiotherapy and chemotherapy for locally advanced cervical cancer. *N Engl J Med.* 1995;15:1144.

95. Fiorica J, Holloway R, Ndubisi B, et al. Phase II trial of topotecan and cisplatin in persistent or recurrent squamous and nonsquamous carcinoma of the cervix. *Gynecol Oncol.* 2002;85:89–94.

96. Buxton EJ, et al. Combination bleomycin, ifosfamide, and cisplatin chemotherapy in cervical cancer. *J Natl Cancer Inst.* 1989;81:359–361.

97. Murad AM, Triginelli SA, Ribalta JC. Phase II trial of bleomycin, ifosfamide, and carboplatin in metastastic cervical cancer. *J Clin Oncol.* 1994;12:55–59.

98. Whitney CW, et al. Randomized comparison of fluorouracil plus cisplatin versus hydroxyurea as an adjunct to radiation therapy in stage IIB-IVA carcinoma of the cervix with negative para-aortic lymph nodes: a Gynecologic Oncology Group and Southwest Oncology Group study. *J Clin Oncol.* 1999;17:1339–1348.

99. Pignata S, Silvestro G, Ferrari E, et al. Phase II study of cisplatin and vinorelbine as firstline chemotherapy in patients with carcinoma of the uterine cervix. *J Clin Oncol.* 1999;17:756–760.

100. Chitapanarux I, et al. Phase II clinical study of irinotecan and cisplatin as first-line chemotherapy in metastatic or recurrent cervical cancer. *Gynecol Oncol.* 2003;89:402–407.

101. Vogl SE, Moukhtar M, Calon A, et al. Chemotherapy for advanced cervical cancer with bleomycin, vincristine, mitomycin-C, and cisplatinum (BOMP). *Cancer Treat Rep.* 1980;64:1005–1007.

102. Alberts DS, Garcia DJ. Salvage chemotherapy in recurrent or refractory squamous cell cancer of the uterine cervix. *Semin Oncol.* 1994;21(Suppl 7):37–46.

103. Levy T, et al. Advanced squamous cell cancer (SCC) of the cervix: a phase II study of docetaxel (taxotere) 100 mg/m^2 intravenously (IV) over 1 h every 21 days: a preliminary report. *Proc Am Soc Clin Oncol.* 1996;15:292a.

104. Thigpen T, et al. The role of paclitaxel in the management of patients with carcinoma of the cervix. *Semin Oncol.* 1997;24(Suppl 2):41–46.

105. Verschraegen CF, et al. Phase II study of irinotecan in prior chemotherapy-treated squamous cell carcinoma of the cervix. *J ClinOncol.* 1997;15:625–631.

106. Lacava JA, et al. Vinorelbine as neoadjuvant chemotherapy in advanced cervical carcinoma. *J Clin Oncol.* 1997;15:604–609.

107. Muderspach LI, et al. A phase II study of topotecan in patients with squamous cell carcinoma of the cervix: a Gynecologic Oncology Group study. *Gynecol Oncol.* 2001;81:213–215.

108. Sauer R, Becker H, Hohenberger W, et al. Preoperative versus postoperative chemoradiotherapy for rectal cancer. *N Engl J Med.* 2004;351:1731–1740.

109. Minsky BD. Combined modality therapy of rectal cancer with oxaliplatin-based regimens. *Clin Colorectal Cancer.* 2004;4(Suppl 1):S29–36.

110. O'Connell MJ, et al. Controlled trial of fluorouracil and low-dose leucovorin given for 6 months as postoperative adjuvant therapy for colon cancer. *J Clin Oncol.* 1997;15:246–250.

111. Wolmark N, et al. The benefit of leucovorin-modulated fluorouracil as postoperative adjuvant therapy for primary colon cancer: results from National Surgical Adjuvant Breast and Bowel Project Protocol C-03. *J Clin Oncol.* 1993;11:1879–1887.

112. Benson AB, et al. NCCN practice guidelines for colorectal cancer. *Oncology.* 2000;14:203–212.

113. deGramont A, et al. Oxaliplatin/5-FU/LV in adjuvant colon cancer: results of the international randomized mosaic trial. *Proc Am Soc Clin Oncol.* 2003;22:253 (abstract 1015).

114. Cassidy J, et al. Capecitabine (X) vs. bolus 5-FU/leucovorin (LV) as adjuvant therapy for colon cancer (the X-ACT study): positive efficacy results of a phase III trial. *Proc Am Soc Clin Oncol.* 2004;23:(abstract 3509).

115. Saltz LB, Cox JV, Blanke C, et al. Irinotecan plus fluorouracil and leucovorin for metastatic colorectal cancer. *N Engl J Med.* 2000;343:905–914.

116. Hurwitz H, et al. Bevacizumab plus irinotecan, fluorouracil, and leucovorin for metastatic colorectal cancer. *N Engl J Med.* 2004;350:2335–2342.

117. Hwang JJ, et al. Capecitabine-based combination chemotherapy. *Am J Oncol Rev.* 2003;2(Suppl 5): 15–25.

118. Douillard JY, et al. Irinotecan combined with fluorouracil compared with fluorouracil alone as first-line treatment for metastatic colorectal cancer: a multicentre randomized trial. *Lancet.* 2000;355:1041–1047.

119. Andre T, et al. CPT-11 (irinotecan) addition to bimonthly, highdose leucovorin and bolus and continuous-infusion 5-fluorouracil (FOLFIRI) for pretreated metastatic colorectal cancer. GERCOR. *Eur J Cancer.* 1999;35:1343–1347.

120. de Gramon A, et al. Leucovorin and fluorouracil with and without oxaliplatin as first-line treatment in advanced colorectal cancer. *J Clin Oncol.* 2000;18: 2938–2947.

121. Tournigand C, et al. FOLFIRI followed by FOLFOX versus FOLFOX followed by FOLFIRI in metastatic colorectal cancer (MCRC): final results of a phase III study. *Proc Am Soc Clin Oncol.* 2001;20:124a(abstract 494).

122. Andre T, et al. FOLFOX7 compared to FOLFOX4. Preliminary results of the randomized optimox study. *Proc Am Soc Clin Oncol.* 2003;22:253(abstract 1016).

123. Cunningham D, et al. Cetuximab monotherapy and cetuximab plus irinotecan in irinotecan-refractory

metastatic colorectal cancer. *N Engl J Med*. 2004;351: 337–345.

124. Scheithauer W, et al. Randomized multicenter phase II trial of two different schedules of capecitabine plus oxaliplatin as first-line treatment in advanced colorectal cancer. *J Clin Oncol*. 2003;21:1307–1312.

125. Kerr D. Capecitabine/irinotecan in colorectal cancer: European early-phase data and planned trials. *Oncology*. 2002;16(Suppl 14):12–15.

126. Goldberg RM, Sargent DJ, Morton RF, et al. A randomized controlled trial of fluorouracil plus leucovorin, irinotecan, and oxaliplatin combinations in patients with previously untreated metastatic colorectal cancer. *J Clin Oncol*. 2004;22:23–30.

127. Poon MA, et al. Biochemical modulation of fluorouracil: evidence of significant improvement of survival and quality of life in patients with advanced colorectal carcinoma. *J Clin Oncol*. 1989;7:1407–1418.

128. Petrelli N, et al. The modulation of fluorouracil with leucovorin in metastatic colorectal carcinoma: a prospective randomized phase III trial. Gastrointestinal Tumor Study Group. *J Clin Oncol*. 1989;7:1419–1426.

129. Kabbinavar F, et al. Results of a randomized phase II controlled trial of bevacizumab in combination with 5-fluorouracil and leucovorin as first-line therapy in subjects with metastatic CRC. *Proc Am Soc Clin Oncol*. 2004;23:(Abstract 3516).

130. Jager E, et al. Weekly high-dose leucovorin versus low-dose leucovorin combined with fluorouracil in advanced colorectal cancer: results of a randomized multicenter trial. Study Group for Palliative Treatment of Metastatic Colorectal Cancer Study Protocol 1. *J Clin Oncol*. 1996;14:2274–2279.

131. de Gramont A, et al. Randomized trial comparing monthly low-dose leucovorin and fluorouracil bolus with bimonthly high-dose leucovorin and fluorouracil bolus plus continuous infusion for advanced colorectal cancer: a French Intergroup study. *J Clin Oncol*. 1997;15:808–815.

132. Mitchell EP, et al. High-dose bevacizumab in combination with FOLFOX4 improves survival in patients with previously treated advanced colorectal cancer: results from the Eastern Cooperative Oncology Group (ECOG) study E3200. Presented at the 2005 American Society of Clinical Oncology Gastrointestinal Cancers Symposium; January 27–29, 2005 Hollywood, FL (abstract 169a).

133. Hochster HS, et al. Bevacizumab (B) with oxaliplatin (O)-based chemotherapy in the first-line therapy of metastatic colorectal cancer (mCRC): Preliminary results of the randomized "TREE-2" trial. Presented at the American Society of Clinical Oncology Gastrointestinal Cancers Symposium; January 27–29, 2005 Hollywood, FL (abstract 241).

134. Blanke, CD, Kasimis B, Schein P, Capizzi R, Kurman M. Phase II study of trimetrexate, fluorouracil, and leucovorin for advanced colorectal cancer. *J Clin Oncol*. 1997;15:915–920.

135. Kemeny N, et al. Phase II study of hepatic arterial floxuridine, leucovorin, and dexamethasone for unresectable liver metastases from colorectal carcinoma. *J Clin Oncol*. 1994;12:2288–2295.

136. Hoff P, et al. Comparison of oral capecitabine versus intravenous fluorouracil plus leucovorin as first-line treatment in 605 patients with metastatic colorectal

137. Pitot HC, et al. Phase II trial of irinotecan in patients with metastatic colorectal carcinoma. *J Clin Oncol*. 1997;15:2910–2919.

138. Ulrich-Pur H, et al. Multicenter phase II trial of dose-fractionated irinotecan in patients with advanced colorectal cancer failing oxaliplatin-based first-line combination chemotherapy. *Ann Oncol*. 2001;12: 1269–1272.

139. Rougier P, et al. Phase II study of irinotecan in the treatment of advanced colorectal cancer in chemotherapy-naïve patients and patients pretreated with fluorouracil-based chemotherapy. *J Clin Oncol*. 1997;15: 251–260.

140. Saltz LB, et al. Phase II trial of cetuximab in patients with refractory colorectal cancer that expressed the epidermal growth factor receptor. *J Clin Onco*. 2004; 22:1201–1208.

141. Leichman CG, et al. Phase II study of fluorouracil and its modulation in advanced colorectal cancer: a Southwestern Oncology Group study. *J Clin Oncol*. 1995;13: 1303–1311.

142. Leichman CG. Schedule dependency of 5-fluorouracil. *Oncology*. 1999;13(Suppl 3):26–32.

143. Hoskins PJ, Swenerton KD, Pike JA, et al. Paclitaxel and carboplatin alone or with radiation in advanced or recurrent endometrial cancer: a phase II study. *J Clin Oncol*. 2001;19:4048–4053.

144. Thigpen JT, et al. A randomized comparison of doxorubicin alone versus doxorubicin plus cyclophosphamide in the management of advanced or recurrent endometrial carcinoma: a Gynecologic Oncology Group study. *J Clin Oncol*. 1994;12:1408–1414.

145. Deppe G, et al. Treatment of recurrent and metastatic endometrial carcinoma with cisplatin and doxorubicin. *Eur J Gynecol Oncol*. 1994;15:263–266.

146. Fiorica JV. Update on the treatment of cervical and uterine carcinoma: focus on topotecan. *Oncologist*. 2002;7(Suppl 5):36–45.

147. Fleming GF, et al. Phase III trial of doxorubicin plus cisplain with or without paclitaxel plus filgrastim in advanced endometrial carcinoma: a Gynecologic Oncology Group Study. *J Clin Oncol*. 2004;22:2159–2165.

148. Burke TW, et al. Postoperative adjuvant cisplatin, doxorubicin, and cyclophosphamide (PAC) chemotherapy in women with high-risk endometrial carcinoma. *Gynecol Oncol*. 1994;55:47–50.

149. Muss HB. Chemotherapy of metastatic endometrial cancer. *Semin Oncol*. 1994;21:107–113.

150. Thigpen JT, et al. Oral medroxyprogesterone acetate in the treatment of advanced or recurrent endometrial carcinoma: a dose-response study by the Gynecologic Oncology Group. *J Clin Oncol*. 1999;17:1736–1744.

151. Ball H, et al. A phase II trial of paclitaxel with advanced or recurrent adenocarcinoma of the endometrium: a Gynecologic Oncology Group study. *Gynecol Oncol*. 1996;62:278–282.

152. Wadler S, et al. Topotecan is an active agent in the first-line treatment of metastatic or recurrent endometrial carcinoma: Eastern Cooperative Oncology Group Study E3E93. *J Clin Oncol*. 2003;21:2110–2114.

153. Ramirez PT, et al. Hormonal therapy for the management of grade1 endometrial adenocarcinoma, a literature review. *Gynecol Onc*. 2004;95(1):133–138.

154. Herskovic A, et al. Combined chemotherapy and radiotherapy compared with radiotherapy alone in patients with cancer of the esophagus. *N Engl J Med.* 1992;326:1593–1598.

155. Heath EI, et al. Phase II evaluation of preoperative chemoradiation and postoperative adjuvant chemotherapy for squamous cell and adenocarcinoma of the esophagus. *J Clin Oncol.* 2000;18:868–876.

156. Kies MS, et al. Cisplatin and 5-fluorouracil in the primary management of squamous esophageal cancer. *Cancer.* 1987;60:2156–2160.

157. Ilson DH, et al. Phase II trial of weekly irinotecan plus cisplatin in first line advanced esophageal cancer. *J Clin Oncol.* 1999;17:3270–3275.

158. Ilson DH, et al. Phase II trial of paclitaxel, fluorouracil, and cisplatin in patients with advanced carcinoma of the esophagus. *J Clin Oncol.* 1998;16:1826–1834.

159. Lin LL, Edward H, Lozano R, Karp D. *Color-Matrix Cancer Staging and Treatment Handbook.* 3rd ed. Houston, TX: University of Texas MD Anderson. 2004;75.

160. Ajani JA, et al. Paclitaxel in the treatment of carcinoma of the esophagus. *Semin Oncol.* 1995;22(Suppl 6):35–40.

161. MacDonald JS, Smalley SR, Benedetti J, et al. Chemoradiotherapy after surgery compared with surgery alone for adenocarcinoma of the stomach or gastroesophageal junction. *N Engl J Med.* 2001;345:725–730.

162. Ajani JA, et al. Docetaxel (D), cisplatin, 5-fluorouracil compare to cisplatin (C) and 5-fluorouracil (F) for chemotherapy-naïve patients with metastatic or locally recurrent, unresectable gastric carcinoma (MGC): interim results of a randomized phase III trial (V3325). *Proc Am Soc ClinOncol.* 2003;22:249 (abstract 999).

163. Wilke M, et al. Preoperative chemotherapy in locally advanced and non-resectable gastric cancer: a phase II study with etoposide, doxorubicin, and cisplatin. *J Clin Oncol.* 1989;7:1318–1326.

164. Findlay M, et al. A phase II study in advanced gastroesophageal cancer using epirubicin and cisplatin in combination with continuous infusion 5-fluorouracil (ECF). *Ann Oncol.* 1994;5:609–616.

165. Wilke M, et al. Preliminary analysis of a randomized phase III trial of FAMTX versus ELF versus cisplatin/FU in advanced gastric cancer. A trial of the EORTC astrointestinal Tract Cancer Cooperative Group and the AIO. *Proc Am Soc Clin Oncol.* 1995;14:206a.

166. Shirao K, Shimada Y, Kondo H, et al. Phase I–II study of irintoecan hydrochloride combined with cisplatin in patients with advanced gastric cancer. *J Clin Oncol.* 1997;15:921–927.

167. MacDonald JS, et al. 5-Fluorouracil, doxorubicin, and Mitomycin (FAM) combination chemotherapy for advanced gastric cancer. *Ann Intern Med.* 1980;93:533–536.

168. Kelsen D, et al. FAMTX versus etoposide, doxorubicin, and cisplatin: a random assignment trial in gastric cancer. *J Clin Oncol.* 1992;10:541–548.

169. Cullinan SA, et al. Controlled evaluation of three drug combination regimens versus fluorouracil alone for the therapy of advanced gastric cancer. North Central Cancer Treatment Group. *J Clin Oncol.* 1994;12:412–416.

170. Ajani JA, et al. Multinational randomized trial of docetaxel, cisplatin with or without 5-fluorouracil in patients with advanced gastric or GE junction adenocarcinoma. *Proc Am Soc Clin Oncol.* 2000;20:165a (abstract 657).

171. O'Connell MJ. Current status of chemotherapy for advanced pancreatic and gastric cancer. *J Clin Oncol.* 1985;3:1032–1039.

172. Ajani JA. Docetaxel for gastric and esophageal carcinomas. *Oncology.* 2002;16(Suppl 6):89–96.

173. Demetri GD, von Mehren M, Blanke CD, et al. Efficacy and safety of imatinib mesylate in advanced gastrointestinal stromal tumors. *N Engl J Med.* 2002;347:472–480.

174. Sutent [package insert]. New York: Pfizer Inc.; 2006 Available at: http://www.pfizer.com/pfizer/download/uspi_sutent.pdf. Accessed March 1, 2006.

175. Shin DS, et al. Phase II trial of paclitaxel, ifosfamide, and cisplatin in patients with recurrent head and neck squamous cell carcinoma. *J Clin Oncol.* 1998;16:1325–1330.

176. Posner M, et al. Multicenter phase I–II trial of docetaxel, cisplatin, and fluorouracil induction chemotherapy for patients with locally advanced squamous cell cancer of the head and neck. *J Clin Oncol.* 2001;19:1096–1104.

177. Shin DM, et al. Phase II study of paclitaxel, ifosfamide, and carboplatin in patients with recurrent or metastatic head and neck squamous cell carcinoma of the head and neck (SCCHN). *Cancer.* 1999;91:1316–1323.

178. Fountzilas G, et al. Paclitaxel and carboplatin in recurrent or metastatic head and neck cancer: a phase II study. *Semin Oncol.* 1997;24(Suppl 2):65–67.

179. Hitt R, et al. A phase I/II study of paclitaxel plus cisplatin as firstline therapy for head and neck cancer. *Semin Oncol.* 1995;22(Suppl 15):50–54.

180. Kish JA, et al. Cisplatin and 5-fluorouracil infusion in patients with recurrent and disseminated epidermoid cancer of the head and neck. *Cancer.* 1984;53:1819–1824.

181. Vokes EE, Schilsky RL, Weichselbaum RR, et al. Cisplatin, 5-fluorouracil, and high-dose oral leucovorin for advanced head and neck cancer. *Cancer.* 1989;63(Suppl 6):1048–1053.

182. Veterans Affairs Laryngeal Cancer Study Group. Induction chemotherapy plus radiation compared with surgery plus radiation in patients with advanced laryngeal cancer. *N Engl J Med.* 1991;324:1685–1690.

183. Forastiere AA, et al. Concurrent chemotherapy and radiotherapy for organ preservation in advanced laryngeal cancer. *N Engl J Med.* 2003;349:2091–2098.

184. Al-Sarraf M, et al. Chemoradiotherapy versus radiotherapy in patients with advanced nasopharyngeal cancer: phase III randomized intergroup study 0099. *J Clin Oncol.* 1998;16:1310–1317.

185. Forastiere AA, et al. Randomized comparison of cisplatin plus fluorouracil and carboplatin plus fluorouracil versus methotrexate in advanced squamous-cell carcinoma of the head and neck: a Southwest Oncology Group study. *J Clin Oncol.* 1992;10:1245–1251.

186. Gebbia V, et al. Vinorelbine plus cisplatin in recurrent or previously untreated unresectable squamous cell carcinoma of the head and neck. *Am J Clin Oncol.* 1995;18:293–296.

187. Dreyfuss A, et al. Taxotere for advanced, inoperable squamous cell carcinoma of the head and neck (SCCHN). *Proc Am Soc Clin Oncol.* 1995;14:875a.

188. Forastiere AA. Current and future trials of Taxol (paclitaxel) in head and neck cancer. *Ann Oncol.* 1994;5(Suppl 6):51–54.

189. Hong WK, et al. Chemotherapy in head and neck cancer. *N Engl Jmed.* 1983;308:75–79.

190. Degardin M, et al. An EORTC-ECSG phase II study of vinorelbine in patients with recurrent and/or metastatic squamous cell carcinoma of the head and neck. *Ann Oncol.* 1998;9:1103–1107.

191. Chua DT, et al. A phase II study of capecitabine in patients with recurrent and metastatic nasophryngeal cancer pretreated with platinum-based chemotherapy. *Oral Oncol.* 2003; 39(4):361–366.

192. Venook AP. Treatment of hepatocellular carcinoma: too many options? *J Clin Oncol.* 1994;12:1323–1334.

193. Okada S, et al. A phase 2 study of cisplatin in patients with hepatocellular carcinoma. *Oncology.* 1993;50: 22–26.

194. Aguayo A, et al. Nonsurgical treatment of hepatocellular carcinoma. *Semin Oncol.* 2001;28:503–513.

195. Ireland-Gill A, et al. Treatment of acquired immunodeficiency syndrome-related Kaposi's sarcoma using bleomycin-containing combination chemotherapy regimens. *Semin Oncol.* 1992;19(Suppl 5):32–37.

196. Laubenstein LL, et al. Treatment of epidemic Kaposi's sarcoma with etoposide or a combination of doxorubicin, bleomycin, and vinblastine. *J Clin Oncol.* 1984;2:1115–1120.

197. Gill PS, Wernz J, Scadden DT, et al. Randomized phase III trial of liposomal daunorubicin versus doxorubicin, bleomycin, and vincristine in AIDS-related Kaposi's sarcoma. *J Clin Oncol* 1996;14:2353–2364.

198. Northfelt DW, et al. Efficacy of pegylated-liposomal doxorubicin in the treatment of AIDS-related Kaposi's sarcoma after failure of standard chemotherapy. *J Clin Oncol.* 1997;15:653–659.

199. Gill PS, et al. Paclitaxel is safe and effective in the treatment of advanced AIDS-related Kaposi's sarcoma. *J Clin Oncol.* 1999;17:1876–1880.

200. Gill PS, et al. Multicenter trial of low-dose paclitaxel in patients with advanced AIDS-related Kaposi's sarcoma. *Cancer.* 2002;95:147–154.

201. Real FX, Oettgen HF, Krown SE. Kaposi's sarcoma and the acquired immunodeficiency syndrome: treatment with high and low dose of recombinant leucocyte A interferon. *J Clin Oncol.* 1986;4:544–551.

202. Groopman JE, et al. Recombinant alpha-2 interferon therapy for Kaposi's sarcoma associated with the acquired immunodeficiency syndrome. *Ann Intern Med.* 1984;100:671–676.

203. Linker CA, Levitt LS, O'Donnell M, et al. Improved results of treatment of adult acute lymphoblastic leukemia. *Blood.* 1987;69:1242–1248.

204. Linker CA, et al. Treatment of adult acute lymphoblastic leukemia with intensive cyclical chemotherapy: a follow-up report. *Blood.* 1991;78:2814–2822.

205. Larson R, et al. A five-drug regimen remission induction regimen with intensive consolidation for adults with acute lymphoblastic leukemia: Cancer and Leukemia Group B Study 8811. *Blood.* 1995;85: 2025–2037.

206. Kantarjian H, et al. Results of treatment with hyper-CVAD, a dose intensive regimen in adult acute lymphoblastic leukemia. *J Clin Oncol.* 2000;18:547–561.

207. Faderl S, et al. The role of clofarabine in hematologic and solid malignancies-development of a next generation nucleoside analog. *Cancer.* 2005;103:1985-1995.

208. Yates JW, et al. Cytosine arabinoside (NSC-63878) and daunorubicin (NSC-83142) in acute nonlymphocytic leukemia. *Cancer Chemother Rep.* 1973;57:485–488.

209. Preisler H, et al. Comparison of three remission induction regimens and two postinduction strategies for the treatment of acute nonlymphocytic leukemia: a Cancer and Leukemia Group B study. *Blood.* 1987;69:1441–1449.

210. Preisler H, et al. Adriamycin-cytosine arabinoside therapy for adult acute myelocytic leukemia. *Cancer Treat Rep.* 1977;61:89–92.

211. Mandelli F, et al. Molecular remission in PML/RAR alpha-positive acute promyelocytic leukemia by combined all-trans retinoic acid and idarubicin (AIDA) therapy. *Blood.* 1997;90:1014–1021.

212. List A, et al. Opportunities for Trisenox (arsenic trioxide) in the treatment of myelodysplastic syndromes. *Leukemia.* 2003;17:1499–1507

213. Ho AD, Lipp T, Ehninfer G, Meyer P, Freund M, Hunstein W. Combination therapy with mitox-antrone and etoposide in refractory acute myelogenous leukemia. *Cancer Treat Rep.* 1986; 70:1025–1027.

214. Montillo M, Mirto S, Petti MC, et al. Fludarabine, cytarabine, and G-CSF (FLAG) for the treatment of poor risk acute myeloid leukemia. *Am J Hematol.* 1998;58:105–109.

215. Wiernik PH, et al. Cytarabine plus idarubicin or daunorubicin as induction and consolidation therapy for previously untreated adult patients with acute myeloid leukemia. *Blood.* 1992;79:313–319.

216. Santana VM, et al. 2-Chlorodeoxyadenosine produces a high rate of complete hematologic remission in relapsed acute myeloid leukemia. *J Clin Oncol.* 1992; 10:364–369.

217. Mayer RJ, et al. Intensive postremission chemotherapy in adults with acute myeloid leukemia. Cancer and Leukemia Group B. *N Engl J Med.* 1994;331:896–903.

218. Degos L, et al. All-trans retinoic acid as a differentiating agent in the treatment of acute promyelocytic leukemia. *Blood.* 1995;85:2643–2653.

219. Sievers EL, et al. Selective ablation of acute myeloid leukemia using antibody-targeted chemotherapy: a phase I study of an anti CD33 calicheamycin immunoconjugate. *Blood.* 1999;11:3678–3684.

220. Trisenox© (package insert). Seattle, WA: Cell Therapeutics; 2003. Trisenox© (arsenic trioxide) injection Nursing Advisory Board Meeting Summary April 2004. Seattle, WA: Cell Therapeutics, Inc.; 2004.

221. Raphael B, et al. Comparison of chlorambucil and prednisone versus cyclophosphamide, vincristine, and prednisone as initial treatment for chronic lymphocytic leukemia: long-term follow-up of an Eastern Cooperative Oncology Group randomized clinical trial. *J Clin Oncol.* 1991;9:770–776.

222. Keating MJ, et al. Long-term follow-up of patients with chronic lymphocytic leukemia (CLL) receiving fludarabine regimens as initial therapy. *Blood.* 1998; 92:1165–1171.

223. O'Brien S, et al. Results of fludarabine and prednisone therapy in 264 patients with chronic lymphocytic leukemia with multivariate analysis-derived prognostic model for response to treatment. *Blood.* 1993;82:1695–1700.

224. Byrd JC, Peterson BL, Morrison VA, et al. Randomized phase 2 study of fludarabine with concurrent versus sequential treatment with rituximab in symptomatic untreated patients with B-cell chronic lymphocytic leukemia: results from Cancer and Leukemia Group B9712. *Blood.* 2003;101:6–14.

225. Keating M, et al. Early results of a chemoimmunotherapy regimen of fludarabine, cyclophosphamide, and rituximab as initial therapy for CLL. *J Clin Oncol.* 2005;22:4079–4088.

226. Osterborg A, et al. Phase II multicenter study of human CD52 antibody in previously treated chronic lymphocytic leukemia. *J Clin Oncol.* 1997;15:1567–1574.

227. Dighiero G, et al. Chlorambucil in indolent chronic lymphocytic leukemia. French Cooperative Group on Chronic Lymphocytic Leukemia. *N Engl J Med.* 1998;338:1506–1514.

228. Saven A, et al. 2-Chlorodeoxyadenosine activity in patients with untreated chronic lymphocytic leukemia. *J Clin Oncol.* 1995;13:570–574.

229. Keating MJ, Kantarjian H, Talpaz M, et al. Fludarabine: a new agent with major activity against chronic lymphocytic leukemia. *Blood.* 1989;74:19–25.

230. Sawitsky A, Rai KR, Glidewell O, Silver RT. Comparison of daily versus intermittent chlorambucil and prednisone therapy in the treatment of patients with chronic lymphocytic leukemia. *Blood.* 1977;50:1049.

231. Guilhot F, et al. Interferon α-2b combined with cytarabine versus interferon alone in chronic myelogenous leukemia. *N Engl J Med.* 1997;337:223–229.

232. Druker BJ, et al. Efficacy and safety of a specific inhibitor of the BCR-ABL tyrosine kinase in chronic myelogenous leukemia. *N Engl J Med.* 2001;344:1031–1037.

233. Hehlmann R, et al. Randomized comparison of busulfan and hydroxyurea in chronic myelogenous leukemia: prolongation of survival by hydroxyurea. The German CML Study Group. *Blood.* 1993;82:398–407.

234. Hehlmann R, Heimpel H, Hasford J, et al. Randomized comparison of interferon-alpha with busulfan and hydroxyurea in chronic myelogenous leukemia. The German CML Study Group. *Blood.* 1994;84:4064–4077.

235. The Italian Cooperative Study Group on Chronic Myelogenous Leukemia. Interferon alfa-2a as compared with conventional chemotherapy for the treatment of chronic myeloid leukemia. *N Engl J Med.* 1994;330:820–825.

236. Saven A, Piro LD. Treatment of hairy cell leukemia. *Blood.* 1992;79:111–1120.

236a. www.emedicine.com/MED/topics371.htm. Besa, Emmanual, July 12, 2006.

236b. Sprycel package insert. Sprycel (dastinib) tablets. Bristol-Myers Squibb Company. Princeton, NJ.

237. Cassileth PA, et al. Pentostatin induces durable remission in hairy cell leukemia. *J Clin Oncol.* 1991;9:243–246.

238. Ratain MJ, et al. Treatment of hairy cell leukemia with recombinant alpha-2 interferon. *Blood.* 1985;65:644–648.

239. Strauss GM, et al. Randomized clinical trial of adjuvant chemotherapy with paclitaxel and carboplatin following resection in stage IB non-small cell lung cancer. CALGB 9633. *J Clin Oncol.* 2004;621S(abstract 7019).

240. Winton T, Livingston R, Johnson D, et al. Vinorelbine plus cisplatin versus observation in resected non-small cell lung cancer. *N Engl J Med.* 2005;352:2589–2597.

241. Langer CJ, et al. Paclitaxel and carboplatin in combination in the treatment of advanced non-small cell lung cancer: a phase II toxicity, response, and survival analysis. *J Clin Oncol.* 1995;13:1860–1870.

242. Giaccone G, et al. Randomized study of paclitaxel-cisplatin versus cisplatin-teniposide in patients with advanced non-small cell lung cancer. The European Organization for Research and Treatment of Cancer Lung Cancer Cooperative Group. *J Clin Oncol.* 1998;16:2133–2141.

243. Fossella F, et al. Randomized, multinational, phase III study of docetaxel plus platinum combinations versus vinorelbine plus cisplatin for advanced non-small cell lung cancer: the TAX 326 Study Group. *J Clin Oncol.* 2003;21:3016–3024.

244. Belani CP, Bonomi P, Dobbs TW, et al. Docetaxel and cisplatin in patients with advanced non-small cell lung cancer (NSCLC): a multicenter phase II trial. *Clin Lung Cancer* 1999;1:144–150.

245. Georgoulias V, et al. Platinum-based and non-platinum-based chemotherapy in advanced non-small cell lung cancer: a randomized multicentre trial. *Lancet.* 2001;357:1478–1484.

246. Abratt RP, Bezwoda WR, Goedhals L, Hacking DJ. Weekly gemcitabine with monthly cisplatin: effective chemotherapy for advanced non-small cell lung cancer. *J Clin Oncol.* 1997;15:744–749.

247. Langer CJ, et al. Gemcitabine and carboplatin in combination: an update of phase I and phase II studies in non-small cell lung cancer. *Semin Oncol.* 1999;26(Suppl 4):12–18.

248. Frasci G, et al. Gemcitabine plus vinorelbine versus vinorelbine alone in elderly patients with advanced non-small cell lung cancer. *J Clin Oncol.* 2000;18:2529–2536.

249. Smith TJ, et al. Economic evaluation of a randomized clinical trial comparing vinorelbine, vinorelbine plus cisplatin, and vindesine plus cisplatin for non-small cell lung cancer. *J Clin Oncol.* 1995;13:2166–2173.

250. Cremonesi M, et al. Vinorelbine and carboplatin in operable nonsmall lung cancer: a monoinstitutional phase II study. *Oncology.* 2003;64(2):97–101.

251. Longeval E, et al. Combination chemotherapy with cisplatin and etoposide in bronchogenic squamous cell carcinoma and adenocarcinoma. A study by the EORTC lung cancer working party. *Cancer.* 1982;50:2751–2756.

252. Gandara D, et al. Consolidation docetaxel after concurrent chemoradiotherapy in stage IIIB non-small cell lung cancer: phase II Southwest Oncology Group Study S9504. *J Clin Oncol.* 2003;21:2004–2010.

253. Lilenbaum RC, et al. Single-agent versus combination chemotherapy in advanced non-small cell lung cancer: the Cancer and Leukemia Group B (study 9730). *J Clin Oncol.* 2005;23:190–196.

254. Tester WJ, et al. Phase II study of patients with metastatic nonsmall cell carcinoma of the lung treated

with paclitaxel by 3-hour infusion. *Cancer.* 1997;79: 724–729.

255. Miller VA, et al. Docetaxel (Taxotere) as a single agent and in combination chemotherapy for the treatment of patients with advanced non-small cell lung cancer. *Semin Oncol.* 2000;27(Suppl 3):3–10.

256. Hainsworth JD, et al. Weekly docetaxel in the treatment of elderly patients with advanced non-small cell lung cancer. *Cancer.* 2000;89:328–333.

257. Hanna N, et al. Randomized phase III trial of pemetrexed versus docetaxel in patients with non-small cell lung cancer previously treated with chemotherapy. *J Clin Oncol.* 2004;22:1589–1597.

258. Manegold C, et al. Single-agent gemcitabine versus cisplatin-etoposide: early results of a randomized phase II study in locally advanced or metastatic non-small cell lung cancer. *Ann Oncol.* 1997;8:525–529.

259. Perez-Soler R, et al. Phase II study of topotecan in patients with advanced non-small cell lung cancer previously untreated with chemotherapy. *J Clin Oncol.* 1996;14:503–513.

260. Furuse K, et al. Randomized study of vinorelbine (VRB) versus vindesine (VDS) in previously untreated stage IIIB or IV non-small cell lung cancer (NSCLC). The Japan Vinorelbine Lung Cancer Cooperative Study Group. *Ann Oncol.* 1996;7:815–820.

261. Herbst RS. Dose-comparative monotherapy trials of ZD1839 in previously treated non-small cell lung cancer patients. *Semin Oncol.* 2003;30(Suppl 1):30–38.

262. Shepherd FA, et al. A randomized placebo-controlled trial of erlotinib in patients with advanced non-small cell lung cancer (NSCLC) following failure of 1st and 2nd line chemotherapy. A National Cancer Institute of Canada Clinical Trials Group (NCIC CTG) trial. *J Clin Oncol.* 2004;22(Suppl 1):14S (abstract 7022).

263. Ihde DC, et al. Prospective randomized comparison of high-dose and standard-dose etoposide and cisplatin chemotherapy in patients with extensive-stage small cell lung cancer. *J Clin Oncol.* 1994;12:2022–2034.

264. Viren M, et al. Carboplatin and etoposide in extensive small cell lung cancer. *Acta Oncol.* 1994;33:921–924.

265. Noda K, et al. Irinotecan plus cisplatin compared with etoposide plus cisplatin for extensive small-cell lung cancer. *N Engl J Med.* 2002;346:85–91.

266. Hainsworth JD, et al. Paclitaxel, carboplatin, and extended-schedule etoposide in the treatment of small cell lung cancer: comparison of sequential phase II trials using different dose-intensities. *J Clin Oncol.* 1997;15:3464–3470.

267. Roth BJ, et al. Randomized study of cyclophosphamide, doxorubicin, and vincristine versus etoposide and cisplatin versus alternation of these two regimens in extensive small cell lung cancer: a phase III trial of the Southeastern Cancer Study Group. *J Clin Oncol.* 1992;10:282–291.

268. Aisner J, et al. Doxorubicin, cyclophosphamide, etoposide and platinum, doxorubicin, cyclophosphamide and etoposide for small cell carcinoma of the lung. *Semin Oncol.* 1986;(Suppl 3):54–62.

269. Johnson DH. Recent developments in chemotherapy treatment of small cell lung cancer. *Semin Oncol.* 1993;20:315–325.

270. Johnson DH, et al. Prolonged administration of oral etoposide in patients with relapsed or refractory small-

cell lung cancer: a phase II trial. *J Clin Oncol.* 1990;8:1013–1017.

271. Hainsworth JD, et al. The current role and future prospects of paclitaxel in the treatment of small cell lung cancer. *Semin Oncol.* 1999;26(Suppl 2):60–66.

272. Ardizzoni A, et al. Topotecan, a new active drug in the second-line treatment of small cell lung cancer: a phase II study in patients with refractory and sensitive disease. The European Organization for Research and Treatment of Cancer Early Clinical Studies Group and New Drug Development Office, and the Lung Cancer Cooperative Group. *J Clin Oncol.* 1997;15:2090–2096.

273. Bonadonna G, et al. Combination chemotherapy of Hodgkin's disease with adriamycin, bleomycin, vinblastine, and imidazole carboxamide versus MOPP. *Cancer.* 1975;36:252–259.

274. DeVita VT, Jr, et al. Combination chemotherapy in the treatment of advanced Hodgkin's disease. *Ann Intern Med.* 1970;73:881–895.

275. Klimo P, et al. MOPP/ABV hybrid program: combination chemotherapy based on early introduction of seven effective drugs for advanced Hodgkin's disease. *J Clin Oncol.* 1985;3:1174–1182.

276. Bartlett NL, et al. Brief chemotherapy, Stanford V, and adjuvant radiotherapy for bulky or advanced-stage Hodgkin's disease: a preliminary report. *J Clin Oncol* 1995;13:1080–1088.

277. Diehl V, et al. BEACOPP, a new dose-escalated and accelerated regimen is at least as effective as COPP/ABVD in patients with advanced-stage Hodgkin's lymphoma. *J Clin Oncol.* 1998;16:3810–3821.

278. Tesch H, et al. Moderate dose escalation for advanced Hodgkin's disease using the bleomycin, etoposide, adriamycin, cyclophosphamide, vincristine, procarbazine, and prednisone scheme and adjuvant radiotherapy: a study of the German Hodgkin's Lymphoma Study Group. *Blood.* 1998;15:4560–4567.

279. Radford JA, et al. Results of a randomized trial comparing MVPP chemotherapy with a hybrid regimen, ChlVPP/EVA, in the initial treatment of Hodgkin's disease. *J Clin Oncol.* 1995;13:2379–2385.

280. Longo DL. The use of chemotherapy in the treatment of Hodgkin's disease. *Semin Oncol.* 1990;17:716–735.

281. Colwill R, et al. Mini-BEAM as salvage therapy for relapsed or refractory Hodgkin's disease before intensive therapy and autologous bone marrow transplantation. *J Clin Oncol.* 1995;13:396–402.

282. Santoro A, et al. Gemcitabine in the treatment of refractory Hodgkin's disease: results of a multicenter phase II study. *J Clin Oncol.* 2000;18:2615–2619.

283. Bagley CM, Jr, et al. Advanced lymphosarcoma: intensive cyclical combination chemotherapy with cyclophosphamide, vincristine, and prednisone. *Ann Intern Med.* 1972;76:227–234.

284. Sonnevald P, et al. Comparison of doxorubicin and mitoxantrone in the treatment of elderly patients with advanced diffuse non-Hodgkin's lymphoma using CHOP versus CNOP chemotherapy. *J Clin Oncol.* 1995;13:2530–2539.

285. McLaughlin P, et al. Fludarabine, mitoxantrone, and dexamethasone: an effective new regimen for indolent lymphoma. *J Clin Oncol.* 1996;14:1262–1268.

286. Hochster H, et al. Efficacy of cyclophosphamide (CYC) and fludarabine (FAMP) as first-line therapy of

low-grade non-Hodgkin's lymphoma (NHL). *Blood.* 1994;84 (Suppl 1):383a.

287. McKelvey EM, et al. Hydroxydaunomycin (Adriamycin) combination chemotherapy in malignant lymphoma. *Cancer.* 1976;38:1484–1493.

288. Vose JM, et al. Phase II study of rituximab in combination with CHOP chemotherapy in patients with previously untreated, aggressive non-Hodgkin's lymphoma. *J Clin Oncol.* 2001;19:389–397.

289. Wilson WH, et al. EPOCH chemotherapy: toxicity and efficacy in relapsed and refractory non-Hodgkin's lymphoma. *J Clin Oncol.* 1993;11:1573–1582.

290. Wilson WH. Chemotherapy sensitization by rituximab: experimental and clinical evidence. *Semin Oncol.* 2000;27 (Suppl 12):30–36.

291. Klimo P, et al. MACOP-B chemotherapy for the treatment of diffuse large-cell lymphoma. *Ann Intern Med.* 1985;102:596–602.

292. Shipp MA, et al. Identification of major prognostic subgroups of patients with large-cell lymphoma treated with m-BACOD or M-BACOD. *Ann Intern Med.* 1986;104:757–765.

293. Longo DL, et al. Superiority of ProMACE-CytaBOM over Pro-MACE-MOPP in the treatment of advanced diffuse aggressive lymphoma: results of a prospective randomized trial. *J Clin Oncol.* 1991;9:25–38.

294. Magrath I, Janus C, Edwards BK, et al. An effective therapy for both undifferentiated lymphomas and lymphoblastic lymphomas in children and young adults. *Blood.* 1984;63:1102–1111.

295. Magrath I, et al. Adults and children with small non-cleaved-cell lymphoma have a similar excellent outcome when treated with the same chemotherapy regimen. *J Clin Oncol.* 1996;14:925.

296. Berstein JI, et al. Combined modality therapy for adults with small non-cleaved cell lymphoma (Burkitt's and non-Burkitt's types). *J Clin Oncol* 1986;4:847–858.

297. Goy AH, et al. Report of a phase II study of proteosome inhibitor bortezomib in patients with relapsed or refractory indolent and aggressive B-cell lymphomas. *Proc Am Soc Clin Oncol.* 2003;22:570 (abstract 2291).

298. Coiffier B, et al. Rituximab plus CHOP in combination with CHOP chemotherapy in patients with diffuse large B-cell lymphoma: an update of the GELA study. *N Engl J Med.* 2002;346:235–242.

299. Vose JM, et al. CNOP for diffuse aggressive non-Hodgkin's lymphoma: the Nebraska lymphoma study group experience. *Leuk Lymphoma.* 2002;43:799–804.

300. Velasquez WS, et al. ESHAP-an effective chemotherapy regimen in refractory and relapsing lymphoma: a 4-year follow-up study. *J Clin Oncol.* 1994;12:1169–1176.

301. Velasquez WS, et al. Effective salvage therapy for lymphoma with cisplatin in combination with high-dose ara-C and dexamethasone. *Blood.* 1988;71:117–122.

302. Moskowitz C, et al. Ifosfamide, carboplatin, and etoposide: a highly effective cytoreduction and peripheral blood progenitor cell mobilization regimen for transplant-eligible patients with non-Hodgkin's lymphoma. *J Clin Oncol.* 1999;17:3776–3785.

303. Rodriguez MA, et al. A phase II trial of mesna/ifosfamide, mitoxantrone, and etoposide for refractory lymphoma. *Ann Oncol.* 1995;6:609–611.

304. Abrey LE, et al. Treatment for primary CNS lymphoma: the next step. *J Clin Oncol.* 2000;18:3144–3150.

305. McLaughlin P, et al. Rituximab chimeric anti-CD20 monoclonal antibody therapy for relapsed indolent lymphoma: half of patients respond to a four-dose treatment program. *J Clin Oncol.* 1998;16:2825–2833.

306. Witzig TE, et al. Randomized controlled trial of yttrium-90-labeled ibritumomab tiuxetan radioimmunotherapy versus rituximab immunotherapy for patients with relapsed or refractory low-grade follicular, or transformed B-cell non-Hodgkin's lymphoma. *J Clin Oncol.* 2002;20:2453–2463.

307. Falkson CI. A phase II trial in patients with previously treated lowgrade lymphoma. *Am J Clin Oncol.* 1996;19:268–270.

308. Betticher DC, von Rohr A, Ratschiller D, et al. Fewer infections but maintained antitumor activity with lower-dose versus standard-dose cladribine in pretreated low-grade non-Hodgkin's lymphoma. *J Clin Oncol.* 1998;16:850–858.

309. Kirkwood JM, et al. Interferon alfa-2b adjuvant therapy of high risk resected cutaneous melanoma: the Eastern Cooperative Oncology Trial EST 1684. *J Clin Oncol.* 1996;14:7–17.

309a. Bexxar package insert. Oct 2005. Glaxo SmithKline. Research Triangle Park, NC.

310. Creagen ET, et al. Phase III clinical trial of the combination of cisplatin, dacarbazine, and carmustine with or without tamoxifen in patients with advanced malignant melanoma. *J Clin Oncol.* 1999;17:1884–1890.

311. DelPrete SA, Maurer LH, O'Donnell J, et al. Combination chemotherapy with cisplatin, carmustine, dacarbazine, and tamoxifen in metastatic melanoma. *Cancer Treat Rep.* 1984;68:1403–1405.

312. Legha SS, et al. A prospective evaluation of a triple-drug regimen containing cisplatin, vinblastine, and DTIC (CVD) for metastatic melanoma. *Cancer.* 1989;64:2024–2029.

313. Falkson CI, et al. Phase III trial of dacarbazine vs dacarbazine with interferon α-2b vs dacarbazine with tamoxifen vs dacarbazine with interferon α-2b and tamoxifen in patients with metastatic malignant melanoma. *J Clin Oncol.* 1998;16:1743–1751.

314. Eton O, Legha SS, Bedikian AY, et al. Sequential biochemotherapy versus chemotherapy for metastatic melanoma: results from a phase III randomized trial. *J Clin Oncol.* 2002;20:2045–2052.

315. Hwu WJ, et al. Temozolomide plus thalidomide in patients with advanced melanoma: results of a dose finding trial. *J Clin Oncol.* 2002;20:2607–2609.

316. Luce JK, et al. Clinical trials with the antitumor agent 5-(3,3-dimethyl-1-triazeno)imidazole-4-carboxamide (NSC-45388). *Cancer Chemother Rep.* 1970;54:119–124.

317. Pritchard KI, et al. DTIC therapy in metastatic malignant melanoma: a simplified dose schedule. *Cancer Treat Rep.* 1980;64:1123–1126.

318. Kirkwood JM, et al. Advances in the diagnosis and treatment of malignant melanoma. *Semin Oncol.* 1997;24(Suppl 4):1–48.

319. Parkinson DR, et al. Interleukin-2 therapy in patients with metastatic malignant melanoma: a phase II study. *J Clin Oncol.* 1990;8:1650–1656.

320. Middleton MR, et al. Randomized phase II study of temozolomide versus dacarbazine in the treatment of

patients with advanced metastatic malignant melanoma. *J Clin Oncol.* 2000;18:158–166.

321. Ardizzoni A, Rosso R, Salvati F, et al. Activity of doxorubicin and cisplatin combination chemotherapy in patients with diffuse malignant pleural mesothelioma. *Cancer.* 1991;67:2984–2987.

322. Shin DM, et al. Prospective study of combination chemotherapy with cyclophosphamide, doxorubicin, and cisplatin for unresectable or metastatic malignant pleural mesothelioma. *Cancer.* 1995;76:2230–2236.

323. Nowak AK, et al. A multicentre phase II study of cisplatin and gemcitabine for malignant mesothelioma. *Br J Cancer.* 2002;87:491–496.

324. Favaretto AG, et al. Gemcitabine combined with carboplatin in patients with malignant pleural mesothelioma: a multicentric phase II study. *Cancer.* 2003; 97:2791–2797.

325. Vogelzang NJ, et al. Phase III study of pemetrexed in combination with cisplatin versus cisplatin alone in patients with malignant pleural mesothelioma. *J Clin Oncol.* 2003;21:2636–2644.

326. Southwest Oncology Group Study. Remission maintenance therapy for multiple myeloma. *Arch Intern Med* 1975;135:147–152.

327. Barlogie B, Smith L, Alexanian R. Effective treatment of advanced multiple myeloma refractory to alkylating agents. *N Engl J Med.* 1984;310:1353–1356.

328. Rajkumar SV, et al. Combination therapy with thalidomide plus dexamethasone for newly diagnosed myeloma. *J Clin Oncol.* 2002;20:4319–4323.

329. Case DC, Jr, et al. Improved survival times in multiple myeloma treated with melphalan, prednisone, cyclophosphamide, vincristine, and BCNU. *Am J Med.* 77;63:897–903.

330. Oken MM, et al. Comparison of melphalan and prednisone with vincristine, carmustine, melphalan, cyclophosphamide and prenisone in the treatment of multiple myeloma: results of Eastern Cooperative Oncology Group Study E2479. *Cancer.* 1997;79(8): 1561–1567.

331. Alexanian R, Barlogie B, Dixon D. High-dose glucocorticoid treatment of resistant myeloma. *Ann Intern Med.* 1986;105:8–11.

332. Cunningham D, et al. High-dose melphalan for multiple myeloma: long-term follow-up data. *J Clin Oncol.* 1994;12:764–768.

333. Singhal S, et al. Antitumor activity of thalidomide in refractory multiple myeloma. *N Engl J Med.* 1999;341: 1565–1571.

334. Richardson P, et al. A phase II study of bortezomib in relapsed, refractory myeloma. *N Engl J Med.* 2003;348: 2609–2617.

335. Browman GP, et al. Randomized trial of interferon maintenance in multiple myeloma: a study of the National Cancer Institute of Canada Clinical Trials Group. *J Clin Oncol.* 1995;13:2354–2360.

336. Richardson, et al. A phase II open-label study of single-agent Revlimid® in relapsed and refractory myeloma. *Haematologica.* 2005;90(suppl. 1):154(Abstract PO. 737.)

337. Swenerton K, et al. Cisplatin-cyclophosphamide versus carboplatincyclophosphamide in advanced ovarian cancer: a randomized phase III study of the National Cancer Institute of Canada Clinical Trials Group. *J Clin Oncol.* 1992;10:718–726.

338. Alberts D, et al. Improved therapeutic index of carboplatin plus cyclophosphamide versus cisplatin plus cyclophosphamide: final report by the Southwestern Oncology Group of a phase III randomized trial in stages III and IV ovarian cancer. *J Clin Oncol.* 1992; 10:706–717.

339. McGuire WP, et al. Cyclophosphamide and cisplatin compared with paclitaxel and cisplatin in patients with stage III and stage IV ovarian cancer. *N Engl J Med.* 1996;334:1–6.

340. Ozols RE. Combination regimens of paclitaxel and the platinum drugs as first-line regimens for ovarian cancer. *Semin Oncol.* 1995;22(Suppl 15):1–6.

341. Markman M, et al. Combination chemotherapy with carboplatin and docetaxel in the treatment of cancers of the ovary and fallopian tube and primary carcinoma of the peritoneum. *J Clin Oncol.* 2001;19:1901–1905.

342. D'Agostino G, Ferrandina G, Ludovsisi M, et al. Phase II study of liposomal doxorubicin and gemcitabine in the salvage treatment of ovarian cancer. *Br J Cancer.* 2003;89:1180–1184.

343. Nagourney RA, et al. Phase II trial of gemcitabine plus cisplatin repeating doublet therapy in previously treated relapsed ovarian cancer patients. *Gynecol Oncol.* 2003;88:35–39.

344. Markman M. Altretamine (hexamethylmelamine) in platinum-resistant and platinum-refractory ovarian cancer: a Gynecologic Oncology Group phase II trial. *Gynecol Oncol.* 1998;69:226–229.

345. Gordon AN, Granai CO, Rose PG, et al. Phase II study of liposomal doxorubicin in platinum- and paclitaxel-refractory epithelial ovarian cancer. *J Clin Oncol.* 2000;18(17):3093–3100.

346. McGuire WP, Rowinsky EK, Rosenshein NB, et al. Taxol: a unique antineoplastic agent with significant activity in advanced ovarian epithelial neoplasms. *Ann Intern Med.* 1989;111:273–279.

347. Kudelka AP, et al. Phase II study of intravenous topotecan as a 5-day infusion for refractory epithelial ovarian carcinoma. *J Clin Oncol.* 1996;14:1552–1557.

348. Lund B, Hansen OP, Theilade K, Hansen M, Neijt NP. Phase II study of gemcitabine (2'2'-difluorodeoxycytidine) in previously treated ovarian cancer patients. *J Natl Cancer Inst.* 1994;86:1530–1533.

349. Ozols RF. Oral etoposide for the treatment of recurrent ovarian cancer. *Drugs.* 1999;58(Suppl 3):43–49.

350. Dimopoulos MA, et al. Treatment of ovarian germ cell tumors with a 3-day bleomycin, etopside, and cisplatin regimen: a prospective multicenter study. *Gynecol Oncol.* 2004;95:695–700.

351. Gastrointestinal Tumor Study Group. Comparative therapeutic trial of radiation with or without chemotherapy in pancreatic carcinoma. *Int J Radiat Oncol Biol Phys.* 1979;5:1643–1647.

352. DeCaprio JA, et al. Fluorouracil and high-dose leucovorin in previously untreated patients with advanced adenocarcinoma of the pancreas: results of a phase II trial. *J Clin Oncol.* 1991;9:2128–2133.

353. Hess V, et al. Combining capecitabine and gemcitabine in patients with advanced pancreatic carcinoma: a phase I/II trial. *J Clin Oncol.* 2003;21:66–68.

354. Fine RL, et al. The GTX regimen: a biochemically synergistic combination for advanced pancreatic cancer (PC). *Proc Am Soc Clin Oncol.* 2003;22:281(abstract 1129).

355. Heinemann V. Randomized Phase III of Gemcitabine plus cisplatin compared with Gemcitabine alone in advanced pancreatic cancer. *J Clin Oncol.* 2006; 24:3946–3951.

356. Epelbaum K, et al. Gemcitabine and cisplatin with advanced pancreatic cancer. *Proc J Clin Oncol.* 2003; 22:1202.

357. Ko AH, et al. Phase II study of fixed dose rate gemcitabine with cisplatin formetastatic adenocarcinoma of the pancreas. *J Clin Oncol.* 2006;24:327–329.

358. Poplin E, Levy DE, Berlin J, et al. Phase III trial of gemcit-abine (30-minute infusion) versus gemcitabine (fixed-dose-rate infusion [FDR]) versus gemcitabine + oxaliplatan (GEMOX) in patients with advanced pancreatic cancer. *Proc Am Soc Clin Oncol.* 2006;24: 1805.

359. Louvet C, et al. Gemcitabine combined with oxaliplatin in advanced pancreatic adenocarcinoma: final results of a GERCOR multicenter phase II study. *J Clin Oncol.* 2002;20:1512–1518.

360. Rocha-Lima C, Savarese D, Bruckner H, et al. Irinotecan plus gemcitabine induces both radiographic and CA19-9 tumor marker responses in patients with previously untreated advanced pancreatic cancer. *J Clin Oncol.* 2002;20:1182–1191.

361. Leonard RC, et al. Chemotherapy prolongs survival in inoperable pancreatic carcinoma. *Br J Cancer.* 1994;81:882–885.

362. Moore MJ, et al. Erlotinib plus gemcitabine compared to gemcitabine alone in patients with advanced pancreatic cancer. A phase III trial of the NCIC-CTG. *J Clin Oncol.* 2005;23:16S(abstract 1).

363. No authors listed. Phase II studies of drug combinations in advanced pancreatic carcinoma 5-fluorouracil plus doxorubicin plus mitomycin C and 2 regimens of streptozotocin plus mitomycin C plus 5-fluorouracil. The Gastrointestinal Study Goup. *J Clin Oncol.* 1986;4(12)1794–1798.

364. Burris HA, et al. Improvements in survival and clinical benefit with gemcitabine as first-line therapy for patients with advanced pancreas cancer: a randomized trial. *J Clin Oncol.* 1997;15:2403–2413.

365. Brand R, et al. A phase I trial of weekly gemcitabine administered as a prolonged infusion in patients with pancreatic cancer and other solid tumors. *Invest New Drugs.* 1997;15:331–341.

366. Cartwright TH, et al. Phase II study of oral capecitabine in patients with advanced or metastatic pancreatic cancer. *J Clin Oncol.* 2002;20:160–164.

367. Eisenberger MA, et al. Prognostic factors in stage D2 prostate cancer: important implications for future trials; results of a cooperative intergroup study (INT.0036). The National Cancer Institute Intergroup Study #0036. *Semin Oncol.* 1994;21:613–619.

368. Jurincic CD, et al. Combined treatment (goserelin plus flutamide) versus monotherapy (goserelin alone) in advanced prostate cancer: a randomized study. *Semin Oncol.* 1991;18(Suppl 6):21–25.

369. Pienta KJ, Redman B, Hussain M, et al. Phase II evaluation of oral estramustine and oral etoposide in hormone-refractory adenocarcinoma of the prostate. *J Clin Oncol.* 1994;12:2005–2012.

370. Hudes GR, Greenberg R, Krigel RL, et al. Phase II study of estramustine and vinblastine, two microtubule inhibitors, in hormone-refractory prostate cancer. *J Clin Oncol.* 1992;11:1754–1761.

371. Hudes GR, et al. Paclitaxel plus estramustine in metastatic hormone-refractory prostate cancer. *Semin Oncol.* 1995;22(Suppl 12):41–45.

372. Tannock IF, et al. Chemotherapy with mitoxantrone plus prednisone or prednisone alone for symptomatic hormone-resistant prostate cancer: a Canadian randomized trial with palliative end points. *J Clin Oncol.* 1996;14:1756–1764.

373. Copur MS, et al. Weekly docetaxel and estramustine in patients with hormone-refractory prostate cancer. *Semin Oncol.* 2001;28:16–21.

374. Eisenberger MA, DeWit R, Berry W, et al. A multicenter phase III comparison of docetaxel (D) + prednisone (P) and mitoxantrone (MTZ) + P in patients with hormone-refractory prostate cancer (HRPC). *Proc Am Soc Clin Oncol.* 2004;23:2(abstract 4).

375. Roth BJ, et al. Taxol in advanced, hormone-refractory carcinoma of the prostate. A phase II trial of the Eastern Cooperative Oncology Group. *Cancer.* 1993;72: 2457–2260.

376. Ahmed S, et al. Feasibility of weekly 1 hour paclitaxel in hormone refractory prostate cancer (HRPC): a preliminary report of a phase II trial. *Proc Am Soc Clin Oncol.* 1998;17:325a.

377. Petrylak DP. Docetaxel (Taxotere) in hormone-refractory prostate cancer. *Semin Oncol.* 2000;27(Suppl 3):24–29.

378. Murphy GP, et al. Use of estramustine phosphate in prostate cancer by the National Prostatic Cancer Project and by Roswell Park Memorial Institute. *Urology.* 1984;23:54–63.

379. Dijkman GA, Debruyne FM, Fernandez del Moral P, et al. A randomized trial comparing the safety and efficacy of the Zoladex 10.8-mg depot, administered every 12 weeks, to that of the Zoladex 3.6-mg depot, administered every 4 weeks, in patients with advanced prostate cancer. The Dutch South East Cooperative Urological Group. *Eur Urol.* 1995;27:43–46.

380. The Leuprolide Study Group. Leuprolide versus diethylstilbestrol for metastatic prostate cancer. *N Engl J Med.* 1984;311:1281–1286.

381. Sharifi R, et al. Leuprolide acetate 22.5 mg 12-week depot formulation in the treatment of patients with advanced prostate cancer. *Clin Ther.* 1996;18:647–657.

382. Schellhammer PF, et al. Clinical benefits of bicalutamide compared with flutamide in combined androgen blockade for patients with advanced prostatic carcinoma: final report of a double-blind, randomized, multi-center trial. Casodex Combination Study Group. *Urology.* 1997;50:330–336.

383. McLeod DG, et al. The use of flutamide in hormone-refractory metastatic prostate cancer. *Cancer.* 1993;72: 3870–3873.

384. Janknegt RA, et al. Orchiectomy and nilutamide or placebo as treatment of metastatic prostatic cancer in a multinational doubleblind randomized trial. *J Urol.* 1993;149:77–82.

385. Johnson DE, et al. Ketoconazole therapy for hormonally refractive metastatic prostate cancer. *Urology.* 1988;31:132–134.

386. Havlin KA, et al. Aminoglutethimide: theoretical considerations and clinical results in advanced prostate cancer. *Cancer Treat Res.* 1988;39:83–96.

387. Atzpodien J, et al. European studies of interleukin-2 in metastatic renal cell carcinoma. *Semin Oncol.* 1993;20(Suppl 9):22.

388. Rini BI, et al. Phase II trial of weekly intravenous gemcitabine with continuous infusion fluorouracil in patients with metastatic renal cell cancer. *J Clin Oncol.* 2000;18:2419–2426.

389. Fyfe G, et al. Results of treatment of 255 patients with metastatic renal cell carcinoma who received high-dose recombinant interleukin-2 therapy. *J Clin Oncol.* 1995;13:688–696.

390. Minasian LM, et al. Interferon alfa-2a in advanced renal cell carcinoma: treatment results and survival in 159 patients with long-term follow-up. *J Clin Oncol.* 1993;11:1368–1375.

391. Motzer RJ, et al. Prognostic factors for survival in previously treated patients with metastatic renal cell carcinoma. *J Clin Oncol.* 2004;223:454–463.

392. Motzer RJ, et al. Activity of SU11248, a multitargeted inhibitor of vascular endothelial growth factor receptor and platelet-derived growth factor receptor, in patients with metastatic renal cell carcinoma. *J Clin Oncol.* 2006; 24:16–24.

393. Antman K, et al. An intergroup phase III randomized study of doxorubicin and dacarbazine with or without ifosfamide and mesna in advanced soft tissue and bone sarcomas. *J Clin Oncol.* 1993;11:1276–1285.

394. Elias A, et al. Response to mesna, doxorubicin, ifosfamide, and dacarbazine in 108 patients with metastatic or unresectable sarcoma and no prior chemotherapy. *J Clin Oncol.* 1989;7:1208–1216.

395. Santoro A, et al. Doxorubicin versus CYVADIC versus doxorubicin plus ifosfamide in first-line treatment of advanced soft tissue sarcomas: a randomized study of the European Organization for Research and Treatment of Cancer Soft Tissue and Bone Sarcoma Group. *J Clin Oncol.* 1995;13:1537–1545.

396. Grier HE, Krailo MD, Tarbell NJ, et al. Addition of ifosfamide and etoposide to standard chemotherapy for Ewing's sarcoma and primitive neuroectodermal tumor of bone. *N Engl J Med.* 2003;348:694–701.

397. Merimsky O, et al. Gemcitabine in soft tissue or bone sarcoma resistant to standard chemotherapy: a phase II study. *Cancer Chemother Pharmacol.* 2000;45: 177–181.

398. Heymach JV, Desai J, Manola J, et al. Phase II study of the antiangiogenic agents U5416 in patients with advanced soft tissue sarcomas. *Clin Cancer Res.* 2004; 10:5732–5740.

399. Einhorn LH, et al. Evaluation of optimal duration of chemotherapy in favorable-prognosis disseminated germ cell tumors: a Southeastern Cancer Study Group Protocol. *J Clin Oncol.* 1989;7:387–391.

400. Williams SD, et al. Treatment of disseminated germ-cell tumors with cisplatin, bleomycin, and either vinblastine or etoposide. *N Engl J Med.* 1987;316: 1435–1440.

401. Bosl G, et al. A randomized trial of etoposide + cisplatin versus vinblastine + bleomycin + cisplatin + cyclophosphamide + dactinomycin in patients with good-prognosis germ cell tumors. *J Clin Oncol.* 1988;6:1231–1238.

402. Einhorn LH, et al. Cis-diamminedichloroplatinum, vinblastine, and bleomycin combination chemotherapy in disseminated testicular cancer. *Ann Intern Med.* 1977;87:293–298.

403. Vugrin D, et al. VAB-6 combination chemotherapy in disseminated cancer of the testis. *Ann Intern Med.* 1981;95:59–61.

404. Motzer RJ, et al. Salvage chemotherapy for patients with germ cell tumors. The Memorial Sloan-Kettering Cancer Center experience. *Cancer.* 1991;67: 1305–1310.

405. Loehrer PJ, et al. Salvage therapy in recurrent germ cell cancer: ifosfamide and cisplatin plus either vinblastine or etoposide. *Ann Intern Med.* 1988;109: 540–546.

406. Loehrer PJ, et al. Cisplatin plus doxorubicin plus cyclophosphamide in metastatic or recurrent thymoma: final results of an intergroup trial. *J Clin Oncol.* 1994;12:1164–1168.

407. Giaccone G, et al. Cisplatin and etoposide combination chemotherapy for locally advanced or metastatic thymoma. A phase II study of the European Organization for Research and Treatment of Cancer Lung Cancer Cooperative Group. *J Clin Oncol.* 1996;14: 814–820.

408. Fornasiero A, et al. Chemotherapy for invasive thymoma. *Cancer.* 1991;68:30–33.

409. Shimaoka K, et al. A randomized trial of doxorubicin versus doxorubicin plus cisplatin in patients with advanced thyroid carcinoma. *Cancer.* 1985;56: 2155–2160.

410. Kaminskas E, Farrell A, Abraham S, et al. Approval summary: azacitidine for treatment of myelodysplastic syndrome subtypes. *Clin Cancer Res.* 2005;11: 3604–3608.

411. List A, Beran M, DiPersio J, et al. Opportunities for trisenox (arsenic trioxide) in the treatment of myelodysplastic syndromes. *Leukemia.* 2003;17:1499–1507.

412. List A, Dewald G, Bennett J, et al. Lenalidomide in the myelodysplastic syndrome with chromosome 5q deletion. *N Engl J Med.* 2006;355:1456–1465.

413. Dacogen (decitabine for injection) Package insert. MGI Pharma, INC. Bloomington, MN: May, 2006.

414. Kantarjian HM, Issa JP. Decitabine dosing schedules. *Semin Hematol.* 2005;42(3 Suppl 2):S17-22.

Index

C

F

G

H

N